The Latest Evolution in learning.

Evolve provides online access to free learning resources and activities designed specifically for the textbook you are using in your class. The resources will provide you with information that enhances the material covered in the book, and much more.

Visit the Web address listed below to start your learning evolution today!

▶▶ **LOGIN:** *http://evolve.elsevier.com/LaFleur/HUC/*

Evolve Student Learning Resources for LaFleur Brooks/Gillingham: *Health Unit Coordinating, 5th edition,* offer the following features:

• Content Updates
The latest content updates from the authors of the textbook to keep you current with recent developments in the field of Health Unit Coordinating.

• Weblinks
Organized by chapter, these links can help you harness the power of the World Wide Web to expand your knowledge beyond this textbook and stay abreast of the very latest news and developments in the health care field.

• Mock Certification Exam
This invaluable study tool consists of 80 questions and is written in the same format used for the national certification exam. Gain practice in taking the exam, then check your knowledge and score by reviewing the answers that are provided.

• NAHUC Web Link
Easily link to the National Association of Health Unit Coordinators (NAHUC) Web site to obtain information about the benefits of professional membership and to register for the national certification exam.

Think outside the book...*evolve.*

Health Unit
COORDINATING

formerly Unit Secretary

Fifth Edition

Health Unit
COORDINATING

formerly Unit Secretary

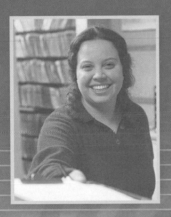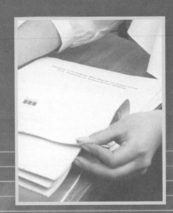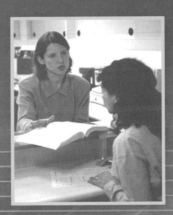

Myrna LaFleur Brooks, RN, BEd, CHUC
Founding President,
National Association of Health Unit Coordinators
Faculty Emeritus,
Maricopa County Community College District
Phoenix, Arizona

Elaine A. Gillingham, AAS, BA, CHUC
Program Director,
Health Unit Coordinator Program
GateWay Community College
Phoenix, Arizona

SAUNDERS
An Imprint of Elsevier

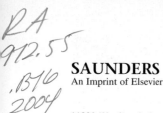

SAUNDERS
An Imprint of Elsevier

11830 Westline Industrial Drive
St. Louis, Missouri 63146

HEALTH UNIT COORDINATING

ISBN 0-7216-0099-9

NOTICE

Medicine is an ever-changing field. Standard safety precautions must be followed, but as new research and clinical experience broaden our knowledge, changes in treatment and drug therapy may become necessary or appropriate. Readers are advised to check the most current product information provided by the manufacturer of each drug to be administered to verify the recommended dose, the method and duration of administration, and contraindications. It is the responsibility of the licensed prescriber, relying on experience and knowledge of the patient, to determine dosages and the best treatment for each individual patient. Neither the publisher nor the author assumes any liability for any injury and/or damage to persons or property arising from this publication.

Previous editions copyrighted 1998, 1993, 1986, 1979

Library of Congress Cataloging-in-Publication Data

LaFleur-Brooks, Myrna.
   Health unit coordinating / Myrna LaFleur-Brooks, Elaine Gillingham.—5th ed.
     p. cm.
   Includes bibliographical references and index.
   ISBN 0-7216-0099-9
    1. Hospital ward clerks. 2. Medical records. 3. Medicine—Terminology. I. Gillingham, Elaine Tight. II. Title.

   RA972.55.B76 2003
   651.5′04261—dc22

                      2003065151

Executive Editor: Adrianne Cochran
Developmental Editors: Helaine Tobin, Rose Foltz
Publishing Services Manager: Pat Joiner
Designer: Kathi Gosche

Printed in the United States of America

Last digit is the print number: 9 8 7 6 5 4 3 2 1

EDITORIAL REVIEW BOARD

To all the health unit coordinator students,
working health unit coordinators,
and educators who have inspired
and contributed to this text.

■ A CAREER IN HEALTH UNIT COORDINATING

Welcome to the exciting and challenging career of health unit coordinating. Individuals practicing as health unit coordinators soon realize that they have far-reaching effects on the delivery of care to patients. Health unit coordinators manage all nonclinical tasks on hospital nursing units, making them essential members of the health care team. Responsibilities include transcribing physicians' orders for patient treatment, preparing patient charts, maintaining statistical reports, dealing with visitors, and much more. It's no surprise that the health unit coordinator's role has been called one of the most important positions on the nursing unit.

As a recognized health care profession, health unit coordinating has its own national organization, the National Association of Health Unit Coordinators (NAHUC), which offers certification to individuals who meet certain standards of excellence.

■ NEW TO THIS EDITION

Instructors and students using the 5th edition of *Health Unit Coordinating* will benefit from all of the quality pedagogical elements in the previous edition, plus these new features:

■ *Attractive, two-color design* enhances interest and easily leads students through exercises and boxed information and instruction

---

100 ▲ Section 2 · PERSONAL AND PROFESSIONAL SKILLS

supplies or medication as needed. When the code or crash cart is completely checked and restocked, as needed, the nurse will again lock the cart after documenting the date and his or her signature on a form attached to the cart. When the cart is used for a code, it is vital that the cart be restocked and replaced per hospital policy.

Other emergency equipment includes fire extinguishers and fire doors. Because of the nature of emergency equipment, it must be checked frequently and immediately after use and be restored as soon as possible to be readied for future emergencies. The health unit coordinator must know the following information regarding emergencies:

1. The emergency equipment and supplies that are stored on the nursing unit and where they are located
2. How to call a code and what his or her responsibilities are during a code
3. The location of the nursing unit fire extinguishers
4. The emergency procedures for the nursing unit
5. The signal codes and procedures for fire, behavioral alarms, disaster codes, and evacuation procedures
6. The procedures for dealing with a hazardous materials spill, although you may not be directly responsible, knowing the procedures allows you to support timely and safe removal of hazardous materials

During a crisis, the hospital personnel often approach the nurses' station and ask the health unit coordinator to locate emergency equipment and initiate emergency procedures. Frequent fire and disaster drills are conducted in hospitals to prepare personnel in the case of a fire or disaster. The health unit coordinator and all hospital personnel must know what to do when there is a fire or disaster; these drills must be taken seriously.

Ignorance of code procedure or the location of nursing unit emergency equipment may cause a delay in the delivery of emergency treatment and result in serious consequences to patients.

■ MANAGEMENT OF THE ACTIVITIES AT THE NURSES' STATION

In Chapter 1 we stated that the health unit coordinator, through his or her communication responsibilities, coordinates the activities involving the doctor, the nursing staff, the other hospital departments, the patients, and the visitors to the nursing unit. Good management techniques are necessary to coordinate these activities effectively.

The following guidelines may be of assistance in managing the activities at the nurses' station.

Patient Activity and Information

The most efficient method for tracking patients and their activities is to use a census worksheet. A census worksheet is a list of the names, rooms, and bed numbers of patients located on a nursing unit, with blank spaces next to each name. A census worksheet may be printed from a computer menu. Print or prepare the sheet at the beginning of each shift. Use information on the patients' Kardex forms (see Chapter 10) or the change-of-shift report to record each patient activity pertinent next to his or her name.

Record only patient activities pertinent to the health unit coordinator job, which includes scheduled diagnostic procedures,

surgeries, planned discharges, transfers, and so forth. Record the time of each activity, if known (Fig. 7–4).

Record other data that you may need to refer to during the shift, such as (1) DNR (do not resuscitate) or no code, (2) NINP (no information, no publication), (3) no visitors allowed, (4) no phone calls to the patient's room, (5) the patient is in respiratory isolation, (6) the patient is out on a temporary pass, (7) the nurse who is assigned to patient, and (8) the resident or attending physician assigned to the patient.

Tape the census worksheet onto the surface area of your desk next to the telephone and near the computer for quick reference. During the shift, update the information as changes occur.

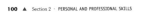
STUDENT ACTIVITY

To practice preparing a unit census worksheet, complete Activity 7–1 in the *Skills Practice Manual*.

The health unit coordinator is also responsible for maintaining the unit census board (as discussed in Chapter 4), which indicates patient names and their room numbers, and the names of doctors and nurses assigned to each patient. This board may not be in plain sight to visitors, to protect patient confidentiality.

Patients and Patients' Charts That Leave the Unit

When a patient leaves the nursing unit for surgery, a diagnostic study, to visit the cafeteria with a relative, or for one of numerous other reasons, record the time the patient leaves the nursing unit and the destination beside the patient's name on the census worksheet. When the patient returns to the nursing unit, draw a line through the recording. Trying to locate charts for doctors, nurses, and other professionals wastes a lot of time. Chart tracking is essential for the efficient use of time for all those involved.

Increasingly, patient-centered or patient-focused nursing units are being designed so that diagnostic technicians come to the patient on the unit whenever possible. This practice is more convenient for the patient and also reduces the number of times the chart is off the unit.

Health personnel, doctors, and visitors are constantly asking the health unit coordinator the whereabouts of patients and/or the patients' charts. By maintaining the census worksheet you can find the answer at a glance.

Addressing Visitors' Requests, Questions, and Complaints

As a health unit coordinator you probably have more contact with the visitors than any of the other nursing unit personnel, since visitors usually stop at the nurses' station for information or

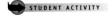
★ INFORMATION ALERT!

Many nursing units average 25 to 40 patients, and so it would be impossible to mentally log the whereabouts of each patient.

Chapter 7 · Management Techniques and Problem-Solving Skills for Health Unit Coordinating ▲ **101**

Room #	Patient Name	Activities
301	Breath, Les	DC Today
302	Pickens, Slim	Surg 11⁰⁰ x ray to be sent ⊼ patient
303-1	Kats, Kitty	
303-2		
304	Bee, Mae	~~Call Dr. James ⊼ ABG results~~ Called Sue 9⁰⁰
305	Honey, Mai	NPO for heart cath @ 9⁰⁰
306-1		
306-2		
307	Pack, Fanny	No calls to room
308	Bugg, June	DC today
309	~~Lynde, Bee~~	Trans to ICU 11³⁰
310-1	Cider, Ida	DNR
310-2	Soo, Ah	Surg 8⁰⁰ Back @ 1³⁰
311-1	Bear, Harry	Resp isolation
311-2	Bread, Thad	
312-1	Kream, Kris	NINP
312-2	Pat, Peggy	Surg 8³⁰ Back @ 2⁰⁰

FIGURE 7–4 ▲ A census worksheet.

some other type of communication regarding the patient's hospitalization. As a visitor approaches the nurses' station, immediately acknowledge that person's presence and provide assistance as soon as possible. At this moment, you represent the entire nursing unit, and the manner in which you respond to the visitor helps shape his or her attitude about the care the patient is receiving and about the hospital as a whole. It is your management responsibility to (1) communicate pertinent information to visitors, (2) respond to visitors' questions and requests, (3) initially handle visitors' complaints, and (4) locate the patient's nurse when necessary.

Communicate pertinent information to the visitor, such as the time for visiting hours, the number of visitors that may be in a patient's room at one time, isolation restrictions, and what items may or may not be taken into the patient's room. Examples of restricted items in the intensive care unit include flowers and plants. Rubber balloons are banned in most hospitals because of latex allergies and the risk of children aspirating broken pieces of

the rubber. Refer to the policy manual for the visitor regulations practiced at your hospital.

The visitor may ask the health unit coordinator such questions as, "May I take the patient to the cafeteria?" or "May the patient have a milkshake?" or "When can the patient go home?" Many questions may be answered by checking information on the patient's Kardex form or by referring to the nursing unit policy or procedure manual. However, if you are in doubt about the answer, check with the nurse.

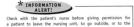
★ INFORMATION ALERT!

Check with the patient's nurse before giving permission for a patient to leave the nursing unit, to go outside, or to the cafeteria.

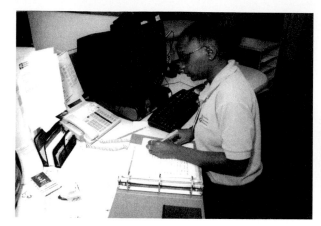

■ *Updated photographs* help students envision their expected role and responsibilities on the job

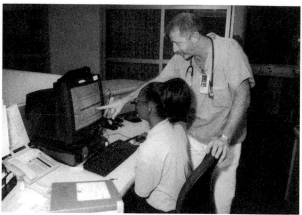

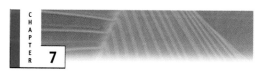

■ *In-depth outlines* at the beginning of each chapter introduce the material to be covered and enable students to see the connections among topics

CHAPTER 7

Management Techniques and Problem-Solving Skills for Health Unit Coordinating

Outline	Chapter Objectives
Chapter Objectives	*Upon completion of this chapter, you will be able to:*
Vocabulary	1. Define the terms in the vocabulary list.
Abbreviations	2. Write the meaning of the abbreviations in the abbreviations list.
Exercise 1	
Exercise 2	3. List five areas of management.
Introduction	4. Briefly discuss the management responsibilities for the nursing unit supplies and equipment.
Management of the Nursing Unit Supplies and Equipment	
Nursing Unit Supplies	5. Explain the contents and purpose of four reference books and manuals that are available on the nursing unit.
Patient Rental Equipment	
Nursing Unit Emergency Equipment	6. Briefly explain a method to record the location of patients and patients' charts and discuss why it is necessary to keep a record of this information.
Management of the Activities at the Nurses' Station	
Patient Activity and Information	7. Explain the necessity of keeping a note pad next to the telephone that is used by the health unit coordinator.
Patients and Patients' Charts That Leave the Unit	
Addressing Visitors' Requests, Questions, and Complaints	8. List three management responsibilities concerning visitors on the nursing unit.
Management Related to the Performance of Health Unit Coordinator Tasks	9. List three steps to follow when dealing with visitors' complaints.
Prioritizing Tasks	10. Given a list of several health unit coordinator tasks, identify those that would have a higher priority and those that would be of lower priority.
Use of a Note Pad	
Ergonomics for the Health Unit Coordinator	
Guidelines for the Prevention of Workplace Injuries	11. Explain the importance of the change-of-shift report.
Organization of the Nurses' Station	12. List eight time-management tips for the health unit coordinator.
Time Management	
Stress Management	13. Define two types of stress and provide an example of each.
Continuous Quality Improvement	14. List five techniques for dealing with stress on the job.
The Five-Step Problem-Solving Model	
Exercise 3	15. Discuss the purpose of continuous quality improvement.
Summary	16. Identify and apply the five-step problem-solving model.
Review Questions	17. Identify two common work-related injuries.
Topics for Discussion	
Web Site of Interest	

95

■ TOTAL EDUCATIONAL PACKAGE

The 5th edition of *Health Unit Coordinating* is part of a total educational package for health unit coordinating offered by W. B. Saunders. Supplemental materials include the following:

Skills Practice Manual to Accompany Health Unit Coordinating, 5th edition

This printed manual contains practice activities to reinforce skills taught in the text, such as transcribing doctors' orders, communicating with co-workers, assembling a patient's chart, documenting lab values, and recording telephoned doctors' orders. Generic hospital forms and actual physicians' orders provide hands-on examples of tasks students will need to perform on the job. Also included is a clinical skills evaluation record, designed to help students objectively record and evaluate their performance during hospital rotations.

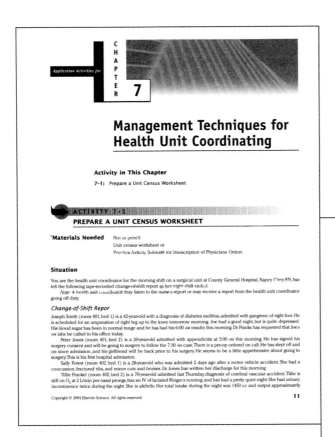

Application Activities for

C
H
A
P
T
E
R

7

Management Techniques for Health Unit Coordinating

Activity in This Chapter

7-1: Prepare a Unit Census Worksheet

ACTIVITY 7-1

PREPARE A UNIT CENSUS WORKSHEET

Materials Needed Pen or pencil
Unit census worksheet or
Practice Activity Software for Transcription of Physicians Orders

Situation

You are the health unit coordinator for the morning shift on a surgical unit at County General Hospital. Nancy Clary, RN, has left the following tape-recorded change-of-shift report as her night shift ended.

Note: A health unit coordinator may listen to the nurse's report or may receive a report from the health unit coordinator going off duty.

Change-of-Shift Report

Joseph Smith (room 401, bed 1) is a 42-year-old with a diagnosis of diabetes mellitus, admitted with gangrene of right foot. He is scheduled for an amputation of right leg up to the knee tomorrow morning. Joe had a good night, but is quite depressed. His blood sugar has been in normal range and he has his 6:00 AM insulin this morning. Dr. Franks has requested that Joe's AM labs be called to his office today.

Peter Jones (room 401, bed 2) is a 20-year-old admitted with appendicitis at 3:00 AM this morning. He has signed his surgery consent and will be going to surgery to follow the 7:30 AM case. There is a pre-op ordered on call. He has slept off and on since admission, and his girlfriend will be back prior to his surgery. He seems to be a little apprehensive about going to surgery. This is his first hospital admission.

Sally Forest (room 402, bed 1) is a 28-year-old who was admitted 2 days ago after a motor vehicle accident. She had a concussion, fractured ribs, and minor cuts and bruises. Dr. Jones has written her discharge for this morning.

Tillie Frankel (room 402, bed 2) is a 70-year-old admitted last Thursday, diagnosis of cerebral vascular accident. Tillie is still on O₂ at 2 L/min per nasal prongs, has an IV of lactated Ringer's running, and has had a pretty quiet night. She had urinary incontinence twice during the night. She is afebrile. Her total intake during the night was 1450 cc and output approximately

Copyright © 2004 Elsevier Science. All rights reserved.   **11**

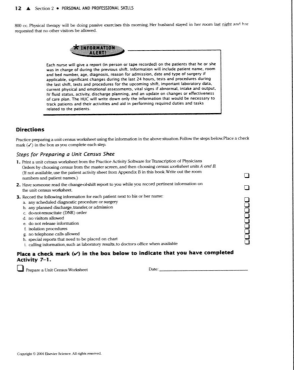

12 ▲ Section 2 • PERSONAL AND PROFESSIONAL SKILLS

800 cc. Physical therapy will be doing passive exercises this morning. Her husband stayed in her room last night and has requested that no other visitors be allowed.

★ INFORMATION ALERT!

Each nurse will give a report (in person or tape recorded) on the patients that he or she was in charge of during the previous shift. Information will include patient name, room and bed number, age, diagnosis, reason for admission, date and type of surgery if applicable, significant changes during the last 24 hours, tests and procedures during the last shift, tests and procedures for the upcoming shift, important laboratory data, current physical and emotional assessments, vital signs if abnormal, intake and output, IV fluid status, activity, discharge planning, and an update on changes or effectiveness of care plan. The HUC will write down only the information that would be necessary to track patients and their activities and aid in performing required duties and tasks related to the patients.

Directions

Practice preparing a unit census worksheet using the information in the above situation. Follow the steps below. Place a check mark (✓) in the box as you complete each step.

Steps for Preparing a Unit Census Sheet

1. Print a unit census worksheet from the Practice Activity Software for Transcription of Physicians Orders by choosing census from the master screen, and then choosing *census worksheet units A and B.* (If not available, use the patient activity sheet from Appendix B in this book. Write out the room numbers and patient names.) ☐

2. Have someone read the change-of-shift report to you while you record pertinent information on the unit census worksheet. ☐

3. Record the following information for each patient next to his or her name:
   a. any scheduled diagnostic procedure or surgery ☐
   b. any planned discharge, transfer, or admission ☐
   c. do-not-resuscitate (DNR) order ☐
   d. no visitors allowed ☐
   e. do not release information ☐
   f. isolation procedures ☐
   g. no telephone calls allowed ☐
   h. special reports that need to be placed on chart ☐
   i. calling information, such as laboratory results, to doctors office when available ☐

Place a check mark (✓) in the box below to indicate that you have completed Activity 7-1.

☐ Prepare a Unit Census Worksheet   Date: _____

Copyright © 2004 Elsevier Science. All rights reserved.

Practice Activity Software for Transcription of Physicians' Orders

This **new**, state-of-the art Windows-based CD—bound free into the *Skills Practice Manual*—simulates a hospital's computer ordering system to be used in the classroom for practice in transcribing doctors' orders, and contains printable hospital forms. The software includes mock nursing units with lists of patients, doctors' rosters, diagnostic test results, and more, offering realistic practice of transcription of doctors' orders to enhance students' skills and confidence.

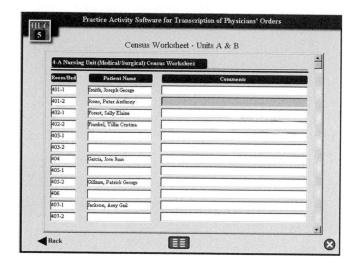

Health Unit Coordinating Certification Review

Following the content organization of *Health Unit Coordinating, 5th edition*, this printed study guide offers multiple-choice review questions and a mock certification exam to help students assess their knowledge and prepare for the NAHUC certification examination. Questions are similar in style to those used on the actual exam. Correct answers and rationales are provided for all questions, along with reference page numbers from *Health Unit Coordinating, 5th edition*, so students can easily obtain more information on topics of interest.

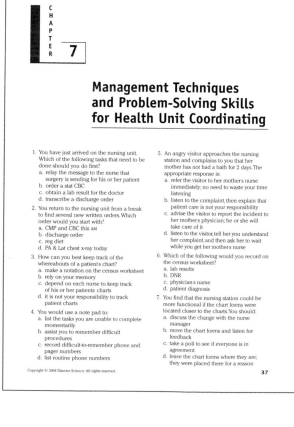

Health Unit Coordinating Pocket Guide

New to this edition, *Health Unit Coordinating Pocket Guide* provides, in a portable, easy-to-read format, the material from the text that is most commonly used and referred to. Special features include a glossary, a list of abbreviations, and the clinical skills evaluation record from the *Skills Practice Manual.* Personal management pages allow users to record information that is unique to their practice situations. Students as well as practicing health unit coordinators can use this tool as a quick and easy reference in clinical rotations or on the job.

Chapter 2 ● Ensuring Effective Interpersonal Communication ▲ 1

Room #	Patient Name	Activities
301	Breath, Lee	DC Today
302	Pickens, Slim	Surg 11^{00} x ray to be sent patient
303-1	Katt, Kitty	
303-2		
304	Bee, Mae	~~Call Dr. James 5 ABG results~~ Called Sue 9^{00}
305	Honey, Mai	NPO for heart cath @ 9^{00}
306-1		
306-2		
307	Pack, Fanny	No calls to room
308	Bugg, June	DC today
309	~~Kynda, Bee~~	Trans to ICU 11^{30}
310-1	Cider, Ida	DNR
310-2	Soo, Ah	~~Surg 8^{00}~~ Back @ 1^{30}
311-1	Bear, Harry	Resp isolation
311-2	Bread, Thad	
312-1	Kream, Kris	NINP
312-2	Pat, Peggy	~~Surg 9^{30}~~ Back @ 2^{00}

FIGURE 2-4 ▲ A census worksheet.

Managing Patient Activities and Information

Through your communication duties as a health unit coordinator, you are responsible for managing patient activities and information. A census worksheet is a tool that can help you accomplish this task efficiently. A census worksheet includes each patient's name, room, and bed number, and blank spaces in which to record pertinent data (Fig 2-4). Maintaining an up-to-date census worksheet allows you to quickly answer frequent questions from doctors, health care personnel, and visitors about patients.

Using a Census Worksheet to Manage Patient Activities and Information

- Print a census worksheet at the beginning of your shift
- Record pertinent patient activities (e.g., scheduled diagnostic procedures, surgeries, planned discharges, transfers, etc.)
- Note the time the patient leaves the unit and destination, and the time he or she returns
- List other important information (e.g., DNR, NINP, etc.)
- Tape a copy of the census worksheet to your desktop
- Update information during your shift

Sample slide

Instructor's Curriculum Resource to Accompany Health Unit Coordinating, 5th edition, with CD-ROM

This invaluable resource now contains both a printed and electronic component to assist instructors in various educational activities. The printed resource includes a 16-week syllabus, classroom activities, and individual and collaborative learning projects, a list of PowerPoint slides on the CD-ROM, and a test bank with over 500 questions. The **new** CD-ROM contains all of the printed materials in Word format, plus more than 500 PowerPoint slides to help instructors with classroom presentations, and a test bank in the ExamView format that will help instructors quickly and easily prepare quizzes and exams.

EVOLVE Web site to Accompany Health Unit Coordinating, 5th edition

This **new** feature provides free materials for both students and instructors, and includes a scored mock certification examination as well as Web links, including a link to the NAHUC Web site for further information about certification. All instructor materials are also available to faculty only for download, including the ExamView testbank, PowerPoint slides, and individual, detailed chapter lesson activities.

An EVOLVE Course Management System (CMS) is also available free to instructors who adopt this textbook. This platform gives instructors yet another resource to facilitate learning, and to make the health unit coordinating content available to their students. In addition to the Evolve Learning Resources available to students and instructors, there is an entire suite of tools available that allows for communication between instructors and students, including a discussion board, e-mail, chat rooms, and more.

To access this comprehensive online resource, go to the EVOLVE home page at **http://evolve.elsevier.com** and enter your user name and password provided to you by your instructor. If your instructor has not set up a Course Management System, you can still access the learning resources available free with this textbook by going to **http://evolve. elsevier.com/LaFleur/HUC/**

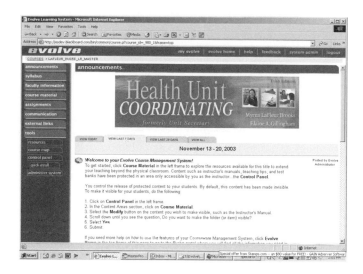

■ MARKET-LEADING TEXTBOOK

Health Unit Coordinating, 5th edition, by Myrna LaFleur Brooks and Elaine A. Gillingham, is the best-selling textbook of its kind on the market. It provides comprehensive coverage of the theory and practice underpinning the health unit coordinator's responsibilities, introduces students to hospitals and health care, and explains nonclinical management of the nursing unit. It also offers a complete module on anatomy, physiology, and medical terminology, enabling students to learn the language of medicine so they can interact confidently with doctors, nurses, and other health care workers. Exercises in each chapter reinforce newly learned material and test students' retention and critical thinking abilities. Abundant photographs, diagrams, and illustrations further enhance understanding of the material. Students studying in programs using this text will be able to master everything they need to know to begin their career performing at a competent level.

■ TO THE STUDENT

How to Use This Text

This text is organized to provide theory in conjunction with hands-on activities in the *Skills Practice Manual to Accompany Health Unit Coordinating* to prepare you to work as a health unit coordinator. The text is divided into five sections:

Section 1, *Orientation to Hospitals, Medical Centers, and Health Care,* provides a fundamental understanding of health care, including the health unit coordinator position.

Section 2, *Personal and Professional Skills,* presents guidelines to use for effective interpersonal and intercultural communication, and management skills. Workplace behavior and appearance, confidentiality as mandated by the Privacy Rule contained the Health Insurance Portability and Accountability Act (HIPAA), and other ethical and legal issues are discussed.

Section 3, *The Patient's Chart and Transcription of Doctors' Orders,* provides information needed to understand written doctors' orders and enhances understanding of the various departments that carry out the orders. Activities are included that provide hands-on experience transcribing doctors' orders by using the *Skills Practice Manual to Accompany Health Unit Coordinating* and the *Practice Activity Software for Transcription of Physicians' Orders to Accompany Health Unit Coordinating.*

Section 4, *Health Unit Coordinator Procedures,* provides information regarding emergencies, infection control, recording vital signs, and admission, preoperative, postoperative, discharge, postmortem, and transfer procedures.

Section 5, *Introduction to Anatomic Structures, Medical Terms, and Illnesses,* presents a basic overview of human anatomy and medical terminology.

Working Your Way Through a Chapter

Read the Objectives

The objectives outline what you are expected to know when you have completed all of the exercises for the chapter. When you have read the chapter and completed the exercises, return to the objectives and quiz yourself to ensure that you have mastered the material.

Read the Vocabulary Lists

Each chapter introduces a list of words related to the material covered in that chapter. When reading the chapter, note the words in the vocabulary list to enhance your understanding of their meanings. Return to the vocabulary list after you have read the chapter and complete the exercises to quiz yourself on the definitions of the words.

Complete the Exercises that Follow the Abbreviation Lists

Most chapters include a list of abbreviations that relate to the material covered in that chapter. Exercises are included to assist you in learning those abbreviations. The abbreviations are also used throughout the chapter. It may be helpful to create flash cards for the abbreviations.

Complete the Review Questions

The review questions are written from the objectives and will assist you in learning and understanding the skills necessary to be successful as a health unit coordinator.

Information Alert! Boxes

Pay special attention to the information provided in the *Information Alert!* boxes, as this information is especially important in performing your job accurately and efficiently. This information is emphasized to reduce the risk of errors while working as a health unit coordinator.

Topics for Discussion

Discussion questions related to chapter material are included at the end of chapters 1 through 22 to increase understanding of health care issues and to promote critical thinking and problem-solving skills. Discuss the questions with your classmates, friends, and family to gain others' perspectives on the topics.

Hands-On Activities

Most chapters in *Health Unit Coordinating* include references to activities found in *Skills Practice Manual to Accompany Health Unit Coordinating*. Chapters 4 and 7 have activities related to communication and management skills. Chapter 8 has activities that will familiarize you with patient chart forms and chart assembly. Chapters 10 through 19 include doctors' orders that relate to material discussed in each chapter. *Practice Activity Software for Transcription of Physicians' Orders to Accompany Health Unit Coordinating* enables you to practice the transcription of the doctors' orders on a simulated hospital computer program. Activities are provided in Chapter 21 for other routine health unit coordinator tasks, such as charting vital signs.

Use of Appendixes

Appendix A, *Word Elements,* assists you in finding the definition of a word part while defining or building a medical term. You may need to find a prefix or suffix that you recognize from Chapter 23 but for which you have forgotten the definition.

Appendix B, *Abbreviations,* helps refresh your memory when you cannot recall the meaning of an abbreviation used in a doctors' order.

Appendix C, *The National Association of Health Unit Coordinators Standards of Practice,* provides the standards of practice for your profession.

Appendix D, *Task and Knowledge Statements from the National Association of Health Unit Coordinators,* lists the competencies and skills required to work as a health unit coordinator.

Appendix E, *National Association of Health Unit Coordinators Code of Ethics,* provides the Code of Ethics for your profession.

Appendix F, *Comprehensive List of Laboratory Studies and Blood Components,* enables you to determine which division of the laboratory would perform a particular lab test.

Answers

Check your answers after completing exercises and review questions to ensure that you have answered them correctly.

■ FROM THE AUTHORS

Congratulations—you have opened the door to the health care world. By using *Health Unit Coordinating* as a learning tool, you may obtain a career in health care. Our hope is that you will become a valuable member of the health care field and feel the pride and satisfaction that comes with helping others. The authors invite students and faculty to contact them with questions and comments, using the "Feedback and Suggestions" form on the Evolve Web site at: http://evolve.elsevier.com/LaFleur/HUC/

ACKNOWLEDGMENTS

Preparing the fifth edition of *Health Unit Coordinating* required the expertise of many, since changes in the health care delivery system and advancement in medical technology demand new knowledge for the health unit coordinator and change in the health unit coordinating practice.

We are grateful for the invaluable expert advice and experience of Margi Schultz, HUC, RN, BSN, MSN, who revised Chapter 13, *Medication Orders,* and Chris Costa, who revised Chapter 23, *Medical Terminology, Basic Human Structure, Diseases, and Disorders.*

Margi Schultz started her health care career working as a health unit coordinator while continuing her education to become an RN. She then worked as a RN in an intensive care unit, while earning her BSN and MSN. Currently, Margi is employed as the Assistant Director of Nursing and full-time faculty member at Gateway Community College in Phoenix, Arizona. Margi is a Doctoral Candidate in the School of Education at Capella University.

Chris Costa has held a variety of positions in the health care field, including health unit coordinator, cardiac monitor technician, supervisor of health unit coordinators, assistant director of patient business office, and director of patient affairs, and has held every office for the Arizona Chapter of Admitting Managers. Chris has been a geriatric care manager and a Medicare community lecturer through the years and writes an e-mail newsletter, "Medical Quotes, Quips, Jokes, and Joules."

We thank the reviewers who helped to ensure that this was the most up-to-date revision it could be. We would also like to express our appreciation for the cooperation we received from Phoenix Children's Hospital, Phoenix Baptist Hospital, Boswell Memorial Hospital, Del Webb Hospital, John C Lincoln Hospital, Good Samaritan Regional Medical Center, and Gateway Community College in Phoenix, Arizona, who allowed access to their various departments to obtain information to prepare the manuscript. In addition, we wish to thank the following individuals for their assistance:

Edith Baie
Assistant Director
Boswell Memorial Hospital Clinical Laboratory
Sun City, Arizona

Clare Boyle, MS, RD
Administrative Dietitian
Boswell Memorial Hospital
Sun City, Arizona

Edward Hoskins, AA, BA, RT
Faculty, Respiratory Therapy Program
GateWay Community College
Phoenix, Arizona

John Lampignano, AA, BS, MEd, RT
Faculty, Diagnostic Imaging Program
GateWay Community College
Phoenix, Arizona

Beckie Schad
Health Unit Coordinator
Del Webb Hospital
Sun City, Arizona

Mickee Southwell
Health Unit Coordinator
Boswell Memorial Hospital
Sun City, Arizona

Peter Zawicki, BS, MS, PT
Division Chair, Health Sciences Division
Faculty, Physical Therapy Assistant Program
GateWay Community College
Phoenix, Arizona

A special thanks to the following staff of W. B. Saunders: Adrianne Cochran, Executive Editor, Helaine Tobin, Developmental Editor, and all the experts from W.B. Saunders for their support and encouragement during the revision of this edition.

Myrna LaFleur Brooks received her diploma in Nursing from the Grey Nuns Hospital in Regina, Saskatchewan, Canada, in 1962 and her Bachelor's degree in Education from Northern Arizona University in 1977. After working as a staff nurse in medical-surgical nursing, she became an instructor and then director in Staff Development at Doctor's Hospital in Phoenix. In 1970 she began her 25-year career with GateWay Community College as a faculty member in the Health Unit Coordinator Program. Frustrated by the lack of textbooks and the lack of recognition of health unit coordinating as a health profession, she and Winnie Starr, Program Director, set out to make changes. They welcomed the offer from W. B. Saunders to write a textbook titled *Unit Clerking*, published in 1979. Its publication opened networking nationwide, which led to the formation of a national association for health unit coordinators. The first organizational meeting was held in Phoenix on August 23, 1980, the date that has since become National Health Unit Coordinator Day, celebrated by unit coordinators and health care facilities alike throughout the nation. The National Association of Health Unit Coordinators (NAHUC), through the dedication of its leaders and members, has brought about the many changes necessary to establish unit coordinating as a health care profession. During her tenure at GateWay Community College, Ms. LaFleur Brooks served as Director of the Health Unit Coordinating and Health Services Management Program and as Chair of the Health Science Division. For the past eight years she has devoted her time to writing and consulting.

Elaine Gillingham started her health care career in Sandusky, Ohio, working after school at a local hospital, and was on-the-job-trained as a health unit coordinator. In 1977, she moved to Phoenix, Arizona, where she met Myrna LaFleur Brooks. Encouraged by Ms. LaFleur Brooks, she obtained a certificate of completion in Health Unit Coordinating and an Associate Degree in Health Services Management from GateWay Community College. She later obtained a Bachelor's degree in education from Ottawa University. Ms. Gillingham served as president of the Phoenix chapter of the National Association of Health Unit Coordinators and sat on the National Board for 2 years. In 1983, she wrote questions for and sat for the first National Certification exam sponsored by the National Association of Health Unit Coordinators. Ms. Gillingham has been teaching in the Health Unit Coordinator Program at GateWay Community College since 1987 and has served as Program Director since 1993. She began reviewing, consulting, and writing for the Health Unit Coordinating books in 1993.

CONTENTS

SECTION 5

Introduction to Anatomic Structures, Medical Terms, and Illnesses 441

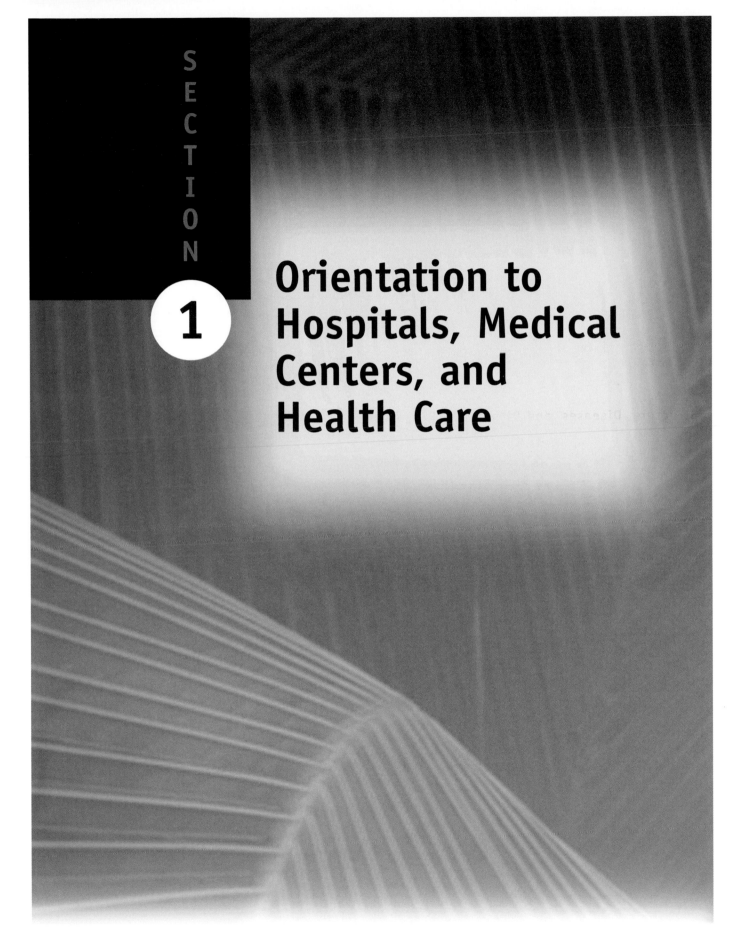

S E C T I O N

1

Orientation to Hospitals, Medical Centers, and Health Care

1

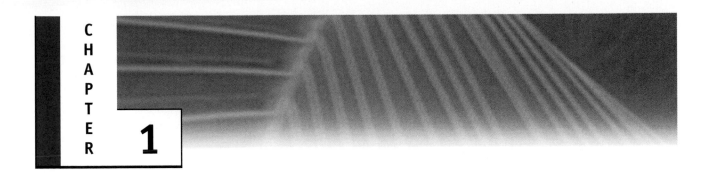

Health Unit Coordinating

An Allied Health Career

 Outline

▶ **Chapter Objectives**

Upon completion of this chapter, you will be able to:

1. Define the terms in the vocabulary list.
2. Write the meaning of the abbreviations in the abbreviations list.
3. Describe the four stages of evolution of health unit coordinating.
4. List three tasks the health unit coordinator may perform that relate to the nursing staff, to doctors, to other hospital departments, and to visitors.
5. List three reasons to become a member of the National Association of Health Unit Coordinators.
6. List the steps of the health services management career path for non-clinical practice.
7. List three reasons to become certified.

▶ **Vocabulary**

Career Ladder ▲ A pathway of upward mobility

Certification ▲ The process of testifying to or endorsing that a person has met certain standards

Certified Health Unit Coordinator (CHUC) ▲ A health unit coordinator who has passed the national certification examination sponsored by the National Association of Health Unit Coordinators (NAHUC)

Clinical Tasks ▲ Tasks performed at the bedside or in direct contact with the patient

Doctor ▲ A person licensed to practice medicine (used interchangeably with the term *physician* throughout this textbook)

Doctors' Orders ▲ The health care a doctor prescribes in writing for a hospitalized patient

Health Unit Coordinator (HUC) ▲ The nursing team member who performs the non-clinical patient care tasks for the nursing unit (also may be called unit clerk or unit secretary)

Hospital Departments ▲ Divisions within the hospital that specialize in services, such as the dietary department, which plans and prepares meals for patients, employees, and visitors

Independent Transcription ▲ The health unit coordinator assumes full responsibility for transcription of doctors' orders; cosignature by the nurse is not required

Non-Clinical Tasks ▲ Tasks performed away from the bedside

Nurses' Station ▲ The desk area of a nursing unit

Nursing Team ▲ A group of nursing staff members who care for patients on a nursing unit

Nursing Unit ▲ An area within the hospital with equipment and nursing personnel to care for a given number of patients (also may be referred to as a wing, floor, pod, strategic business unit, ward, or station)

Patient ▲ A person receiving health care, including preventive, promotion, acute, chronic, and all other services in the continuum of care

Policy and Procedure Manual ▲ A handbook with such information as guidelines for practice, hospital regulations, and job descriptions for hospital personnel

Recertification ▲ A process for certified health unit coordinators to exhibit continued personal and professional growth and current competency to practice in the field

Transcription ▲ A process used to communicate the doctors' orders to the nursing staff and other hospital departments; computers or handwritten requisitions are used

Abbreviations

Abbreviation	Meaning
CHUC	certified health unit coordinator
HUC	health unit coordinator
SHUC	student health unit coordinator
pt	patient

EXERCISE 1

Write the abbreviation for each term listed below.

1. certified health unit coordinator _____

2. health unit coordinator _____

3. student health unit coordinator _____

4. patient _____

EXERCISE 2

Write the meaning of each abbreviation listed below.
1. *CHUC*

_____

2. *HUC*

_____

3. *SHUC*

_____

4. *pt*

_____

■ INTRODUCTION TO HEALTH UNIT COORDINATING

Whether you are a student beginning an educational program or a health care employee, you probably have experienced difficulty in trying to explain to a relative or a friend what you do or will be doing as a health unit coordinator. Why? Because the public is aware of doctors, nurses, dentists, and possibly a few other health professions, but most people do not understand the important role of the health unit coordinator in the delivery of health care.

By contrast, understanding of your profession is much different within the health care community. When you share with another health professional that you are a health unit coordinator or that you are studying to become one, the comments include: "It's one of the most important positions on the nursing unit," "We are so disorganized if the unit coordinator is not there," "The unit coordinator creates the attitude for the entire unit," "The unit coordinator sets the pace for the day's work," and "Ask the unit coordinator—he or she knows everything."

Comments such as these are heard because the health unit coordinator organizes the activities for the nursing unit and manages its non-clinical functions. Therefore, the health unit coordinator can enhance or inhibit the delivery of health care to the patients on the nursing unit.

The overall job is usually non-clinical in nature. The work area is the nurses' station. Many health care facilities require health unit coordinators to wear scrubs, sometimes in a particular color. Some facilities opt for professional, non-clinical wear, such as shown in Figure 1–1.

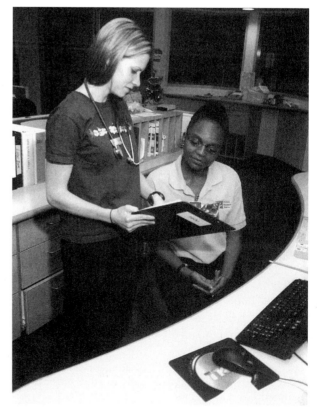

FIGURE 1–1 ▲ The health unit coordinator's work area is the nurses' station.

HISTORY OF HEALTH UNIT COORDINATING

Traditionally, health professions have evolved through four stages: on-the-job training, formal education, the formation of a national association, and certification or licensure. Health unit coordinating is no exception to the tradition.

On-The-Job-Training

During World War II hospitals experienced a drastic shortage of registered nurses. To compensate for this shortage, auxiliary personnel were trained on the job to assist the registered nurse. The health unit coordinator was trained to assist the nurse with the non-clinical tasks, whereas the nursing assistant was trained to assist the nurse at the bedside.

Following World War II, the nursing shortage was not as critical; however, the duties of the nurses were expanding. Advancement in technology was increasing the workload of the doctor, which resulted in the shifting of many tasks, such as taking blood pressure and starting intravenous therapy, to the nursing staff. Federally sponsored health programs required more detailed record-keeping, hospitals were becoming larger and more complex, and increasing numbers of specialists were required to carry out the new tests and treatments. The non-clinical demands of every hospitalized patient increased proportionally; therefore, the need for employing health unit coordinators continued. Today a 500-bed hospital has approximately 50 to 60 health unit coordinating positions. The role continues to change and expand.

Health unit coordinators were trained on the job for more than 20 years. The first record of health unit coordinating is found in an article published in *Modern Hospital* in 1940, which discussed the implementation of health unit coordinating at Montefiore Hospital in Pittsburgh, Pennsylvania. The author, Abraham Oseroff, a hospital administrator, stated "a new helper was introduced to the nursing unit to take care of the many details of secretarial nature that formerly made demands on the limited time of the nurse." The title of the new helper was "floor secretary." Interestingly, the author wrote, "the idea of floor secretary was first met with skepticism, but it proved to be worthwhile from the beginning."

Formal Education

In 1966, one of the first educational programs for health unit coordinating was offered in a vocational school in Minneapolis (Fig. 1–2, *A–C*). An article published in *Nursing Outlook* in 1966 described a research project that led to the implementation of this program. The most popular title for "floor secretary" had become "ward" or "unit clerk." The article's author, Ruth Stryker, recommended that the title be changed to "station coordinator" because the data showed that the unit clerk "did a great deal of managing in the form of coordinating activities." Ruth Stryker wrote one of the first textbooks for health unit coordinating, *The Hospital Ward Clerk*, which was published by the C. V. Mosby Company in 1970. Today, prior to employment, most health unit coordinators are educated in one of the many community colleges or vocational technical schools nationwide that offer health unit coordinator educational programs.

Professional Association

The occupation of health unit coordinator existed and grew for 40 years without the guidance of a professional association. The purpose of a professional association is to set standards of education and practice by peers to be enforced by peers for the protection of the public. Altruistic in nature, it is designed to enlighten its members and guide the profession to better serve the public. The constitution states the basic laws and principles of the association, and elected officers carry out the purpose listed in the constitution. By 1980, several educational programs were well established across the nation, and the educators in these programs began to discuss the possibility of forming a national association.

The first organizational meeting was held in Phoenix, Arizona, on August 23, 1980 (Fig. 1–2, *D*). This date has since been proclaimed National Health Unit Coordinating Day by the national association. The 10 founding members represented both education and practice. In attendance were Kathy Jordan, Winnie Starr, Connie Johnston, Estelle Johnson, and Myrna LaFleur from Arizona; Kay Cox from California; Helga Hegge from Minnesota; Jane Pedersen from Wisconsin; Carolyn Hinken from New Mexico; and Velma Kerschner from Texas. During this first meeting the founding members declared the formation of a national association for health coordinators to be called the *National Association of Health Unit Coordinators* (NAHUC) (Fig. 1–2, *F*). The founding members recognized the need to update the title and to have a uniform title used nationwide; "health unit coordinator" was chosen. The association has worked tirelessly since then to have this adopted in hospitals nationwide. Because "unit clerk" was the most popular title nationwide in 1980, it was included in the title of the national association with the intent that it would be dropped from the title when "coordinator" became recognized. In 1990, the national association changed its name to the "National Association of Health Unit Coordinators," dropping "clerk" from its name.

At the second organizational meeting, held in San Juan Capistrano, California, the constitution was ratified and the officers were elected. Today, the association has approximately 3000 members. Standards of practice (see Appendix C), including educational requirements and a code of ethics (see Appendix E), have been adopted. The association has three boards that govern various branches of the association. The Certification Board is responsible for offering the certification exam and maintaining records. The Education Board is responsible for activities related to educational aspects of the profession. The Accreditation Board is responsible for determining and evaluating standards of educational programs nationwide (see the Box *NAHUC Membership Information*).

NAHUC MEMBERSHIP INFORMATION

To receive an NAHUC or certification test application:
- Phone
  Toll-free: 888-22-NAHUC (62482)
  Locally: 815-633-4351
- Address: 1947 Madron Road
                  Rockford, IL 61107
- Fax: 815-633-4438
- Web site: www.nahuc.org
- E-mail: office@nahuc.org

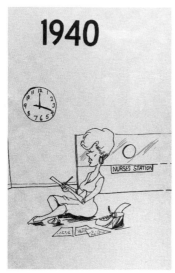

A

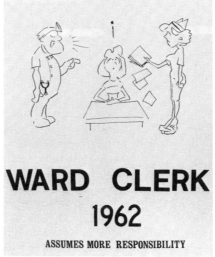

B

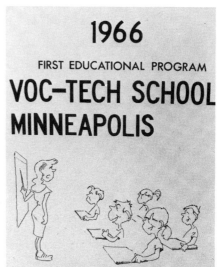

C

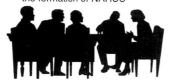

D

1980

August 23rd: First meeting for the formation of NAHUC

This date has been set aside as National Health Unit Coordinator Day

1983

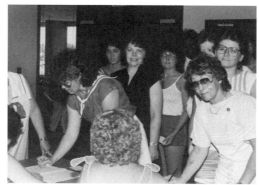

E   First certification exam

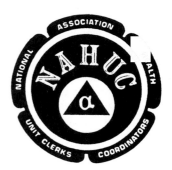

Logo prior to 1990 showing "unit clerk"

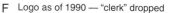

F   Logo as of 1990 — "clerk" dropped

FIGURE 1–2 ▲ History of health unit coordinating. *A,* In 1940, health unit coordinating was first introduced as a health care occupation. The first job title was "floor secretary." *B,* In 1962, the more common title was "ward clerk." More responsibilities were added to the job. *C,* In 1966, the first vocational educational program for health unit coordinating was established. *D,* On August 23, 1980, the first meeting for the formation of the National Association of Health Unit Coordinators (Clerks) was held in Phoenix, Arizona. *E,* In 1983, the first certification exam was offered by the National Association of Health Unit Coordinators (Clerks). *F,* The logo for the National Association of Health Unit Coordinators. The five outer segments represent doctors, nursing staff, patients, visitors, and hospital departments. The circle connecting the segments is symbolic of the health unit coordinator's role in coordinating the activities of these five groups. In 1990, "Clerk" was dropped from the name of the association now known as the National Association of Health Unit Coordinators.

✳ INFORMATION ALERT!

Evolution of Job Title

Following is an outline of the evolution of the job title from floor secretary to health unit coordinator.

1940	Floor Secretary
1966	Ward or Unit Clerk
1970	Ward or Unit Secretary
1979	Ward or Unit Secretary, Ward or Unit Clerk, Service Coordinator (all were used throughout the country)
1980	Health Unit Coordinator

Certification

Certification and/or licensure is the final step in the evolution of a health profession. Certification is a process of testifying to or endorsing that a person has met certain standards. The first certification examination was offered by NAHUC in May 1983. American Guidance Service, a professional testing company, was employed to administer the test. Nearly 5000 people took the first exam. Today, the examination is administered nationwide at testing sites using an electronic system. Questions are answered on a touch-sensitive computer screen, and test results are given immediately on completion of examination. The test is offered to anyone with a graduate equivalent degree (GED) or high school diploma.

It is not necessary to be a member of NAHUC or to have completed an educational program to sit for the examination (some health unit coordinators have been trained on the job and have years of experience). The goal of every student of health unit coordinating should be to become certified. Passing the national certification examination indicates that you have met a standard of excellence and that you are competent to practice health unit coordinating (see the Box *Five Reasons to Become Certified*).

Recertification is a process for certified health unit coordinators to exhibit continued personal and professional growth and current competency to practice in the field. The National Association of Health Unit Coordinators requires certified health unit coordinators to be recertified to ensure that they stay current in their field of practice. Recertification may be achieved by taking the test every 3 years or by obtaining continuing education unit (CEU) hours. NAHUC offers various opportunities for obtaining continuing education units. Also, employers often offer seminars and workshops that provide CEUs to the health unit coordinators in their health care facility and/or the community.

For a group to become a profession they must have the following credentials:

- A national association
- A formal education
- Certification or licensure
- A code of ethics
- An identified body of systematic knowledge and technical skill
- Members who function with a degree of autonomy and authority under the assumption that they alone have the expertise to make decisions in their area of competence

Formation of the national association and the dedication of health unit coordinators nationwide to developing and implementing the previously mentioned structure and practices have advanced health unit coordinating to the professionalism it deserves.

Students are encouraged to join the NAHUC (see the Box *Five Reasons to Become a Member of NAHUC*). For general information or information on membership or certification testing

sites, write to NAHUC, 1947 Madron Road, Rockford, Illinois 61107; call toll free: 888-22-NAHUC (62482); locally: 815-633-4351; fax: 815-633-4438; e-mail: office@nahuc.org; or visit the web site: www.nahuc.org.

■ HEALTH UNIT COORDINATING TODAY

Although health unit coordinating began as a clerical job to assist the nurse, today it is a position that consists of many responsibilities that vary among hospitals. These responsibilities include coordinating the activities of the nursing staff, the doctors, the hospital departments, the patients, and the visitors to the nursing unit (Fig. 1–3). Health unit coordinators also may be employed in doctors' offices, clinics, and long-term care facilities to assist the nurse with clerical duties related to the patients' health records.

Responsibilities of the Health Unit Coordinator

Responsibility to the Nursing Staff

Responsibilities vary among health care facilities. The health unit coordinator is a member of the health care team (Fig. 1–4) and usually functions under the direction of the nurse manager or unit manager. Responsibilities include (1) communicating all new doctors' orders to the patient's nurse (Fig. 1–5); (2) maintaining the patient's chart; (3) performing the non-clinical tasks for admission, discharge, and transfer of a patient; (4) preparing the patient's chart for surgery; and (5) handling all telephone communication for the nursing unit.

Interaction with the Doctor

The health unit coordinator greets the doctors on their arrival at the nurses' station and helps them, if necessary, to obtain the patients' charts and to procure equipment for patients' examina-

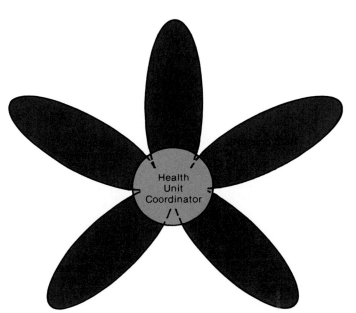

FIGURE 1–3 ▲ The health unit coordinator coordinates the activities of the doctors, the nursing staff, the hospital departments, the patients, and the visitors for the nursing unit.

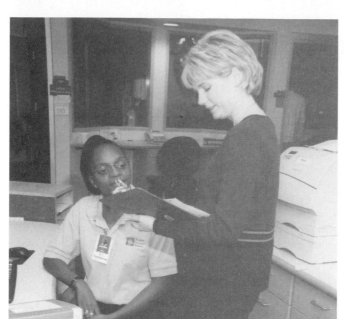

FIGURE 1–4 ▲ The health unit coordinator is a member of the nursing team and usually functions under the direction of the nurse manager or unit manager.

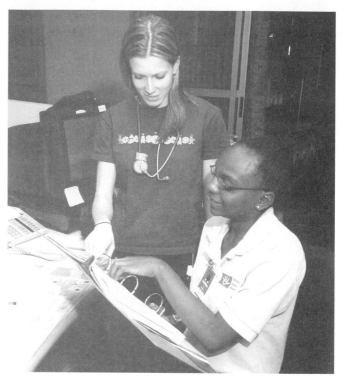

FIGURE 1–5 ▲ The health unit coordinator works closely with the nursing staff.

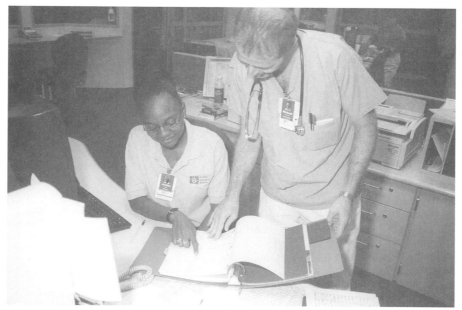

FIGURE 1–6 ▲ The health unit coordinator assists the doctor with obtaining charts and equipment stored in the nursing unit.

tions (Fig. 1–6). Other responsibilities include (1) transcribing the doctors' orders (Fig. 1–7), (2) placing calls to and receiving calls from the doctors' offices, and (3) obtaining information for the physician as to whether previously ordered procedures have been completed.

Relationship with Hospital Departments

The health unit coordinator is the communicator between the doctor and nursing personnel and other hospital departments. Responsibilities include (1) scheduling diagnostic procedures and treatments; (2) requesting services from mainte-

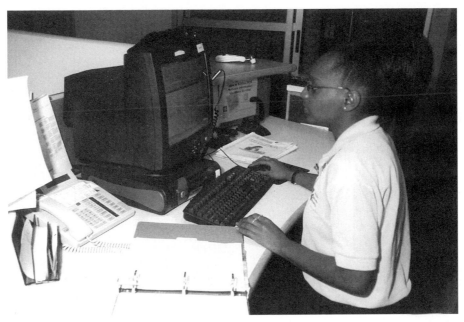

FIGURE 1–7 ▲ A major responsibility of the health unit coordinator is transcribing doctors' orders.

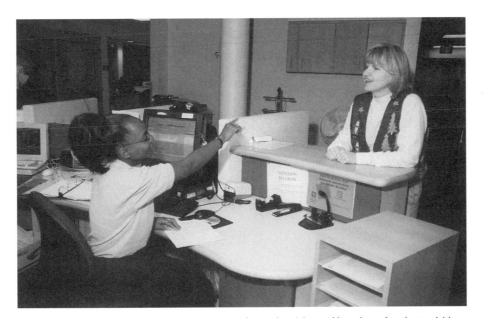

FIGURE 1–8 ▲ The health unit coordinator informs the visitors of location of patients, visiting hours, and any special precautions needed.

nance and other service departments; (3) working closely with the admitting department to admit, transfer, and discharge patients; and (4) ordering the supplies for the nursing unit ranging from food to paper products and patient care supplies.

Interaction with the Patient

The health unit coordinator greets new patients when they arrive on the nursing unit and may accompany them to their rooms. By use of the intercom in each patient's room, the health unit coordinator relays patients' requests to the nursing personnel. The health unit coordinator usually has little bedside contact with the patients.

Interaction with Hospital Visitors

The health unit coordinator (1) finds and advises visitors of patient location; (2) provides information on location of bathrooms, visitors' lounge, cafeteria, etc.; (3) informs visitors of the visiting rules and of any special precautions regarding their visit to a patient's room; (4) receives telephone calls from relatives or friends inquiring about the patient's condition; and (5) is often the first person to handle visitor complaints (Fig. 1–8).

EXAMPLE OF COMPETENCIES FOR AN EDUCATIONAL PROGRAM

STATEMENT OF COMPETENCY FOR HEALTH UNIT COORDINATOR

Upon completion of the program, the student demonstrated the ability to:

- Perform the health unit coordinator responsibilities and accountability to the nursing personnel, to the medical staff, to other hospital departments, and to the patients and visitors
- Operate the nursing unit communication systems: computer terminal, telephone, fax machine, intercom, pager, shredder, label printer, and conveyor system
- Record diagnostic test values, vital signs, and census data
- Order daily diets and daily laboratory tests
- File reports on the patients' charts
- Transcribe doctors' orders utilizing basic knowledge of anatomy and physiology, disease processes, medical terminology, and accepted abbreviations (competent to perform this task without the checking and cosignature of the registered nurse)
- Perform the non-clinical tasks for patient admission, transfer, discharge, preoperative and postoperative procedures
- Plan and execute a daily routine for the performance of non-clinical tasks for the nursing unit
- Manage the non-clinical functions of the nursing unit
- Maintain the nursing unit supplies
- Prepare patient consent forms
- Maintain the patients' charts
- Coordinate scheduling of patients' tests and diagnostic procedures
- Transcribe medication orders, utilizing concepts of drug categories, automatic stop dates, automatic cancellations, time scheduling, and routes of administration
- Practice within the professional ethical framework of health unit coordinating
- Schedule radiologic procedures that require patient preparation
- Communicate effectively with patients, visitors, and members of the health care team

Job Description

The tasks that may be performed by the health unit coordinator are many and vary among facilities. Appendix D lists health unit coordinator task and knowledge statements compiled from a nationwide research project done in 1996 by NAHUC's Job Analysis Study.

Hospitals outline the responsibilities for each category of employee in a formal written statement called a job description. Because health unit coordinating practice varies from hospital to hospital, it is important to look at the hospital's job description for health unit coordinating to find out what the responsibilities will be during employment. Job descriptions are a part of the hospital's policy and procedure manual, which usually is located on all nursing units.

Educational programs also outline the competencies or job skills that students are expected to know on completion of the program (see the Box *Example of Competencies for an Educational Program*).

■ CAREER LADDER OPPORTUNITIES IN HEALTH UNIT COORDINATING

A career ladder is a pathway of upward mobility and is a popular concept in health care facilities. Most facilities offer opportunities to assist employees to advance, such as prepaid on-campus education programs, college tuition reimbursement, and flexible work schedules. Many hospitals provide additional training for the health unit coordinator to acquire skills in cardiac monitoring, coding, and admitting duties (see the Box *Example of Job Descriptions and a Career Ladder for Health Unit Coordinating*).

■ CAREER PATHS

Health unit coordinating is recognized as the entry-level job in the non-clinical career path. On acquiring experience and the education needed, the health unit coordinator can advance to a health unit management position. A health unit manager's position includes performing the following duties for one or more nursing units:

- Establishing policies and procedures for the nursing units
- Planning departmental organization
- Hiring, motivating, and supervising health unit coordinators
- Providing staff development programs
- Preparing the nursing unit budget
- Participating in research

Figure 1–9 gives an example of career advancement for nonclinical practice.

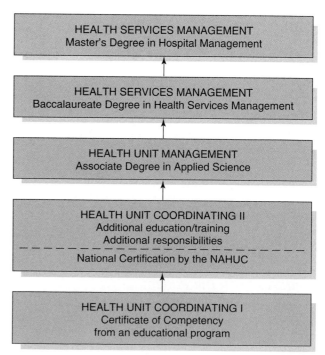

FIGURE 1–9 ▲ Career path for non-clinical practice.

EXAMPLE OF JOB DESCRIPTIONS AND CAREER LADDER FOR HEALTH UNIT COORDINATING

HEALTH UNIT COORDINATOR 1

Education
- Must be a graduate of a recognized educational program or be a certified health unit coordinator

Overall Responsibilities
- Manages supplies and equipment on a nursing unit
- Manages and performs the receptionist role for a nursing unit
- Uses discretion and protects the confidentiality of patient information
- Sets priorities and organizes the workload on a nursing unit

Job duties
- Performs the telephone communications for the nursing unit
- Transcribes the doctors' orders
- Performs patient admission, transfer, and discharge procedures
- Enters patient admission data into the computer
- Performs non-clinical preoperative and postoperative procedures
- Operates nursing unit equipment: pneumatic tube system, intercom system, fax machine, shredder, computer, and printer
- Maintains the daily census sheet and census board
- Maintains each patient's chart: files patient data in chart holder, labels and places standard forms in the chart holder as needed, and records the whereabouts of the chart if it is removed from the nursing unit
- Enters patient acuity into the computer
- Recaptures lost SPD charges
- Determines need for and orders unit supplies from the purchasing department
- Maintains up-to-date bulletin board

- Communicates pertinent data and hospital procedure to the patients' visitors
- Assists as directed during emergency situations
- Maintains reference books and policy/procedure manuals
- Assists doctors and other health personnel at the nurses' station

Job Relationships
- Usually functions under the supervision of the nurse manager

HEALTH UNIT COORDINATOR 2

Education
- Must have 3 years' experience and be NAHUC certified

Job Duties
- Performs all functions listed for Health Unit Coordinator 1
- Completes the time schedule for nursing personnel assigned to the nursing unit
- Collects and records nursing unit data and statistics under the direction of the nurse manager
- Supervises health unit coordinator 1 employees assigned to the health unit
- Oversees the orientation of health unit coordinators and newly hired nursing personnel to the health unit coordinator skills
- Acts as a liaison between patients, visitors, and nursing personnel

Other Duties That Would Require Additional Education
- Cardiac monitoring
- Admitting responsibilities
- Coding

Job Relationships
- Functions under the supervision of the nurse manager

■ SUMMARY

Health unit coordinating is a recognized health care profession. Individuals practicing as health unit coordinators soon realize that they have far-reaching effects on the delivery of care to the patients. The job can be stressful at times, but it is very rewarding. The career ladder concept and the increased technology used in health care facilities have added extra excitement to the field of non-clinical practice.

REVIEW QUESTIONS

1. Label the following tasks as clinical or non-clinical:

    a. assisting a patient to the bathroom _____

    b. transcribing doctors' orders _____

    c. filing reports in patients' charts _____

    d. feeding a patient _____

    e. answering the unit telephone _____

    f. changing a patient's dressing _____

    g. answering a patient's request on the intercom _____

2. The four stages of evolution of a health profession are listed below. Write the year that each stage began for health unit co-ordinating, and describe the events surrounding the dates.

    a. on-the-job training _____

    _____

    b. formal education _____

    _____

    c. professional association _____

    _____

    d. certification or licensure _____

    _____

3. List three health unit coordinating tasks that relate to the:

    a. nursing personnel

        i. _____

        ii. _____

        iii. _____

    b. doctor

        i. _____

        ii. _____

        iii. _____

    c. hospital departments

        i. _____

        ii. _____

        iii. _____

    d. patient's visitors

        i. _____

        ii. _____

        iii. _____

4. Describe what is meant by *transcription*.

    _____

5. Explain what *independent transcription* means.

_____

6. List three reasons to become a member of the National Association of Health Unit Coordinators.

a. _____

b. _____

c. _____

7. List three reasons to become certified.

a. _____

b. _____

c. _____

8. The steps of the health services management career path for non-clinical practice are:

a. _____

b. _____

c. _____

d. _____

9. Your job description can be found in the _____ .

TOPICS FOR DISCUSSION

1. Visit the NAHUC web site at www.nahuc.org. (If you do not have access to the web at home, use a school computer or go to a library.)
   a. Locate the on-line Health Unit Coordinator Certification Handbook. Discuss the sample questions listed.
   b. Locate and print the NAHUC Standards of Practice, and discuss the significance of each standard listed.
   c. Locate the list of NAHUC representatives and copy the name, telephone number, and e-mail address of the representative for your area. Discuss the advantages of knowing the name of your local NAHUC representative.
2. Discuss the reasons why recertification is required by the National Association of Health Unit Coordinators.

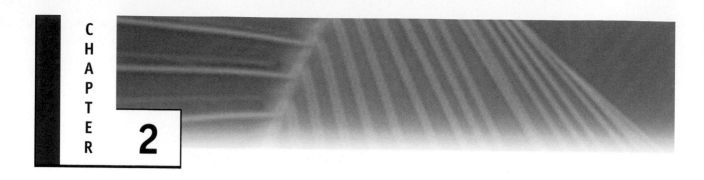

Health Care Today

Chapter Objectives

Upon completion of this chapter, you will be able to:

1. Define the terms in the vocabulary list.
2. Write the meaning of the abbreviations in the abbreviations list.
3. List five functions a hospital may perform.
4. List three ways in which hospitals may be classified.
5. List three annual in-services required by JCAHO.
6. Describe the general structure of a typical hospital.
7. Identify the respective roles of an attending physician and a hospital resident.
8. Identify the title of physicians serving in a specialty.
9. Explain the function of the departments in finance, diagnostic and therapeutic services, additional services, and operational services.
10. Describe other health care delivery systems and services.
11. Define managed care and why it was created.
12. Describe four major health care payment sources and the types of populations they serve.
13. List three components of health care delivery systems, and identify examples of each component.
14. List three resources that may be used for finding job opportunities.

Vocabulary

Accreditation ▲ Recognition that a health care organization has met an official standard

Acute Care ▲ Short-term care for serious illness or trauma

Attending Physician ▲ The term applied to a physician who admits and is responsible for a hospital patient

Capitation ▲ A payment method whereby the provider of care receives a set dollar amount per patient, regardless of services rendered

Case Manager ▲ A health care professional and expert in managed care who assists patients in assessing health and social service systems to assure that all required services are obtained; coordinates care with doctor and insurance companies

Chief Executive Officer ▲ The individual in direct charge of a hospital who is responsible to the governing board

Chronic Care ▲ Care for illnesses of long duration, such as diabetes or emphysema

Community Health ▲ Concerned with the members of a community with emphasis on prevention and early detection of disease

Governing Board ▲ A group of community citizens at the head of the hospital organizational structure

Health Maintenance Organization ▲ An organization that has management responsibility for providing comprehensive health care services on a prepayment basis to voluntarily enrolled persons within a designated population

Home Health ▲ Equipment and services are provided to patient in-home to provide comfort and care

Hospice ▲ Supportive care for terminally ill patients and their families

Hospitalist ▲ A full-time, acute care specialist whose focus is exclusively on hospitalized patients.

Inpatient ▲ A patient who has been admitted to a health care facility at least overnight for treatment and care

Integrated Delivery Networks ▲ Health care organization merged into systems that can provide all needed health care services under one corporate umbrella

Managed Care ▲ The use of a planned and systematic approach to providing health care, with the goal of offering quality care at the lowest possible cost

Medicaid ▲ A federal and state program that provides medical assistance for the indigent

Medicare ▲ Government insurance; enacted in 1965 for individuals older than age 65 and any person with a disability who has received Social Security for 2 years (some disabilities are covered immediately)

Merger ▲ The combining of individual physician practices and small, stand-alone hospitals into larger networks

Primary Care Physician ▲ Sometimes referred to as "gatekeepers," these general practitioners are the first physicians to see a patient for an illness

Proprietary ▲ For profit

Resident ▲ A graduate of a medical school who is gaining experience in a hospital

Surfing the Web ▲ Using different web sites on the Internet to locate information

Voluntary ▲ Not for profit

Web Address ▲ (URL, or uniform resource locator) Keywords that when entered after http://www. on the Internet will take user to specified location, referred to as a *web site*

Abbreviations

Abbreviation	Meaning
CEO	chief executive officer
CFO	chief financial officer
COO	chief operating officer
DSU	day surgery unit
DO	doctor of osteopathy
DRG	diagnosis-related groups
ECF	extended care facility
ED	emergency department
ER	emergency room
HMO	health maintenance organization
HO	house officer
JCAHO	Joint Commission on Accreditation of Healthcare Organizations
LTC	long-term care
MD	medical doctor
Neuro	neurology
OB	obstetrics
OR	operating room
Ortho	orthopedics
PACU	postanesthesia care unit
Peds	pediatrics
PPO	preferred provider organization
Psych	psychiatry
RR	recovery room
SAD	save a day (patient admitted the day of surgery)
SDS	same-day surgery (patient admitted the day of surgery)
SNF	skilled nursing facility
Surg	surgical
UCR	usual, customary, and reasonable
www	World Wide Web

EXERCISE 1

Write the correct abbreviation for each term listed below.

1. chief executive officer _____

2. chief financial officer _____

3. chief operating officer _____

4. day surgery unit _____

5. doctor of osteopathy _____

6. diagnosis-related grouping _____

7. extended care facility _____

8. emergency department _____

9. emergency room _____

10. health maintenance organization _____

11. house officer _____

12. Joint Commission on Accreditation of Healthcare Organizations _____

13. long-term care _____

14. medical doctor _____

15. neurology _____

16. obstetrics _____

17. operating room _____

18. orthopedics _____

19. postanesthesia care unit _____

20. pediatrics _____

21. preferred provider
    organization   _____

22. psychiatry   _____

23. recovery room   _____

24. save a day   _____

25. same day surgery   _____

26. skilled nursing facility _____

27. surgical   _____

28. usual, customary, and
    reasonable   _____

29. World Wide Web   _____

EXERCISE ❷

Write the meaning of each abbreviation below.

1. CEO

    _____

2. CFO

    _____

3. COO

    _____

4. DSU

    _____

5. DO

    _____

6. DRG

    _____

7. ECF

    _____

8. ED

    _____

9. ER

    _____

10. HMO

    _____

11. HO

    _____

12. JCAHO

    _____

13. LTC

    _____

14. MD

    _____

15. Neuro

    _____

16. OB

    _____

17. OR

    _____

18. Ortho

    _____

19. PACU

    _____

20. *Peds*

_____

21. *PPO*

_____

22. *Psych*

_____

23. *RR*

_____

24. *SAD*

_____

25. *SDS*

_____

26. *SNF*

_____

27. *Surg*

_____

28. *UCR*

_____

29. *www*

_____

▉ HEALTH CARE DELIVERY SYSTEMS AND SERVICES

History of Hospitals

The history of early Egyptian and Indian civilizations records that crude hospitals were in existence six centuries before Christ. The early Greeks and Romans used their temples to the gods as refuges for the sick.

During the Crusades, *hospitea* were established for pilgrims to rest from their travels. The word *hospital* comes to us originally from the Latin noun *hospes,* which means "guest" or "host." The term hospice, which relates to family-centered care for the terminally ill, also is derived from *hospes.*

As Christianity progressed, the care of the sick, although remaining an important part of the work of the church, was moved out of the temples into separate buildings. During the 12th and 13th centuries, there was great hospital growth in England and France. Members of religious orders cared for the needs of the ill. An organizational structure similar to that of the modern hospital began to emerge.

The earliest hospital in what is now the United States served sick soldiers on Manhattan Island in 1663. However, the first established hospitals were founded in Philadelphia in the early 18th century.

The development of hospitals continued worldwide as more inventions and discoveries were brought to light. The middle 19th and early 20th centuries were important to hospital growth because during this period the foundations were laid for modern biology, and books on the subject began to be written. The early 20th century also saw substantial advances in the education of nurses and doctors and an increase in the number of people being trained for these professions.

Through the centuries people's interest in the welfare of their fellow human beings continued to grow. The hospital of today continues to serve those in need during illness or injury with modern technologies, improved medical knowledge, and compassion.

Hospital Functions

The primary function of the hospital is the care and treatment of the sick. This is true of all hospitals regardless of size. Other functions are the education of physicians and other health care personnel, research, and prevention of disease. Especially in smaller communities, the hospital also serves as a local health center.

Only large hospitals may find it possible to perform all five functions. The functions the hospital performs depend on many factors, including the hospital's location, the population it serves, and the size of the facility.

The care and treatment of the sick or injured necessitate proper accommodations for the patient, with adequate medical and nursing care. Services performed take into account the patient's comfort and safety. The care and treatment of each patient call for a team effort. Each department involved with the patient plays an important role in assisting the patient to return to a better state of health.

Some hospitals maintain schools in various health services, such as radiology, clinical laboratory, and respiratory care. Other hospitals provide practical experience for students enrolled in university or community college educational programs in all levels of nursing, diet therapy, hospital administration, health unit coordinating, and other hospital-related fields. A hospital may have a residency program for doctors, and it also may provide additional experiences for medical students.

The type of research carried on in hospitals may depend on specific services rendered by the hospital. A hospital specializing in the care of cancer patients would do research in cancer, whereas a hospital that specializes in the care of patients with skeletal deformities would perform research in that area.

The trend today is toward the prevention of disease. The hospital may serve as a community health center, providing low-cost or free clinics for detection of symptoms of beginning disease conditions and for immunization programs. Doctors and other health care personnel also provide counseling and instruction in health care.

Hospital Classifications

There are many ways of classifying hospitals. The three most common classifications are (1) the type of patient service offered, (2) the ownership of the hospital, and (3) the type of accreditation the hospital has been given.

"Type of service offered" refers to the distinction between general hospitals and specialized hospitals. General hospitals—the most common type—render various services for patients suffering from many disease conditions and injuries. Not all general hospitals in a community offer identical services because it would prove too costly. Specialized hospitals provide services to a particular body part (e.g., an eye hospital), a particular segment of the population (e.g., a children's hospital), or for a particular type of care (e.g., a psychiatric or rehabilitation hospital).

The ownership of the hospital is the second type of classification. The federal government maintains hospitals for veterans and for personnel in the Navy and Air Force. The government also provides health services in hospitals for Native Americans. States, counties, and cities are also owners of hospitals. Churches and fraternal organizations may own and control general or specialized hospitals, which are usually nonprofit agencies. Proprietary hospitals (operated for profit and owned by a group of individuals or corporations) are also in operation.

The hospital of today is often part of a health care system. The health care system usually has a "parent" corporation that oversees the other companies within the system. The hospital is one of the subsidiary companies. Subsidiaries are designated either as profit or nonprofit. Each has its own board of directors. Other companies in the system, aside from the hospital, could be a company providing durable medical equipment, another providing home care to the community, another operating parking facilities or linen services, and so forth. Most health care systems have a component called a foundation, whose purpose is to focus on donations and fundraising activities that benefit the entire system.

The third type of hospital classification—by accreditation—refers to recognition that a hospital has met an official standard. For example, a JCAHO-accredited hospital means that the hospital has been surveyed, graded, and approved by the Joint Commission on the Accreditation of Healthcare Organizations. Participation in JCAHO accreditation is voluntary. Several other accrediting agencies also conduct surveys, according to the services provided by the hospital. All facilities receiving Medicare reimbursement require JCAHO accreditation.

The hospital's license to operate usually is granted by the Department of Health Services of the individual state.

The American Hospital Association (AHA) and the JCAHO determine the hospital operational guidelines. AHA guidelines address confidentiality, privacy, informed consents, patient rights, and the like. JCAHO guidelines address quality of care and dimensions of performance. JCAHO-required annual in-services include cardiopulmonary resuscitation, infectious disease control, fire and safety, and universal (standard) precautions (tuberculosis skin test and possibly hepatitis screen, rubella testing, and urine drug testing are required).

Hospital Organization

Administrative Personnel

The governing board is at the top of the organizational structure of a hospital. The governing board also may be referred to as the board of trustees or the board of directors. Three of the main responsibilities of the board include establishing policy, providing adequate financing, and overseeing personnel standards. The board is composed of persons from the business and professional communities as well as concerned citizens from all socioeconomic groups. The number of hospital board members varies with the size of the hospital. In hospitals that are part of a health care system, the hospital's governing board is responsible to the board of the parent corporation of the system.

In direct charge of the hospital, responsible to the governing board, is the chief executive officer (CEO). He or she plans for the implementation of policies set forth by the governing board. The chief operating officer (COO) is responsible for the day-to-day operations of the hospital and reports directly to the CEO. The chief financial officer (CFO) is responsible for the fiscal aspects of the hospital administration and reports directly to the CEO. A vice president or a director supervises each service within the hospital. Vice presidents report to the hospital COO (Fig. 2–1).

The board delegates the supervision of the quality of patient care and the conduct of the physicians practicing in the hospital to a committee representative of the medical staff.

The Medical Staff

Because the health unit coordinator transcribes doctors' orders and acts as the receptionist for the nursing unit, he or she has a great deal of interaction with the medical staff. Therefore, it is helpful to know the different roles of the doctors in a hospital.

The hospital governing board has a duty to the community to exercise care in the selection of doctors appointed to the medical staff. A doctor who has submitted his or her credentials to the state medical board and has a license to practice in the state may submit an application for appointment to the staff of a hospital or hospitals.

A physician who has been appointed to the medical staff and sends patients to the hospital for admission is known as the patient's attending physician. The attending physician prescribes the care and treatment (doctor's orders) for his or her patients during their hospital stay. A doctor caring for hospital patients may be a doctor of medicine (MD) or a doctor of osteopathy (DO). Both pursue identical approved programs of study, but colleges of osteopathic medicine place special emphasis on the relationship of organs and the musculoskeletal system. Structural problems are corrected by manipulation. Attending physicians are not hospital employees and receive no salary from the hospital. A hospitalist is a full-time acute care specialist whose focus is exclusively on hospitalized patients. This position was created in 1991 to enable family physicians to effectively manage their inpatient practices and treat more people in their outpatient prac-

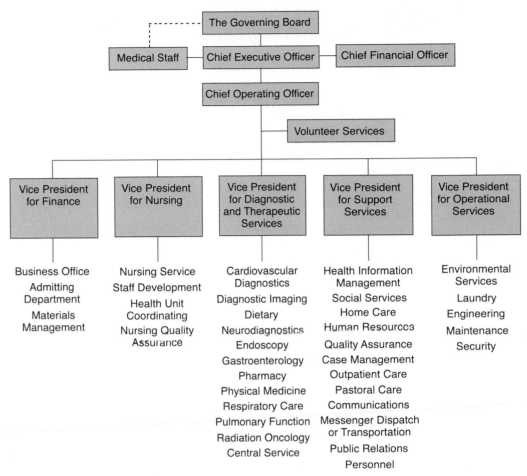

FIGURE 2-1 ▲ An example of a typical hospital organizational structure.

tices. Hospitalists are employed by the hospital and receive a salary from the hospital. There may be other doctors on the staff (such as the director of medical education, the hospital pathologist, or the director of radiation oncology) who are salaried hospital employees.

Large hospitals may have an educational program for medical school graduates to apply their knowledge in the practice of medicine. The term *intern* rarely is used in reference to the medical school graduate. The term *resident* is applied to all medical school graduates gaining hospital experience. These graduates frequently are referred to as postgraduate year 1 (PGY-1) or first-year resident. Residents may be referred to as house staff or house officers (HO).

Physicians who specialize in a particular aspect of medicine, such as pediatrics, internal medicine, or general surgery, spend 3 to 5 years in a specific residency program. After completing the residency and passing a specific exam, the physician is said to be certified. Often after residency there is a 1- to 2-year fellowship period to gain more familiarity in a specific area, such as cardiology. These practitioners are referred to as fellows. Some attending physicians serve as teachers for the hospital residents.

Many physicians have chosen to practice in special fields and are known by their specialties. It is common to refer to a doctor by his or her specialty, as in the terms cardiologist, gynecologist, or pediatrician.

In the course of your work at the hospital, you may be required to use medical specialty terms when referring to doctors (see the Box *Common Medical Specialties*).

Hospital Departments and Services

As a coordinator for the nursing unit you interact daily with many hospital departments either during the transcription of doctor's orders or when requesting services provided by the department. Therefore, it is important for you to have an overall view of the departments and their functions as they relate to your role as the health unit coordinator. See the Box *Hospital Departments* for a brief description of their services. The services are divided into business services, diagnostic and therapeutic services, support services, and operational services. It is important to remember that not all hospitals have each of the departments listed, nor may the department in each hospital use the same name as used in this text.

Business Services

Business services deal with the financial aspect of the hospital. The health unit coordinator works closely with the admitting department during the patient's admission to, transfer within, and discharge from the hospital. The health unit coordinator also orders all the unit supplies from the purchasing department.

COMMON MEDICAL SPECIALTIES

PHYSICIAN'S SPECIALTY	SPECIALTY DESCRIPTION
Allergist	Treats patients who have hypersensitivity to pollens, foods, medications, and other substances
Anesthesiologist	Administers drugs or gases to produce loss of consciousness or sensation in the patient; care during surgery and recovery from anesthetic is included
Cardiologist	Diagnoses and treats diseases of the heart and blood vessels
Dermatologist	Diagnoses and treats disorders of the skin
Emergency room physician	Diagnoses and treats patients in trauma and emergency situations
Endocrinologist	Diagnoses and treats diseases of the internal glands that secrete hormones
Family practitioner	Specializes in primary health care for all family members
Gastroenterologist	Diagnoses and treats diseases of the digestive tract
Geriatrist	Diagnoses and treats diseases and problems of aging
Gynecologist	Diagnoses and treats disorders and diseases of the female reproductive tract
Hospitalist	Provides acute care exclusively to hospitalized patients
Internist	Diagnoses and treats medically diseases and disorders of the internal organs of adults
Neonatologist	Diagnoses and treats disorders of the newborn
Neurologist	Diagnoses and treats diseases of the nervous system
Obstetrician	Cares for women during pregnancy, labor, delivery, and following delivery
Oncologist	Diagnoses and treats cancerous conditions
Ophthalmologist	Diagnoses and treats diseases and defects of the eye
Orthopedist	Diagnoses and treats diseases or fractures of the musculoskeletal system
Otolaryngologist	Diagnoses and treats diseases of the ear, nose, and throat
Pathologist	Studies cell changes and other alterations of the body caused by disease
Pediatrician	Provides preventive care and diagnoses and treats diseases of children
Physiatrist	Diagnoses and treats diseases of the neuromusculoskeletal system with physical elements to restore the individual to participation in society
Proctologist	Diagnoses and treats diseases of the rectum and anus
Psychiatrist	Diagnoses and treats mental illness
Radiation oncologist	Treats cancer through the use of radiation
Radiologist	Diagnoses and also treats some diseases by using various methods of imaging such as x-ray, ultrasound, radioactive materials, and magnetic resonance
Surgeon	Treats diseases and injuries by operative methods; may specialize in a particular areas, such as heart, eye, or pediatric surgery
Urologist	Diagnoses and treats diseases of the male and female urinary tracts and of the male reproductive system

The *business office* is in charge of patient accounts, budget planning, employee payroll, and payment of bills incurred by the hospital. This office determines the ability of the patient to pay through hospitalization insurance and Medicare or Medicaid. The business office also provides a place for safekeeping of patient valuables. In the area of budget planning, each department and nursing unit is issued a cost-control-center number. For example, the dietary department may be given number 4622. All purchases, maintenance fees, and other expenses must have the cost-control-center number on the request for recordkeeping purposes.

The *admitting department*, sometimes called patient services, admits new patients to the hospital, transfers patients within the hospital, and discharges patients from the hospital. On admission, the admitting department obtains pertinent information from patients or their relatives, witnesses the signing of the admission agreement by the patient or his or her representative, and prepares the identification bracelet and labels.

The *materials management department*, or purchasing department, is responsible for obtaining all supplies and equipment to be used by hospital departments. Sometimes small hospitals band together to have greater purchasing power and save one another money.

Diagnostic and Therapeutic Services

The following departments relate to the direct care of the hospitalized patient. During the transcription procedures, the health unit coordinator orders tests, treatments, or supplies from these departments, according to the doctors' orders.

The *cardiovascular diagnostics department* performs tests related to cardiac (heart) and blood-vessel function. The diagnostic procedure ordered most often is the electrocardiogram, which is performed at the patient's bedside. Cardiac catheterization is carried out in the department.

The *diagnostic imaging department* includes the radiology, nuclear medicine, and ultrasound departments. Diagnostic studies are performed by using x-ray, ultrasound, computed tomography, magnetic resonance imaging, and radioactive element scanners. A radiologist, a medical doctor qualified in the use of x-ray and other imaging devices, is in charge of this department. The

HOSPITAL DEPARTMENTS

DEPARTMENT	SERVICE
Business:	
Business office	Patient accounts
Admitting	Admission of new patients
Purchasing	Obtains supplies and equipment
Central services	Storage and distribution of supplies and equipment used for client care
Diagnostic and therapeutic:	
Cardiovascular diagnostics	Tests related to heart and blood vessels
Diagnostic imaging	X-rays, nuclear medicine, and ultrasound studies
Dietary	Meals
Neurodiagnostics	Studies of the brain
Endoscopy	Diagnostic procedures using endoscopes
Gastroenterology	Studies related to the digestive system
Pathology/clinical laboratory	Diagnostic procedures on specimens from the body
Pharmacy	Medications
Physical medicine	Rehabilitation
Respiratory care	Treatment related to respiratory function
Diagnostic and therapeutic:	
Radiation oncology	Treatment of cancer growths
Support services:	
Health information management	Patient records
Quality assurance	Quality care
Social service	Assistance to patients and families
Case management	Coordinates patient care with insurance companies
Home care or discharge planning	Transition from hospital to home
Outpatient	Services to patients outside the hospital
Pastoral care	Spiritual support
Patient advocate	Available to patients who have concerns about their care or environment
Communications	Switchboard
Transportation	Delivery
Public relations	Provides information to the public
Volunteer services	A variety of services provided by volunteers
Operational services:	
Environmental	Housekeeping duties
Mechanical	Keeps equipment in working condition
Laundry	Maintains linens
Human resources	Recruitment, records, and benefits
Security	Protection

radiographer, a graduate of a 2- or 4-year educational program, performs many of the technical procedures.

The *dietary department,* which is under the direction of a registered dietitian who is a graduate of a 4-year college program, plans and prepares meals for patients, employees, and visitors. Personnel within the department deliver meals and nourishment to the nursing care units. The dietitian also instructs patients in proper nutrition and in the use of special diets when they are ordered by the doctor. Some hospitals participate in an internship program for college students enrolled in a hospital dietitian curriculum.

The *neurodiagnostics department* performs diagnostic studies of the brain. Electroencephalography (EEG) records the electric impulses of brain waves. An EEG technician performs the test. A physician, usually a neurologist, interprets the brain-wave tracings.

The *endoscopy department* performs diagnostic procedures by using endoscopes. These instruments permit the visual examination of a body cavity or hollow organ, such as the stomach. A specialist employed by the hospital or in private practice may perform endoscopies. Registered nurses or licensed practical nurses usually assist the doctors with these procedures.

The *gastroenterology department,* or GI lab, performs studies to diagnose disease conditions of the digestive system. Tests are usually performed on an outpatient basis. Tests are related to problems of the esophagus, stomach, pancreas, gallbladder, and small intestine. A gastroenterologist, a doctor with additional education related to disease of the gastrointestinal system, is in charge of the department. A laboratory technologist or registered nurse may assist with these procedures.

The *pathology department,* or clinical laboratory, is concerned with diagnostic procedures performed on specimens from the body, such as blood, tissues, urine, stools, sputum, and bone marrow. This department may be separated into several divisions named for the tests or substances to be examined, such as hematology, urinalysis, microbiology, chemistry, and blood bank. The pathologist also examines specimens removed during surgery. Autopsies are performed under the direction of this department. The laboratory functions under the direction of a pathologist and employs medical technologists and medical laboratory technicians who have graduated from a recognized school for laboratory personnel.

The *pharmacy* provides the medications used by the patient within the hospital or in the clinics. The pharmacist fills the prescription ordered by the doctor. The pharmacy also may provide lotions and mouthwashes for patient use. Intravenous solutions to which medications have been added also are prepared in the pharmacy under sterile conditions. A registered pharmacist is in charge of the pharmacy.

The *physical medicine department* is composed of several smaller departments related to the rehabilitation of the patient. The physical medicine department is under the direction of a physiatrist. Physical therapy and occupational therapy are the two most common therapeutic areas within the physical medicine department. Small hospitals may have only a physical therapy department. The physical therapy department provides treatment by the use of exercise, massage, heat, light, water, and other methods. Registered physical therapists (graduates of a 4-year college program) and physical therapy technicians (graduates of a 2-year community college program) carry out the prescribed evaluations and treatments.

The *occupational therapy department* provides patients with purposeful activities that are designed to evaluate and treat those who are impaired physically, mentally, and developmentally. These activities help prevent deformities, restore function to affected body parts, and preserve morale. Registered occupational therapists, graduates of a 4-year college program, are employed in the occupational therapy department.

The *respiratory care department* performs diagnostic tests to determine lung function, provides treatment related to respiratory function, and assists in maintaining patients on ventilators (breathing machines). The department also administers respiratory physical therapy. The respiratory care therapist and the respiratory care technician, graduates of 1- to 4-year educational programs, are employed here. In many hospitals the respiratory care department is called the cardiopulmonary department.

The *radiation oncology department,* or radiation therapy department, may be a division within the diagnostic imaging department or a separate department. Its primary purpose is to treat cancerous growths. Cobalt-beam units and linear accelerators are examples of equipment used in these departments. The radiation oncologist, a physician with additional education in the use of radiation for the treatment of disease, is the head of the radiation oncology department.

Support Services

The following departments are also very important in the concept of caring for all patients' needs. The health unit coordinator interacts with most of the following departments by requesting services, supplies, and/or equipment for the patients on the nursing unit.

The *central service department* is the distribution area for supplies and equipment used by nursing personnel to perform treatments on patients. Enema kits, dressing trays, bandages, and other supplies used most frequently by the nursing unit personnel may be kept on the nursing unit. Central service department technicians replenish the unit supply daily. Packs of supplies used by the operating and delivery rooms may be processed and sterilized by the central service department personnel.

The *health information management department,* also called the health or medical records department, cares for the patient's record after the patients are discharged from the hospital. Records are stored here and may be retrieved for the doctor if the patient is readmitted. The records also may be used for research. This department is also responsible for coding medical and surgical conditions of patients on discharge. This coding is related to the system of Medicare reimbursement, involving diagnosis-related groupings (DRGs), whereby payment is based on the type of illness. Accurate coding of the patient's diagnosis using the International Classification of Disease (ICD) system is a critical function within the department. If coding is not exact, the direct result can be financial loss for the hospital. Medical transcription (not related to transcription as used in the transcription of a doctor's orders) is another service of the health records department that is available to doctors for the dictation of patient's histories, physical examination findings, and so forth. The transcriptionist prepares typewritten reports from the dictated tapes. The reports are placed on the hospitalized patients' chart.

The *quality assurance department* provides information to various departments within the hospital for the purpose of assisting those departments to provide quality care. Through analysis of actual occurrences and practices against standards set by various departments, quality assurance continuously uses ongoing activities to suggest improvements. Individual departments, such as nursing, may have their own quality assurance component, which coordinates with the hospital-wide quality assurance department. Risk management is a system of ensuring appropriate nursing care and can be part of the quality assurance manager's responsibilities. Risk management includes identifying possible risks, analyzing them, acting to reduce the risks, and evaluating the steps taken.

The *social service department* provides services to patients and to their families when emotional and environmental difficulties impede the patient's recovery. The social worker's knowledge of the community and of the agencies providing a variety of services aids in lifting emotional and financial burdens caused by the illness. This department also can arrange nursing home and extended care facility placement. The department head holds an advanced degree in social work.

The *case manager* is an individual who works in health care facilities, usually under the social services department, to coordinate the patient's care with insurance companies. The case manager is an expert in managed care and acts as an advocate for the patient to most appropriately utilize the benefits and coverage of his or her health policy.

The *home care department* assists patients in preparing for the transition from the hospital to home. A registered nurse with a public health background usually heads the department. The needs of the patient returning to the home environment are identified. Plans for care by the visiting nurse service and rental of needed equipment may be arranged before the patient is discharged. Follow-up studies also are provided for the doctor.

The *outpatient department* or clinic provides services to patients outside the hospital. Clinics for various disease conditions, such as diabetes, allergies, and gynecologic problems, may be open weekly. Prenatal care and dental care also may be offered. Visits are usually by appointment. The outpatient area also provides clinical experiences for resident doctors.

The *pastoral care department* provides spiritual support to the patient and family in time of need. There are hospitals that maintain a chaplaincy program for members of the clergy interested in becoming hospital chaplains.

The *communications department* may be called the telephone switchboard in many hospitals. The telephone operators process incoming and outgoing telephone calls and operate the doctor paging system. In emergencies, such as a fire, disaster, or cardiac arrest, communications personnel alert the hospital personnel in code, such as Code 1000, to announce a fire in the hospital. In some hospitals the telephone operator also may serve as an information station for visitors to the hospital.

The *messenger, dispatch,* or *transportation department* performs multiple tasks throughout the hospital. Delivery of interdepartmental mail, carrying of specimens to the laboratory, assisting with the discharge or admission of patients, and transporting of patients from one area of the hospital to another are all carried out by personnel of this department.

The *public relations department* serves to provide the public with information concerning the hospital's activities. This may be accomplished by means of the community newspaper. Many hospitals publish a weekly, bimonthly, or monthly newspaper for patients and/or employees.

The *volunteer services department* is made up of people from the community. The members of the women's auxiliary or its counterpart, the men's auxiliary, give generously of their time and talents to staff the patient library or gift shop. Many perform tasks for the various hospital departments or on the nursing unit. High school students also may have an auxiliary organization.

Operational Services

The following services are not related to the direct care of the hospitalized patient but are concerned with the patient's hospital environment. It is the health unit coordinator's task to request services from these departments as needed by the nursing unit.

The main responsibility of *environmental services,* sometimes called the housekeeping department, is to maintain a clean hospital through proper cleaning methods aimed at preventing the spread of infection. Daily cleaning of the hospital is provided by environmental services. Environmental services is responsible for cleaning the individual patient unit after a patient has been discharged and preparing it for a new admission. Another duty that this department may perform is the changing of draperies and the cubicle curtains around the patient's bed. In some hospitals, environmental services also have the responsibility of delivering isolation equipment to the unit.

The *mechanical services department* of the hospital is responsible for keeping all equipment in working condition. In a large hospital, this department may be divided into various branches, such as engineering, maintenance, and electronic equipment repair. The engineering division is concerned with heating, lighting, air conditioning, power systems, water, and sewage. The maintenance division is responsible for keeping the hospital and its surroundings, equipment, and furnishings in tip-top condition. Services rendered include painting, maintenance of televisions, carpentry, and pneumatic tube systems repairs. Gardeners and groundskeepers are also members of this department. *Hospital information systems* personnel repair and maintain electronic equipment, including telephones, computers, printers, and so on.

The *laundry department* maintains the linen supply for the hospital, which may include the washing, drying, and repairing of the linens. Many hospitals send the laundry out to a commercial laundry under the coordination of the hospital laundry department. Some hospitals may join together in ownership of a laundry service, which more economically serves the needs of all. Laundry personnel may deliver the linen to the nursing care units.

The *human resources department* organizes recruitment programs, interviews new employees, conducts employee termination interviews, and maintains records for each employee. Employee benefits and retirement records are also the responsibility of the human resource department.

An employee fitness center is available in many hospitals to assist employees with their own health maintenance. Some hospitals may have counseling services available to employees to assist them in coping with personal and employment problems.

The *security department* is responsible for protecting the hospital, patients, visitors, and employees. Thefts and disturbances on the premises should be reported to this department. Whenever a threat of violence is perceived, you must notify security and the nurse in charge immediately.

Other Health Care Delivery Systems

Health care services often are provided in nonhospital settings. This is particularly true for long-term care. *Extended care facilities (ECFs)* provide care for patients who are not acutely ill and cannot be cared for at home. These facilities can provide either skilled or intermediate levels of care. The following facilities are providers of long-term care and provide employment opportunities for health unit coordinators. Nursing homes are licensed by the state and may be classified by ownership and accreditation. Nursing homes provide care for those who are so sick or functionally disabled that they require ongoing nursing and support services provided in a formal health care institution. They generally are classified as custodial care; however, another level of nursing home is the *skilled nursing facility (SNF),* which provides care for those too sick to go home or to a nursing home but who are not so acutely ill that they require the technologic and professional intensity of a hospital. Many hospitals also operate an SNF.

Physical medicine and rehabilitation facilities also may be classified as ECFs, although such care may be given to outpatients as well. Individuals receiving care in such facilities primarily require special support services in addition to varying levels of nursing care.

Long-term care also may be provided in the home through a home health agency. These agencies provide such services as skilled nursing, rehabilitation (for such problems as speech or language pathology or for physical or occupational therapy), pharmacy, and medical social work. *Hospice* is another form of care sometimes classified as long term. It provides palliative and supportive care for terminally ill patients and their families. Emphasis is placed on the control of symptoms and preparation for and support before and after death. The hospice can be freestanding, hospital-based, or home-based. A hospice is really not a type of facility but a new concept of providing health care services where necessary.

■ MANAGED CARE

People are living longer because of advancements in health care technology, early diagnosis, improved sanitation, improved food choices, greater emphasis on health lifestyle choices, better pharmacologic agents, more advanced surgical procedures, and a decrease in infectious diseases. This increase in the older population and the cost of increased technology has caused a crisis in health care, resulting in the emergence of managed health care. Managed health care is the use of a planned and systematic approach to providing quality health care for the lowest possible cost.

Managed care systems most often are associated with health maintenance organizations (HMOs), organizations that have management responsibility for providing comprehensive health care services on a prepayment basis (capitation) to voluntarily enrolled persons within a designated population. There are several models of HMOs, and each is unique in the way it contracts for the services of physicians.

- The *staff model HMO* is a multispecialty group of physicians practicing at a facility that is an HMO and whose physicians are salaried employees
- The *group model HMO* is similar to the staff model, but there is no specific facility called an HMO; physicians contract with the HMO to provide nearly all the services to members
- The *individual practice association model (IPA)* is used when the HMO contracts with an association of individual physicians to provide services for members in their private offices; physicians are able to contract with large patient populations and still maintain independence (except for emergencies, members must be referred by physicians in the HMO before receiving services outside the facility; failure to do so may result in the HMO not paying for the care)
- The *preferred provider organization (PPO)* is an independent group of physicians or hospitals that provide health care for fees 15% to 20% lower than customary rates. It is more like a traditional insurance plan (no capitation), because there is a "participating physician list," and patients usually do not need referrals.

In 1983, Congress authorized the creation of Medicare's prospective payment system (PPS) for hospitals. This changed the way physicians and hospitals receive payment in that they no longer established their own prices. The policy required Medicare to fix prices in advance on a cost-per-case basis, using as a measure 467 DRGs.

■ COMPONENTS OF THE HEALTH CARE DELIVERY SYSTEM

The three major components of the health care delivery system include the following:

1. *Primary:* Originates with the primary care physician and provides outpatient/ambulatory service (physician's office, dentist office, surgical center, health clinics, and pharmacies).
2. *Secondary:* Implies care by a specialist, provides intermediate services (routine surgery, emergency treatment, diagnostic and therapeutic radiology). Examples include outpatient facilities, urgent care facilities, clinics, and ambulatory surgery).
3. *Tertiary:* Center of American health system (highly complex services and therapy). Examples include acute care hospitals, nursing homes, rehabilitation settings, and intermediate and extended nursing care.

■ HEALTH CARE PAYMENT SOURCES

There are many sources for health care payment; several are listed below.

- *Third-party payers* are insurance companies or government programs that pay for health care services on behalf of the patient.
- *Medicare* is government insurance that was enacted in 1965 for individuals older than age 65 or any person with a disability who has received Social Security for 2 years (some disabilities, such as end-stage renal disease, are covered immediately). Two types of coverage are Type A, which is hospital insurance, and Type B, which is medical insurance (premium and deductible).
- *Medicaid* is a federal and state program that provides medical assistance for the indigent. There are no entitlement features; recipients must prove their eligibility. Funds come from federal grants and are administered by the state, and benefits are closely associated to the economic status of the beneficiary. Benefits cover inpatient care, outpatient and diagnostic services, skilled nursing facilities, physician, and home health care.
- *Indemnity insurance* is a fee-for-service plan. The patient may use any licensed physician, other health care providers, or an accredited hospital and the plan will pay for a certain portion (usually 80% of the cost). There is an annual deductible of $100 to $500. The charges in excess of the eligible charges (usual, customary and reasonable, or UCR) are not covered by the plan.
- *Worker's compensation* pays the medical bills and significant portion of the lost wages when an on-the-job accident or illness results in injury or disability. The employer pays a premium to an insurance carrier to meet the worker's compensation policy. The injured worker must fill out a claim form and send it to the insurance carrier. The injured worker receives no bill, pays no deductible, and is covered 100% for medical expenses related to that injury or illness.

■ EMPLOYMENT IN THE HEALTH CARE FIELD

U.S. government statistics indicate that health care is the fastest growing industry, employing more than 98 million workers. Health care is delivered in hospitals, clinics, physician's offices, HMOs, surgi-centers, rehabilitation facilities, ECFs, mental health facilities, home care agencies, and hospice settings. There are more than 200 health careers identified, and it is a $2 billion-a-day business (see the Box *Current Health Care Professionals*).

There are several ways to research job and job-training opportunities. One way is by surfing the web. There are many national sites, and each state has local web sites for careers online that you can search for information in your location.

Internet general national web sites include the following:

www.careerbuilder.com
www.monster.com
www.jobsinhealthcare.com

You also can search the Internet by specific profession by using various search sites and typing in key words such as "health unit coordinator."

Other resources include the following:

Newspaper classified advertisements
Job placement/career counselors
Employment agencies
Health care facility bulletin boards
Networking with professionals in the field
Instructors
Health care hotlines
Library resources

CURRENT HEALTH CARE PROFESSIONALS

1. Ambulance attendant
2. Animal health technologist
3. Art therapist
4. Athletic trainer
5. Audiologist/speech–language pathologist
6. Cardiovascular technologist
7. Chiropractor
8. Clinical laboratory scientist
9. Clinical laboratory technician
10. Counselor
11. Cytotechnologist
12. Dental assistant
13. Dental hygienist
14. Dentist
15. Diagnostic medical sonographer
16. Dialysis technician
17. Dietetic technician
18. Dietitian/nutritionist
19. Electrocardiograph technician
20. Electroneurodiagnostic technician
21. Emergency medical technician/paramedic
22. Health information (medical records) administrator
23. Health information clerk
24. Health information technician
25. Health unit coordinator
26. Histotechnologist
27. Home health aide
28. Homeopath
29. Hospital admitting clerk
30. Hospital central service worker
31. Licensed practical nurse
32. Medical assistant
33. Medical biller
34. Medical coder
35. Medical illustrator
36. Medical radiation technologist
37. Medical transcriptionist
38. Midwife
39. Music therapist
40. Naturopath
41. Nuclear medicine technologist
42. Nurse anesthetist
43. Nurse practitioner
44. Nursing assistant
45. Occupational therapist
46. Occupational therapist assistant
47. Ophthalmic dispensing optician
48. Ophthalmic laboratory technician
49. Ophthalmic medical technician
50. Optician
51. Optometrist
52. Orthotist
53. Patient care technician
54. Perfusionist
55. Perioperative nurse
56. Pharmacist
57. Pharmacist assistant
58. Phlebotomist
59. Physical therapist
60. Physical therapy assistant
61. Physician
62. Physician's assistant
63. Physician specialist
64. Physiotherapist
65. Podiatrist
66. Prosthetist
67. Psychologist
68. Psychology technician
69. Radiology technician
70. Radiology technologist
71. Registered nurse
72. Rehabilitation counselor
73. Respiratory therapist
74. Respiratory therapy technician
75. Surgical technician first assistant
76. Surgical technologist
77. Therapeutic recreation specialist
78. Ultrasonographer
79. Veterinarian
80. Others as identified

■ SUMMARY

You will find that administrative organization, job titles, and job descriptions differ in many aspects among health care facilities. The health unit coordinator needs to have knowledge of the hospital, its personnel, and the services that it renders to carry out his or her assigned tasks. Managed health care is the principal form of health care delivery in the United States today. Its purpose is to provide quality care at the lowest cost possible. Managed care will continue to grow in response to employers' demands for lower-cost health care.

REVIEW QUESTIONS

1. The primary function of the hospital is:

   _____

2. Four other functions of a hospital are:

   a. _____

   b. _____

   c. _____

   d. _____

3. The doctor who may admit and care for patients in the hospital is known as the patient's:

   _____

4. A doctor who is a medical school graduate gaining experience in the hospital is called a:

   _____

5. Hospitals may be classified according to:

   a. _____

   b. _____

   c. _____

6. Match the specialists listed in the left-hand column with their area of expertise by filling in the appropriate letter from the right-hand column.

_____ 1. Internist

_____ 2. Cardiologist

_____ 3. Gynecologist

_____ 4. Dermatologist

_____ 5. Allergist

_____ 6. Neonatologist

_____ 7. Pediatrician

_____ 8. Psychiatrist

_____ 9. Anesthesiologist

_____ 10. Otolaryngologist

_____ 11. Geriatrist

_____ 12. Endocrinologist

_____ 13. Pathologist

_____ 14. Hospitalist

a. disorders of the newborn

b. treatment of mental disorders

c. diseases of ear, nose, and throat

d. study of cell changes and other alterations of the body caused by disease

e. administration of drugs or gases that cause loss of feeling or sensation

f. glandular diseases

g. hypersensitivity to foods, pollens, or medicines

h. focus is exclusively on hospitalized patients

i. problems and diseases of the aged

j. disease of adults

k. diseases of children

l. diseases of the female reproductive tract

m. heart disease

n. diseases of the skin

7. Match the specialists listed in the left-hand column with their area of expertise by filling in the appropriate letter from the right-hand column.

_____ 1. Surgeon

_____ 2. Urologist

_____ 3. Orthopedist

_____ 4. Neurologist

_____ 5. Physiatrist

_____ 6. Radiologist

_____ 7. Oncologist

_____ 8. Obstetrician

_____ 9. Radiation oncologist

_____ 10. Proctologist

_____ 11. Ophthalmologist

_____ 12. Emergency room physician

a. use of x-rays, ultrasound, and radioactive element scanners

b. diseases of the nervous system

c. diagnosis and treatment of cancerous conditions

d. treats trauma patients

e. eye diseases

f. treatment of cancer by radiation

g. diseases of the male reproductive tract

h. diseases of the rectum

i. use of operative methods

j. diseases of the skeletal system

k. care of pregnant women

l. treatment of disease by use of physical elements

8. Name the hospital department in charge of each of the following tasks.

   a. patient accounts

   _____

   b. transfer, discharge, and admissions

   _____

   c. performing blood, urine, and tissue studies

   _____

   d. diagnostic tests using computed tomography, ultrasound, radioactive element scanners, and radiant energy

   _____

   e. treatment for cancerous growths

   _____

   f. providing medications for patients

   _____

   g. treatment by use of exercise, heat, and light

   _____

   h. evaluation, treatment, and preservation of morale by using purposeful activities

   _____

   i. treatment related to respiratory function

   _____

   j. food preparation and treatment using foods

   _____

   k. diagnosis by use of instruments to view body cavities or hollow organs such as esophagus and bronchi

   _____

   l. diagnostic procedures for diseases of the GI tract

   _____

   m. diagnostic studies of the heart

   _____

   n. brain studies

   _____

   o. the patient's record on discharge

   _____

   p. supplies and equipment for treatment of patients

   _____

   q. services to patients outside the hospital

   _____

   r. providing service for financial and social problems

   _____

   s. planning the transition from hospital to home

   _____

   t. maintaining a clean hospital

   _____

   u. supplies and equipment for all hospital departments

   _____

   v. spiritual services

   _____

   w. keeping the hospital repaired

   _____

   x. maintaining the linen supply

   _____

   y. telephone and paging services

   _____

   z. protecting patients, visitors, employees, and hospital

   _____

   aa. repairing computers

   _____

9. Recognition that a hospital has met an official standard is called:

_____

10. List four annual in-services required by JCAHO.

   a. _____

   b. _____

   c. _____

   d. _____

11. Name the citizen group that is at the head of the hospital's organizational structure.

_____

12. The individual in direct charge of a hospital who is responsible to the governing board is the·

_____

13. List three resources to access employment opportunities.

   a. _____

   b. _____

   c. _____

14. The case manager is an expert in _____ and acts as the patient's

_____ .

15. Define the following terms/abbreviations:

   a. acute care _____

   b. merger _____

   c. proprietary _____

   d. HMO _____

   e. URL _____

   f. capitation _____

16. _____ provides supportive care for terminally ill patients and their families.

17. _____ provides equipment and services to the patient in their home.

18. Explain the purpose of managed care.

_____

_____

19. Medicare type A is: _____

20. Medicare type B is: _____

21. Label the following health care providers as working in a primary, secondary, or tertiary health care delivery system.

    a. specialist _____

    b. physician's office _____

    c. acute care hospital _____

    d. dentist's office _____

22. _____ pays the medical bills and a significant portion of lost wages when on-the-job accident or illness results in injury or disability.

TOPICS FOR DISCUSSION

1. Does managed care cause health care providers to have a conflict of interest?

2. What factors should be considered in choosing a health care plan?

3. Would you interview a new physician or health care provider before choosing care for yourself or family?

4. Discuss problems that you have encountered with your health care provider, and discuss some ways that could improve interaction between the consumer and health care providers.

5. Using the Internet or other employment resources, find two job openings. Discuss which one you would choose, and why.

3

The Nursing Department

Chapter Objectives

Upon completion of this chapter, you will be able to:

1. Define the terms in the vocabulary list.

2. Write the meaning of the abbreviations in the abbreviations list.

3. List three personnel commonly employed in the nursing units and special care units and briefly describe the role of each.

4. Identify the services provided by each of the nursing and special units listed in this chapter.

5. Describe the responsibilities of the nursing service department.

6. Discuss the various nursing care delivery models presented in this chapter.

7. List three services that come under the general heading of perioperative services and give a description of each.

Vocabulary

Acuity ▲ Level of care a patient would require based on his or her medical condition; used to evaluate staffing needs

Assignment Sheet ▲ A form completed at the beginning of each work shift that indicates the nursing staff member(s) assigned to each patient on that nursing unit

Assistant Nurse Manager ▲ A registered nurse who assists the nurse manager in coordinating the activities on the nursing unit

Certified Nursing Assistant ▲ A health care giver who performs basic nursing tasks and has been certified by passing a required certification examination

Clinical Pathway ▲ A method of outlining a patient's path of treatment for a specific diagnosis, procedure, or symptom

Director of Nurses ▲ A registered nurse in charge of nursing services (may be called director of patient services, nursing administrator, or vice president of nursing services)

Licensed Practical Nurse ▲ A graduate of a 1-year school of nursing, who is licensed in the state in which he or she is practicing; provides direct care and functions under the direction of the registered nurse

Nurse Manager ▲ A registered nurse who assists the director of nursing in carrying out administrative responsibilities and is in charge of one or more nursing units (also may be called unit manager, clinical manager, or patient care manager)

Nursing Service Department ▲ The hospital department responsible for all the nursing care administered to the patients

Nursing Unit Administration ▲ A division within the hospital responsible for non-clinical patient care

Patient Support Associate ▲ Job description as well as title varies among hospitals; may include some patient-admitting responsibilities, coding, or stocking nursing units

Perioperative Services ▲ A department of the hospital that provides care before (preoperative), during (intraoperative), and after (postoperative) surgery. It encompasses total care of the patient during the surgical experience

Primary Care Nursing ▲ One nurse provides total care to assigned patients

Registered Nurse ▲ A graduate of a 2- or 4-year college-based school of nursing or a 3-year hospital-based program, who is licensed in the state in which he or she is practicing; may give direct patient care or supervise patient care given by others

Shift Manager ▲ A registered nurse who is responsible for one or more units during his or her assigned shift (also may be called nursing coordinator)

Staff Development ▲ The department responsible for both orientations of new employees and continuing education of employed nursing service personnel (also may be called educational services)

Team Leader ▲ A registered nurse who is in charge of a nursing team (also may be called pod leader)

Team Nursing ▲ Consists of a charge nurse and two to three team leaders with four to five team members working under the supervision of each team leader

Abbreviations

Abbreviation	Meaning
CCU	coronary care unit
CNA	certified nursing assistant
CVICU	cardiovascular intensive care unit
Gyn	gynecology
ICU	intensive care unit
L&D	labor and delivery
LPN	licensed practical nurse
Med	medical
MICU	medical intensive care unit
Neuro	neurology
NICU	neonatal intensive care unit
Ortho	orthopedics
PICU	pediatric intensive care unit
PSA	patient support associate
Psych	psychiatry
RN	registered nurse
SICU	surgical intensive care unit
SSU	short-stay unit
TICU	trauma intensive care unit

EXERCISE ⬤1

Write the correct abbreviation for each term listed below.

1. coronary care unit _____

2. certified nursing assistant _____

3. cardiovascular intensive care unit _____

4. gynecology _____

5. intensive care unit _____

6. labor and delivery _____

7. licensed practical nurse _____

8. medical _____

9. medical intensive care unit _____

10. neurology _____

11. neonatal intensive care unit _____

12. orthopedics _____

13. pediatric intensive care unit _____

14. patient support associate _____

15. psychiatry _____

16. registered nurse _____

17. surgical intensive care unit _____

18. short-stay unit _____

19. trauma intensive care unit _____

EXERCISE ⬤2

Write the meaning of each abbreviation listed below.

1. CCU

_____

2. CNA

_____

3. CVICU

_____

4. Gyn

_____

5. ICU

_____

6. L&D

_____

7. LPN

_____

8. Med

_____

9. MICU

_____

10. Neuro

_____

11. NICU

_____

12. Ortho

_____

13. PICU

_____

14. PSA

_____

15. Psych

_____

16. RN

_____

17. SICU

_____

18. SSU

_____

19. TICU

_____

■ NURSING SERVICE ORGANIZATION

The Nursing Service Department

The *nursing service department* is responsible for ensuring the physical and emotional care of the hospitalized patient, performing nursing treatment, and evaluating and coordinating treatment and diagnostic studies performed by other hospital departments. Other responsibilities include patient assessment and recording, planning and implementing patient care plans, and patient teaching. As you can see, nursing service is the single largest component of the hospital. Often 50% of all hospital personnel are employed in the nursing service department.

■ NURSING SERVICE ADMINISTRATIVE PERSONNEL

The *director of nurses*, also called the *vice president of nursing*, is responsible for the overall administration of nursing service. Setting nursing practice standards and staffing are two examples of the responsibilities of the director of nursing. The director of nursing is responsible to the chief executive officer of the health care facility.

The *nurse manager* (also called the *clinical manager* or the *patient care manager*) assists the director of nursing in carrying out administrative responsibilities and is usually in charge of one or more nursing units. The nurse manager reports to the director of nurses. The assistant nurse manager assists the manager in coordinating the activities of the nursing units.

The *director of staff development* is responsible for the orientation and evaluation of new nursing service employees and for the continuing education—including Joint Commission on Accreditation of Healthcare Organizations, or JCAHO, requirements—of all employed nursing service personnel. He or she usually reports to the director of nursing.

■ HOSPITAL NURSING UNITS

As you should recall from Chapter 1, the health unit coordinator works at the nurses' station on the nursing unit. The hospital is divided into nursing units according to the type(s) of service(s) provided to the patients.

Many methods are used to name the nursing units within the hospital. Sometimes the units are named according to the service offered, such as pediatrics; or the name may be derived from the floor level and direction of the hospital wing (e.g., 4 East).

Regular Nursing Units

Most nursing units are designed to accommodate 18 to 50 hospitalized patients. A regular nursing unit may provide one of the following services:

Behavioral health: Includes psychiatry (psych), which is the care of patients hospitalized for treatment of disorders of the mind or having difficulty coping with life situations; also may include programs for treatment of alcohol and drug abuse and programs related to changing destructive behaviors such as eating disorders
Cardiovascular: Care of patients who are hospitalized for treatment of diseases of the circulatory system
Gynecology surgery (Gyn): Care of women who are hospitalized for surgery of the female reproductive tract
Medical (Med): Care of patients who are hospitalized for medical treatment
Neurology (Neuro): Care of clients who are hospitalized for treatment of diseases of the nervous system
Obstetrics (OB), labor and delivery (L&D), and nursery: Care of mothers before, during, and after labor and care of newborn infants
Oncology: Care of patients who are hospitalized for treatment of cancer
Orthopedics (Ortho): Care of patients who are hospitalized for treatment of diseases or fractures of the musculoskeletal system
Pediatrics (Peds): Care of children (12 and younger) who are hospitalized for medical or surgical treatment
Rehabilitation (Rehab): Care of patients who are hospitalized for physical handicaps; usually these patients need long-term treatment and care
Stepdown unit: Care of patients who require more specialized care than that given at regular nursing units but who do not require intensive care (also called intermediate or transitional care unit)
Surgical (Surg): Care of patients who are hospitalized for general surgical treatment
Telemetry: Care of patients with cardiac arrhythmias and other heart problems, whose electrocardiogram readings are monitored at the nurses' station
Urology: Care of patients who are hospitalized for treatment of disease of the male reproductive or urinary systems or of the female urinary system

Intensive Care Units

Another type of nursing unit found in the modern hospital is the *intensive care unit (ICU)* (also called special care units). Its purpose is to provide constant specialized nursing care to critically ill patients. As the condition of the critically ill patient improves, he or she is transferred to the *stepdown unit* for less intense nursing care. The personnel employed in the intensive care units are specially qualified for the type of nursing care offered by the unit.

Intensive care units are identified by the type of care they provide. For example, the *surgical intensive care unit (SICU)* cares for surgical patients, the *medical intensive care unit (MICU)* cares for medical patients, the *coronary care unit (CCU)* cares for patients with heart disease, the *trauma intensive care unit (TICU)* cares for patients involved in trauma, the *neonatal intensive care unit (NICU)* cares for premature and ill newborns, and the *pediatric intensive care unit (PICU)* cares for pediatric patients.

Specialty Units

Specialty areas within the hospital that are usually a part of nursing service and employ various categories of nursing personnel include the following:

Day surgery or outpatient surgery unit or ambulatory surgery: Care of patients who are having surgery or examinations but who do not require overnight hospitalization; may be referred to as save a day (SAD) or same-day surgery (SDS)
Emergency department: Care of patients who need emergency treatment; after emergency treatment is administered, the patient either is admitted to the hospital or discharged home, according to his or her medical needs

Perioperative services include the following:

Preoperative area: Area in the hospital where patients are prepared for surgery
Intraoperative area: Operating room/area in the hospital where surgery is performed
Postoperative area: Postanesthesia care unit or recovery room/area in the hospital where patients are cared for immediately after surgery until they have recovered from the effects of the anesthesia

■ NURSING UNIT PERSONNEL

To maintain 24-hour coverage, nursing service personnel usually are scheduled in two shifts, divided into 7:00 AM to 7:30 PM (day shift) and 7:00 PM to 7:30 AM (night shift). Three shifts also may be used; the shifts then are usually 7:00 AM to 3:30 PM, 3:00 PM to 11:30 PM, and 11:00 PM to 7:30 AM. Shifts overlap one-half hour to allow communication between personnel.

The *nurse manager* (also called clinical manager, patient care manager, or unit manager) is a registered nurse (RN) who usually is responsible for the patients and nursing personnel on his or her unit for 24 hours a day. The nurse manager reports to the director of nurses. Managerial responsibilities include the planning and coordinating of quality nursing care for patients hospitalized on the unit. Selecting, supervising, scheduling, and evaluating personnel employed on the unit are other managerial responsibilities of the nurse manager. The nurse manager works closely with the physicians to coordinate nursing care with the care prescribed by the physician. Usually an RN, titled charge nurse, shift manager, nursing care manager, or assistant nurse manager oversees the nursing unit in the absence of the nurse manager.

Nursing personnel other than the health unit coordinator who may be employed on the nursing unit and who function under the supervision of the nurse manager are discussed in the following paragraphs. The job descriptions also may be found in your hospital's policy manual.

The *registered nurse* is a graduate of a 2- to 4-year college-based program or a 3-year hospital-based program and currently is licensed in the state in which he or she is practicing. The RN performs all types of treatments, and it is usually hospital policy that only the RN can perform complex procedures, such as administering intravenous (IV) medication. The RN is responsible for applying the nursing process. This encompasses the assessment, nursing diagnosis, planning, implementation, and evaluation of patient care. He or she also participates in patient/family teaching as well as teaching staff members.

```
Registered       Registered       Registered
nurse            nurse            nurse
Health unit      Health unit      Health unit
coordinator      coordinator      coordinator
8-hour shift     8-hour shift     8-hour shift
```

Patient care
The registered nurse plans,
organizes, and performs all care

FIGURE 3-1 ▲ Total patient care (case nursing) model.

The *licensed practical nurse (LPN)* is a graduate of a 1-year school of nursing and is licensed in the state in which he or she is practicing. The LPN functions under the direction of the RN and gives direct patient care; performs technical skills, such as discontinuing an IV; and administers medication to the patients, as prescribed by the physician.

The *certified nursing assistant (CNA)* is either trained on the job or has completed a short training course 6 to 12 weeks in length at a vocational school. A state examination is required for the nursing assistant to be certified. Nursing assistants perform bedside tasks, such as bathing and feeding patients. They also perform basic treatments, such as taking vital signs and giving enemas. The CNA functions under the supervision of the RN or LPN.

NURSING CARE DELIVERY MODELS

Because health unit coordinators frequently need to communicate information to the nurse caring for a patient, they need to be aware of the types of patient care assignments used by the nursing unit.

Total Patient Care Model

The *total patient care model* sometimes is referred to as case nursing. In total patient care, the registered nurse assigned to a patient is responsible for planning, organizing, and performing all care, including providing personal hygiene, medications, treatments, emotional support, and education required for a group of

patients during an assigned shift. An example of a total patient care model is shown in Figure 3-1.

Functional Nursing Care Model

The *functional nursing model* evolved during the 1940s as a result of the shortage of nurses caused by World War II, and continues today. Staff members were assigned to complete certain tasks for a group of patients rather than for specific patients. For example, the RN performs all assessments and administers all IV medications; the LPN gives all oral medications; and the CNA performs hygiene tasks, takes vital signs, and performs other clinical tasks. A nurse manager makes the assignments. An example of a functional nursing model is shown in Figure 3-2.

Team Nursing Care Model

The *nursing team care model* is made up of the charge nurse who oversees the nursing unit, two to- three team leaders (RNs), and three to four team members who work under the supervision of each team leader. Members of the team may be RNs, LPNs, and/or CNAs. The team leader assigns patients for each team member based on patient acuity to care for during a shift. Each team member performs the particular tasks for his or her patients that he or she is qualified to perform. The team leader is responsible for both the patients and the members of his or her team. A team usually cares for 15 or fewer patients; thus a nursing unit may have one to three teams. Many hospitals use modified forms of the team nursing method. An example of a team nursing model is shown in Figure 3-3.

Primary Nursing Care Model

The *primary nursing care model* is a type of total patient care in which one nurse is responsible for planning, implementing, and evaluating the patient's care for a 24-hour period throughout the patient's hospital stay. When the primary nurse is off duty, an associate nurse who follows the care plan established by the primary nurse provides care. The primary nurse is notified if any problems or complications develop and directs alterations in the plan of care. A fundamental responsibility for the primary nurse is to maintain clear communication among the patient, family,

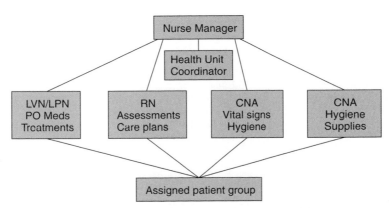

FIGURE 3-2 ▲ Functional nursing care model.

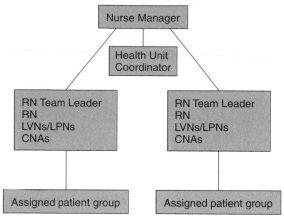

FIGURE 3–3 ▲ Team nursing care model.

FIGURE 3–5 ▲ Patient-centered (patient-focused) care model.

physician, associate nurses, and any other members of the health care team. An example of a primary nursing care model is shown in Figure 3–4.

Patient-Centered Care or Patient-Focused Care Model

The *patient-centered care model*, sometimes referred to as the patient-focused care model, is a recent development in nursing care and is a result of work redesign in health care organizations in an effort to become more patient oriented rather than hospital or department oriented. Patient-centered care involves all departments that deal with the patient (Fig. 3-5), such as respiratory care, other ancillary departments, and the nursing department working together on the nursing unit to provide care to the patients, and it is a multidisciplinary approach. A typical patient-centered team may include, in addition to a nurse manager, RNs, patient support assistants, and CNAs. The CNAs support RNs and are trained to perform multiple duties, including bedside care, oxygen set up, and phlebotomy. The patient support assistants perform various tasks in the unit, including housekeeping, stocking supplies, transporting patients, and assisting with patient care duties. The health unit coordinator performs non-clinical aspects of patient care, including medical recordkeeping, admitting and discharge, and clerical tasks. The job roles and titles used in the patient-centered model vary among health care facilities as they determine how patient needs are best met. An example of a patient-centered model is shown in Fig. 3–5.

■ CLINICAL PATHWAYS

Clinical pathways, also called critical paths, are used as a method of outlining a patient's path of treatment for a specific diagnosis, procedure, or symptom. Doctors' orders are usually preprinted with options that the doctor may choose to meet a specific patient's needs. Examples of preprinted doctors' orders include surgical as well as medical orders. See Figure 3–6 for an example of a clinical pathway for a patient with a diagnosis of pneumonia. Each physician develops his or her protocol into the orders. The health unit coordinator will label the appropriate preprinted doctor's orders and place them in the patient's charts. After the doctor chooses his or her options and signs the orders, the health unit coordinator will transcribe the orders.

The goals for developing and using clinical pathways are the following: (1) Identify patient and family needs. (2) Determine realistic patient outcomes and the frames required to achieve those outcomes. (3) Reduce length of stay and inappropriate use of resources. (4) Clarify the appropriate care setting, providers, and timelines of intervention. The "pathway" can be viewed as a road map the patient and health care team should follow to guide the patient's care management and recovery. As the patient progresses along the path, specified goals should be accomplished. If a patient's progress deviates or leaves the planned path, a variance has occurred. A positive variance occurs when the patient's progress is ahead of schedule. A negative variance is when a predicted goal is not accomplished.

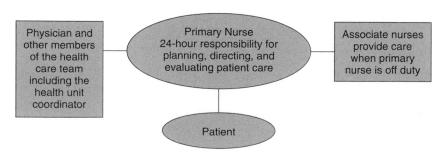

FIGURE 3–4 ▲ Primary nursing care model.

Diagnosis: _____

Comorbidities: ☐Angina ☐Atrial Fibrillation ☐Cardiomyopathy ☐COPD ☐CHF ☐Dehydration ☐Malnurtition
☐ Diabetes w/ manifestations ☐ Diabetes, Insulin Dependent ☐ Diabetes, Uncontrolled
☐ Other: _____

Condition:

Consults:

Treatments:
O2 via nasal prongs, titrate to maintain sats ≥ 90%, decrease as tolerated.
Vital signs q 4hrs. x 24hrs., then routine.
I&O
Incentive spirometer q 2hrs. while awake, cough and deep breathe.

Activity:
Ambulate QID, if possible.

Diet:
☐4gm Na, Low in Saturated Fat.
☐If patient is diabetic, 1800-2400 ADA.
☐Regular

Laboratory Requests: (Do not repeat if done in ER)
Stat blood culture x 2
Sputum culture
CBC, CMP, UA
☐Other:

Diagnostics: (Do not repeat if done in ER)
☐ Chest x-ray
☐ Other:

IV Fluids:
IV lock

Medications:
Antibiotics for community-acquired pneumonia (give first dose within 2hrs. of orders being noted, even if blood or sputum cultures not done). Antibiotic recommendations per updated Infectious Disease Society of America guidelines, 2000. *Please use choices from either one column or the other, not both.*

For those with low risk for complications or resistant organisms:
☐ Ceftriaxone (Rocephin) 1gm IV q 24hrs.
☐ Doxycycline (Vibramycin) 100mg IV q 12hrs.
(Combination therapy optimal for streptococcal and atypical organism coverage).
☐ MD aware of Penicillin allergy, OK to give Rocephin.

For those with frequent hospitalizations where resistant organisms are suspected:
☐ Levofloxacin (Levaquin) 500mg IV q 24hrs.
(monotherapy)

If patient taking **scheduled oral medications**, will **receive oral Levaquin starting on Day 2** (per P&T decision, May 2001)

☐ Albuterol inhaler with spacer _____ puffs q _____hours.
☐ Atrovent inhaler with spacer _____ puffs q _____hours.
☐ Medication/inhaler/spacer teaching per Respiratory if on metered-dose inhaler (MDI)
SVN's with Albuterol 2.5mg/3ml unit dose q 4hrs.
☐ Include Atrovent in SVN 500mcg/2.5ml unit dose q 4hrs.
☐ Self administer SVN's
☐ Other:

Discharge Planning:

Physician signature to activate per path: | **Date:**

Opportunity Medical Center

**PNEUMONIA
ORDER SET**

FIGURE 3–6 ▲ Clinical pathway for a diagnosis of pneumonia.

ASSIGNMENT SHEET

Nursing Unit 3 West   **Date** 00/00/00   **Shift** 7 A – 7 P

Nurse	Pager #	Lunch	Breaks
Sara	17–8234	12:30	9A & 4P

Patient Name	Rm #
Tony Garcia	321–1
Frank Gerod	321–2
Pat Smith	322
Jody Hackenheimer	327–1

Nurse	Pager #	Lunch	Breaks
Cheryl	17–8222	1:00	10A & 4:30P

Patient Name	Rm #
Carl Patell	318–1
Frances Conners	319–1
Penny Packer	319–2

	Name	Office ext	Pager #
Nurse Manager	Pat Lawson	3249	17–6000
Residents on call	Julie		17–2244
	David		17–2238
Case Managers	Jan	3245	17–5525
	Stan	3245	17–5528

A

FIGURE 3–7 ▲ *A*, An example of an assignment sheet for the total care nursing delivery model.

■ ASSIGNMENT SHEET

An assignment sheet is a form completed at the beginning of each work shift that indicates the nursing staff assigned to each patient on that nursing unit. The form also may include lunch times and break times for the nursing personnel. The health unit coordinator keeps the assignment sheet near his or her work area to refer to when necessary to locate the nurse caring for a particular patient. Information on the assignment sheet may vary depending on the nursing delivery system used. Refer to Figure 3–7 for an example of an assignment sheet used for the total care and team nursing models.

ASSIGNMENT SHEET

Nursing Unit 3 West   **Date** 00/00/00   **Shift** 7 A — 7 P

Team 1		Pager #	Lunch	Breaks	Assignment	Rm #
TL	Sara	17—8234	12:30	9A & 4P		321—327
LPN	Elaine	17—3749	1:30	10A & 3:30P	medications	318—327
CNA	John		2:00	9A & 4P	T. Garcia	321—1
					F. Gerod	321—2
					P. Smith	322
					J. Hackenheimer	327—1
CNA	Julie		2:30	11A & 4:30P	C. Patell	318—1
					F. Conners	319—1
					P. Packer	319—2

Team 2		Pager #	Lunch	Breaks	Assignment	Rm #
	Peter	17—8222	2:30	10A & 5P	TL	316—320
CNA	Jane		1:00	9A & 4P	T. Johns	316—1
					T. Pratt	317—2
					P. Smith	318—1
					C. Luctzu	318—2
CNA	Cynthia		2:30	11A & 4:30P	M. Peterson	318—1
					I. Hayes	319—1
					M. Baker	319—2

	Name	Office ext	Pager #
Nurse Manager	Pat Lawson	3249	17—6000
Resident on call	Julie		17—2244
Case Manager	Jan	3245	17—5525

B

FIGURE 3–7, cont'd ▲ *B,* An example of an assignment sheet for the team nursing delivery model.

■ NURSING UNIT ADMINISTRATION

Some hospitals have a division of nursing unit administration that is responsible for non-clinical patient care functions. Nursing unit administration is made up of two categories of workers: the health unit coordinator and the health unit manager. We already have discussed the role of the health unit coordinator; however, in nursing unit administration the health unit coordinator usually is supervised by the health unit manager rather than by the nurse manager. The health unit coordinator continues to work very closely with the nursing unit team.

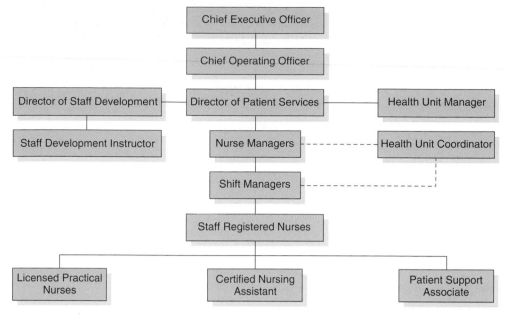

FIGURE 3–8 ▲ Organizational structure for the nursing service department and nursing unit administration.

The *health unit manager* performs supervisory and administrative non-clinical functions, such as budgeting, research, and training new employees, for several nursing units. As mentioned in Chapter 1, health unit management is the second step of the service management career path for health unit coordinators.

Health unit managers also may be RNs or hold degrees in other disciplines. Unit management usually functions under administration rather than under the nursing service department. See Figure 3–8 for an organizational chart that includes nursing unit administration.

■ SUMMARY

Health care delivery is continually undergoing changes to provide the most efficient and cost-effective patient care. In fact, by the time this text is published some of this information may be obsolete. It will be your responsibility to keep up and to adapt to changes as they occur in your place of employment. Although the health unit coordinator does not give direct patient care, his or her performance greatly influences the quality of care delivered by other nursing team members.

REVIEW
QUESTIONS

1. Match the appropriate nursing unit from the right-hand column to which patients with the conditions listed in the left-hand column would likely be admitted.

_____ 1. Cardiac arrhythmia	a. GYN
_____ 2. Drug abuse	b. urology
_____ 3. Surgical treatment	c. behavioral health
_____ 4. Was critically ill, still requires specialized care, but no longer needs intensive care	d. surgical
_____ 5. Disease of the circulatory system	e. telemetry
_____ 6. Disease of the urinary system	f. neurology
_____ 7. 10 years old	g. cardiovascular
_____ 8. Long-term treatment and care	h. pediatrics

_____ 9. Cancer   i. orthopedics

_____ 10. Fractured hip   j. oncology

_____ 11. Surgery of the female reproductive tract   k. obstetrics

_____ 12. Medical treatment   l. medical

_____ 13. Disease of the nervous system   m. rehabilitation

_____ 14. Pregnant and about to deliver   n. stepdown unit

2. Briefly describe the responsibilities of the nursing service department.

   _____

   _____

3. List three nursing personnel commonly employed on a nursing unit, and briefly describe the role of each.

   a. _____

   _____

   b. _____

   _____

   c. _____

   _____

4. List three services that come under the general heading of perioperative services and give a brief description of each.

   a. _____

   _____

   b. _____

   _____

   c. _____

   _____

5. Explain why a patient would be admitted to an ICU and why he or she would be transferred to a stepdown unit.

   _____

   _____

6. Compare the primary nursing care delivery model with the team nursing care delivery model.

_____

_____

7. The level of care required by a patient's medical condition is referred to as the

_____ and is used by nursing when making nursing team
member assignments.

8. _____ is the hospital department responsible for both orientation of
new employees and continuing education, including JCAHO requirements.

9. Define "patient-centered" or "patient-focused" care.

_____

_____

10. List three nursing personnel that could work on a nursing team.

a. _____

b. _____

c. _____

11. Explain the use of clinical pathways.

_____

_____

TOPICS FOR DISCUSSION

1. Have you ever visited a patient who was in an ICU? Discuss how it was different from visiting a patient on a regular nursing unit.

2. Do you know someone who is a nurse? Discuss how his or her responsibilities have changed in the past 5 years.

3. Have you been admitted to a hospital or visited someone in the last 2 years? Discuss how you would rate the care that you (or the person you visited) received.

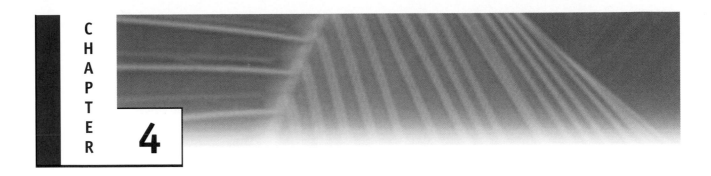

Communication Devices and Their Uses

▶ Chapter Objectives

Upon completion of this chapter, you will be able to:

1. Define the terms in the vocabulary list.
2. Write the meaning of the abbreviations in the abbreviation list.
3. State three circumstances that would require use of the hold button.
4. List and apply eight rules of telephone etiquette.
5. Describe briefly how to plan a telephone call to a doctors' office regarding a patient.
6. List six items to be recorded when taking a telephone message, and explain why it is important to accurately record messages.
7. List two methods of paging within the health care facility.
8. Discuss why a redial option should not be used on a fax machine in the nursing station.
9. Discuss the health unit coordinator's responsibility in the maintenance of the unit bulletin board.
10. List three uses of the computer terminal located on the nursing unit.
11. List four guidelines to use when leaving a voice mail message.
12. Identify two guidelines for use of e-mail in the workplace and list two examples of misuse of e-mail.

▶ Vocabulary

Cell Phone ▲ Wireless phone that may be carried by some hospital personnel and doctors

Computer ▲ An electronic machine capable of accepting, processing, and retrieving information

Computer Terminal ▲ Combination of three components: a keyboard, a viewing screen, and a printer

Copy Machine ▲ A machine used for making duplicates of typed or written materials

Cursor ▲ A flashing indicator that identifies the area on the viewing screen that will receive the information

Doctors' Roster ▲ Alphabetic listing of names, telephone numbers, and directory telephone numbers of physicians on staff (most hospitals have made this available on computer as well).

Downtime Requisition ▲ A requisition (paper order form) used to process information when the computer is not available for use

Dumbwaiter ▲ A mechanical device for transporting food or supplies from one hospital floor to another

E-mail (electronic mail) ▲ A method of sending and receiving messages via the computer to anyone with an e-mail address

Fax Machine ▲ A telecommunication device that transmits copies of written material over a telephone wire from one site to another

Keyboard ▲ A computer component used to type information into the computer

Label Printer ▲ A machine that prints patient labels; located near the health unit coordinator's area

Menu ▲ A list of options that is projected on the viewing screen of the computer

Modem ▲ A device that enables a computer to send and receive data over regular phone lines

Patient Call System Intercom ▲ A device used to communicate between the nurses' station and patient rooms on the nursing unit

Pneumatic Tube System ▲ A system in which air pressure transports tubes carrying supplies, requisitions, or *some* lab specimens from one hospital unit or department to another

Pocket Pager ▲ A small electronic device that when activated by dialing a series of telephone numbers delivers a message to the carrier of the pager

Shredder ▲ A machine located in most nursing stations that shreds confidential material (chart forms that have a patient's label affixed with patient name, room number, patient account number, medical record number, and the like)

Tower ▲ The system unit of the computer; houses internal components

Viewing Screen ▲ A computer component that displays information; it resembles a television, and it also may be called a monitor, a cathode ray tube, or a VDT (video display terminal)

Voice Paging System ▲ The system on which the hospital telephone operator pages a message for a doctor or makes other announcements; the system reaches all hospital areas (only used when absolutely necessary to keep noise level down)

EXERCISE 1

Write the correct abbreviation for the following terms.

1. Floppy drive   _____

2. Hard drive stored inside the computer   _____

3. Central processing unit   _____

4. Personal computer   _____

5. Video display terminal   _____

EXERCISE 2

Write the meaning of each abbreviation below:

1. *A Drive*

   _____

2. *C Drive*

   _____

3. *CPU*

   _____

4. *PC*

   _____

5. *VDT*

   _____

Abbreviations

Abbreviation	Meaning
A Drive	usually the drive closest to the top of the computer; also called the floppy drive
C Drive	hard drive stored inside the computer
CPU	central processing unit; the microprocessor, often called the computer's brain
PC	personal computer
VDT	video display terminal

In health care facilities, the health unit coordinator has an opportunity to use many devices to communicate. They will be discussed here so you will have a better understanding of how you will use these devices on the job.

■ THE TELEPHONE

The telephone is probably the most used communications device at the nurses' station (Fig. 4–1). Because we are so familiar with using the telephone, often we fail to use it in a professional manner in the workplace. Speaking on the telephone requires a different interaction than speaking face-to-face (Fig. 4–2). A good

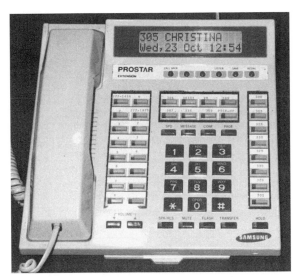

FIGURE 4–1 ▲ Telephone with several lines and a hold button.

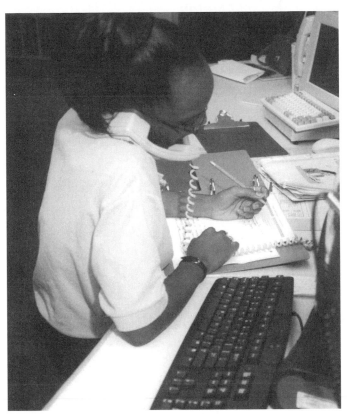

FIGURE 4–2 ▲ The health unit coordinator handles the telephone communication for the nursing unit.

attitude about telephone transactions will result in more positive customer (includes patients, patients' relatives and friends, doctors, and others) relationships for you and your hospital. Proper telephone etiquette is essential in the health care setting to promote effective communication.

Telephone Etiquette

- Answer the telephone promptly and kindly, preferably prior to the third ring. If you are engaged in a conversation at the nurses' station, excuse yourself to answer the telephone (Fig. 4–3).
- Identify yourself properly by stating your location, your name, and your status. For example: "4 East, Stacey Smith, health unit coordinator." The manner in which you identify yourself and address the caller is the caller's first clue about your professional identity, your self-esteem, your mood, your expectations, and your willingness to continue the communication. At this time you are conveying to the caller an image of the hospital. By correctly identifying yourself, you save the caller time and eliminate confusion.
- Speak into the telephone—be sure the mouthpiece is not under your chin, making it difficult for the caller to hear you.
- Give the caller your undivided attention—it is difficult to focus on the telephone conversation if you are attempting to do something else while you are listening.
- Speak clearly and distinctly—do not eat food or chew gum while talking on the telephone.
- Always be courteous—say please or thank you.
- When you do not know, state that you will locate someone who can help the caller.
- If necessary to step away or answer another call, place the caller on hold after asking permission to do so and waiting for an answer. For example: "May I put you on hold, Mr. Phillips, while I find Jane to speak to you?"

Each time you use the telephone for communication, you are creating an image of your nursing unit for your customers. Realize this and handle each telephone conversation with care.

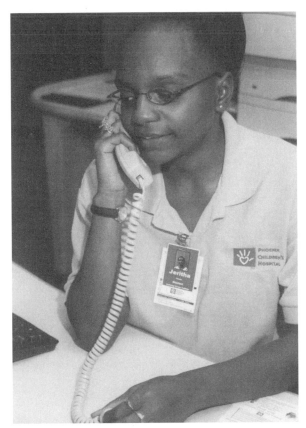

FIGURE 4–3 ▲ Let the tone of your voice communicate with a smile.

Use of the Hold Button

Telephones on hospital nursing units may have several incoming telephone lines plus a hold button. The hold button allows a caller to stay on the line while other calls are answered. Use the hold button:

■ To locate information or a person for the caller. Always return to the person on hold every 30 to 60 seconds to ask if they wish to remain on hold or leave a number for a return call.

■ To answer other phone lines. Return to first caller after asking second caller if they would hold or if you could call them back.

■ To protect patient confidentiality. Conversations held in the nursing station often involve confidential patient information and should not be overheard.

When communicating a message concerning a call on hold, include the name of the caller, the nature of the call if possible, and which line the call is on. The message may be as follows: "Mr. Barry, Dr. Harrison is on line 1 regarding Mr. Mark's medication order."

 STUDENT ACTIVITY

To practice answering the telephone and placing a caller on hold, complete Activities 4–1 and 4–2 in the *Skills Practice Manual.*

Taking Messages

When taking messages over the telephone or in person, be sure you get all the information needed for the person for whom the call is intended. You must record the following information:

■ Who the message is for
■ The caller's name
■ The date and time of the call
■ The purpose of the call
■ The number to call if a return call is expected
■ Your name

Always write the information down. As a student or a newly employed health unit coordinator, gaining the trust and confidence of the nursing team members is important. Putting messages in writing may be the first important step in gaining the confidence of the unit personnel while guaranteeing accuracy during the communication process. Always have a pad and pencil or pen near each telephone. Deliver messages promptly. Many health care facilities have special telephone message pads (Fig. 4–4).

 STUDENT ACTIVITY

To practice recording messages, complete Activity 4–3 in the *Skills Practice Manual.*

Placing Telephone Calls

When you are asked to place a call to a doctor, to another department, or outside of the health care facility, *plan your call.* If it concerns a patient, have the patient's chart handy so that you can

To_____		
Date_____ Time_____		

WHILE YOU WERE OUT

M_____

of_____

Phone_____

	Area Code	Number	Extension
TELEPHONED		PLEASE CALL	
CALLED TO SEE YOU		WILL CALL AGAIN	
WANTS TO SEE YOU		URGENT	
	RETURNED YOUR CALL		

Message_____

_____

_____

_____

_____

Operator

FIGURE 4–4 ▲ A pad for telephone messages.

look for the facts that you may be asked. Also write down the main facts you wish to discuss, and the telephone number you are calling should the line be busy and the call need to be made later.

Anyone who asks you to place a call regarding a patient should provide you with the patient's name and the reason for the call. You also should write down who requested the call to be made. Before placing a call for a nurse to a doctor, alert the nurse that you are making the call and ask him or her to stay on the unit, if possible, or to designate someone else to take the call in their place.

 STUDENT ACTIVITY

To practice placing a telephone call, complete Activity 4–4 in the *Skills Practice Manual.*

Voice Mail

Many health care facilities, physicians' offices, and homes use voice mail to receive incoming calls. To use voice mail effectively, follow these guidelines.

After listening to the recorded greeting and indicated tone, do the following:

■ Speak slowly and distinctly so the person listening to the message can hear and understand what you are communicating.

■ If you are leaving a message, include the name of the patient and/or the doctor—give the first and last name, and spell the last name.

- If the message includes a telephone number or laboratory values, speak slowly and repeat the numbers twice, allowing time for the listener to record the information.
- Always leave your name and telephone number, and repeat both twice (at the beginning of the message and at the end of the message) so the listener can call you for clarification if necessary.

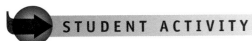

STUDENT ACTIVITY

To practice leaving a voice mail message, complete Activity 4–5 in the *Skills Practice Manual*.

Telephone Directories

Many health care facilities publish a directory of extension numbers for telephones in the hospital. They are alphabetized and easy to use. Both department numbers and key personnel are listed. Hospitals using the individual pocket pager also may publish a directory of pocket pager numbers.

The doctors' roster is another directory frequently used by the health unit coordinator. Most health care facilities have computer access to this information, but they also have a hard copy on the nursing units. The information includes the names of the doctors (in alphabetic order) who have admitting or visiting privileges. It lists their medical specialty, their office telephone number, and the answering service telephone number. When placing a telephone call, select the doctor's number with care because there are often several doctors listed with the same name. If two doctors have the same first and last names, refer to their specialty to select the correct telephone number. To practice placing a telephone call, complete the activities at the end of this chapter.

■ UNIT INTERCOM

The intercom system (Fig. 4–5) is a device used to communicate between the nurses' station and patients' rooms on a nursing unit. The intercom provides a method of taking patients' requests without going into the room. On admission, the patient should receive directions for the use of the call light and intercom from a member of the nursing staff. The importance of this step is emphasized by the following story: A little boy admitted to a hospital room was not told about the intercom system. When the health unit coordinator noted that the child had his light on, she turned on the intercom and asked if he needed help. He replied, "Yes, wall."

A buzzer and/or light on the intercom alert you that someone has activated their call system. The room number button lights up on the intercom console to designate the caller's room. By pressing the appropriate button you may converse with the patient. Always identify yourself and your location. For example, you may say, "This is Kimberly at the nurses' station. May I help you?" When there are two or more patients in the room, ask the patient to identify himself or herself.

The health unit coordinator also may use the intercom to locate nursing personnel. To page personnel on the intercom, depress the button that allows for the message to be heard in each of the rooms. A simple message, such as "Susan, please call the nurses' station," is all that is needed.

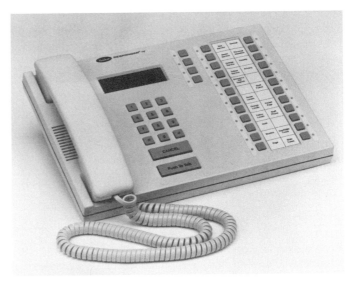

FIGURE 4–5 ▲ A *Responder IV* intercom device. (Courtesy of Rauland-Borg Corporation.)

The health unit coordinator should be selective in the information communicated over the intercom because some types of messages may prove embarrassing to the patient. For example, do not use the intercom to ask a patient if he or she has had a bowel movement. Try to keep the message as brief as possible, and do not communicate any confidential patient information to a nurse over the intercom because other patients may hear the message.

■ POCKET PAGER

The pocket pager (Fig. 4–6) is a small, electronic device that is activated by dialing a series of numbers on a telephone to deliver a message to the carrier of the pager. The pocket pager may be digital or voice. When using a voice pager, dial the pager number and state the message. Always say the message including name and extension number twice. A digital pager is similar in appearance to a voice pager. To contact a person by digital pager, dial the pager number from a touch-tone phone. Listen for a ring followed by a series of beeps. Dial your telephone number followed by the pound sign (#). You will hear a series of fast beeps, which indicates a completed page. The number appears on the pager display. The receiver then calls you back for the message. Allow at least 5 minutes before paging a second time, unless it is a stat (emergency) situation.

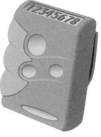

FIGURE 4–6 ▲ A pocket pager. (Courtesy of Motorola Communications and Electronics, Inc.)

Some nursing units use a number code entered at the end of the call back number—the number 1 indicating "stat," number 2 indicating "as soon as possible," and number 3 indicating "at your convenience." Residents, ancillary personnel, and your instructor carry pocket pagers.

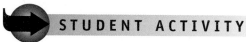

STUDENT ACTIVITY

To practice contacting a person using a digital pager, complete Activity 4–6 in the *Skills Practice Manual*.

■ VOICE PAGING SYSTEM

The voice paging system is a communication system in which the hospital switchboard operator, upon request, pages someone on a speaker that is heard in every area of the hospital. To locate a doctor with this system, dial the hospital switchboard operator, indicate the name of the doctor who is needed, and give the telephone extension number of the unit you are on. The operator announces the name of the doctor needed and the extension number to call.

The operator also uses the voice paging system to locate a doctor for calls from outside the hospital. The health unit coordinator frequently is asked by doctors to listen for their page, especially when they are in a patient's room. When a page for a doctor is announced, the health unit coordinator may contact the operator for the message and deliver it to the doctor.

■ COPY AND SHREDDER MACHINES

Many nursing units have a copy machine available for making copies of written or typed materials. Photocopying of patient records is discussed in Chapter 6. The fax machine also can be used to make a minimal amount of copies.

Patient forms containing confidential information cannot be thrown in the wastebasket. Shredder machines or boxes for materials to be picked up and taken to be shredded are placed on nursing units. Chart forms that have labels with patient name, patient account number, and health record identification number that do not have documentation on them must be shredded.

■ FAX MACHINE

A fax machine is a telecommunication device that transmits copies of written material over a telephone wire from one site to another (Fig. 4–7). Reports and other documents are faxed to and from health care institutions and doctors' offices. Most hospitals, to be cost effective, have eliminated the three part (NCR, or no carbon required) physician order sheets in favor of faxing the orders to the pharmacy. When faxing the pharmacy copy, the health unit coordinator can use the fax machine to make a copy of the orders to give to the appropriate nurse. Fax machines have a redial option, allowing a document to be sent to the location last programmed into the machine. Many health care workers in the nurses' station use the fax machine. Therefore, it is important not to use the redial option that may send a document to the wrong location. Patient information is extremely confidential and if sent to the wrong location could result in an employee being disciplined or terminated. The fax machine is not for personal use, such as sending jokes to coworkers, entries in contests, or the like.

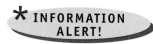

INFORMATION ALERT!

Do not use the redial option when using the fax machine. It may result in medical information being sent to the wrong location.

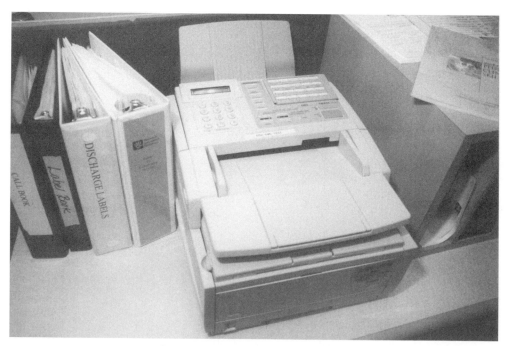

FIGURE 4–7 ▲ A facsimile (fax) machine.

■ PNEUMATIC TUBE

The pneumatic tube is a system in which air pressure transports tubes carrying supplies, requisitions, or messages from one hospital unit or department to another. These items are placed in a special carrying tube, which then is inserted into the pneumatic tube system; a keypad is used to enter the location to where the message is to be sent. Medications that do not break or spill are transported in this manner Do *not* place specimens obtained by a painful procedure in the pneumatic tube. When a tube carrying supplies or other items arrives at the nursing unit, it is the health unit coordinator's responsibility to remove the tube from the pneumatic tube system as soon as possible and disperse the items accordingly. You will be instructed in the operation of your hospital's pneumatic tube system during your hospital orientation.

Some health care facilities have a telelift system that is operated in much the same way and for the same purposes as the tube system. It consists of a small boxcar that is carried on a conveyor belt to designated locations. A keypad is used to program the car to go to a specific unit of a department.

■ COMPUTER

Most hospitals provide two to five computer terminals on each nursing unit so that doctors, residents, and nursing staff have easy access to patient information such as patient location, diagnostic test results, and physicians' orders. A computer terminal is usually made up of three components: the keyboard, the viewing screen, and the printer. The health unit coordinator usually has a separate terminal for ordering diagnostic tests, supplies, and equipment and entering discharges, transfers, and admissions.

Usually three computer components are located at the nurses' station: the keyboard, the viewing screen, and the printer (Fig. 4–8). These may be referred to as a computer terminal The keyboard resembles a typewriter, and the keys are depressed in the same way as typewriter keys to feed information into the

computer. Basic computer knowledge and typing skills are very helpful in performing the ordering and data entry tasks required. A mouse is used to select information to be fed into the computer (Fig. 4–9). The mouse is used to move the *cursor*, which is a flashing indicator showing the user the area on the screen that will receive the information. The cursor may be moved to any area on the screen; once the cursor is at the desired location, the user will click the mouse.

The viewing screen has many names. You may hear it referred to as the *monitor* or the *VDT* (video display terminal). The viewing screen resembles a television. Information typed on the keyboard is displayed on the computer screen. A menu can be brought up on the screen to make a selection of an item or a test to be ordered (Fig. 4–10), or a menu can be recalled for informational purposes only, such as a census (list of room numbers with patients names and their admitting physician's names).

Computers are connected to a printer, and at any given time the user can give the computer a command to print any of the stored information. For instance, when the health unit coordinator uses the computer to order a patient's diet, the diet order prints out on the printer located in the dietary department. The health unit coordinator should be alert to printed material being sent via the printer and remove the printed documents as soon as possible.

Many health care facilities now have bedside computers available in each patient's room (usually in intensive care units) for nursing personnel to record care and treatments performed. These records generally are printed every 24 hours for placement on the patients' chart. The health care facility's computer system contains a great deal of information that is confidential and that must not be tampered with; therefore, a security system is used. On employment, you are assigned an identification code and a password. Each time you use the computer you gain entry to the system by using your password. You probably will be asked to sign a confidentiality statement. Your identification code and identification number should never be given to anyone.

There are times when the computer is shut down for servicing or because of mechanical failure. During these times, down-

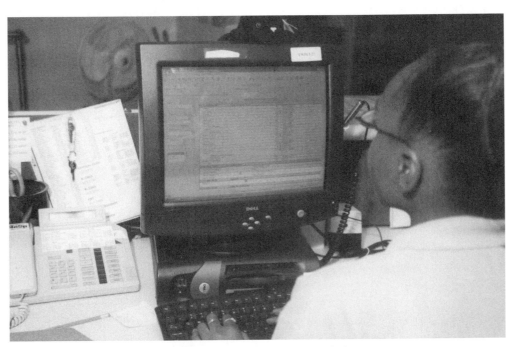

FIGURE 4–8 ▲ A computer terminal.

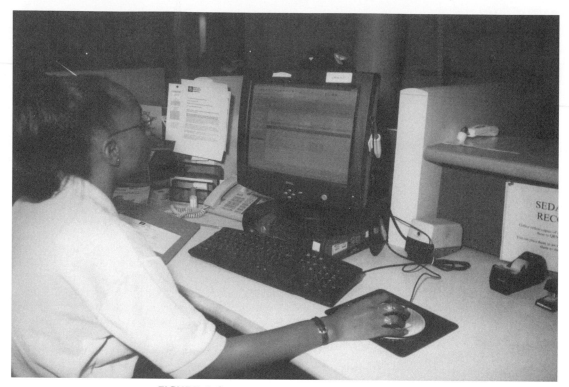

FIGURE 4–9 ▲ A computer terminal with a mouse.

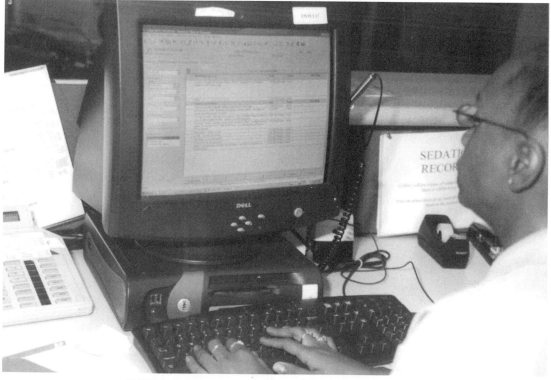

FIGURE 4–10 ▲ A laboratory menu on the computer screen.

time requisitions are used to process information. When computer function returns, the information processed by the paper method must be fed into the computer.

E-mail (electronic mail) is used to send and receive messages using e-mail addresses. Guidelines to be followed when using e-mail in the workplace include: (1) Do not use for personal messages or to send inappropriate material such as jokes; and (2) Send or respond to the necessary person or department only; refrain from "sending to all" or using "reply to all" unless necessary.

A current trend in health care facilities is to eliminate as much paperwork as possible. Some facilities have computerized kardexes, and some have developed a system that enables doctors to enter their orders directly on the computer. Computerized kardexes and doctors' orders will greatly reduce the risk of errors caused by poor handwriting.

Health care facilities use many different types of computer programs, and many have developed special programs to suit their individual needs. The CD included with the *Skills Practice Manual* will provide practice with the basic skills needed to function in a health care setting. Computer training usually is provided for new employees, and some facilities will allow health unit coordinator students to sit in on these classes. Students will be instructed in the specifics of the hospital computer program from an experienced working health unit coordinator during their clinical experience. Application of computer use for transcription and other health unit coordinating procedures will be introduced in their respective chapters.

■ NURSING UNIT CENSUS BOARDS

Many nursing units have small chalkboards or grease boards in the nurses' station area to record census information. The board shows unit room numbers, admitting doctor's names, and the nurse assigned to each patient. The patient's name intentionally may be omitted to maintain patient confidentiality. The health unit coordinator has the responsibility to remove the names of discharged or transferred patients while adding the names of newly admitted or transferred patients. New HIPPA laws (see Chapter 6) may change the current usage of census boards.

■ NURSING UNIT BULLETIN BOARD

The health unit coordinator may have the responsibility to maintain the nursing unit bulletin board. This responsibility includes posting material in an attractive manner and keeping the posted material current. The material to be posted on the bulletin board may be determined by the nurse manager or may be set forth by administration policy. Bulletins regarding changes that will take place in the facility or nursing policies and schedules of staff development classes are examples of materials posted on the bulletin board.

If the date were not indicated on the bulletin, the health unit coordinator would indicate the date posted. Policy changes are very important. It may be requested that each person initial the notice after reading it so the nurse manager will know that all the unit employees have read them. The health unit coordinator then would place the initialed notice on the nurse manager's desk when it is removed from the bulletin board. A neat board with up-to-date notices prompts the unit personnel to read what is posted.

■ SUMMARY

Your ability to use the computer, telephone, intercom, and other communications devices efficiently and effectively contributes to the smooth operation of your nursing unit. Accuracy in taking telephone messages and communicating them to the correct person is a must for an efficiently run nursing unit.

▼ REVIEW QUESTIONS

1. List four guidelines to use when leaving a message on voice mail.

   a. _____

   b. _____

   c. _____

   d. _____

2. List eight rules of telephone etiquette.

   a. _____

   b. _____

   c. _____

d. _____

e. _____

f. _____

g. _____

h. _____

3. List six items to be recorded when taking a telephone message.

a. _____

b. _____

c. _____

d. _____

e. _____

f. _____

4. Define the following terms.

a. menu _____

b. computer terminal _____

c. cursor _____

d. viewing screen _____

e. doctors' roster _____

f. downtime requisition _____

g. shredder _____

h. pneumatic tube system _____

i. label printer _____

5. Three circumstances that require the use of the telephone hold button are:

a. _____

b. _____

c. _____

6. Briefly describe how you would plan a call to a doctor's office regarding a patient.

_____

_____

7. Discuss the health coordinator's responsibility in the maintenance of the unit bulletin board.

   _____

   _____

8. If you are a health unit coordinator working on 4 East, write out what you would say when answering the telephone.

   _____

   _____

9. A. You have received a telephone call from Dr. Johnson for Dr. Taylor, whom you need to locate. You would:
      a. Say nothing, and place the telephone receiver on the desk because it is rude to put a doctor on hold.
      b. Say, "Hold for a minute and I will find her for you."
      c. Say, "Just a minute," and then place the caller on hold.
      d. Say, "May I place you on hold while I find her for you?"

   B. When you find Dr. Taylor, she is talking to a patient and you can't interrupt her. You would:
      a. Wait until Dr. Taylor is finished, and then notify her that she has a call.
      b. Return to the caller and tell him to be patient because it will be a few minutes.
      c. Return to the caller, explain the situation, and ask if he would prefer to remain on hold or leave a number for Dr. Taylor to return the call.
      d. Return to the caller and tell him to call back in a few minutes.

   C. Now Dr. Taylor is available and the caller is still on hold. You would say:
      a. "There is someone on line 1 for you."
      b. "It's Doctor Johnson for you."
      c. "Dr. Johnson is on line 1."
      d. "Dr. Johnson is on line 1 regarding the consultation ordered on Mrs. White."

10. List three uses of the computer terminal located on the nursing unit.

    a. _____

    b. _____

    c. _____

11. _____ It is good practice to state your return telephone number at the beginning as well as at the end of the recorded voice mail message. (True or False)

12. Define the term _e-mail:_

    _____

13. List two guidelines to follow when using e-mail in the workplace.

    a. _____

    b. _____

14. List two examples of misuse of e-mail.

a. _____

b. _____

15. Discuss possible repercussions of using the redial option on the hospital fax machine:

_____

_____

▼ **TOPICS FOR DISCUSSION**

1. Have you ever been placed on hold without your permission or been forgotten and left on hold until you finally hung up? Discuss how you felt when this happened.
2. Discuss telephone experiences that you have had with a person that was discourteous. How could the person have handled each situation in a courteous manner?

3. What are some examples of inappropriate use of e-mail in the workplace? Discuss the possible consequences.

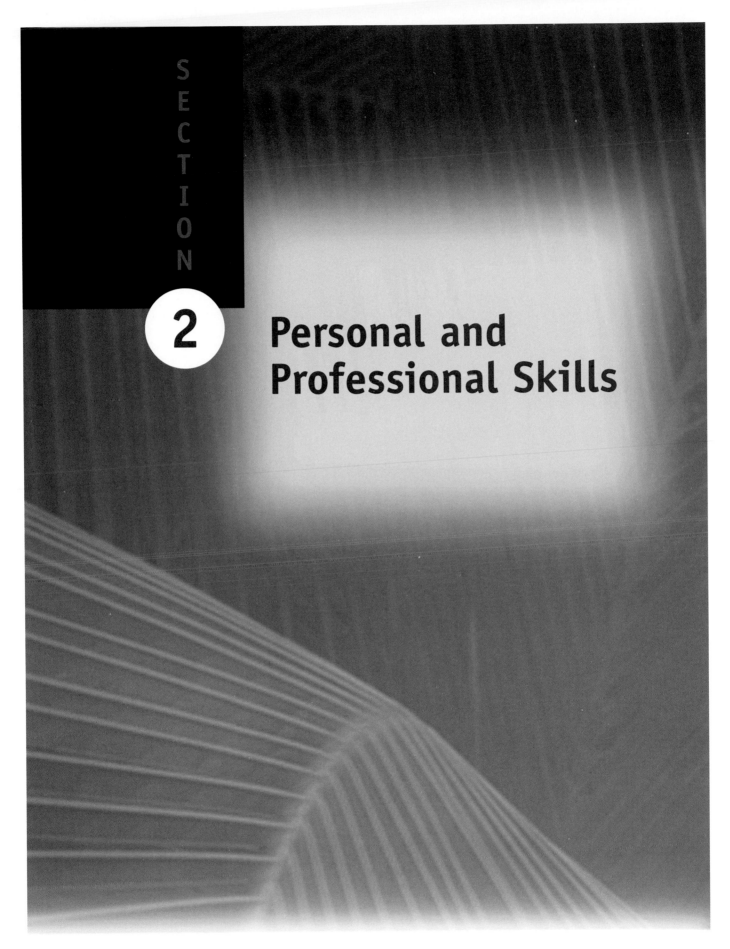

SECTION

2

Personal and Professional Skills

Communication and Interpersonal Skills

Chapter Objectives

Upon completion of this chapter, you will be able to:

1. Define the terms in the vocabulary list.
2. Give instances that exemplify human needs, classify each according to Maslow's hierarchy of human needs, and give appropriate responses to meet the listed needs.
3. List and discuss the four components of the communication process.
4. Interpret and apply the communication model.
5. List examples of verbal and nonverbal communication.
6. Discuss two types of nonverbal communication.
7. Identify causes of unsuccessful communication.
8. List eight ways to improve listening skills.
9. List five ways to improve feedback skills.
10. Describe the importance of culturally sensitive care in the health care setting.
11. List four guidelines to follow that could improve intercultural communication.
12. Identify assertive, nonassertive, and aggressive behaviors.
13. Respond to situations using assertive skills.
14. List six steps to follow when dealing with a person on the telephone who is angry.
15. Identify four ways that communication and interpersonal skills are used in the health care setting.

Vocabulary

Ageism ▲ Discrimination on grounds of age

Aggressive ▲ A behavioral style in which a person attempts to be the dominant force in an interaction

Assertive ▲ A behavioral style in which a person stands up for his or her own rights and feelings without violating the rights and feelings of others

Broken Record ▲ Assertive skill wherein a person repeats his or her stand over and over again

Communication ▲ The process of transmitting feelings, images, and ideas from the mind of one person to the mind of another person for the purpose of obtaining a response

EXAMPLE

Sarah has been hospitalized for 2 weeks. During this time she has been visited only once by her husband. In an attempt to meet her belonging needs, she has been turning on her call light hourly for minor requests.

Esteem Needs

As a person develops satisfying relationships with others, esteem needs and the need for self-respect and for the respect of others emerge. Esteem needs may be met by seeking special status within a group, owning a company, learning a skill very well, or developing a talent to be performed for others. Attainment of self-respect leads to feelings of adequacy, self-confidence, and strength. They result in prestige, recognition, and dignity for the individual.

Hospitalization frequently interferes with the ability to meet esteem needs. Many aspects of hospitalization such as wearing hospital gowns, sharing a room with others, having side rails on the bed, and being referred to as a room number or a disease instead of by name serve to depersonalize the patient. Often busy hospital personnel overlook a patient's past accomplishments and status.

EXAMPLE

Tom has been hospitalized for more than a week. He is walking past the nurses' station and stops and reads the name tag of the health unit coordinator. "You are Jenny Mason. That's a nice name. You know, since I have been in the hospital no one has called me by my name. I feel like a nobody."

Self-Actualization Needs

Once a person feels basic satisfaction of the first four needs, the next step is for him or her is to become "self-actualized." Self-actualization is the developing of a personality to its full potential. Contentment, self-fulfillment, creativity, originality, independence, and acceptance of other people all characterize the self-actualized person. Self-actualization is growth motivated from within you. As Maslow expressed it, "What a man can be, he must be." Thus, self-actualization is the desire to become what one is capable of becoming. It is growing and changing because you feel it is important. A self-actualized person has taken steps to make this happen.

EXAMPLE

Mahatma Gandhi is an example of a self-actualized person. The Indian leader frequently sacrificed his physiologic and safety needs for the satisfaction of other needs when India was striving for independence from Great Britain. In his historic fasts, Gandhi went weeks without nourishment to protest governmental injustices. He was operating at the self-actualization level.

Example of Different Needs in a Conversation

The human needs model can be used to demonstrate interpersonal behavior between health unit coordinators and hospital personnel or between health unit coordinators and patients or visitors.

Health unit coordinator: Mary is in isolation. You need to put this gown on before you go into her room. *(No dominant need expressed.)*

Husband: Mary is in isolation? What for? I want to know exactly what is going on here. *(Safety need expressed.* The husband is concerned about Mary's safety, and is also concerned that he may contract what Mary has.)

Health unit coordinator (defensively): Look, if you don't want to wear the gown, don't go in. I don't make the rules here. *(Esteem need expressed.* The health unit coordinator interprets the husband's request for information as an attack on her competence; self-esteem is at stake. Fighting back is used to try to satisfy self-esteem needs.)

In this example, if the health unit coordinator had perceived that the husband's question was motivated by *safety* needs, she would have responded with understanding rather than with defensiveness and aggression.

EXERCISE ❶

Match the level of need on "Maslow's hierarchy of human needs" listed in Column 2 with the human needs listed in Column 1. Write the letter preceding the level in the space provided to indicate your answer.

	Column 1	Column 2
1. _____	The need for oxygen	a. Physiologic Needs
2. _____	The need for shelter	
3. _____	The need to be safe from danger	b. Safety and Security Needs
4. _____	The need to be loved	c. Belonging and Love Needs
5. _____	The need for respect	d. Esteem Needs
6. _____	The need to feel self-confident	e. Self-Actualization Needs
7. _____	The need for acceptance within a group	
8. _____	The need to belong	
9. _____	The need for exercise	
10. _____	The need for the feeling of security	

COMMUNICATION SKILLS

Most of us spend much of our time communicating, but few of us communicate as effectively as we should. Many factors contribute to communication difficulties. For instance, the English language has grown considerably throughout its history, and there are now more than 600,000 words in the language. It is impossible to know how many words an individual may have in his or her vocabulary, but it is believed that a high-school graduate comprehends 3000 to 5000 words. How does the speaker know which of the 600,000 words are included in the receiver's 5000-word vocabulary? The medical world also has a growing language of its own, which is made up of abbreviations and medical terms. "Remember now, Sidney is NPO," or "Your doctor feels that you may have diverticulitis, so she has scheduled you for a BE tomorrow" may have little meaning to those not familiar with the medical terms. Some words have more than one meaning. For instance, a *chip* in the computer world has a much different meaning than a *chip* used in a poker game.

Communication is 55% facial expression and eye contact, including the length of glance; 38% vocal qualities, including tone, loudness, firmness, hesitations, and pauses; and 7% verbal, actual words (Fig. 5–2). There is often inconsistency between what a person is saying and how he or she appears. ("Of course I'm listening to you, Mother," says the 9-year-old boy as he sits glued to the television set, leaving the mother wondering whether the child is indeed listening to her.)

Another major weakness in the communication process is poor listening skills. Often we are thinking of something else while the speaker is talking to us; we are formulating a response or prejudging what is being said.

Daughter: I have stopped eating breakfast meats.

Mother: But breakfast is the most important meal of the day. You should not give it up.

Instead of listening to what is being said the mother has prejudged that the daughter is skipping breakfast altogether rather than just breakfast meats.

Because the health unit coordinator is the communicator for the nursing unit, effective communication is vital for both job success and proficient operation of the nursing unit.

Communication takes place daily with doctors, nurses, allied health professionals, patients, visitors, and administrators (Fig. 5–3). The health unit coordinator is often the first person seen by the new patient and visitors. The words, gestures, facial expression, and body posture the health unit coordinator uses can be recognized as sounding, looking, and feeling opinionated, supportive, thoughtful, or insecure. The tone of voice, the words spoken, and the facial expressions used during the patient's or visitor's initial contact with the nursing unit leaves a lasting impression.

Components of Communication

Communication is the process of transmitting images, feelings, and ideas from the mind of one person to the minds of one or more people for the purpose of obtaining a response. The communication process consists of four components:

Sender: The person transmitting the message
Message: The images, feelings, and ideas transmitted
Receiver: The person receiving the message
Feedback: The response to the message

Communication seems like a simple process; however, the act of communicating does not guarantee that effective communication has taken place or that the message sent was the same as the message received. For example, a program was developed for a computer to translate one language into another. The computer translated the English phrase "out of sight, out of mind" into Russian, and then translated it back into English as "invisible idiot."

Communication Model

A model is a representation of a process—a map, for instance. We will use a model to take a closer look at the communication process, to identify why so many of us communicate poorly, and to find ways to improve our communication with others (Fig. 5–4).

Sender

The sender must translate mental images, feelings, and ideas into symbols to communicate them to the receiver. The process is called *encoding*. Encoding involves the sender deciding whether to send the message in verbal symbols or in nonverbal symbols (Fig. 5–5). What are the right words to use so the receiver will understand the message? Different words are used if you are speaking to a child, to an adult, or to another health care professional. Nonverbal symbols, such as facial expressions, may be used to communicate the message. Encoding occurs each time we communicate. A poor choice of words or an inconsistency between verbal and nonverbal messages may result in unsuccessful communication.

Message

Once the idea, feeling, or image is encoded, it is sent to the receiver. This step of the communication process is called the *message*.

Communication is...

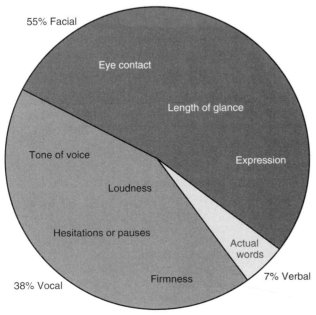

FIGURE 5-2 ▲ Verbal and nonverbal communication.

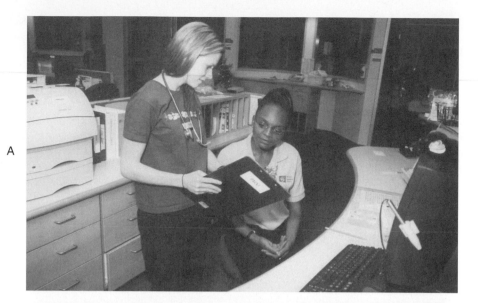

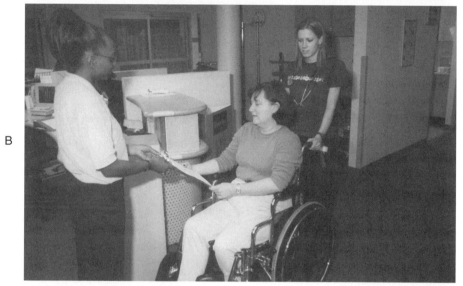

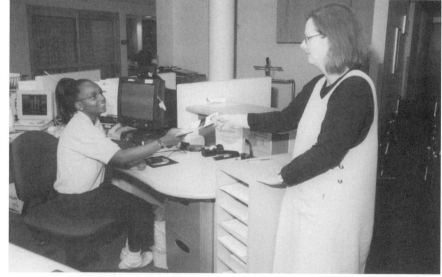

FIGURE 5–3 ▲ The health unit coordinator is the communicator for the nursing unit. *A,* Communicating with hospital staff. *B,* Welcoming a new patient to the unit. *C,* Informing a visitor.

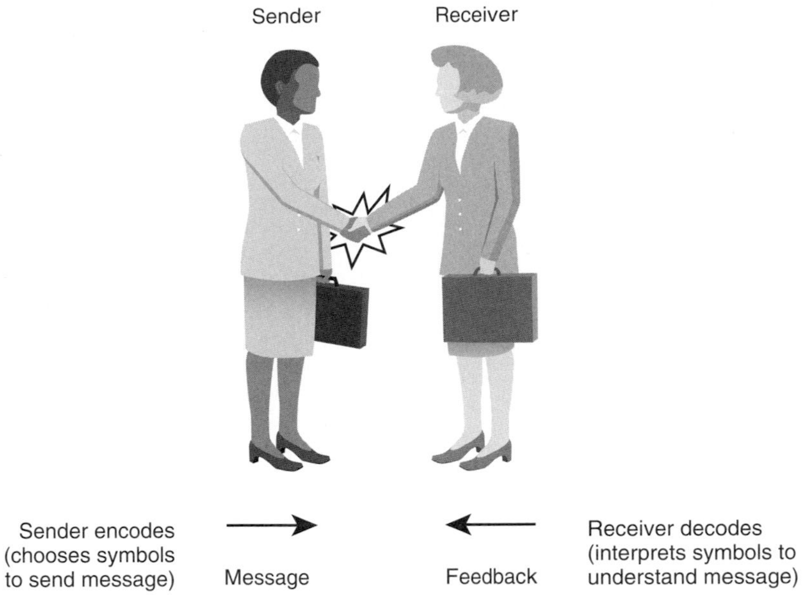

Sender   Receiver

Sender encodes
(chooses symbols   →   ←   Receiver decodes
to send message)   (interprets symbols to
                    Message   Feedback   understand message)

FIGURE 5-4 ▲ The communication model.

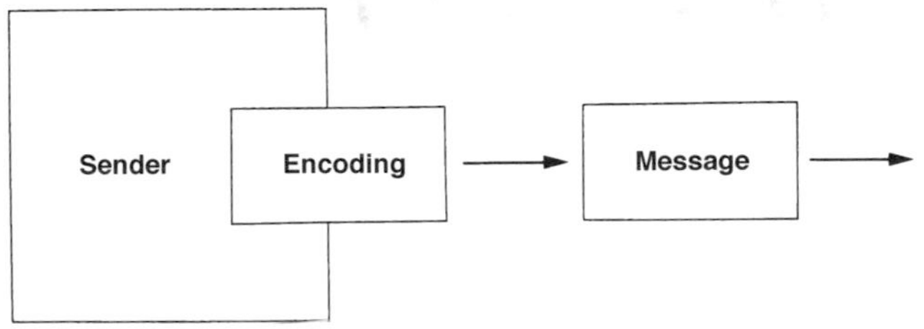

Receiver

As the message reaches the receiver, he or she must decode the verbal and nonverbal symbols. *Decoding* is the process of translating the symbols received from the sender to determine the message. Unsuccessful decoding can be caused by inconsistency in the verbal and nonverbal symbols from the sender. For instance, "Of course I love you," said harshly may be difficult to decode correctly. Lifestyle, age, cultural background, environment, and poor listening habits are other reasons for incorrect decoding. In successful communication the ideas, feelings, and images of the sender match those of the receiver (Fig. 5–6, *A*). In unsuccessful communication, errors occur in encoding or in decoding the message (Fig. 5–6, *B*).

| Sender | Encoding | → | Message | → |

FIGURE 5-5 ▲ The communication process: message sending.

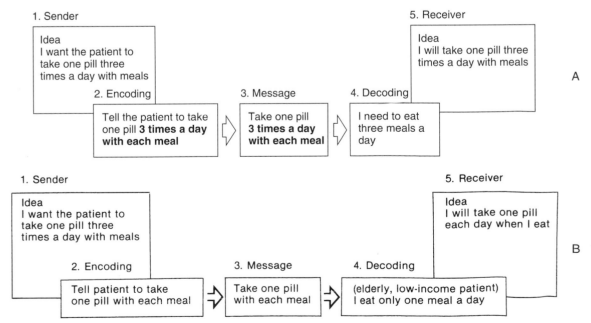

FIGURE 5-6 ▲ *A,* An example of successful communication. *B,* An example of unsuccessful communication.

Verbal and Nonverbal Communication

Two methods of communication are verbal and nonverbal. Verbal communication is the use of language or the actual words spoken, whereas nonverbal communication is the use of eye contact, body language, facial expression, or symbolic expressions such as clothing that communicate a message. Sometimes our verbal and nonverbal communication contradicts each other. For example, when a person is asked, "What is wrong?" and responds, "Oh nothing, I'm just fine" as he shrugs his shoulders, frowns, and turns away, the dejected body language is more believable than the words spoken.

Types of Nonverbal Communication

Nonverbal communication can be separated further into two types: symbolic and body language:

Symbolic	Body Language
clothing	posture
hair	ambulation
jewelry	touching
body art	personal distance
cosmetics	eye contact
automobile	breathing
house	hand gestures
perfume or cologne	facial expressions

Listening Skills

Listening is something we have done all our lives, but most of us have had little or no training in how to do it effectively. We take it for granted. Many of us think of communication as the sender giving us a message, but for successful communication the sender and the receiver both must participate actively in the communication process. Active participation for the receiver requires effective listening skills.

Five Levels of Listening

According to Dr. Steven Covey in his best-selling book, *Seven Habits of Highly Effective People*, we listen at five different levels depending on our interest in what is being said or what we might be doing while we are listening.

1. *Ignoring:* making no effort to listen
2. *Pretend listening:* giving the appearance that you are listening
3. *Selective listening:* hearing only the parts that interest you
4. *Attentive listening* (also called active listening): paying attention and focusing on what the speaker says and comparing it to your own experience
5. *Empathic listening:* listening and responding with both the heart and mind to truly understand, realizing that every person has a right to feel as they do.

Guidelines for Improving Listening Skills

1. *Stop talking.* The first step toward improving listening skills is to stop talking. The maxim that we have two ears and one mouth may indicate that we need to listen twice as much as we speak.
2. *Teach yourself to concentrate.* The average person speaks between 100 and 200 words a minute. The listener can process up to 400 words a minute. Often we find ourselves pretending to listen, listening selectively to the speaker, not listening

for meaning in the message, or hearing only what interests us; in so doing we miss important cues or even words. "We cannot send you any help" has a much different meaning from "We cannot send you any help *right now.*"

3. *Take time to listen.* When someone talks to you, stop what you are doing and look at the speaker. Practice attentive listening by focusing on the meaning of the words and watching for the nonverbal symbols. "I wish I were dead" spoken by an elderly patient may mean "I'm lonely."
4. *Listen with your eyes.* Practice empathetic listening by looking into the eyes of the sender. What is the sender saying? A visitor standing at the desk saying, "My mother is not back from surgery yet" may really be saying, "I'm frightened. She has been in surgery so long there must be complications."
5. *Listen to what is being said, not only how it is being said.* Use both attentive and empathetic listening to fully understand what is being said. Avoid being distracted by a lisp, by how fast the sender is talking, or by what the sender is wearing, for instance. Concentrate on the verbal and nonverbal communication symbols used by the sender.
6. *Suspend judgment.* Often we react emotionally to what is said or what we think is being said. We prejudge what the speaker is saying and unconsciously tune out ideas or beliefs that do not match our own.
7. *Do not interrupt the speaker.* Interrupting the speaker or finishing the sentence discourages the sender and breaks down communication. To break this habit, try apologizing each time you interrupt the sender.
8. *Remove distractions.* Noise, a ringing telephone, and conversations of others are types of distractions that interfere with effective listening.
9. *Listen for both feeling and content* (seek to understand). Use empathetic listening by keeping in mind that every person has a right to feel as they do.

Feedback

Feedback, the response to the message sent, is the final component to the communication process. Effective communication is virtually impossible without it. Feedback tells the sender how much of the message was understood, indicates whether the receiver agrees or disagrees with the message, and helps the sender correct confusing or vague language. Feedback can be as simple as a nod, it may be an answer to a question, or it may be used to encourage further communication and to assist the sender in developing ideas or sharing feelings.

Guidelines for Improving Feedback Skills

1. *Use paraphrasing* (repeat the message to the sender in your own words). Phrases such as "Let me see if I have this right ..." and "This is what you want ..." are acceptable as lines leading into paraphrasing. For example: "Let me repeat that to you. For the dressing change tomorrow you want a dressing tray, size 7 gloves, and three packages of 4 × 4's."
2. *Repeat the last word or words of the message* (to allow the speaker to more fully develop the thought). Be careful not to parrot the whole message or the speaker may respond with "That's what I just said."

Patient: I'm not sure I want to have the myelogram.
Health unit coordinator: Myelogram?

Patient: Yes, I'm scheduled for one this afternoon, and frankly I'm scared stiff. My neighbor had one…

3. *Use specific rather than general feedback.* "Your idea has merit" is more meaningful than "You are so bright."
4. *Use constructive feedback rather than destructive feedback.* Do not use feedback that makes a person feel worse. "Moving your work station to the other counter may work" is better than saying, "That's a dumb idea, it won't work there!"
5. *Do not deny senders' feelings.* The use of statements such as: "Don't worry" to someone who is frightened that he or she has cancer is of no help. Feedback encouraging the person to expound on his or her fears will be much more helpful to the person.

Intercultural Communication Skills

The United States often is referred to as the "melting pot" because of its culturally diverse society. Cultures are developed when groups of people spend an extended time together. Each of us has values, beliefs, habits, and customs as a result of our backgrounds that make up our culture. Subcultures are smaller groups of people with certain ethnic, occupational, religious, or physical characteristics within the larger culture (e.g., elderly people, teens, nurses, Christians, athletes). It is essential for health care workers to understand and evaluate their own values, beliefs, and customs before working with and caring for people of varying cultures in health care. There are many conflicts that occur in the health care delivery systems caused by cultural misunderstandings (e.g., verbal, nonverbal language, lack or courtesy, objectivity). Culturally sensitive care involves taking the time to learn about the cultural backgrounds of patients and may involve incorporating their beliefs and practices into their care. Refer to Table 5–1 to learn about the cultural backgrounds of African Americans, Asians, Hispanics, and Native Americans.

Often people judge others by the standards of their own values and beliefs with their own and find it difficult to accept other cultures. This is referred to as ethnocentrism. Health unit coordinators may have attitudes regarding a patient refusing a treatment because of religious beliefs, a patient admitted for a sex-change surgery, or a patient who is a former alcoholic receiving a liver transplant. These attitudes are based on ethnocentrism and must not affect the care given to these patients. Health unit coordinators must beware of stereotyping and must not make assumptions or draw conclusions about a patient or a coworker based on race or ethnicity. Patients and coworkers deserve to be treated and respected as unique individuals regardless of their gender, age, economic status, religion, sexual status, education, occupation, physical makeup, or limitations or command of the English language.

Guidelines for Speaking to Someone Who Does Not Speak English Well

While working as a health unit coordinator, you may need to speak to someone from a different culture who does not speak English well. Use the following guidelines to assist you in this process:

- Do not shout
- Talk distinctly and slowly
- Emphasize key words
- Let the listener read your lips
- Use printed words and pictures
- Do not use slang or jargon

TABLE 5–1	Variations Among Selected Cultural Groups			
	African Americans	**Asians**	**Hispanics**	**Native Americans**
Verbal communication	Asking personal questions of someone met for the first time is seen as improper and intrusive	High respect for others, especially those in positions of authority	Expression of negative feelings is considered impolite	Speak in a low tone of voice and expect that the listener will be attentive
Nonverbal communication	Direct eye contact in conversation often is considered rude	Direct eye contact among superiors may be considered disrespectful	Avoidance of eye contact usually is a sign of attentiveness and respect	Direct eye contact often is considered disrespectful
Touch	Touching another's hair often is considered offensive	It is not customary to shake hands with persons of the opposite sex	Touching often is observed between two persons in conversation	A light touch of the person's hand instead of a firm handshake often is used when greeting a person
Family organization	Usually have close, extended family networks; women play key roles in health care decisions	Usually have close, extended family ties; emphasis may be on family needs rather than individual needs	Usually have close, extended family ties; all members of the family may be involved in health care decisions	Usually have close, extended family ties; emphasis tends to be on the family rather than on individual needs
Time	Often present-oriented	Often present-oriented	Often present-oriented	Often present-oriented
Alternative healers	"Granny," "root doctor," voodoo priest, spiritualist	Acupuncturist, acupressurist, herbalist	Curandero, espiritualista, yerbo	Medicine man, shaman
Self-care practices	Poultices, herbs, oils, roots	Hot and cold foods, herbs, teas, soups, cupping, burning, rubbing, pinching	Hot and cold foods, herbs	Herbs, corn meal, medicine bundle

Data from Giger JN, Davidhizar, RE: *Transcultural nursing*, ed 3, St. Louis, 1999, Mosby; Spector RE: *Cultural diversity in health and illness*, ed 5, Upper Saddle River, NJ, 2000, Prentice Hall; Payne KT: In Taylor OL, editor: *Nature of communication disorders in culturally and linguistically diverse populations*, San Diego, 1986, College Hill Press.

- Organize your thoughts
- Choose your words carefully
- Construct your sentences to say exactly what you want to say
- Observe body language carefully
- Try to pronounce names correctly
- Ask for feedback to determine understanding

■ ASSERTIVENESS FOR THE HEALTH UNIT COORDINATOR

Have you ever said yes to a request but really wanted to say no or left a conversation wishing you had "stood up for yourself"? If your answer is yes, then you responded to the request in a *nonassertive* behavior style.

Have you ever allowed a situation to get out of control, then "blew up" and later wished you had handled the situation better? If your answer is yes, then you responded to the situation in an *aggressive* behavioral style.

A third type of response is an *assertive* behavior style, in which an individual expresses her or his wants and desires in an honest and appropriate way, while respecting other people's rights.

As a health unit coordinator, you may have to ask patients or visitors to change their behavior to conform to safety regulations and hospital rules or to allow for the comfort of others. For example, you may have to ask a patient's relative not to smoke in the hospital, or you may have to ask a patient to turn down the television volume at the request of the patient's roommate. Asking another person to change his or her behavior can provoke a defensive reaction. Knowing you have a choice of behavior styles and choosing the right way to handle a given situation assists you in communicating more effectively.

Also, as a health unit coordinator, you engage in unlimited encounters during the day that can lead to conflict. Using assertiveness, the art of expressing yourself clearly and concisely; being able to clarify when necessary; and being able to explain and communicate in an open, honest manner enables you to cope more effectively with problems and conflicts as they arise (see the Box *A Bill of Assertive Rights* on page 67).

Behavioral Styles

Nonassertive Behavioral Style

A nonassertive response is typically self-denying and does not express true feelings. The person does not stand up for his or her rights and allows others to choose for him or her. Because of inadequate behavior the individual feels hurt and anxious. A nonassertive health unit coordinator may have strong opinions about things going on at the nurses' station but keeps these feelings to himself or herself.

EXAMPLE

> Kim feels that she is scheduled to work more holidays and 12-hour shifts than the other health unit coordinators on the unit. Instead of saying anything to the nurse manager, she is upset every time she looks at the new work schedule.

A nonassertive choice avoids conflict; therefore, feelings of frustration or anger are not expressed to the person responsible.

EXAMPLE

> Robert spent 15 minutes in the unit lounge complaining to coworkers about how Betsy, a nurse, is condescending toward him and makes disparaging remarks in conversations with him. She expects him to leave what he is working on to run special errands for her. He is angry and frustrated but refuses to talk to her directly about these problems.

A nonassertive approach to requesting behavior change is to use general or apologetic statements or to use words that minimize the message. This low-key approach allows others to easily ignore the request.

EXAMPLE

> Two visitors were relaxing in a visitors' lounge near the nursing station. They both lit cigarettes. A "no smoking" sign is posted nearby. Mary approaches the visitors and says, "I'm sorry, but I have to ask a little favor. This is not my rule, but smoking is not allowed here."

Aggressive Behavioral Style

An aggressive response is typically self-enhancing at the expense of others. The person may express feelings but hurts others in the process. Verbal attacks, disparaging remarks, and manipulations indicate aggressive behavior. An aggressive health unit coordinator uses "you" statements, often followed by personal judgments. Using "you" statements provokes more defensiveness than using "I" statements.

EXAMPLE

> Kim feels she is scheduled to work more holidays and 12-hour shifts than the other health unit coordinators. An aggressive Kim may approach the nurse manager and say, "You are simply unfair, and you don't care about me. I have to work more than the others."

Statements that use *always* and *never* are often part of aggressive communications.

EXAMPLE

> Robert is upset with the nurse, Betsy, because she expects him to leave what he is doing to run errands for her. Robert responds aggressively, "You *always* expect me to stop my work for you; you think what you want is so important and you *never* think about anyone else."

An aggressive health unit coordinator uses demands instead of requests. Demanding does not elicit another's cooperation and generates defensiveness. Disparaging remarks also cause the receiver to feel humiliated.

EXAMPLE

> An aggressive unit coordinator asks the visitors to stop smoking by saying, "Put out your cigarettes. You can't smoke here. Can't you see the 'no-smoking' sign?"

Assertive Behavioral Style

An assertive response includes standing up for your rights without violating the rights of others. Assertive behavior is self-enhancing but not at the expense of others. It involves open, honest communication and being able to express needs, expectations, and feelings. Being assertive also means being able both to accept compliments with ease and to admit errors. It also means taking responsibility for your actions. It is common for a person to assert himself or herself verbally only after frustration builds. At that point it is too late to communicate assertively, and an aggressive response is used instead. It is useful to use assertiveness in all interactions before frustration builds. It is easy for the beginner to confuse assertive behavior with aggressive behavior. To distinguish the difference, remember that with assertive behavior the rights of another are not violated.

An assertive health unit coordinator is able to use clear, direct, nonapologetic expressions of feelings and expectations. Descriptive rather than judgmental criticisms and "I" rather than "you" statements are used.

A BILL OF ASSERTIVE RIGHTS

- You have the right to judge your own behavior, thoughts, and emotions, and to take the responsibility for their initiation and consequences upon yourself.
- You have the right to offer no reasons or excuses to justify your behavior.
- You have the right to judge if you are responsible for finding solutions to other people's problems.
- You have the right to change your mind.
- You have the right to make mistakes—and be responsible for them.
- You have the right to say "I don't know."
- You have the right to be independent of the goodwill of others before coping with them.
- You have the right to be illogical in making decisions.
- You have the right to say "I don't understand."
- You have the right to say "I don't care."

YOU HAVE THE RIGHT TO SAY "NO" WITHOUT FEELING GUILTY.

From Smith, Manual J.: *When I Say No, I Feel Guilty.* New York, Bantam Books, 1975, with permission.

EXAMPLE

> Kim, as an assertive health unit coordinator, chooses to talk to the nurse manager about her feelings. "I feel that I am working more holidays and more 12-hour shifts than the other health unit coordinators. I had to work both Christmas and Easter this year, and last pay period I had to work four 12-hour shifts. I would like to share working the holidays equally with the others. The 12-hour shifts do not work well with my family life; however, if others also do not like the 12-hour shifts I am willing to work my fair share of them."

An assertive health unit coordinator uses concise statements and specific behavioral descriptions.

EXAMPLE

> Robert is assertive in dealing with Betsy when he chooses to talk to her. He begins with using an "I" statement," then describes the incident in which he felt Betsy was condescending. "I felt you were condescending toward me when you said, 'Even you should have been able to see that I needed your help.'" He also mentions the specific remark she made that he found disparaging. Depending on the discussion that follows, it also may be appropriate for him to ask Betsy for a behavior change. Robert also describes an incident in which Betsy asked him to interrupt his work to run errands for her. He describes how he could be more productive if he was allowed to do the task for her when it was convenient to his work schedule.

An assertive health unit coordinator uses requests instead of demands and personalizes statements of concern.

EXAMPLE

> Mary, an assertive health unit coordinator, approaches the visitors and says, "Please stop smoking in this area. There is a designated smoking area located in the outside dining portion of the cafeteria where you can sit down and have a cigarette."

Assertiveness is based on the belief that each individual has the same fundamental human rights; therefore, the doctor is not better than the health unit coordinator or the teacher is not better than the students. In becoming assertive do not focus on changing your personality, but rather on changing your behavior in specific situations. It is highly unlikely that anyone is always assertive; however, once assertiveness is learned, it can be one of your behavioral choices.

Table 5–2 compares nonassertive, aggressive, and assertive behavioral styles.

TABLE 5–2	Comparison of Nonassertive, Aggressive, and Assertive Behavioral Styles		
Components	**Nonassertive**	**Aggressive**	**Assertive**
Rights	Does not stand up for rights	Stands up for rights but violates the rights of others	Stands up for rights without violating rights of others
Choice	Allows others to choose (to avoid conflict)	Chooses for others	Chooses for self
Belief	I'm not OK, you're OK; lose/win	I'm OK, you're not OK; win/lose	I'm OK, you're OK; win/win
Responsibility	Others responsible for behavior Blame themselves for poor results; may blame others for feelings	Responsible for others' behavior Blames others for poor results Feelings aren't important	Responsible for own behavior Assumes responsibility for own errors; assumes responsibility for feelings
Traits	Self-denying, apologetic, timid, emotionally dishonest, difficult to say "no," guilty, whining, "poor me"	Dominates, humiliates, sarcasm Self-enhancing at the expense of others, opinionated	Expresses feelings, feels good about self, candid, diplomatic, listens, eye contact
Goals	Does not achieve goals	Achieves goals at the expense of others	May achieve goals
Word choices	Minimizing words such as "I'm sorry" "I believe" "I think" "Little," "sort of" General instead of specific statements; statement disguised as questions	"You statements" Always/never statements Demands instead of requests	"I understand . . ." "I feel . . ." "I apologize . . ." Neutral language Concise statements
Body language	Lack of eye contact; slumping, downtrodden posture; words and nonverbal messages that don't match	"Looking-through-you" eye contact; tense, impatient posture	Erect, relaxed posture; eye contact; verbal and nonverbal messages match

EXERCISE 2

Identify the behavioral style of each of the following statements by writing AG for aggressive, AS for assertive, and NA for nonassertive in the spaces provided.

1. "I would like to have Monday off." _____

2. "You should know how to order diets. You have been here long enough." _____

3. "I'm sorry. I'm so forgetful. I won't let it happen again." _____

4. "I would kind of like to go on my break now." _____

5. "The next NAHUC chapter meeting is tomorrow at 6:00 PM. I am going. Would you like to go with me?" _____

6. "I know nothing about it. You were here yesterday—you should know." _____

7. "I would like to finish transcribing this set of orders before I take this specimen to the lab." _____

8. "I wish somebody else around here would answer the phone once in a while." _____

9. "Your chart is right here, Dr. James. I would think you could find it on your own." _____

10. "I apologize, I did not order the liver scan. I will order it immediately." _____

11. "You are always late. You never care that I have to stay over and cover for you." _____

12. "I really hate to ask you this, and you don't have to do it, but would you work for me on Saturday?" _____

13. "May I help you find your chart, Dr. McLean?" _____

14. "I don't know what the nurse manager thinks I am, a machine or something. We need more help around here." _____

15. "Mrs. Smith, I would like you to turn your light off so Mrs. Jones can rest." _____

16. "Mary, I would like to switch days off with you." _____

Evaluating Your Assertiveness

Table 5–3 is an assertive inventory developed by Alberti and Emmons. These authors state that the inventory "provides a list of questions which should be useful in increasing your awareness of your own behavior in situations which call for assertiveness. The inventory is not a standardized psychological test. There are no right answers. The only "score" is your own evaluation of how

TABLE 5-3	The Assertiveness Inventory				

The following questions will be helpful in assessing your assertiveness. Be honest with your responses. All you have to do is draw a circle around the number that describes you best. For some questions, the assertive end of the scale is at 0; for others it is at 3.

Key: 0 means *no* or *never;* 1 means *somewhat* or *sometimes;* 2 means *usually* or *a good deal;* and 3 means *practically always* or *entirely.*

Question	0	1	2	3
1. When a person is highly unfair, do you call it to his or her attention?	0	1	2	3
2. Do you find it difficult to make decisions?	0	1	2	3
3. Are you openly critical of others' ideas, opinions, or behavior?	0	1	2	3
4. Do you speak out in protest when someone takes your place in line?	0	1	2	3
5. Do you often avoid people or situations for fear of embarrassment?	0	1	2	3
6. Do you usually have confidence in your own judgment?	0	1	2	3
7. Do you insist that your spouse or roommate take on a fair share of household chores?	0	1	2	3
8. Are you prone to "flying off the handle?"	0	1	2	3
9. When a salesperson makes an effort, do you find it hard to say "no" even though the merchandise is not really what you want?	0	1	2	3
10. When a latecomer is waited on before you, do you call attention to the situation?	0	1	2	3
11. Are you reluctant to speak up in a discussion or debate?	0	1	2	3
12. If a person has borrowed money (or a book, a garment, or something else of value) and is overdue in returning it, do you mention it?	0	1	2	3
13. Do you continue to pursue an argument after the other person has had enough?	0	1	2	3
14. Do you generally express what you feel?	0	1	2	3
15. Are you disturbed if someone watches you at work?	0	1	2	3
16. If someone keeps kicking or bumping your chair in a movie or a lecture, do you ask the person to stop?	0	1	2	3
17. Do you find it difficult to keep eye contact when talking to another person?	0	1	2	3
18. In a good restaurant, when your meal is improperly prepared or served, do you ask the waiter or waitress to correct the situation?	0	1	2	3
19. When you discover merchandise is faulty, do you return it for an adjustment?	0	1	2	3
20. Do you show your anger by name-calling or obscenities?	0	1	2	3
21. Do you try to be a wallflower or piece of furniture in social situations?	0	1	2	3
22. Do you insist that your property manager (mechanic, repairman, etc.) make repairs, adjustments, or replacements that are his or her responsibility?	0	1	2	3
23. Do you often step in and make decisions for others?	0	1	2	3
24. Are you able to express love and affection openly?	0	1	2	3
25. Are you able to ask your friends for small favors or help?	0	1	2	3
26. Do you think you always have the right answer?	0	1	2	3
27. When you differ with a person you respect, are you able to speak up for your own viewpoint?	0	1	2	3
28. Are you able to refuse unreasonable requests made by friends?	0	1	2	3
29. Do you have difficulty complimenting or praising others?	0	1	2	3
30. If you are disturbed by someone smoking near you, can you say so?	0	1	2	3
31. Do you shout or use bullying tactics to get others to do as you wish?	0	1	2	3
32. Do you finish other people's sentences for them?	0	1	2	3
33. Do you get into physical fights with others, especially with strangers?	0	1	2	3
34. At family meals, do you control the conversation?	0	1	2	3
35. When you meet a stranger, are you the first to introduce yourself and begin a conversation?	0	1	2	3

you measure up to what you would like to be able to do." Take time now to respond to the questions in the inventory.

Assertiveness Skills

The goal of using assertiveness in communication is to arrive at an "I win, you win" conclusion—in other words, a workable compromise. A workable compromise is dealing with a conflict in such a way that the solution is satisfactory to all involved parties. Four assertiveness skills that may be used to reach a workable compromise are broken record, fogging, negative assertion, and negative inquiry.

Broken Record

The broken record is an assertiveness skill that allows you to say no over and over again without raising your voice or getting irritated or angry. You must be persistent and not give reasons, excuses, or explanations for not doing what the other person wants you to do. By doing this you can ignore manipulative traps and argumentative baiting.

Jane: Let's go to lunch.

Sue: Thanks for asking; however, *I can't go, I just started a new diet.*

Jane: So what! You start a new diet every week. It has never stopped you from going before.

Sue: Well, thanks anyway, but *I just started a new diet, I can't go to lunch.*

Jane: Well you don't have to eat anything fattening.

Sue: Thanks anyway. *I can't go. I just started a new diet.*

Fogging

Fogging is an assertiveness skill that allows you to accept manipulative criticism and anxiety-producing statements by offering no resistance and by using a noncommittal reply, calmly acknowledging that there may be some truth in what the critic is saying yet retaining the right to remain your own judge. When you use fogging, it is hard for the other person to see exactly what you are saying.

John: You are really a slow worker!

Bill: I can see it may appear that I am a slow worker; however, I have only been here a month. I will speed up once I know the procedures better.

Negative Assertion

Negative assertion is an assertiveness skill that allows you to accept your errors and faults without becoming defensive or resorting to anger. It is a technique of admitting errors without affecting your worth as a human being. It includes not using self-depreciation, such as "that was so stupid of me."

Dr. Smith: You didn't order the CBC on Mr. Jones yesterday.

Sue: You're right. I did not order it, I apologize. Should I order it today?

Negative Inquiry

Negative inquiry is an assertiveness skill that allows you to actively prompt criticism to use the information or, if manipulative, to exhaust it. By doing this you obtain clarification about the criticism and hopefully bring out possible hidden issues that may really be the point.

Nurse manager: Your work is getting sloppy. If you want to stay on this unit you will have to change.

Unit coordinator: You say my work is sloppy. What is it about my work that is sloppy?

EXERCISE 3

Practice writing verbal responses to the situations described in the following exercise. Use the behavioral style indicated. Practice using the assertiveness skills when answering assertively.

1. A coworker comes in at 3:00 PM and finds that there were no admission charts made up for the new admits. She throws a chart down in front of you and storms off. You did not have time to put the charts together.

   Assertive:

   _____

   Nonassertive:

   _____

Aggressive:

_____

2. You have been asked to float to the pediatric unit. You work on orthopedics. When you arrive on Peds, a nurse says to you: "It would really be nice to get someone who knows what he's doing."

   Assertive:

   _____

   Nonassertive:

   _____

   Aggressive:

   _____

3. You forgot to order a CBC yesterday while transcribing Mr. Jones' orders. When the error was discovered by the nurse manager, she said, "You didn't order the CBC on Mr. Jones yesterday!"

   Assertive:

   _____

   Nonassertive:

   _____

   Aggressive:

   _____

4. A local celebrity is a patient on your unit. The doctor has left strict instructions that only relatives can visit the patient and for only short periods. A visitor has just approached the nursing station. He claims he is the local celebrity's manager and must see the patient about some financial matters today.

   Assertive:

   _____

   Nonassertive:

   _____

Aggressive:

_____

_____

5. Your immediate supervisor has just told you that your work is simply sloppy and to improve it or else.

Assertive:

_____

Nonassertive:

_____

Aggressive:

_____

6. It is 9:00 AM, and Dr. Jones has asked you to please locate the CBC results he ordered yesterday on Mr. Smith. You call the lab, and you cannot immediately locate them. When you tell this to Dr. Jones he responds angrily, "What in the hell is going on here? Can't anybody do anything right on this unit?"

Assertive:

_____

Nonassertive:

_____

Aggressive:

_____

■ STEPS TO DEAL WITH AN ANGRY TELEPHONE CALLER

At times the health unit coordinator is confronted with an angry or disgruntled telephone caller. Following the few helpful steps outlined here will assist you in handling the situation effectively.

1. *When answering the telephone always identify yourself by nursing unit, name, and status* (Fig. 5–7). Doing this puts you on a more personal level with the caller. Also, callers may become even more upset if they need to ask questions to determine whom they are talking to.
2. *Avoid putting the person on hold.* Placing an angry person on hold may escalate their anger.
3. *Listen to what the caller is saying.* Do not become defensive. Keep in mind that the caller is not really angry with you.
4. *Write down what the caller is saying.* The notes may come in handy, and they help you control your own anger.
5. *Acknowledge the anger.* Use phrases such as, "I understand that you are angry" and "I hear your frustration."
6. *Do not allow the caller to become abusive.* Say, "I feel you are becoming abusive" or "Please call me back in a few minutes so we can talk about this calmly."

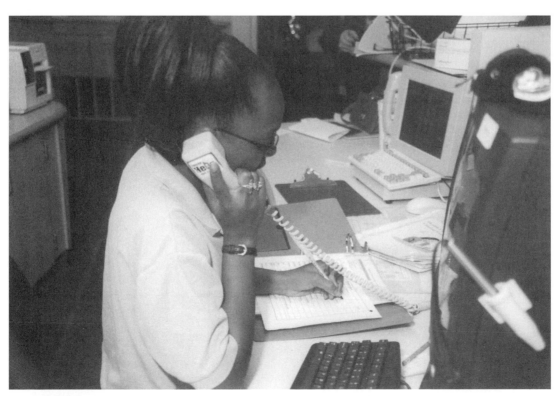

FIGURE 5–7 ▲ When answering the telephone, always identify yourself by nursing unit, name, and status.

■ HOW COMMUNICATION AND INTERPERSONAL SKILLS ARE USED IN THE HEALTH CARE SETTING

Following are five major areas in which the health unit coordinator may use communication and interpersonal skills discussed in this chapter in the health care setting:

1. *Obtaining information.* Often the health unit coordinator must obtain information to communicate a message in a correct and timely manner. Applying assertive skills to ask a question correctly, using appropriate listening skills when receiving the response and when the situation calls for it, and using the guidelines for speaking to a person who does not speak English well will be useful.

2. *Providing information.* The health unit coordinator will be providing information to visitors, doctors, nursing staff, and other hospital departments as well as institutions outside the hospital. Being aware of verbal and nonverbal use of language will be helpful in doing this.

3. *Developing trust.* Trust is vital to a healthy work environment, and assertive communication plays a big role in establishing and maintaining this trust.

4. *Showing understanding.* Understanding the needs of the patients, families, and coworkers will foster successful communication in the work environment. Using Maslow's hierarchy of needs and intercultural communication skills will be of use in this area.

5. *Relieving stress.* Stress in the workplace is a constant; how we manage it makes a difference. Recognizing the three behavioral types and using assertiveness skills can be helpful in this area. Using the communication model of selecting words carefully for communication and using effective listening skills may help avoid or alleviate stressful situations.

■ SUMMARY

Effective communication is essential in the health care setting. Quality patient care requires an efficient, professional, and culturally sensitive team. Health care can be extremely stressful so it is vital that personnel remain calm, exercise assertiveness skills, and have empathy for patients and coworkers. Each member of a health care team is important and necessary.

▼ REVIEW QUESTIONS

1. Write an example of a hospitalized patient's situation that exemplifies each of the first four needs outlined in Maslow's hierarchy of needs.

   a. physiologic

   _____

   b. safety and security

   _____

   c. belonging and love

   _____

   d. esteem

   _____

2. Define the following terms.

   a. sender

   _____

   b. message

   _____

c. receiver

_____

d. feedback

_____

e. encoding

_____

f. decoding

_____

3. Four components of the communication process are:

a. _____

b. _____

c. _____

d. _____

4. Using the communication model, demonstrate a successful communication process and an unsuccessful communication process. Identify at which step of the process the errors occurred.

a. successful communication:

_____

_____

_____

b. unsuccessful communication

_____

_____

_____

5. List two common errors in encoding a message.

a. _____

b. _____

6. List two common errors in decoding a message.

a. _____

b. _____

7. List three examples of *symbolic* nonverbal communication.

    a. _____

    b. _____

    c. _____

8. List three examples of body language used in nonverbal communication.

    a. _____

    b. _____

    c. _____

9. Fill in the percentage used of each of the following verbal and nonverbal communications during the process of communicating messages.

    a. Facial expression and eye contact, including the length of glance   _____ %

    b. Vocal qualities, including tone, loudness, firmness, hesitations, and pauses   _____ %

    c. Verbal, actual words   _____ %

10. List two common causes of unsuccessful communication.

    a. _____

    b. _____

11. Identify the cause(s) of unsuccessful communication in each of the following situations.

    a. A nurse interviewing an Asian patient sits on the side of his bed while making direct eye contact. The patient looks away, avoiding eye contact. The nurse thinks the patient is despondent or is being rude. (Refer to Table 5–1.)

    _____

    _____

    b. Mrs. Fredrick, an elderly female patient who has never been ill before, is admitted to the hospital. Joe, a young male CNA, is assisting her into bed. Joe tells Mrs. Fredrick, "OK, honey, your doctor has ordered that you be NPO because you're going to have a UGI this morning." Mrs. Fredrick begins to cry.

    _____

    _____

    c. Dr. James asks Sue, the health unit coordinator, to answer her calls while she is in the treatment room performing a procedure. Sue receives a call from her boyfriend and doesn't hear the operator paging Dr. James. When Dr. James returns to the nursing station and asks for her message, Sue says, "What message?" Dr. James angrily walks away.

    _____

    _____

d. Cindi, the RN caring for Stan Potter, a homeless man, does not spend as much time with him on admission because he is dirty and doesn't have any social skills.

_____

_____

12. List two listening skills that you feel would most help you improve your interpersonal communication.

a. _____

b. _____

13. List the two feedback skills that you feel would help you improve your interpersonal communication.

a. _____

b. _____

14. Practice identifying the types of human needs listed below. Read each sentence, then write in the space provided the need expressed. Record an appropriate response.

a. *Patient:* "I am having exploratory surgery tomorrow. I hope it's not cancer."

Need expressed:

_____

Appropriate feedback:

_____

b. *Patient:* "Tell the nurse I need something for this pain right away."

Need expressed:

_____

Appropriate feedback:

_____

c. *Health unit coordinator:* "They have asked me to run for office in our local chapter of NAHUC. I said I would."

Need expressed:

_____

Appropriate feedback:

_____

d. *Patient:* "When you get to be my age you won't have many friends who are able to visit you when you are in the hospital."

Need expressed:

_____

Appropriate feedback:

_____

e. *Health unit coordinator:* "I made such a mess out of running that meeting, I feel like a complete idiot."

Need expressed:

_____

Appropriate feedback:

_____

f. *Child:* "Please don't stick me with that needle."

Need expressed:

_____

Appropriate feedback:

_____

g. *Nurse:* "I really like my job, but somehow it isn't enough. I might start looking for something else to do."

Need expressed:

_____

Appropriate feedback:

_____

h. *Patient:* "Just a minute—are you saying that I didn't have the watch with me when I came into the hospital?"

Need expressed:

_____

Appropriate feedback:

_____

15. Describe a time when you felt proud of an accomplishment. What need was being satisfied?

_____

_____

16. Label the following behaviors as assertive, nonassertive, or aggressive.

a. self-denying   _____

b. self-enhancing at the expense of others   _____

c. open, honest, and respectful of others' rights _____

17. Explain the following assertiveness techniques.

    a. Broken record

    _____

    _____

    b. Fogging

    _____

    _____

    c. Negative assertion

    _____

    _____

    d. Negative inquiry

    _____

    _____

18. List at least four steps that you should follow when dealing with an angry caller.

    a. _____

    b. _____

    c. _____

    d. _____

19. Define the following terms.

    a. ethnocentrism

    _____

    b. elitism

    _____

    c. subcultures

    _____

    d. culture

    _____

    e. stereotyping

    _____

TOPICS FOR
DISCUSSION

1. Do you remember a misunderstanding that occurred because someone interpreted something you said differently than you intended it? Discuss how you could have worded the message differently. Discuss what you think caused the misinterpretation.

2. How do you feel when you meet people from other cultures? Does it make you uncomfortable when others are speaking a different language than yours? Discuss how you can communicate with people that do not understand your language.

3. Discuss what the term "culturally sensitive care" means to you.

4. Discuss the importance of effective interpersonal communication for the health unit coordinator.

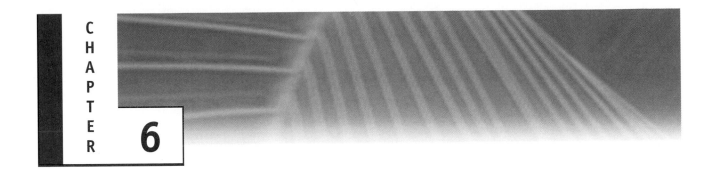

C
H
A
P
T
E
R

6

Workplace Behavior

Ethics and Legal Concepts

Chapter Objectives

Upon completion of this chapter, you will be able to:

1. Define the terms in the vocabulary list.
2. Write the meaning of the abbreviations in the abbreviations list.
3. List four factors that influence a worker's behavior.
4. Explain how personal values could affect interactions in the health care setting.
5. List six behavior traits that make up one's work ethics.
6. List three guidelines to follow to maintain the confidentiality of the contents of a patient's chart.
7. Explain the purpose of the Privacy Rule contained in the Health Insurance Portability and Accountability Act.
8. Explain what is meant by "protected health information."
9. List two responsibilities of the health unit coordinator in maintaining confidentiality of patient protected health information.
10. List four guidelines to follow to achieve a professional appearance.
11. Identify two types of sexual harassment.
12. Discuss four steps to take when reporting sexual harassment.
13. Discuss immediate action to take when witnessing violence or potential for violence.
14. Identify the agencies that investigate abuse of adults and of children.
15. Discuss two purposes of an employee performance evaluation.

16. List two purposes of a patient's bill of rights.

17. Identify three ethical principles for patient care and their application in health unit coordinating.

18. Identify the legal elements necessary to prove medical malpractice.

19. Explain what the standard of care is for a health unit coordinator.

20. Identify two preventive measures that you can take to minimize the risk of malpractice within your own practice.

Vocabulary

Accountability ▲ Taking responsibility for your actions, being answerable to someone for something you have done

Attitude ▲ A manner of thought or feeling expressed in a person's behavior

Autonomy ▲ Independence, personal liberty

Behavior ▲ What people do and say

Code of Ethics ▲ A set of standards for behavior based on values

Confidentiality ▲ Protecting the privacy of any confidential information, either spoken or written

Damages ▲ Monetary compensation awarded by a court for an injury caused by the act of another

Defendant ▲ The person against whom a civil or criminal action is brought

Deposition ▲ Pretrial statement of a witness under oath, taken in question-and-answer form, as it would be in court, with opportunity given to the adversary to be present to cross-examine

Discrimination ▲ Seeing a difference; prejudicial treatment of a person

Empathy ▲ Capacity to share and understand the feelings or ideas of another

Ethics ▲ Behavior that is based on values (beliefs); how we make judgments in regard to right and wrong

Evidence ▲ All the means by which any alleged matter of fact, the truth of which is submitted to investigation at trial, is established or disproved; evidence includes the testimony of witnesses and the introduction of records, documents, exhibits, objects, or any other substantiating matter offered for the purpose of inducing belief in the party's contention by the judge or jury

Expert Witness ▲ A witness who has special knowledge of the subject about which he or she is to testify; the knowledge must generally be such as is not normally possessed by the average person

Fidelity ▲ Doing what one promises

Hostile Environment ▲ A sexually oriented atmosphere or pattern of behavior that is determined to be sexual harassment

Implied Contract ▲ A nonexplicit agreement that impacts some aspect of the employment relationship

Informed Consent ▲ A doctrine that states that before a patient is asked to consent to a risky or invasive diagnostic or treatment procedure he or she is entitled to receive certain information: (1) a description of the procedure, (2) any alternatives to it and their risks, (3) the risks of death or serious bodily disability from the procedure, (4) the probable results of the procedure, including any problems of recuperation and time of recuperation anticipated, and (5) anything else that is generally disclosed to patients asked to consent to the procedure

Liability ▲ The condition of being responsible either for damages resulting from an injurious act or from discharging an obligation or debt

Medical Malpractice ▲ Professional negligence of a health care professional; failure to meet a professional standard of care, resulting in harm to another; for example, failure to provide "good and accepted medical care"

Negligence ▲ Failure to satisfactorily perform one's legal duty, such that another person incurs some injury

Philosophy ▲ Principles; underlying conduct

Plaintiff ▲ The person who brings a lawsuit against another

Principles ▲ Basic truths; moral code of conduct

Quid Pro Quo (Latin) ▲ Involves making conditions of employment (hiring, promotion, retention) contingent on the victim providing sexual favors

Respondeat Superior (Latin) ▲ "Let the master answer." Legal doctrine that imposes liability upon the employer. Note: The employee is also liable for his or her own actions

Respect ▲ Holding a person in esteem or honor; having appreciation and regard for another

Retaliation ▲ Revenge; payback

Scope of Practice ▲ A legal description of what a specific health professional may and may not do

Sexual Harassment ▲ Unwanted, unwelcome behavior; sexual in nature

Standard of Care ▲ The legal duty one owes to another according to the circumstances of a particular case; it is the care that a reasonable and prudent person would have exercised in the given situation

Statute ▲ A law passed by the legislature and signed by the governor at the state level and the president at the federal level

Statute of Limitations ▲ The time within which a plaintiff must bring a civil suit; the limit varies depending upon the type of suit, and it is set by the various state legislatures

Tact ▲ Use of discretion regarding feelings of others

Tort ▲ A wrong against another person or his property that is not a crime but for which the law provides a remedy

Values ▲ Personal beliefs about the worth of a principle, standard, or quality; what one holds as most important

Values Clarification ▲ Examination of our value system

Work Ethics ▲ Moral values regarding work

Abbreviations

Abbreviation	Meaning
APS	Adult Protective Services
CPS	Child Protective Services
HIPAA	Health Insurance Portability and Accountability Act
NINP	no information, no publication

PHI   protected health information
SNAT   suspected nonaccidental trauma

EXERCISE 1

Write the abbreviation for each term listed below.

1. Adult Protective Services   _____

2. Child Protective Services   _____

3. No information, no publication   _____

4. Suspected nonaccidental trauma   _____

5. Health Insurance Portability and Accountability Act   _____

6. Protected health information   _____

EXERCISE 2

Write the meaning of each abbreviation listed below.
1. APS

_____

2. CPS

_____

3. NINP

_____

4. SNAT

_____

5. HIPAA

_____

6. PHI

◼ WORKPLACE BEHAVIOR

There are many factors that influence a person's workplace behavior. What is most important to a person or what each needs or gets from his or her work affects a person's behavior.

Factors That Influence Workplace Behavior

The following are factors that influence a person's behavior in the workplace:

1. Philosophy and standards of the organization
2. Leadership style of supervisors
3. How meaningful or important the work is to the person
4. How challenging the work is for the person
5. How the person fits in with coworkers
6. Personal characteristics of a worker such as abilities, interests, aptitudes, values, and expectations

There are many job options for a health unit coordinator in the health care field. Choose a position that will best satisfy your needs. If you love to be around children, pediatrics may be ideal for you or if you want to be challenged, the emergency room or an intensive care unit may be your best choice. You may want a job that will provide more solitude, such as working in the recovery room, or you may want a more social setting, such as a medical–surgical unit. Choose your job carefully.

Personal values may have a significant impact on how you interact with others on the job. As a health unit coordinator, your job requires that you communicate in a nonjudgmental way. Examining your value system is important when preparing to work in the health care setting.

How Values Influence Interactions in the Health Care Setting

Our values are formed by the age of 6 and are influenced by our parents, siblings, extended family, friends, peers, teachers, and work supervisors. Significant emotional events in our lives and other life experiences may change our values. For example, losing a loved one may cause you to treasure family and value life in a way you had not before. Life experiences can change what we view as most important and also help us gain empathy for others. Our values can have a major impact on how we relate to others and the choices and decisions that we make. Diane Uustal, a well-known nurse and ethicist, describes values as being "a basis for what a person thinks about, chooses, feels for, and acts on." (Uustal, 1992) A health unit coordinator's personal values may cause problems in his or her interactions.

EXAMPLE

Joan, a health unit coordinator, has a father who was an abusive alcoholic. Joan is adamant about her feelings regarding alcoholics and is very much against drinking. Mr. Thomas is admitted because he was in a car accident that was caused by his drunkenness. Whenever Mr. Thomas approaches the desk to talk to Joan, she is very rude to him. Joan is allowing her personal values to influence her behavior. It is important to remain nonjudgmental when dealing with patients and their families and to ensure that personal values do not affect communication with others. At times this may be difficult, especially when communicating with a person identified as an abuser of a child, a spouse, or an elderly person.

A patient's values could also influence our behavior when it conflicts with our own values.

EXAMPLE

> A patient is admitted with internal bleeding; his religion prohibits him from receiving a blood transfusion. Janet, a health unit coordinator, states that she cannot understand how anyone could risk his or her life because of a silly religious belief. The patient has a right to his own values and the right to refuse a treatment.

■ VALUES CLARIFICATION

Values clarification is an important tool for health unit coordinators to use in their preparation to become competent professionals. Examining your values and committing to a virtuous value system will assist you in making ethical decisions. It is essential for health unit coordinators to understand and be aware of their values and to remain nonjudgmental of the values others hold that differ from their own. Value conflicts include cultural, spiritual, social, and ethnic differences.

EXERCISE 3

The purpose of this exercise is to examine your feelings and values related to future employment in health care. Complete the following sentences:

1. A patient has the right to _____

   _____

2. The health care team works best when _____

   _____

3. I fail to show respect for others' values when _____

   _____

4. The most difficult situation to deal with would be _____

   _____

5. When communicating with patients and families, it is

   important to _____

   _____

■ WORK ETHICS

Work ethics are a person's moral values regarding work. It is essential that the health unit coordinator have the following work ethic traits.

Behavior Traits That Make Up a Person's Work Ethics

Dependability: Patients and members of the health care team rely on you to report to work when scheduled and to be on time. You are also depended upon to perform duties and tasks as assigned and to keep obligations and promises. Adequate sleep and abstinence from drugs are essential to maintain your dependability. Lack of sleep, use of illegal drugs, or misuse of prescription drugs would clearly endanger patients.

Accountability: Part of being dependable is being accountable. Accountability is taking responsibility for your actions (i.e., being answerable to someone for something you have done). Health unit coordinators must be aware of and never exceed their scope of practice. If you are unable to report to work or do your job, it is your responsibility to communicate this to the staffing office at least 2 hours before your scheduled shift.

Consideration: Be considerate of the physical condition and emotional state of the patients and your coworkers.

Cheerfulness: Greet and converse with patients and others in a pleasant manner. Health unit coordinators cannot bring personal problems to work. Sarcasm, moodiness, or bad tempers are inappropriate in the workplace.

Empathy: Make every attempt to see things from the viewpoint of patients, families, and coworkers. Keep in mind that stress and worry can affect people's behavior, so refrain from treating a display of anger or frustration as a personal attack.

Trustworthiness: Your employer, patients, and coworkers have placed their confidence in you to keep patient information confidential. Health unit coordinators have access to a lot of information and must not engage in gossip regarding patients, coworkers, physicians, or the hospital.

Respectfulness: Respect is a primary value in health care and can be shown in many ways: tone of voice, body language, attitude toward others, and attitude about work. All life is worthy of respect. We all have a right to our own value system and need to respect that others have a right to theirs. Make every attempt to understand the values and beliefs of your patients and coworkers that may differ from your own.

Courtesy: Be polite and courteous to patients, families, visitors, coworkers, and supervisors. Address people by name (i.e., Mrs. Johnson or Dr. Smith). Other courteous acts include saying "please" and "thank you" and not interrupting when others are speaking.

Tactfulness: Be sensitive to the problems and needs of others. Be aware of what you say and how you say it.

Conscientiousness: Be careful, alert, and accurate in following orders and instructions. Never attempt to perform a procedure or task that you have not been trained or licensed to perform.

Honesty: Be sincere, truthful, and genuine and show a true interest in your relationships with patients, families, visitors, and coworkers. If you make an error, bring it to the attention of the appropriate person(s). Never attempt to cover up an error!

Cooperation: Be willing to work with others, especially in the team-oriented climate of health care. When coworkers work as a team, everyone involved benefits.

Attitude: Attitude is a manner of thought or feeling that can be seen by others when observing your behavior. The tone of your voice and your body language can change the message you are trying to send. Your attitude will be reflected in your work. Be positive about your job and the contribution that you are making.

THE HEALTH INSURANCE PORTABILITY AND ACCOUNTABILITY ACT OF 1996 AND PRIVACY RULE REGARDING CONFIDENTIALITY

The Patient Privacy Rule contained in the Health Insurance Portability and Accountability Act of 1996 was implemented on April 14, 2003. The patient privacy rule protects patient health information and mandates that all patients be provided a copy of privacy policies when treated in a doctor's office or when admitted to any health care facility. When admitted to the hospital a patient will be given a facility directory opt-out form to sign indicating if he or she wishes to be listed in the hospital directory (Fig. 6–1). If the patient chooses not to be listed, his or her chart would be labeled *no information/no publication (NINP)*, meaning that no information would be provided to anyone calling, including stating that the patient is in the hospital.

The health unit coordinator has access to a great deal of *protected health information (PHI)* because of the very nature of the job. Protected health information is information about the patient that includes demographic information (e.g., name, address, phone number) that may identify the individual and relates to his or her past, present, or future physical or mental health and related health care services. This information must be treated with absolute confidentiality by all health personnel. All health care personnel will be required to sign a confidentiality agreement upon employment.

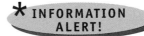

★ INFORMATION ALERT!

The HIPAA Privacy Rule mainly addresses physical safeguards and protecting patient information in paper documents. The Security Rule addresses electronic information solely and will be implemented in April 2005.

FACILITY DIRECTORY OPT OUT FORM

☐ I hereby request that my name, location, general condition, and religious affiliation NOT BE INCLUDED in the facility directory. By invoking this right, I understand that people inquiring by phone or in person will be told, "*I have no information about this patient.*" No deliveries, except U.S. Mail, will be forwarded to me (e.g., flowers).

☐ I hereby request that my name, location, and general condition be released ONLY to those persons listed below. No deliveries, except U.S. Mail, will be forwarded to me (e.g., flowers). (Religious affiliation, if any, will only be provided to clergy.)

_____   _____

_____   _____

☐ I hereby request that my name, location, and general condition be released to anyone EXCEPT those persons listed below. No deliveries, except U.S. Mail, will be forwarded to me (e.g., flowers). (Religious affiliation, if any, will only be provided to clergy.)

_____   _____

_____   _____

☐ I hereby request that my name, location, general condition and religious affiliation BE PLACED in the facility directory.

PRINT PATIENT NAME:_____ DATE:_____

PATIENT SIGNATURE: _____ DATE:_____

WITNESS SIGNATURE:_____

Form to be forwarded or faxed to Admitting Department.

File original in permanent medical record.

FIGURE 6–1 ▲ Facility directory opt-out form.

A health unit coordinator has two responsibilities to ensure the confidentiality of patient information. One is to avoid verbally repeating confidential information, and the other is to control the patient's chart in a manner that ensures confidentiality of the contents.

Following are basic guidelines that will help you establish discipline regarding confidentiality of patient information.

Guidelines for Maintaining Patient Confidentiality

- *Do not discuss patient information* (other than what is necessary to care for the patient). All patient information is confidential. Some information, such as that about sexual preferences or sexually transmitted diseases, is so confidential that it is obvious to treat it as such; however, other information, such as the patient's age, weight, or test results, may be harder to identify as being confidential material. Remember: Never discuss any patient information except when necessary for treatment reasons.

- *Conduct conversations with other health personnel outside of the hearing distance of the patients and visitors.* Never converse about patient information in the hallways, cafeteria, or away from the hospital. Be aware of the identity of others who are at the nurses' station during discussions regarding patients. Often, overheard bits of information may be misconstrued by patients or visitors and result in unnecessary concern for or by the patient. Even if the medical information is factual, it can produce unnecessary worry, anxiety, or even panic in a patient.

- *Do not discuss medical treatment with the patient or relatives* (unless specifically instructed to do so by the doctor or the nurse).

- *Do not discuss general patient information.* Often hospital personnel, other patients, visitors, or your own friends, relatives, or neighbors may ask you questions regarding a specific patient (especially if the patient is a celebrity) out of curiosity. Politely refuse to give out the information, and then quickly change the discussion to another subject.

- *Do not discuss hospital incidents away from the nursing unit.* Discussing code arrest procedures, unexpected death, and similar information with persons other than health professionals or within hearing distance of others may instill fear in them regarding health care; such apprehension may even cause them to delay necessary health treatment in the future.

- *Refer all telephone calls from reporters, police personnel, legal agencies, and other investigative sources to the nurse manager.*

- If in doubt about the authenticity of a telephone caller, obtain information from the caller so you may return the call. After you have had time to confirm the caller's identity, call him or her back.

Guidelines for Maintaining Confidentiality of the Patient Chart

- *Follow the hospital policy for duplicating portions of the patient's chart.* Duplication of the patient's chart forms may be the responsibility of the health unit coordinator or the health records department of the hospital. (Read the hospital policy and procedure manual to determine policy regarding copying a patient's chart.)

- *Control access to the patient's chart.* Only authorized persons, such as doctors and hospital personnel, should have access

to the chart. Always know the status of the person using the chart at the nurses' station. Do not give a chart to someone on request because he or she "looks like a doctor." Should relatives or friends of a patient request to see the chart, do not give it to them under any circumstance. If a patient requests to see his or her chart, advise the patient that you will notify his or her nurse and/or doctor. A patient has a legal right to see his or her chart, but the doctor must write an order and the doctor or the nurse will go over it with the patient.

- *Ask outside agency personnel for picture identification.* Reviewers for insurance companies have the responsibility of examining patient charts to ensure that tests, procedures, and hospital days will be paid for by the patients' insurance. Social workers from protective services also need to review patient charts when investigating possible abuse. It is the responsibility of outside agency personnel to show the health unit coordinator picture identification; if they fail to do this the health unit coordinator must ask to see the identification.

- *Control transportation of the patient's chart.* Never send the patient's chart to another department through the pneumatic tube system. Do not give patients their charts to hold while they are being transported from one area of the hospital to another.

■ WORKPLACE APPEARANCE

Your professional appearance will earn trust, respect, and confidence of your employer, coworkers, patients, and others. A professional appearance also demonstrates self-confidence and sends a message that you respect yourself and your position. Follow the dress code outlined in the policy and procedure manual of the facility where you work. All employees represent the facility for which they work; patients and visitors gain their first impressions of the facility by the appearance of its employees (Fig. 6–2).

Guidelines for Workplace Appearance

Female: Clothes or uniforms should fit well, be modest in length and style, and above all should be clean, mended, and wrinkle free. Color and design of undergarments should not be visible through your clothes or uniform. Where business dress is called for, slacks or skirts are appropriate with a blouse or sweater. Denim is usually not acceptable.

Male: Slacks and shirt or sweater should fit well, and they should be clean and pressed.

Female and Male: Shoes should be clean and appropriate, as defined in the dress code. Most facilities do not allow open-toe or open-heel shoes. Most nursing personnel wear white tennis shoes (not hightops) for comfort.

Female: Socks/stockings should be worn, especially with a skirt or dress.

Male: Socks should be worn.

Female and Male: Jewelry worn should be modest. Body piercing may or may not be acceptable in your chosen place of employment. Some earrings will interfere with talking on the telephone. Good taste is the key.

Female and Male: Tattoos may or may not be acceptable in your chosen place of employment. Again, good taste is called for.

Female and Male: Hair should be clean and well groomed. Control long hair to keep it out of your face and off of your collar.

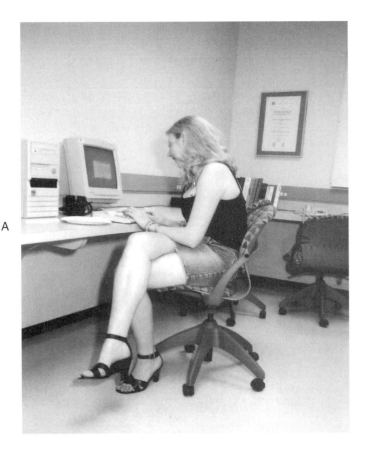

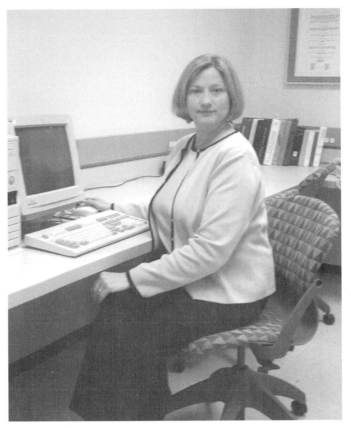

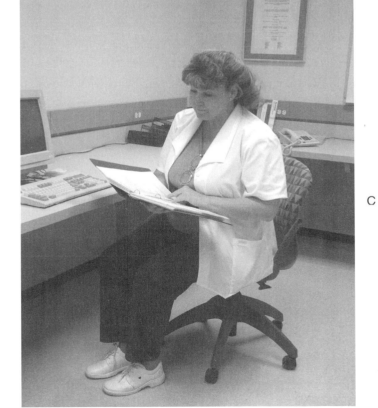

FIGURE 6–2 ▲ *A,* This health unit coordinator is inappropriately dressed. *B,* This health unit coordinator is appropriately dressed in business attire. *C,* This health unit coordinator is appropriately dressed in scrubs.

Female: Sculptured nails and nail polish are not acceptable for health care workers. Sculptured nails and chipped nail polish provide a place for microorganisms to grow.
Female: Make-up should be modest in amount and color.
Female: Perfumes, colognes, and hair spray should be very light or not worn at all.
Male: Aftershave, colognes, and hair spray should be very light or not worn at all. Patients with respiratory problems, allergies, or nausea could have ill effects from the aroma.

▪ EMPLOYMENT ISSUES

Job Responsibilities

Employee job responsibilities are defined in a document called a "job description" and can be found in the hospital policy and procedure manual. Know your responsibilities and do not perform tasks that are out of your scope of practice.

Sexual Harassment

Sexual harassment is defined as unwanted and unwelcome behavior that is sexual in nature. There are two forms of sexual harassment: (1) *quid pro quo*, which involves making conditions of employment (e.g., hiring, promotion, retention) contingent on the victim providing sexual favors, and (2) a hostile working environment, which is an environment that a *reasonable person* would find hostile and abusive.

Victims of harassment may feel intimidated, anxious, angry, ashamed, and/or helpless. Often sexual harassment is not reported because the victim believes "no action would be taken," fears retaliation, or has concern for the abuser.

If you feel you are being harassed, you should (1) advise the person to stop, that you do not like or welcome his or her behavior, (2) document the comments and behavior of the person, and (3) file a complaint with your supervisor or management.

Violence in the Workplace

Violence has increased in our society and in the workplace—perhaps, in part, due to the struggling economy and social conditions. Workplace violence may be defined as violent acts (including physical assaults and threats of assaults) directed toward persons at work or on duty. Physical assaults include attacks ranging from slapping and beating to the use of weapons. Threats are expressions of intent to cause harm and include verbal threats, threatening body language, and written threats.

When a patient is admitted to the hospital as a victim of gang-related or domestic violence, there is often a restraining order to prohibit individuals responsible for the violence from having any contact with the patient. Often the patient has a NINP (no information, no publication) order written on his or her chart. This would require the health unit coordinator or anyone answering the phone to deny any information about that patient, including the patient's presence in the hospital. The patient's name would not be listed on the census board, would not be posted outside his or her room, and would not be written on the outside of the chart. Usually an alias would be used to avoid visitor suspicion. A code word or phrase is given to the patient's family so

the health care worker can know that a person is authorized to visit the patient. All telephone calls from reporters, police personnel, legal agencies, and other investigative sources should be referred to the nurse manager.

The health unit coordinator is able to see most of what is happening on the nursing unit from his or her location at the nurses' station. He or she needs to be alert to signals that may be associated with impending violence. Signals of impending violence may include:

- Verbally expressed anger and frustration
- Body language, such as threatening gestures
- Signs of drug or alcohol use
- Presence of a weapon
- The presence of someone who has a restraining order that prohibits them from being there

The health unit coordinator should not approach the threatening person, but should present a calm attitude and call security immediately.

Agencies That Investigate Abuse

All states have mandatory reporting laws for suspected child or elderly abuse. Some states have mandatory reporting laws for domestic abuse. Child Protective Services (CPS) will be called to investigate suspected child abuse (a SNAT, suspected nonaccidental trauma). Adult Protective Services (APS) will be called in to investigate elderly or domestic abuse. The social workers from these agencies must show the health unit coordinator picture identification prior to looking at a patient's chart. If the social worker fails to do this, it is the responsibility of the health unit coordinator to ask for identification. It is important to keep this information strictly confidential and to remain nonjudgmental when interacting with family members.

Employee Performance Evaluations

After an employee is hired, during and after training, he or she must be evaluated. The performance evaluation (also called a performance appraisal) is the ongoing process of evaluating the employee's job performance. This process should provide both positive feedback and also suggestions on how to improve in areas where needed. The basic purposes of the evaluation process are to provide feedback and to make compensation decisions (concerning salary increases). It would be helpful to the health unit coordinator and also the nurse manager for the employee to keep a diary of accomplishments, classes taken, and in-services attended during the evaluation period. This will eliminate the "what have you done well lately" problem. Performance evaluations are placed in the employee's file.

▪ HEALTH CARE ETHICS

Ethics is that part of philosophy that deals with judgments about what is right or wrong in given situations. Each health care profession has a code of ethics, derived from a set of basic principles that define the concepts of right or wrong for that profession. The National Association of Health Unit Coordinators (NAHUC) has an established code of ethics (see the Box *NAHUC Code of Ethics*).

Patient's Bill of Rights

The American Hospital Association approved the first patient's bill of rights in 1973. The expectation was that observance of these rights would result in more effective patient care and greater satisfaction for the patient, the patient's physician, and the health care organization. The patient's bill of rights has been adopted and modified many times. The Joint Commission on Accreditation of Health Care Organizations now requires that all hospitals have a bill of rights (see the Box *A Patient's Bill of Rights* for an example). A copy must be given to each patient or parent of the patient on admission. Additionally, a copy of the bill of rights should be posted at entrances and other prominent places throughout the hospital. The patient's bill of rights varies in wording among hospitals, but all are based on the following basic ethical principles.

Ethical Principles for Patient Care

Respect

This principle declares that the patient has the right to considerate and respectful care. Respect is to hold in esteem or honor and to show a feeling of appreciation and regard. Health care workers must provide services with respect for human dignity and the uniqueness of each patient, unrestricted by considerations of social or economic status, personal attributes, or the nature of health problems.

Autonomy

This principle means that an individual is free to choose and implement his or her own decisions. From this basic principle, we have derived the rule involved in informed consent.

The patient's bill of rights states that a patient has the right to refuse treatment to the extent permitted by law and to be informed of the medical consequences of that choice. The right does not judge the quality of a decision by a patient to refuse treatment, only that the patient has the right to make the decision. This is the process of autonomy at work.

Veracity

The principle of veracity requires both the health professional and the patient to tell the truth. The health professional must disclose the truth so that the patient can practice autonomy and the

patient must be truthful so that appropriate care can be given. Although there are situations where health professionals may feel justified in lying to a patient to avoid some greater harm, other alternatives must be sought. Lying will almost always harm patient autonomy and cause the potential loss of provider credibility.

Beneficence

This is the principle that any action a health professional takes should benefit the patient. This principle creates an ethical dilemma for clinical practitioners more so than health unit coordinators. The dilemma arises due to the advanced technology available to practitioners today. In cases where a patient is maintained on life support machines and is in a coma or vegetative state, is it of benefit to maintain the patient on the machines?

Nonmaleficence

This principle, which comes from the Hippocratic oath, means that a health professional will never inflict harm on the patient. Although similar to the principle of beneficence, it differs in that beneficence indicates a positive action promoting the good. In nonmaleficence, the principle is to refrain from inflicting harm. Health unit coordinators should always be aware of the seriousness of transcribing doctors' orders, since an error may result in harm to the patient.

Confidentiality

Principle 2 of the NAHUC Code of Ethics and the American Hospital Association's "A Patients' Bill of Rights" outline the individual's right to privacy in health care. Health unit coordinators who breach the confidentiality of a patient's medical record have not only violated ethical standards, but may well have violated the law.

Interconnection between Ethical and Legal Issues

Ethical issues and legal issues often become intertwined in the health care context. An ethical dilemma is a situation that presents a conflicting moral claim—a situation that is at odds with your personal system of values. Sometimes conflicts can occur between what is legal and what is ethical. For example, assume you are working in a gynecology clinic and a patient comes in for an abortion. You may believe that abortions should not be performed and are unethical. However, abortions are legal in our country.

To deal with these situations as a health unit coordinator, you must learn to examine your values and be aware of how they affect your work. All health care professionals must learn methods of reasoning through ethical dilemmas rather than reacting to them emotionally. The issues that may arise and cause conflict are usually situations involving the privacy rights of patients or unprofessional conduct of a fellow health care worker.

In any of the potential problem areas you may run into as a health unit coordinator, you must apply your good judgment, honesty, and reasoning to come up with a moral and ethical way to resolve the conflict.

■ LEGAL CONCEPTS

The law is derived from three sources: (1) the constitution—both federal and state constitutions, (2) statutes—written laws drawn up by the legislature, and (3) common law—a case-by-case determination by a judge of what is fair under a given set of facts. Laws are subject to change, but common law is especially changeable because each case presented to a judge is different. Judges look to cases that have been decided previously for guidance on how to rule in a particular situation. However, a judge is free to interpret the law where no precedent exists or to interpret against precedent. Most medical negligence or medical malpractice law is derived from common law. That means that medical negligence law, like other forms of common law, is constantly in a state of change.

Standard of Practice for the Health Unit Coordinator

While working as a health unit coordinator, you are responsible for performing at the level of competence of other health unit coordinators who work under circumstances similar to your own. This responsibility is your legal duty as a health care professional and is the *standard of practice* to which you will be held. If you do not carry out this duty and a patient is injured as a result, you have been negligent of your duty and you may be held liable for your actions (see the Box *Standards of Practice for Health Unit Coordinators*).

The standard of practice is established by *expert witness* testimony. For our purposes, an expert is a person who is trained in your profession and who testifies at trial as to what a reasonably prudent health unit coordinator would have done under the circumstances in question. Evidence of the standard of care may also be found in textbooks, standards from your professional organization, medical journals, policy and procedure manuals, or standards of the Joint Commission on the Accreditation of Healthcare Organizations. This means that you must keep up with the current practices in your profession, read current literature, be familiar with hospital policies and procedures affecting your job, and know your job description and the duties it details.

The standard of care for which you are responsible becomes higher with your increased experience and education.

STANDARDS OF PRACTICE FOR HEALTH UNIT COORDINATORS

STANDARD 1: EDUCATION

Health unit coordinator personnel shall be prepared through appropriate education and training programs for their responsibility in the provision of non-direct patient care and non-clinical services.

STANDARD 2: POLICY AND PROCEDURE

Written standards of health unit coordinators' practice and related policies and procedures shall define and describe the scope and conduct of non-clinical service provided by the health unit coordinator. These standards, policies, and procedures shall be reviewed annually and revised as necessary. These revisions will be dated to indicate the last review, signed by the responsible authority, and implemented.

STANDARD 3: STANDARDS OF PERFORMANCE

Written evaluation of health unit coordinators shall be criteria based and related to the standards of performance as defined by the health care organization.

STANDARD 4: COMMUNICATION

The health unit coordinator shall appropriately and effectively communicate with nursing and medical staff, all ancillary departments, visitors, guests, and patients.

STANDARD 5: PROFESSIONALISM AND ETHICS

The health unit coordinator shall take all possible measures to ensure the optimal quality of non-direct, non-clinical patient care. The optimal professional and ethical conduct and practices of NAHUC members shall be maintained at all times.

STANDARD 6: LEADERSHIP

The health unit coordinator shall be organized to meet and maintain established standards of non-clinical services.

Your actions will be compared with those of a reasonably prudent health unit coordinator with the same experience and education under the same circumstances.

The role of the health unit coordinator has expanded broadly in the last 5 years. You are now recognized as an essential member of the health care team. Incidental to this greater recognition and expanding responsibility comes increased accountability. There is a liability dimension to accountability. The health unit coordinator may be held legally responsible for judgments exercised and actions taken in the course of practice.

■ MEDICAL MALPRACTICE

Medical malpractice is the professional negligence of a health care professional; the failure to meet a professional standard of care, resulting in harm to another; the failure to provide, for example, "good and accepted medical care." According to the National Academy of Science, approximately 98,000 Americans die from "medical mistakes" each year. Each member of the nursing team is responsible for his or her actions. If the health unit coordinator is not sure about what the doctor has written due to illegible handwriting, the doctor's orders must be clarified before they are transcribed. It may be necessary to call the doctor for clarification.

Negligence

Negligence is a legal term that means that someone failed to perform his or her legal duty satisfactorily, and another person was injured in some way because of that failure. This breach of duty is said to have occurred when something was done that should not have been done, or when something should have been done but was not. Either way, the person responsible for the duty is liable for whatever injury was suffered by the innocent party.

For instance, one of your duties as a health unit coordinator is to transcribe doctors' orders accurately and promptly. If you are negligent in doing so—that is, you don't transcribe the orders properly or don't transcribe them at all—you may be responsible for a patient's injury that results from your negligence.

Liability

Legally, each of you is responsible for your own acts. When those acts are negligent and are done in the course and scope of your employment as a health unit coordinator, they have special ramifications.

As a hospital employee, the hospital is also liable for your negligence on the job because of the legal doctrine *respondeat superior* (which means, "let the master respond"). This means that you and the hospital are held responsible for your negligent acts on the job. Remember that the hospital is liable for your actions only when they occur within the course and scope of your employment. If the negligent act is a result of conduct outside the scope of your employment (i.e., outside of your job description), you alone are held responsible.

The *respondeat superior* doctrine does not take away your personal liability, but rather, creates an additional party for the injured person to hold responsible for the damage he or she has incurred.

■ PERMANENT LEGAL DOCUMENTS

A patient's chart contains his or her medical records and permanent legal documents on file at the hospital. All documentation is written in ink, and no erasures are allowed.

Because the medical record is the legal record of the patient's medical course, you must treat it with special care and confidentiality. Only authorized persons may read patients' charts or have access to them. This protection of the legal record is part of your duty as a health unit coordinator.

Informed Consent

An informed consent documents that the person signing it has been informed of the risks and characteristics of a planned procedure and that he or she understands them. The witness to the patient or guardian signing the consent must date and sign the consent. Telephone consents require that two health care personnel listen to the verbal consent given via the telephone and those personnel sign as witnesses. Preparation of informed consents and other types of consents will be discussed in Chapter 8.

What You Can Do to Avoid Legal Problems

Following are some tips to help you avoid legal problems while working as a health unit coordinator:

- *Know your job description.* Do not engage in activities outside your job description.
- *Keep current with your employer's policy and procedures.* If you believe the policies and procedures are outdated, bring them to your employer's attention and participate in the revisions.
- *Keep current in your practice.* If you are called upon to do something you are not qualified to do, get help and find out how to do it. Remember, a standard of care can be set by medical literature and periodicals. Continued education is a must for all health care workers. Of course, make sure you have the proper training before you assume any professional position.
- *Do not assume anything.* Question orders, policies, and procedures that do not seem appropriate. Do not do something unless you are sure you know how to do it. Your biggest safeguard is to ask questions.
- *Do not perform nursing tasks, even as favors.*
- *Be aware of your relationships with patients.* Patients who truly feel that you care and have tried to help them to the best of your abilities are less likely to see a lawyer if a problem arises.

■ SUMMARY

The modern health care professional is called upon to exercise professional behavior and judgment in many complex situations. By understanding confidentiality, your legal duty, and your ethical responsibility, you will be able to legally and morally fulfill your professional obligations.

REVIEW QUESTIONS

1. List four factors that influence a person's behavior.

   a. _____

   b. _____

   c. _____

   d. _____

2. Describe a situation in which a health unit coordinator's personal values could influence his or her interactions on the job.

   _____

   _____

3. List six behavior traits that make up one's work ethics.

   a. _____

   b. _____

   c. _____

   d. _____

   e. _____

   f. _____

4. Explain the purpose of the Privacy Rule contained in the Health Insurance Portability and Accountability Act.

   _____

   _____

5. Explain what is meant by "protected health information."

   _____

   _____

6. Describe how the health unit coordinator may practice confidentiality in the following situations.

   a. You are having dinner in the cafeteria with several other health workers. A famous television star was admitted to your unit yesterday. The talk turns to the patient. You are asked, "Is she really only 35?" "What is her diagnosis?" and other personal questions. What is your response?

   _____

   _____

b. You are working at the nurses' station and you notice a patient's wife approaching your desk. At the same time, two other members of the hospital staff, unaware of the wife's presence, begin talking about her husband's condition. What do you do?

_____

_____

c. A patient approaches you at the nurses' station and says, "My roommate hasn't eaten anything today. I'm really worried about her. What is she in the hospital for?" How do you answer?

_____

_____

d. A telephone caller says that he is a reporter from the local newspaper and wants to know if a car accident victim was admitted to your nursing unit. What do you tell him?

_____

_____

e. You answer the telephone on the nursing unit. The caller states that he is a relative of the patient, and then asks for personal patient information. The patient is hospitalized for a gunshot wound received during a fight and has "NINP" written in his chart. You are somewhat doubtful about the identity of the caller. How do you handle the situation?

_____

_____

f. You are riding home on the bus after work. Another hospital employee sits down beside you and states, "That was quite a code you had on your unit today. What all happened anyway?" How do you respond?

_____

_____

g. You are out in your yard and your neighbor stops to chat with you. During the conversation, your neighbor tells you her friend is in the hospital where you work, on the same nursing unit. The neighbor asks you what is wrong with her friend and how long she will be in the hospital. What do you tell her?

_____

_____

7. Two health unit coordinator responsibilities for maintaining confidentiality of patient information are:

a. _____

b. _____

8. Three guidelines to follow to maintain confidentiality of the contents of a patient's chart are:

a. _____

b. _____

c. _____

9. Explain why it is important for the health unit coordinator to be professional in his or her appearance.

   _____

   _____

10. Identify two types of sexual harassment.

    a. _____

    b. _____

11. What is the first step to take if you feel someone is making inappropriate, sexually oriented remarks to you?

    _____

12. Explain the action you would take if you witnessed a visitor becoming angry and loud with a nurse on the nursing unit.

    _____

13. List two purposes of an employee performance evaluation.

    a. _____

    b. _____

14. What can you do to prepare for a performance evaluation?

    _____

    _____

15. Match the terms in Column 1 with the phrases in Column 2.

Column 1

_____ 1. accountability

_____ 2. defendant

_____ 3. ethics

_____ 4. expert witness

_____ 5. statute

_____ 6. tort

Column 2

a. judgments of right or wrong

b. having the responsibility to answer for what you have done

c. a wrong, which is not a crime

d. a law

e. a person against whom action is brought

f. a witness having special knowledge

g. a person who brings a lawsuit against another

h. professional negligence

i. responsibility for damages resulting from an injurious act

16. Match the terms in Column 1 with the phrases in Column 2.

Column 1

_____ 1. statute of limitations

_____ 2. damages

_____ 3. *respondeat superior*

_____ 4. deposition

_____ 5. medical malpractice

_____ 6. standard of care

_____ 7. evidence

_____ 8. informed consent

Column 2

a. testimony of a witness

b. values, rules of conduct

c. pretrial statement of a witness under oath

d. time within which a plaintiff must bring a suit

e. information a patient is entitled to before consenting to an invasive treatment

f. failure to provide "good and accepted medical care"

g. "let the master answer"

h. care that a reasonable and prudent person would have given in a similar situation

i. monetary compensation

17. Indicate whether each statement is true or false.

a. _____ You, as a practicing health unit coordinator, are not held legally responsible for your errors in transcription because you are not licensed.

b. _____ It is acceptable procedure to allow all medical personnel to read patients' charts, since they understand the confidential nature of their contents.

c. _____ It is acceptable to help a nurse with his or her tasks as long as the nurse provides close supervision and assumes responsibility for what you do.

18. For each of the following, identify the universal principle of medical ethics that is being applied.

a. The health unit coordinator safeguards the patient's right to privacy by judiciously protecting confidential information.

Principle involved: _____

b. The health unit coordinator maintains competence in health unit coordinating.

Principle involved: _____

c. The health unit coordinator provides services with respect for the patient's right to be informed about his or her medical care.

Principle involved: _____

d. The health unit coordinator reports unethical or illegal professional activities that may harm the patient.

Principle involved: _____

e. The health unit coordinator participates in the profession's efforts to protect patients from misinformation.

Principle involved: _____

19. Write the two purposes of "A Patient's Bill of Rights."

a. _____

b. _____

20. Make a list of what is inappropriate in the appearance of the health unit coordinator pictured in Figure 6–2, *A*.

_____

_____

TOPICS FOR DISCUSSION

1. Discuss what you are looking for in a job.
2. Discuss why you chose a career in health care.
3. Discuss the personal values that guide your daily interactions.

4. Have you experienced a situation that you considered to be sexual harassment? Discuss the action you took and the end result.
5. Discuss possible consequences of a health care worker discussing a patient's protected health information outside the hospital.

WEB SITES OF INTEREST

http://www.naccchildlaw.org/
http://www.nahuc.org/
http://www.oaktrees.org/elder/
http://www.osha.gov/SLTC/workplaceviolence/index.html

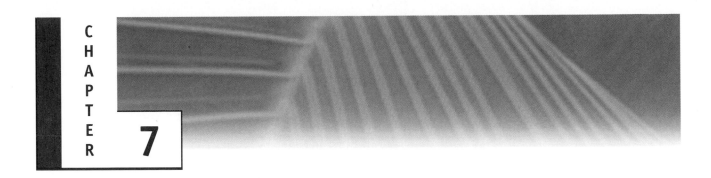

C H A P T E R 7

Management Techniques and Problem-Solving Skills for Health Unit Coordinating

Chapter Objectives

Upon completion of this chapter, you will be able to:

1. Define the terms in the vocabulary list.
2. Write the meaning of the abbreviations in the abbreviations list.
3. List five areas of management.
4. Briefly discuss the management responsibilities for the nursing unit supplies and equipment.
5. Explain the contents and purpose of four reference books and manuals that are available on the nursing unit.
6. Briefly explain a method to record the location of patients and patients' charts and discuss why it is necessary to keep a record of this information.
7. Explain the necessity of keeping a note pad next to the telephone that is used by the health unit coordinator.
8. List three management responsibilities concerning visitors on the nursing unit.
9. List three steps to follow when dealing with visitors' complaints.
10. Given a list of several health unit coordinator tasks, identify those that would have a higher priority and those that would be of lower priority.
11. Explain the importance of the change-of-shift report.
12. List eight time-management tips for the health unit coordinator.
13. Define two types of stress and provide an example of each.
14. List five techniques for dealing with stress on the job.
15. Discuss the purpose of continuous quality improvement.
16. Identify and apply the five-step problem-solving model.
17. Identify two common work-related injuries.

18. Explain five guidelines to follow that could prevent workplace injuries.

19. List four items that should be within reaching distance of the health unit coordinator's desk area.

Vocabulary

Brainstorming ▲ A structured group activity that allows three to ten people to tap into the creativity of the group to identify new ideas. Typically in quality improvement, the technique is used to identify probable causes and possible solutions of quality problems.

Cardiopulmonary Resuscitation (CPR) ▲ The basic life-saving procedure of artificial ventilation and chest compressions done in the event of a cardiac arrest (all health care workers are required to be certified in CPR)

Census Sheet ▲ A list of patients' names, room and bed numbers, ages, acuity (level of care), and physicians' names located on a nursing unit (may be printed from a computer menu)

Census Worksheet ▲ Located on a nursing unit; a list of each patient's name, room number, and bed number, with blank spaces next to each name. May be used by the health unit coordinator to record patient activities. Also called a patient information sheet or patient activity sheet.

Central Service Department Charge Slip ▲ A form that is initiated to charge a discharged patient for any items that were not charged to him or her at the time of use

Central Service Department Credit Slip ▲ A form that is used to credit a patient for items found in the room unused after patient's discharge or if it is found that a patient was mistakenly charged for an item not used for that patient

Central Service Department Discrepancy Report ▲ A list of items that are missing from nursing unit patient supply cupboard or closet that were not charged to a patient. A discrepancy report is sent to the nursing unit each day from the central service department.

Change-of-Shift Report ▲ The communication process between shifts, in which the nursing personnel going "off duty" report the nursing unit activities to the personnel coming "on duty." (Health unit coordinators may give the report to each other or may listen to the nurse's report.)

Code Blue ▲ A term used in hospitals to announce when a patient has stopped breathing or his or her heart has stopped beating, or both

Code or Crash Cart ▲ A cart stocked by the nursing and pharmacy staff with emergency medication, advanced breathing supplies, intravenous solutions and appropriate tubing, needles, a heart monitor and defibrillator, an oxygen tank, and a suction machine (used when a patient stops breathing or his or her heart stops beating, or both)

Continuous Quality Improvement (CQI) ▲ The practice of continuously improving quality of each function at each level of every department of the health care organization (also called total quality management—or TQM)

Crisis Stress ▲ A profound effect experienced by individuals, resulting from common, uncontrollable, often unpredictable life experiences (death, divorce, illness, and others)

Ergonomics ▲ A branch of ecology concerned with human factors in the design and operation of machines and the physical environment

Perennial Stress ▲ The wear and tear of day-to-day living, with the feeling that one is a square peg trying to fit in a round hole

Proactive ▲ To take action prior to an event; to use the power, freedom, and ability to choose responses to whatever happens to us, based on our values (circumstances do not control us; we control them)

Reactive ▲ To take action or respond after an event happens; circumstances are often in control

Standard Supply List ▲ A computerized or written record of the quantity of each item that the nursing unit currently needs to last until the next supply order date (separate lists are found taped inside cabinet doors, supply drawers, and on code or crash cart)

Stress ▲ A physical, chemical, or emotional factor that causes bodily or mental tension and may be a factor in disease causation

Supply Needs Sheet ▲ A sheet of paper used by all the nursing unit personnel to jot down items that need reordering

Abbreviations

Abbreviation	Meaning
CPR	cardiopulmonary resuscitation
CQI	Continuous Quality Improvement

EXERCISE 1

Write the correct abbreviation for each term listed below.

1. Cardiopulmonary resuscitation _____

2. Continuous Quality Improvement _____

EXERCISE 2

Write the meaning of each abbreviation below.
1. CPR

_____

2. CQI

_____

■ INTRODUCTION

Webster's defines *manage* as "to control or guide." The health unit coordinator who learns to "manage or guide" certain facets within his or her job is able to realize the full potential of health unit coordinating.

In order to implement the management techniques discussed in this chapter, you must (1) understand the philosophy of your health care facility, and (2) know and understand the health unit coordinating job description for your nursing unit. Upon employment, study these areas carefully.

Although the health unit coordinator position does not include the direct management of people, how the health unit coordinator manages certain aspects of the job indirectly affects the other nursing unit personnel and the patients. Management can be divided into the following five areas:

1. Management of the nursing unit supplies and equipment
2. Management of the activities at the nurses' station
3. Management related to the performance of tasks
4. Management of time
5. Management of stress

■ MANAGEMENT OF THE NURSING UNIT SUPPLIES AND EQUIPMENT

Your responsibility for the control of the equipment and supplies used on the nursing unit will vary greatly among hospitals. However, this function definitely falls in the non-clinical category of tasks and may very well be part of your job description.

Proper management of the nursing unit supplies and equipment greatly enhances the delivery of patient care. Improper management, on the other hand, can result in minor annoyances, such as the doctor discovering that the batteries are burned out when attempting to use the unit's ophthalmoscope to examine a patient's eyes. Serious hindrances in the delivery of health care can also occur, such as failure to locate the emergency equipment during a code blue. Management of the nursing unit supplies and equipment takes you into all areas of the nursing unit. Besides the nurses' station and the patients' rooms, the nursing unit may also include the following areas:

Unit kitchen or galley: Used to store food items and to prepare beverages and snacks for the patients
Linen room or cart: Used to store linens
Employee lounge: Used by the nursing unit personnel for conferences, coffee breaks, and other activities
Report room: A room that is used by nursing personnel going off duty to give a change-of-shift report to the personnel who are coming on duty (report may be in person or tape-recorded)
Medication room: Used to store medications and used by the nurse to prepare medications for administration
Treatment room: A room that is used to perform invasive procedures such as lumbar punctures
Utility room: Used for the storage and care of equipment and supplies. Some hospitals have two utility rooms. One is referred to as a contaminated or dirty utility room, an area where used equipment is stored until "pick up" by the supply department where it is cleaned, sterilized, and repackaged for distribution as needed. The other storage room is an area where unused supplies and equipment are stored, such as IV poles.
Visitor waiting room: Used as a visiting area for the patients' relatives and friends
Conference room: Used for patient care conferences or for a doctor or pastor to speak to family members in private

The following suggestions may assist you in the management of the nursing unit supplies and equipment.

Nursing Unit Supplies

Ordering of the nursing unit supplies is discussed in Chapter 21. The health unit coordinator's management responsibilities for supplies relate to the amount of supplies needed and their location on the nursing unit. Supplies that the health unit coordinator may be directly responsible for maintaining include chart forms, office supplies, batteries, dietary supplies, and other miscellaneous items. Supplies stocked on a unit will vary depending on unit specialty; for example, a pediatric unit will stock diapers, baby bottles, and similar items, while an orthopedic unit will stock slings, sandbags, and other orthopedic items.

Only the needed amount of supplies should be maintained on the nursing unit. Overstocking may result in waste, since some items become outdated and are no longer useful. Understocking may result in a waste of both time and energy; in the long run this may be costly. Most hospitals use a standard supply list (Fig. 7–1), a computerized or written record of the quantity of each item currently needed by the nursing unit, to last until the next supply order date.

Standard supply lists are sometimes taped inside cupboard doors or on the bottom of drawers where supplies are stored. To determine and order the number of supplies needed, simply compare the quantity on the standard supply list with the quantity of the item on the shelf and requisition the difference. Keep in mind that the standard supply for many items may change, and therefore the standard supply list must be updated accordingly.

Another suggestion is to maintain a supply needs list for items (other than those maintained by the central service department) on the nursing unit bulletin board and request all the nursing unit personnel to record supplies that are running low (Fig. 7–2). Use the list as a reference for items needed when ordering supplies for the nursing unit.

Standard Supply List

Form	Amount
Doctors' order forms	10 pks
CABG orders	5 pks
Doctors' progress notes	10 pks
Nurses' admission notes	10 pks
Allergy adverse reaction documentations	10 pks
Patient valuables check list	10 pks
Patient care documentation records	10 pks
Kardexes	5 pks
Medication administration records	5 pks
Graphic records	5 pks
Surgical consents	8 pks
Blood transfusion consents	8 pks
Reviewer communication records	5 pks
IV therapy records	5 pks
Home instructions	10 pks
Coding summary forms	10 pks
Health information checklist	10 pks
Anticoagulant therapy records	8 pks
Diabetic records	5 pks

FIGURE 7–1 ▲ An example of a standard supply list.

supplies or medication as needed. When the code or crash cart is completely checked and restocked, as needed, the nurse will again lock the cart after documenting the date and his or her signature on a form attached to the cart. When the cart is used for a code, it is vital that the cart be restocked and replaced per hospital policy.

Other emergency equipment includes fire extinguishers and fire doors. Because of the nature of emergency equipment, it must be checked frequently and immediately after use and be restored as soon as possible to be readied for future emergencies.

The health unit coordinator must know the following information regarding emergencies:

1. The emergency equipment and supplies that are stored on the nursing unit and where they are located
2. How to call a code and what his or her responsibilities are during a code
3. The location of the nursing unit fire extinguishers
4. The emergency procedures for the nursing unit
5. The signal codes and procedures for fire, behavioral alarms, disaster codes, and evacuation procedures
6. The procedures for dealing with a hazardous materials spill; although you may not be directly responsible, knowing the procedures allows you to support timely and safe removal of hazardous materials

During a crisis, the hospital personnel often approach the nurses' station and ask the health unit coordinator to locate emergency equipment and initiate emergency procedures. Frequent fire and disaster drills are conducted in hospitals to prepare personnel in the case of a fire or disaster. The health unit coordinator and all hospital personnel must know what to do when there is a fire or disaster; these drills must be taken seriously.

Ignorance of code procedure or the location of nursing unit emergency equipment may cause a delay in the delivery of emergency treatment and result in serious consequences to patients.

■ MANAGEMENT OF THE ACTIVITIES AT THE NURSES' STATION

In Chapter 1 we stated that the health unit coordinator, through his or her communication responsibilities, coordinates the activities involving the doctor, the nursing staff, the other hospital departments, the patients, and the visitors to the nursing unit. Good management techniques are necessary to coordinate these activities effectively.

The following guidelines may be of assistance in managing the activities at the nurses' station.

Patient Activity and Information

The most efficient method for tracking patients and their activities is to use a census worksheet. A census worksheet is a list of the names, rooms, and bed numbers of patients located on a nursing unit, with blank spaces next to each name. A census worksheet may be printed from a computer menu. Print or prepare the sheet at the beginning of each shift. Use information on the patients' Kardex forms (see Chapter 10) or the change-of-shift report to record each patient's information next to his or her name.

Record only patient activities pertinent to the health unit coordinator job, which includes scheduled diagnostic procedures,

surgeries, planned discharges, transfers, and so forth. Record the time of each activity, if known (Fig. 7–4).

Record other data that you may need to refer to during the shift, such as (1) DNR (do not resuscitate) or no code, (2) NINP (no information, no publication), (3) no visitors allowed, (4) no phone calls to the patient's room, (5) the patient is in respiratory isolation, (6) the patient is out on a temporary pass, (7) the nurse who is assigned to patient, and (8) the resident or attending physician assigned to the patient.

Tape the census worksheet onto the surface area of your desk next to the telephone and near the computer for quick reference. During the shift, update the information as changes occur.

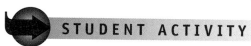

To practice preparing a unit census worksheet, complete Activity 7–1 in the *Skills Practice Manual*.

The health unit coordinator is also responsible for maintaining the unit census board (as discussed in Chapter 4), which indicates patient names and their room numbers, and the names of doctors and nurses assigned to each patient. This board may not be in plain sight to visitors, to protect patient confidentiality.

Patients and Patients' Charts That Leave the Unit

When a patient leaves the nursing unit for surgery, a diagnostic study, to visit the cafeteria with a relative, or for one of numerous other reasons, record the time the patient leaves the nursing unit and the destination beside the patient's name on the census worksheet. When the patient returns to the nursing unit, draw a line through the recording. Trying to locate charts for doctors, nurses, and other professionals wastes a lot of time. Chart tracking is essential for the efficient use of time for all those involved.

Increasingly, patient-centered or patient-focused nursing units are being designed so that diagnostic technicians come to the patient on the unit whenever possible. This practice is more convenient for the patient and also reduces the number of times the chart is off the unit.

Health personnel, doctors, and visitors are constantly asking the health unit coordinator the whereabouts of patients and/or the patients' charts. By maintaining the census worksheet you can find the answer at a glance.

Addressing Visitors' Requests, Questions, and Complaints

As a health unit coordinator you probably have more contact with the visitors than any of the other nursing unit personnel, since visitors usually stop at the nurses' station for information or

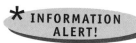

Many nursing units average 25 to 40 patients, and so it would be impossible to mentally log the whereabouts of each patient.

Room #	Patient Name	Activities
301	Breath, Les	DC Today
302	Pickens, Slim	Surg 11^{00} x ray to be sent $\overline{c}$ patient
303-1	Katt, Kitty	
303-2		
304	Bee, Mae	~~Call Dr. James $\overline{c}$ ABG results~~ Called Sue 9^{00}
305	Honey, Mai	NPO for heart cath @ 9^{00}
306-1		
306-2		
307	Pack, Fanny	No calls to room
308	Bugg, June	DC today
309	~~Kynde, Bee~~	Trans to ICU 11^{30}
310-1	Cider, Ida	DNR
310-2	Soo, Ah	~~Surg 8^{00}~~ Back @ 1^{30}
311-1	Bear, Harry	Resp isolation
311-2	Bread, Thad	
312-1	Kream, Kris	NINP
312-2	Pat, Peggy	~~Surg 9^{30}~~ Back @ 2^{00}

FIGURE 7–4 ▲ A census worksheet.

some other type of communication regarding the patient's hospitalization. As a visitor approaches the nurses' station, immediately acknowledge that person's presence and provide assistance as soon as possible. At this moment, you represent the entire nursing unit, and the manner in which you respond to the visitor helps shape his or her attitude about the care the patient is receiving and about the hospital as a whole. It is your management responsibility to (1) communicate pertinent information to visitors, (2) respond to visitors' questions and requests, (3) initially handle visitors' complaints, and (4) locate the patient's nurse when necessary.

Communicate pertinent information to the visitor, such as the time for visiting hours, the number of visitors that may be in a patient's room at one time, isolation restrictions, and what items may or may not be taken into the patient's room. Examples of restricted items in the intensive care unit include flowers and plants. Rubber balloons are banned in most hospitals because of latex allergies and the risk of children aspirating broken pieces of

the rubber. Refer to the policy manual for the visitor regulations practiced at your hospital.

The visitor may ask the health unit coordinator such questions as, "May I take the patient to the cafeteria?" or "May the patient have a milkshake?" or "When can the patient go home?" Many questions may be answered by checking information on the patient's Kardex form or by referring to the nursing unit policy or procedure manual. However, if you are in doubt about the answer, check with the nurse.

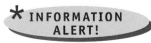

★ INFORMATION ALERT!

Check with the patient's nurse before giving permission for a patient to leave the nursing unit, to go outside, or to the cafeteria.

Never discuss aspects of the patient's medical condition with the patient's visitors. Refer all of these questions to the doctor or nurse (Fig. 7–5). If you do not know the answer to a question or feel the question should be referred to the nurse, respond to the visitor by saying, "I'll ask his or her nurse to come talk with you," or something similar, rather than saying, "I don't know" or "I'm not allowed to give out that information."

The health unit coordinator is often confronted by visitors' complaints, some justified and some unjustified. Visitors, especially the relatives of a critically ill patient, are under a great deal of stress. The uncertainty of the course of the illness, unfamiliarity with the hospital routine, and many other factors contribute to their feelings of uneasiness and insecurity. Also, they are often dealing with emotions, such as guilt and/or anger. Often these feelings are expressed in the form of complaints regarding the patient's care. How you respond to the visitor's initial remarks may make the difference in whether the problem is solved at the nursing unit level or whether it escalates up through the nursing administration to the chief executive officer. Follow these steps when dealing with visitor complaints.

1. Listen carefully and attentively to what the person is saying (Fig. 7–6). If the person's voice is raised, or is angry in tone, remember that the hostility is not being directed to you personally. It is important for you to understand that the person is upset and that to listen carefully to what he or she is saying is the first step toward dealing with a challenging situation.

2. Ask pertinent, objective questions and gather as many facts as possible. Demonstrate a caring attitude when gathering information. Whether or not the complaint is justified is not important at this time.

3. Respond to the complaint accordingly. Respond verbally with such phrases as, "I understand what you are telling me" or "I understand how you feel." Do not respond defensively with statements such as, "I wasn't here yesterday" or "That's not my job." If the complaint needs the attention of the nurse, say, "Please wait here; I will get the nurse to talk with you about this matter." If visitors appear even the least bit anxious or angry, refer them to the nurse immediately, since time often exaggerates a situation out of proportion (Fig. 7–7). You may wish to acknowledge the anger by saying, "I can see you're angry" or something similar prior to referring the person to the nurse. Doing this demonstrates a caring attitude.

4. Refrain from eating or chewing gum when communicating with visitors; it may send an "I don't care" message.

5. Try to avoid answering the phone, but if you must, ask the person on the phone to hold, then return to handling the complaint.

■ MANAGEMENT RELATED TO THE PERFORMANCE OF HEALTH UNIT COORDINATOR TASKS

Prioritizing Tasks

As a health unit coordinator you will often experience situations in which there are several tasks to be performed at the same time. Management involves being able to determine which task takes priority over another. Awareness and experience are necessary to develop skill in determining priorities.

Situations dictate priorities; a task that is normally of lower priority sometimes becomes a high-priority task; for example, filing a report in a patient's chart may become a high priority if that patient is scheduled for surgery in a short time. Some of these tasks can be performed simultaneously, such as ordering stat laboratory tests while conveying a message to the nurse regarding a patient returning from surgery. Below is a list of the usual priority order of tasks.

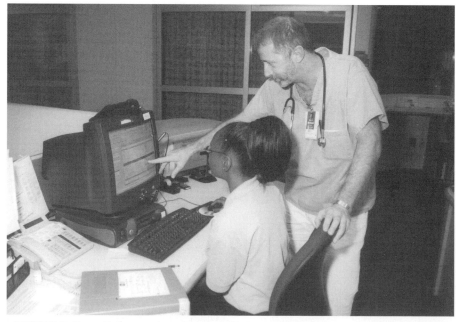

FIGURE 7–5 ▲ Refer questions about a patient's medical condition to the doctor or nurse.

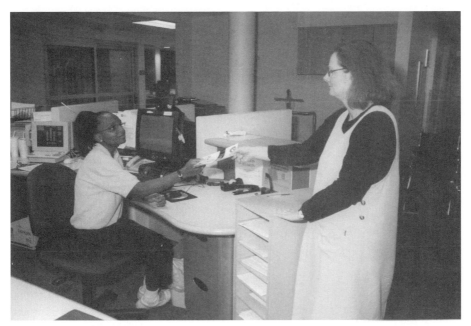

FIGURE 7–6 ▲ Listen carefully and attentively to a visitor's complaints.

1. Orders involving a patient in a medical crisis take priority over all other tasks
2. Transcribing stat orders
3. Answering the nursing unit telephone (preferably prior to third ring)
4. Communicating a telephoned message to the nurse that a patient needs to be prepared to go to surgery, is now out of surgery and in the recovery room, or is returning from surgery back to his or her room.
5. Notifying the patient's nurse and doctor of stat laboratory results
6. Transcribing pre-op and post-op orders
7. Transcribing new admission orders and daily routine orders
8. Transcribing discharge and transfer orders, so that the clerical work can be processed by the time the patient is ready to leave or be transferred
9. Performing the routine tasks at the scheduled times

The following techniques may assist you in managing your workload:

1. Ask for assistance when necessary.
2. If you return to the nursing unit from a break and find several charts lying about, open each chart and check for new orders, place charts that do not have new orders in the chart rack, read all new orders, notify the patient's nurse of any stats and provide him or her with a copy of the orders, fax or send copies to the pharmacy, then proceed to transcribe all other orders one chart at a time.
3. Always complete a set of orders that you have started transcribing prior to taking a break.
4. Follow the ten steps of transcription (outlined in Chapter 9) and never sign off on orders until you are sure that you have completed each step.

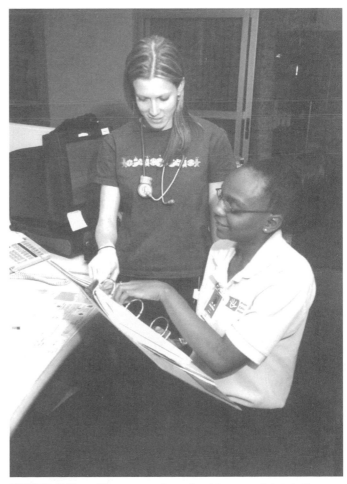

FIGURE 7–7 ▲ You may need to refer visitor complaints to the nurse.

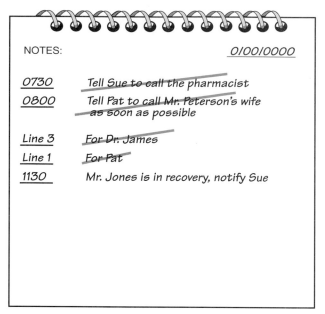

NOTES: 0/00/0000

0730   ~~Tell Sue to call the pharmacist~~

0800   ~~Tell Pat to call Mr. Peterson's wife~~
          ~~as soon as possible~~

Line 3   ~~For Dr. James~~

Line 1   ~~For Pat~~

1130   Mr. Jones is in recovery, notify Sue

FIGURE 7–8 ▲ A note pad used as a memory sheet.

Use of a Note Pad

Keep a note pad next to the telephone to jot down the names and line numbers when you place more than one caller on hold and to list tasks that you are unable to complete momentarily (Fig. 7–8). You often need to communicate information that is not urgent to a member of the nursing team. Consider the following two examples: (1) You receive a telephone message for Mary to call the pharmacy at her convenience. Rather than wasting time trying to locate Mary, record this information on the note pad. When Mary returns to the nurses' station, communicate the message to her. Draw a line through the message on the memory sheet to indicate you have communicated the message; (2) You need to call the doctor's office and you are unable to complete the call because the line is busy. Record the task on the note pad, along with the doctor's telephone number and other pertinent data so that you will have it available when you are able to place the call. When you complete the call, cross it off on the note pad. During an 8- or 12-hour shift there are countless items to record on the note pad. Near the end of your shift, check that all the items listed have been completed and take care of any that remain.

Ergonomics for the Health Unit Coordinator

Ergonomics is the study of work for the purpose of making the workplace more comfortable and to improve both health and productivity. There are two types of common work-related injuries: (1) acute, which consist of fractures, crushing, or low back strain injuries, and (2) cumulative, which occur over time due to repetitive motion activity. Cumulative injuries include carpal tunnel syndrome, tendonitis, or low back pain. Discomfort and fatigue, whether personal or work related, can cause inefficiency in your work as well as cumulative injuries. A comprehensive approach to ergonomics addresses three areas of work: physical, environmental, and emotional.

The following guidelines in each area may be of assistance in reducing injury risks for the health unit coordinator.

Guidelines for the Prevention of Workplace Injuries

■ The computer terminal should be located where it will reduce awkward head and neck postures; position the terminal so that you must look slightly downward to look at the middle of the screen. The preferred viewing distance is 18–24 inches (Fig. 7–9).

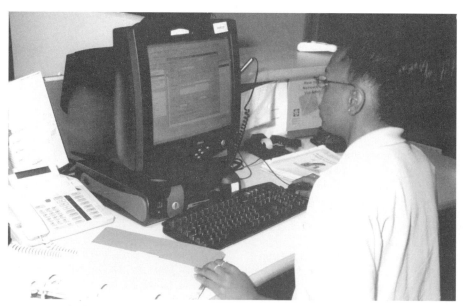

FIGURE 7–9 ▲ Proper body positioning when using a computer terminal.

- Adjust your chair so that you sit straight yet in a relaxed position, with a backrest supporting the small of your back and your feet flat on the floor
- Adjust your chair back to a slightly backward position and extend your legs out slightly so there are no sharp angles that cause pressure to be placed on your hip or knee joints as you work
- Your wrists should be straight as you type, with forearms level and elbows close to your body—reduce bending of the wrists by moving the entire arm
- Use a computer wrist pad
- Eliminate situations that would require constant bending over to complete your tasks
- Shift your weight in your chair frequently
- Use proper body mechanics when lifting—don't bend over with legs straight or twist while lifting and avoid trying to lift above shoulder level
- Take frequent mini-stretches of your neck (lean your head down in each direction for a 5-second count)
- Stand, walk, and stretch your back and legs at least every hour. These small breaks in position help avoid neuromuscular strain and alleviate the tension of job stress

Organization of the Nurses' Station

A well-organized and neat nurses' station gives the appearance of a well-run nursing unit. First use the Box *Organizing Items within Your Reaching Distance* to check your working area at the nurses' station.

Note: Prior to initiating changes in the work area, discuss the changes with all of your co-workers and the nurse manager. Frequently take the time to stand back and observe the nurses' station area. Is it cluttered and unorganized in appearance? If so, take a moment to restore all items to their original places. Return charts to the chart rack.

ORGANIZING ITEMS WITHIN YOUR REACHING DISTANCE

- Counter space should provide enough space so that you are not cramped and people will not have to lean over you to obtain charts, office supplies, or other items
- Label printer should be in close proximity to your work space
- Frequently used forms should be stored within reaching distance
- Charts should be located in an area where they can be easily reached
- The telephone should be within easy reach
- The fax machine should be in close proximity to your work space
- The unit shredder should be in close proximity to your work space
- The unit reference books and manuals should be kept within reaching distance

Time Management

The ability to manage your time may be the single most important factor toward successful health unit coordinating. However, it is not easy to learn how to effectively use your time. Experience, awareness, flexibility, and motivation are all necessary to achieve the goal of using your time to its full potential.

William Rochti in *Leadership in the Office* (1963) tells a story that superbly demonstrates how the day tends to "go" when there is no plan for managing time:

> A farmer told his wife, "I'll plow the south 40 tomorrow." The next morning he went out to lubricate the tractor. But he needed oil; so he went to the shop to get it. On the way he noticed that the pigs hadn't been fed. He started for the bin to get them some feed, but some sacks there reminded him that the potatoes needed sprouting. He walked over toward the potato bin. En route, he spotted the woodpile and remembered that he'd promised to carry some wood to the house. But he had to chop it first, and he'd left his ax behind the chicken coop. As he went for the ax, he met his wife, feeding the chickens. With surprise she asked, "Have you finished the south 40 already?" "Finished!" the farmer bellowed. "I haven't even started."

Like the farmer, the health unit coordinator engaged in one part of his or her job is constantly seeing other tasks that need to be done. Knowing how to plan your day to make the best use of your time helps you avoid the pitfalls of the farmer. The following time-management techniques may be of assistance to the health unit coordinator.

Time-Management Techniques

1. Plan for rush periods. Take time at the beginning of each day to prepare for anticipated rush periods. For example, since it is always busy in the morning while the doctors are making rounds, allow time to assist the doctors in locating their charts and other items they may need. If several surgery patients are scheduled for your unit, you can anticipate a rush in the afternoon when they arrive on the unit from the postanesthesia care unit (PACU); if there are several empty beds on the nursing unit in the morning when you arrive on duty, you can anticipate a rush during the admitting time in the afternoon.
2. Plan a daily schedule for the routine health unit coordinator tasks; schedule the routine tasks to be done at the time of day that produces the best outcome. Plan to perform the regular tasks, such as transcribing doctors' orders and placing telephone calls, according to demand between the scheduled routine tasks. Follow your plan to make changes as you discover ways to improve the use of your time.
3. Group activities. Save time by grouping activities together, such as delivering specimens to the laboratory on your way to lunch, or checking the patients' charts to see if new forms are needed, at the same time you file reports.
4. Complete one task before beginning another. This is not always possible because a stat order always takes precedence over whatever else you are doing. However, apply this principle as consistently as possible.

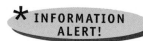
INFORMATION ALERT!

Your greatest contribution to the function of the nursing unit as a whole is to know your job and to perform your job to the best of your ability. If you are asked by other health personnel to perform tasks that are part of their job description, politely refuse to do so.

5. Know your job and perform your job. A nursing unit is made up of many people working together to perform the overall function of caring for the patients. For the nursing unit to function effectively, each person must first know his or her job description and, second, must perform the tasks outlined in the job description. It is important that you stay within the boundaries of the job and not drift over into performing the tasks assigned to other health personnel. For example, on a busy day it may seem appropriate for you to "help out" the nursing staff by feeding a patient or passing out food trays. We caution you against this practice for two reasons: first, you are not educationally prepared to perform clinical tasks, and second, you are thereby leaving your own tasks unattended.

6. Take the breaks assigned to you. Often on a busy day the immediate solution to getting the job done may appear to be to skip lunch, coffee breaks, or both. Do not be tempted to do so. Often a few minutes away from the pressure allows you to recoup and return to handle the situation with renewed vigor and speed.

7. Delegate tasks to volunteers. Determine which of your tasks the volunteers have been trained to do and are allowed to do. Filing records in the chart is a time-consuming task that can usually be performed by volunteer workers. Work out a plan to have a volunteer assist you each day at the times that are most helpful to you. Remember that volunteer workers volunteer because they want to work.

8. Avoid unnecessary conversation. Often there are many other health professionals within the nurses' station, and thus it is very easy to be drawn into unnecessary conversation. Be aware of this and avoid it when possible.

Stress Management

Stress is a physical, chemical, or emotional factor that causes bodily or mental tension and may be a factor in disease causation. There are two types of stress: (1) perennial stress—the wear and tear of day-to-day living with the feeling that one is a square peg trying to fit in a round hole, and (2) crisis stress resulting from common, uncontrollable, often unpredictable life experiences that have a profound effect on individuals (e.g., death, divorce, illness). Hospital units are often very stressful and the personnel dealing with life-and-death situations often become extremely stressed. The health unit coordinator is in the center of all the activity at the nursing station and is often said to be in the hot seat. The following stress-management techniques may assist the health unit coordinator in dealing with stress.

Stress-Management Techniques

1. Effective time management is the first step in managing stress
2. Realize that the nurses, doctors, and other health care workers may be working under a lot of stress and do not take their expressions of frustration personally
3. Say "no" tactfully when asked to do additional work if you truly do not have time
4. Ask for help when you need it
5. Keep your sense of humor. Humor is a great stress reliever as long as it is timely and appropriate. "You grow up the first day you laugh at yourself"—Ethel Barrymore
6. Take your scheduled breaks

Remember, 10% of stress is what happens to you and 90% is your reaction to it.

■ CONTINUOUS QUALITY IMPROVEMENT

Continuous quality improvement (CQI), a requirement of JCAHO, is the practice of continuously improving quality at every level of every department of every function of the health care organization. Most hospitals have CQI committees to oversee the assessment and improvement of work processes in addition to focusing on what patients want and need.

How does this translate to the health unit coordinator? Quality improvement will remain an important part of your work. Learn the language of quality. The quality movement is global because CQI results in products and services of better quality. Competition to provide the best product and service in the most efficient manner has increased worldwide. Find out who has the "best practices" in health unit coordinating and put those methods to work in your unit whenever you can. The health unit coordinator is often asked to serve on a committee to solve quality improvement problems dealing with the nursing unit clerical processes. A committee in this process may use two techniques—application of the following problem-solving model, and brainstorming.

The Five-Step Problem-Solving Model

1. Identify and analyze the problem.
2. Identify alternative plans for solution.
3. Choose the best plan.
4. Put plan for solution in place.
5. Evaluate plan after in place for a given time.

Application of the Five-Step Problem-Solving Model and Brainstorming

The admitting department reported to the nursing department that when patients are discharged, there is a long delay before the health unit coordinator provides the information to the admitting department. This causes inconvenience to the patients going home and also to patients waiting for beds. The nurse manager asked Cynthia, a health unit coordinator, to join a committee (consisting of two admitting personnel, one nurse manager, and two health unit coordinators) assigned to find the cause and a solution to this problem. The committee met several times and used the five-step problem-solving model and brainstorming, as outlined below.

1. *Identify and analyze the problem:* The problem was discussed and it was determined that (a) discharged patients had to wait for their paperwork to be processed because the admitting department was not notified of the discharge in time, and (b) new admissions had to wait for beds to be admitted. The group identified possible causes of the problem and recorded them on slips of paper that Cynthia collected to share later with the entire group. The probable cause of the problem was determined to be that the nursing unit personnel wanted to get caught up with their work before getting a new admission, so they asked the health unit coordinator to delay notifying the admitting department of discharges.

2. *Identify alternative plans for the solution:* The brainstorming technique was used to identify alternative solutions to resolve the problem. Cynthia again collected the papers to share with the group as a whole. Some suggested solutions that were listed on a white board were to: (a) ask the doctor to notify admitting when he or she discharges a patient, (b) have a mandatory meeting with all health unit coordinators to discuss the problem again, and (c) create a policy requiring that a discharge order be sent to the admitting department within 20 minutes after it is written.

3. *Choose the best plan:* The committee members chose (c) as the best solution and planned the next meeting to create the policy.

4. *Put the plan for the solution in place:* The policy was created, approved, and implemented. The committee agreed to meet in 6 weeks to evaluate the solution.

5. *Evaluate the plan after it is in place for a given time:* The committee met a last time to evaluate the plan and concluded that there had been a great improvement in the discharge process.

EXERCISE 3

Use the problem-solving model and the brainstorming technique to solve the following problem:

A doctor complained that when he arrives early in the morning to make rounds, he cannot find his patients' charts. He has to ask for help to locate laboratory results, and the patients'

temperatures are seldom charted. He stated that no one seems willing to assist him.

1. *Identify and analyze the problem.*

_____

_____

2. *Identify alternative plans for the solution.*

_____

_____

3. *Choose the best plan.*

_____

_____

4. *Put the plan for the solution in place.*

_____

_____

5. *Evaluate plan after it is in place for a given time.*

_____

_____

SUMMARY

To meet the challenge of management requires more effort and motivation on the part of the health unit coordinator than just "getting the job done"; however, the effort and motivation are rewarding. Job success is self-made. We hope you take the step beyond "getting the job done" and employ the management techniques necessary to develop your career to its potential. Use of the ergonomic suggestions and the time- and stress-management techniques will help make your job a more pleasurable experience.

REVIEW
QUESTIONS

1. List five areas of management.

   a. _____

   b. _____

   c. _____

   d. _____

   e. _____

2. Briefly discuss your management responsibilities regarding:

   a. nursing unit supplies

   _____

   b. equipment stored at the nurses' station

   _____

   c. nursing unit reference material

   _____

   d. maintenance of the nursing unit

   _____

   e. the patient's rental equipment

   _____

   f. nursing unit emergency equipment

   _____

3. List five items that you would record for quick reference during a shift on the census worksheet.

   a. _____

   b. _____

   c. _____

   d. _____

   e. _____

4. Discuss how you may keep a record of which patients and which of the patients' charts are temporarily away from the nursing unit.

   _____

   _____

5. Why is it necessary to keep a written record of the whereabouts of each patient and each patient chart?

_____

_____

6. List three management responsibilities concerning visitors.

    a. _____

    b. _____

    c. _____

7. List three steps to follow when dealing with visitor complaints.

    a. _____

    b. _____

    c. _____

8. List three tasks that are usually the highest priority for the health unit coordinator.

    a. _____

    b. _____

    c. _____

9. You have just arrived on the nursing unit and you are ready to begin the day. The following tasks need to be done. Indicate the order in which you would perform the tasks by numbering them in the spaces provided.

    _____ a. two discharge orders must be processed

    _____ b. a nurse comes out of a room and asks you to call a code arrest on a patient

    _____ c. the telephone is ringing

    _____ d. a doctor has placed an order for a chest x-ray today

    _____ e. the surgical patients' charts must be checked to see that the necessary reports are included in preparation for surgery

    _____ f. two tubes have just arrived in the pneumatic tube system

10. List eight steps you may follow to make the best use of your time:

    a. _____

    b. _____

    c. _____

    d. _____

e. _____

f. _____

g. _____

h. _____

11. Define the following terms:

    a. standard supply list

    _____

    b. census worksheet

    _____

    c. change-of-shift report

    _____

    d. central service department credit slip

    _____

    e. central service department charge slip

    _____

12. Describe how you would respond to the following situations.
    a. Mrs. Robert Frances, whose husband has been hospitalized for 3 weeks with a cerebral hemorrhage, walks up to the nurses' station and in a loud, angry voice states, "No one is taking care of my Robert. When I came in today his lunch tray was just sitting there, cold, and no one was feeding him, and his bed is wet."

    _____

    _____

    b. The visiting-hours policy for your hospital states that children may visit the patients only on weekends. A female visitor with a small child and a baby asks you what room Mr. Blair is in. It is Tuesday afternoon.

    _____

    _____

    c. The patient, Mr. Christine in Room 365-1, complains to you that the other patient in his room has six people visiting him at this time and he finds this very upsetting.

    _____

    _____

    d. You have been employed for a month on a very busy surgical nursing unit. The label maker is located so far from your working area that each time you need to use it, you must get up from your chair and walk to where it is located.

    _____

    _____

e. It is a very busy day; the beds are all full, and two nursing personnel have called in sick and cannot be replaced. At the moment you are all "caught up" with your tasks. A nurse approaches you and asks, "Would you please help Mr. Tiesen to the restroom for me? His room is close to the nurses' station so you will be able to hear the telephone ring."

_____

_____

13. List five informational items that the health unit coordinator going off duty should communicate to the health unit coordinator coming on duty during the shift report.

a. _____

b. _____

c. _____

d. _____

e. _____

14. List two examples of information that you would write on a note pad next to your telephone and explain the importance of using a note pad.

a. _____

b. _____

15. Discuss four guidelines to assist you in managing your workload.

a. _____

b. _____

c. _____

d. _____

16. Define the term "ergonomics."

_____

17. Identify two types of work-related injuries.

a. _____

b. _____

18. List five guidelines that you can follow to avoid workplace injury.

a. _____

b. _____

c. _____

d. _____

e. _____

19. List two types of stress and provide an example of each.

a. _____

b. _____

20. List five techniques for dealing with stress on the job.

a. _____

b. _____

c. _____

d. _____

e. _____

21. Explain the purpose of Continuous Quality Improvement. _____

_____

22. List four items that should be within reaching distance of the health unit coordinator's desk area.

a. _____

b. _____

c. _____

d. _____

23. Explain what steps you would take if, upon arriving on the nursing unit, you found several charts flagged that have new orders written on them.

_____

_____

TOPICS FOR DISCUSSION

1. Have you or someone you know had a workplace injury? Discuss how the injury could have been avoided.
2. Think of a time when you were upset regarding the way you or a family member was treated in a health care setting.

How was it resolved? Discuss how it could have been handled in a more professional manner.
3. Discuss your most effective technique for relieving stress.

■ WEB SITE OF INTEREST

http://www.osha.gov

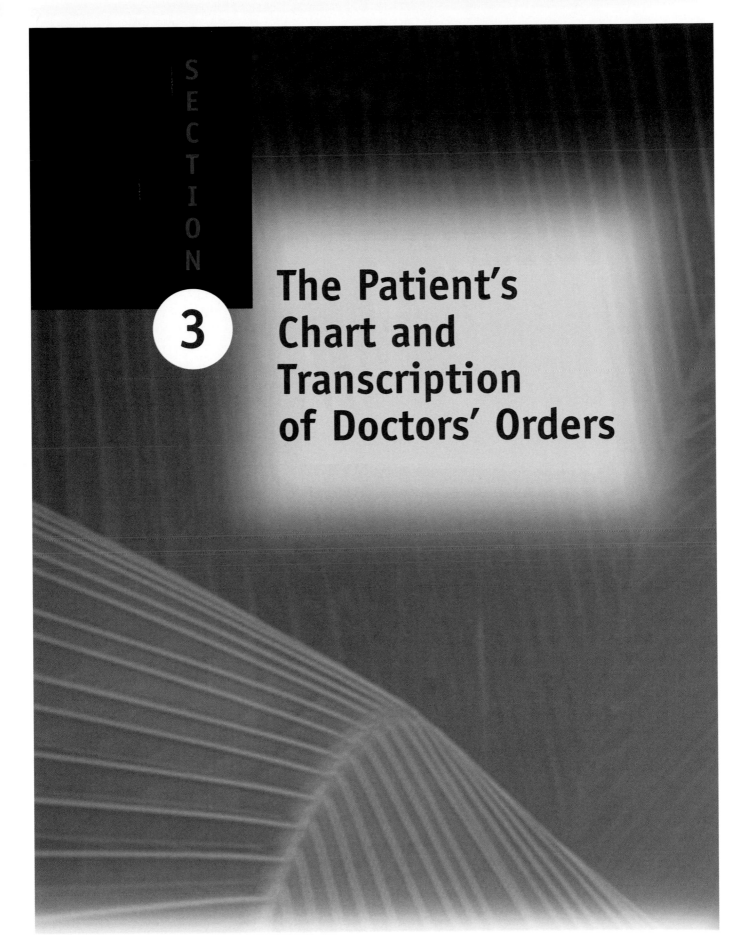

The Patient's Chart and Transcription of Doctors' Orders

The Patient's Chart

Chapter Objectives

Upon completion of this chapter, you will be able to:

1. Define the terms in the vocabulary list.
2. Write the meaning of the abbreviations in the abbreviations list.
3. List six purposes of a patient's chart.
4. List five guidelines to be followed by all personnel when writing on a patient's chart.
5. Identify three standard patient chart forms that are initiated in the admitting department.
6. Name eight patient standard chart forms included in the admission packet and describe the purpose of each form.
7. Name eight patient supplemental chart forms and describe the purpose of each form.
8. List eight health unit coordinator duties in the maintenance of a patient's chart.
9. List five guidelines to follow in the preparation of a consent form.
10. List four types of permits or release forms a patient may be required to sign during his or her hospital stay.
11. Describe the methods for correcting a labeling error and a written entry error on a patient chart form.
12. Read and write military times.

Vocabulary

Admission Packet ▲ A preassembled packet of standard chart forms to be used on the admission of a client to the nursing unit

Allergy ▲ An acquired, abnormal immune response to a substance that does not normally cause a reaction; could include medications, food, tape, and many others

Allergy Labels ▲ Labels affixed to the front cover of a patient's chart that indicate a patient's allergies

Allergy Bracelet ▲ A red plastic bracelet that is worn by a patient that indicates his or her allergies

Identification Labels ▲ Preprinted labels containing individual patient information to identify patient records

Inpatient ▲ A patient who has been admitted to a health care facility at least overnight for treatment and care

Name Alert ▲ A method of alerting staff when two or more patients with the same or similarly spelled last names are located on a nursing unit

Old Record ▲ The patient's record from previous admissions stored in the health records department that may be retrieved for review when a patient is admitted to the emergency room, nursing unit, or outpatient department; older microfilmed records may also be requested by the patient's doctor.

Outpatient ▲ A patient receiving care by a health care facility but not admitted to the facility or staying overnight

"Split" or Thinned Chart ▲ Portions of the patient's current chart that are removed when the chart becomes so full that it is unmanageable

Standard Chart Forms ▲ Forms for regularly entering information about patients; they are included in all inpatient charts

Stuffing Charts ▲ Placing extra chart forms in patients' charts on a nursing unit so they will be available when needed

Supplemental Chart Forms ▲ Patient chart forms used only when specific conditions or events dictate their use

Walla Roo ▲ A chart rack located on the wall outside of a patient's room that stores the patient's chart and when unlocked forms a shelf to write upon

Abbreviations

Note: These abbreviations are listed as they are commonly written; however, you may also see some in upper case and lower case letters and with or without periods.

Abbreviation	Meaning
COA or C of A	conditions of admission
H&P	history and physical
Hx	history
ID labels	identification labels
MAR	medication administration record
NKA	no known allergies
NKFA	no known food allergies
NKMA	no known medication allergies
NKDA	no known drug allergies

EXERCISE 1

Write the abbreviation for each term listed below.

1. history _____

2. no known allergies _____

3. conditions of admission _____

4. identification labels _____

5. history and physical _____

6. medication administration record _____

7. no known medication allergies _____

8. no known drug allergies _____

9. no known food allergies _____

EXERCISE 2

Write the meaning of each abbreviation listed below.

1. *COA* or *C of A*

_____

2. *ID labels*

_____

3. *NKFA*

_____

4. *MAR*

_____

5. *NKA*

_____

6. *NKDA*

_____

7. *H&P*

_____

8. *Hx*

_____

9. *NKMA*

_____

■ PURPOSES OF A PATIENT'S CHART

The patient's chart serves many purposes, but as a health unit coordinator you will see the chart used mainly as a means of communication between the doctor and the hospital staff.

The chart is also used for planning patient care, for research, and for educational purposes. As a legal document, the chart protects the patient, the doctor, the staff, and the hospital or health care facility. Careful notations by the doctors and personnel provide a written record of the patient's illness, care, treatment, and the outcomes from the hospitalization. If the patient is readmitted to the hospital or health care facility, the chart may be retrieved from the health records department to provide a history of past illnesses and treatment that was given for them.

The Patient Chart as a Legal Document

When a patient is discharged, his or her chart is sent to the health records department. The health records department personnel analyze and check the chart for completeness. When there are records that are not complete or have signatures missing, those chart forms are flagged and the appropriate nurses and/or doctors are notified that they must come to the health records department to complete or sign the chart forms. Completed charts are indexed and stored where they are available for retrieval as needed. Older records are microfilmed (documents are placed on film in reduced scale), and stored. The health records personnel upon request may retrieve the microfilmed records. The length of time the record must be stored depends upon the laws of the state. The record may serve as evidence in a court of law. As a legal document, it must be maintained in an acceptable manner. Unless a patient has been readmitted to the hospital, the health records department will not send old records to nursing units.

■ GUIDELINES TO FOLLOW WHEN WRITING ON A PATIENT CHART

All persons writing on the chart follow the same guidelines. As a health unit coordinator, you have minor charting tasks, but since you are responsible for the chart, you should learn the following basic rules:

1. All chart form entries must be made in ink. This is to ensure permanence of the record. Black ink is preferred by many health care facilities because it produces a clearer picture

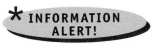

✴ INFORMATION ALERT!

Purposes of a Patient's Chart

Means of communication
Planning patient care
Research
Education
Legal document
History of patient illnesses, care, treatment, and outcomes

when the record is microfilmed, faxed, or reproduced on a copier.
2. The written entries on the chart forms must be legible and accurate. Entries may be either in script or printed. Diagnostic reports, history and physical examination reports, and surgery reports are usually typewritten.
3. Recorded entries on the chart may not be obliterated or erased. The method for correcting errors is outlined later on in this chapter.
4. All written entries on the chart forms must include the date and time (military or traditional) the entry is made.
5. Abbreviations may be used according to the health care facility's list of "approved abbreviations."

■ MILITARY TIME

Military time is a system that utilizes all 24 hours in a day (each hour has its own name) rather than repeating hours and using AM and PM. For example, 1:45 AM is recorded as 0145 and 1:45 PM is recorded as 1345; the colon is not needed when using military time (Table 8–1). The hours after midnight are recorded as 0100, 0200, and so forth. Twelve noon is recorded as 1200 and the hours that follow are arrived at by adding the hours after noon to 1200. Thus, 1:00 PM is 1200 + 1 = 1300, 2 PM is 1200 + 2 = 1400, and so forth. See Figure 8–1 for a comparison of standard and military times. The use of military time eliminates confusion because hours are not repeated and AM or PM is unnecessary.

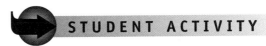

STUDENT ACTIVITY

To practice converting standard time to military time, complete Activity 8–1 in the *Skills Practice Manual*.

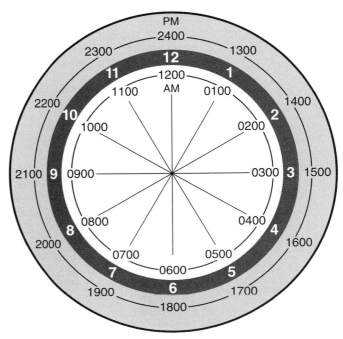

FIGURE 8–1 ▲ The 24-hour clock showing military time.

■ THE CHART IS CONFIDENTIAL

As discussed in Chapter 6, the chart is confidential and the health unit coordinator is a custodian of all patient records on the unit. Any information provided by the patient to the health care facility and the medical staff is confidential.

■ THE CHART BINDER

The forms that constitute the patient's chart are usually kept together in a three-ring binder. The binder may open from the bottom, or it may be a notebook that opens from the side or the bottom (Fig. 8–2).

The chart forms in the binder are sectioned off by dividers placed in the chart according to the sequence set forth by the health care facility (Fig. 8–3).

TABLE 8-1	Standard and Military Time Comparisons		
Standard Time	Military Time	Standard Time	Military Time
12:15 AM	0015	1:00 PM	1300
12:30 AM	0030	1:15 PM	1315
12:45 AM	0045	1:30 PM	1330
1:00 AM	0100	1:45 PM	1345
2:00 AM	0200	2:00 PM	1400
3:00 AM	0300	3:00 PM	1500
4:00 AM	0400	4:00 PM	1600
5:00 AM	0500	5:00 PM	1700
6:00 AM	0600	6:00 PM	1800
7:00 AM	0700	7:00 PM	1900
8:00 AM	0800	8:00 PM	2000
9:00 AM	0900	9:00 PM	2100
10:00 AM	1000	10:00 PM	2200
11:00 AM	1100	11:00 PM	2300
12:00 noon	1200	12:00 midnight	2400

The charts are identified for each patient by a label containing the patient's name and the doctor's name (Fig. 8–4). The room and bed numbers also appear on the outside of the chart binder. Many health care facilities use colored tape on the outside of the chart to assist the doctors in identifying their patients' charts. The chart binders are often used to alert the hospital staff of special situations. For example, "name alert," a piece of red tape with "name alert" recorded on it, may be placed on the chart binder to remind staff that more than one patient with the same or similarly spelled last name is housed on the unit. Or NINP is often recorded on the chart binder to remind the staff that no information and no publication are to be issued on a particular patient.

■ THE CHART RACK

There are many types of chart racks on the market. One type allows patient charts to be placed in a chart rack in which each slot on the rack holds one patient's chart. The slots are labeled with the room and bed numbers, usually numbered in the same sequence as the rooms on the unit (Fig. 8–5). Another type of chart storage is a Walla Roo, a locked chart rack located on the wall outside of the patient's room. It stores one patient's chart and when unlocked forms a shelf to write upon (Fig. 8–6).

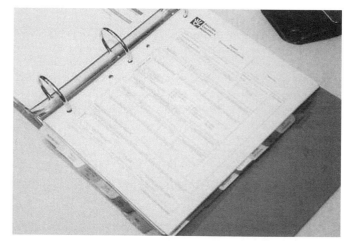

FIGURE 8–3 ▲ Patient's chart with dividers.

FIGURE 8–2 ▲ Chart binder.

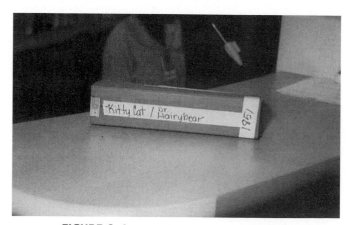

FIGURE 8–4 ▲ Chart binder properly labeled.

■ PATIENT IDENTIFICATION LABELS

A packet of patient identification labels is printed from the computer when the patient is admitted and as needed during his or her hospital stay. Information on the identification labels may include the patient's name, age, sex, account number, health record number, room number, admission date, and attending physician's name (Fig. 8–7). These identification labels are kept on the unit in the patient's chart and are used to label chart forms, requisitions, specimens, clothing, and other belongings.

■ STANDARD PATIENT CHART FORMS

Standard patient chart forms are forms that are included in all inpatients' charts and may vary in different hospitals. A new trend is to have paperless records (completely computerized) in place of many of the paper chart forms. The following thirteen chart forms are the most commonly used presently.

Standard Patient Chart Forms Initiated in the Admitting Department

1. Face Sheet or Information Form

The face sheet or information form (Fig. 8–8) contains information about the patient, such as name, address, telephone number, name of employer, the admission diagnosis, health care insurance policy information, and next of kin. In most health care facilities, the form originates in the admitting department and is then sent to the unit to be placed in the patient's chart. Several copies (at least five) should be maintained in the patient's chart to be taken by the attending physician and by consulting physicians to be used for billing purposes. The health unit coordinator can order copies of the face sheet on the computer. The face sheet is used to locate in-

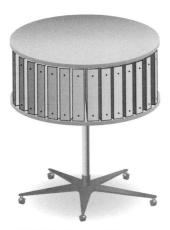

FIGURE 8–5 ▲ Chart rack.

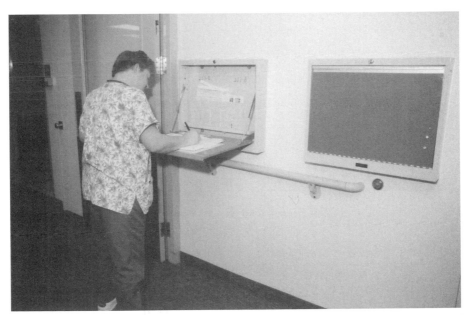

FIGURE 8–6 ▲ A Walla Roo located on the wall outside each patient's nursing bedside room to store patient charts.

Patient name _____	Name Cat, Kitty	MR #2223401	_____ Medical record #
Date of admission _____	DOA 01/12/03	DOB 11/11/64	_____ Date of birth
Patient account # _____	ACCT # 02350103	Fe 39	_____ Sex–age
Admitting doctor _____	Dr. Harry Bear	Surg	_____ Type of service
		BCBS	_____ Insurance

FIGURE 8–7 ▲ Patient ID label.

1	PATIENT HOSP.NO.(M.R.#) 987-654	INFO STATUS							ACCOUNT NO. (BUS. OFF.) 123-456
2	PATIENT NAME LAST Andrews	FIRST Iver		MIDDLE S.	ADM. DATE MO. 8 / DAY 7 / YR. XX		ADM. TIME 1345		HOW BROUGHT TO HOSPITAL Amb.

3	PATIENT'S CURRENT ADDRESS 701 East Danish Lane	STREET, P.O. BOX, APT. NO.	CITY Carpenterville, AZ	STATE	ZIP CODE 85013	TELEPHONE NO. 246-XXXX
4	PATIENT'S PERMANENT ADDRESS Same	STREET, P.O. BOX, APT. NO.	CITY	STATE	ZIP CODE	TELEPHONE NO.

5	SEX 1. MALE 2. FEMALE [1]	MARITAL STATUS 1. SINGLE 4. DIVORCED 2. MARRIED 5. WIDOWED 3. SEPARATED [5]	RACE 1. WHITE 4. ORIENTAL 2. BLACK 5. OTHER 3. INDIAN [1]	RELIGION 1. CATHOLIC 2. JEWISH 3. PROTESTANT 4. OTHER 5. LDS [3]	AREA OF RESIDENCE

6	BIRTHDATE 10/6/XX	AGE 69	PLACE OF BIRTH N.J.	MAIDEN NAME	SOC. SEC. NO./MEDICARE NO. 151-18-XXXX

7	PATIENT'S OCCUPATION Retired	UNION & LOCAL NO.	PATIENT'S EMPLOYER	ADDRESS	TELEPHONE NO.

8	PREVIOUSLY TREATED HERE? ☒ YES ☐ NO NAME USED Same			PREV. ADM. DATE	MO. DA. YR. 2/3/XX	PREV. ADMISSION 1. INPATIENT 2. OUTPATIENT [1]	IF NEWBORN, MOTHER'S HOSP. NO.

9	UNIT A5	ROOM NO.	ACCOM. CODES	1. PRI 2. SEMI 3. NURSERY 4. PREMIE 5. ICU 6. RCU 7. CCU 8. VIP [2]	ROOM RATE	PAY STATUS	CLASS OF ADMISSION 1. EMERGENCY 3. URGENT 2. ELECTIVE 4. OTHER [3]

10	ADMITTING DIAGNOSIS Cerebrovascular accident

11	PHYSICIAN NAME I.M. Human	PHYSICIAN NO. 432	ADM. SERVICE Med.	INFORMATION OBTAINED FROM: daughter

12	SPOUSE OR NEAREST RELATIVE (NEXT OF KIN) Kay Ellis	RELATIONSHIP daugh	ADDRESS 301 West Restful Dr. Phoenix	TELEPHONE NO. 258-XXXX
13	SECOND RELATIVE OR FRIEND Marie Darrow	RELATIONSHIP sister	ADDRESS 12 Center St. Danstown, CA	TELEPHONE NO. 837-XXXX
14	RESPONSIBLE PARTY NAME Self		RELATIONSHIP	SOC. SEC. NO.

15	RESP. PARTY ADDRESS	STREET P.O. BOX APT. NO.	CITY	STATE	ZIP CODE	TELEPHONE NO.
16	RESP. PARTY OCCUPATION	NO. YRS. IN THIS EMPLOY	RESP. PARTY EMPLOYER	ADDRESS		TELEPHONE NO.

17	LENGTH OF TIME IN ARIZ. 10 yrs.	1. OWN HOME 2. RENT HOME [1]	TYPE OF HOME Single	BANK NAME & BRANCH Desert National - Camelhead	1. SAVINGS 2. CHECKING [1]
18	CREDIT REFERENCES	1. NAME Deep River S&L	ADDRESS 9832 N. LasVegas Pl. Phoenix		TELEPHONE NO. 943-XXXX
19		2. NAME Yucca Federal	ADDRESS 1903 W. Bottletree Ave. Phoenix		TELEPHONE NO. 246-XXXX

20	INDUSTRIAL INJURY	DATE: MO. DA. YR.	CLAIM NO.	EMPLOYER'S NAME AND ADDRESS AT TIME OF INJURY		
21	BLUE CROSS	NAME OF PLAN	GROUP NO.	IDENTIFICATION	EFFECTIVE DATE MO. DA. YR.	CITY	STATE
22	CHAMPUS DATA	PATIENT'S ID NO.	CARD EFFECTIVE MO. DA. YR.	CARD EXPIRES MO. DA. YR.	PATIENT OR SPONSORS BRANCH OF SERVICE	SERVICE CARD NO.
23		SPONSORS NAME		RANK-SERVICE NO.	DUTY STATION	
24	OTHER INSURANCE (INC. BLOOD BANK & BLUE SHIELD)	INS. CO. NO. 1000	COMPANY NAME Desert State	POLICY HOLDER NAME Iver Andrews	POLICY NO. A657483	DATE ISSUED MO. DA. YR. 2/17/XX	CITY	STATE AZ
25		INS. CO. NO.	COMPANY NAME	POLICY HOLDER NAME	POLICY NO.	DATE ISSUED MO. DA. YR.	CITY	STATE

26	NAME OF HEALTH FACILITY DISCHARGED FROM WITHIN LAST 60 DAYS None		ADDRESS

27	OTHER INFO.	V. A. ☐	COORDINATION OF BENEFITS ☐	INTERVIEWED BY G. Talker	TYPED BY W.K.S.

28 REMARKS:

FIGURE 8–8 ▲ Face sheet or information form.

formation when calling the family or when calling consulting physicians.

2. Conditions of Admission Form

The conditions of admission form (Fig. 8–9) is signed by the patient in the admitting department and then sent to the unit to be placed in the patient's chart. The form provides legal permission to the hospital/doctor to treat the patient and also serves as a financial agreement.

3. Advance Directive Checklist Form

An advance directive checklist form (Fig. 8–10) documents that a patient was informed of his or her choice to declare his or her health care decisions. Advance directives are discussed in Chapter 19. The Self Determination Act of 1990 mandates that each

patient admitted to a health care facility be asked if he or she has or wishes to have an advanced directive. An advance directive checklist is placed in patients' charts to document that they were advised of their choice.

Standard Patient Chart Forms Included in the Admission Packet

1. Physician's Order Form

The physician's order form, or doctor's order sheet (Fig. 8–11) is the form on which the doctor requests the care and treatment procedures for the patient. All orders should be dated and must be signed by the physician giving the order. This form may be in duplicate or triplicate, may be printed on specially treated paper

Text continues on page 127

CONDITIONS OF ADMISSION / MEDICAL TREATMENT AGREEMENT

1. **GENERAL DUTY NURSING:** Hospital provides only general nursing care. If the patient needs special or private nursing, it must be arranged by the patient or physician treating the patient.

2. **CONSENT TO TREATMENT:** The patient is under the control of the attending physician and the undersigned consents to x-ray examinations, laboratory procedures, anesthesia, medical and surgical treatment or hospital services rendered under the general and special instructions of the physician. Many of the physicians of medicine furnishing services to the patient, including radiologists, pathologists, anesthesiologists are independent contractors and are not employees of the hospital. Patient or the undersigned consents to treatment being rendered by these and other physicians.

3. **RELEASE OF INFORMATION:** The hospital may disclose all or any part of the patient's medical record and or hospital charges (Including information regarding alcohol or drug abuse, psychiatric illness or communicable disease related information including HIV related information) to any person or corporation which is or may be liable or under contract to the hospital for reimbursement on this admission and/or hospital service, including but not limited to, hospital/medical service companies, insurance companies, worker's compensation carriers, welfare funds, governmental agencies and/or any health care provider for continued patient care. The hospital may also disclose on an anonymous basis any information concerning my case which is necessary or appropriate for the advancement of medical science, medical education, medical research, for the collection of statistical data or pursuant to State or Federal law, statute or regulation.

4. **PERSONAL PROPERTY:** The hospital has a safe in which to keep MONEY/VALUABLES. The hospital is not responsible for any loss or damage to personal property not deposited in the safe. The hospital specifically will not be responsible for loss or damage to glasses, dentures, hearing aids, contact lenses and prosthetic devices.

5. **PRICE QUOTES:** I understand that any price quotations given may not include physicians' fees or services and are based on averages which may vary significantly from actual charges based on physician practice patterns, secondary or tertiary medical conditions and professional interpretations of a physician's order(s).

6. **PHYSICIAN BILLS:** Your attending/consulting physicians may be billing you separately from the hospital. These physicians may or may not participate with the same insurance plans as the hospital which may result in reduced reimbursement from your insurance company for physician fees.

7. **TEACHING PROGRAMS:** The Hospital participates in programs for training of health care personnel. Some services may be provided to the patient by persons in training under the supervision and instruction of physicians or hospital employees. These persons may also observe care given to the patient by physicians and hospital employees. Photos or video tapes may be made of surgical procedures by physicians or hospital personnel.

8. **FINANCIAL AGREEMENT:** I agree that in return for the services provided to the patient by the hospital or other health care providers, I will pay the account of the patient, or prior to discharge or make financial arrangements satisfactory to the hospital or any other providers for payment. If an account is sent to an attorney for collection, I agree to pay reasonable attorney's fees and collection expenses. The amount of the attorney's fee shall be established by the Court and not by a jury in any court action. A delinquent account may be charged interest at the legal rate. I request that payment of any authorized Medicare benefits be made on my behalf, I assign the benefits payable for physician services to the physician or organization furnishing the services or authorize such physician or organization to submit a claim to Medicare for payment. If any signer is entitled to benefits of any type under any policy of Insurance insuring the patient, or any other party liable to the patient, that benefit is hereby assigned to hospital or to the provider group rendering service, for application to patient's bill. **HOWEVER, IT IS UNDERSTOOD THAT THE UNDERSIGNED AND THE PATIENT ARE PRIMARILY RESPONSIBLE FOR PAYMENT OF THE PATIENT'S BILL. EMERGENCY CARE WILL BE PROVIDED WITHOUT REGARD TO THE ABILITY TO PAY.**

I HAVE READ AND UNDERSTAND THESE CONDITIONS AND I HAVE RECEIVED A COPY. I AM THE PATIENT OR AM AUTHORIZED TO ACT ON BEHALF OF THE PATIENT TO SIGN THIS AGREEMENT.

_____   _____   _____
Witness   (circle one)   Patient   Parent   Authorized Party   Date

I HAVE PREVIOUSLY EXECUTED:

POWER OF ATTORNEY FOR HEALTH CARE   YES   NO   (CIRCLE ONE)

LIVING WILL   YES   NO   (CIRCLE ONE)

POWER OF ATTORNEY FOR HEALTH CARE UNDER A.R.S. 14-5501:   I appoint

_____   _____   _____
Name   Address   Phone #

as my agent to act in all matters relating to health care, including full power to give or refuse consent to all medical, surgical and hospital care. This power of attorney shall become effective upon my disability or incapacity or when there is uncertainty whether I am dead or alive and shall have the same effect as if I were alive, competent and able to act for myself.

_____   _____
Witness   Patient

_____   (Two witnesses required unless notarized)
Witness

COPY 1 - Chart
COPY 2 - Billing
COPY 3 - Patient

MR-684 3/95   **CONDITIONS OF ADMISSION / MEDICAL TREATMENT AGREEMENT**

FIGURE 8–9 ▲ Condition of admission form (COA or C of A).

ADVANCE DIRECTIVE CHECKLIST

Patient Name: _____

❏ Advance Directives Brochure Provided   ❏ Advance Directives Brochure Refused

The Following Information Was Obtained From: ❏ Patient   ❏ Other: _____

❏ **Patient HAS executed the following Advance Directive(s):**	COPY RECEIVED		COPY REQUESTED
	THIS ADMIT	PRIOR ADMIT	
❏ Declaration for Health Care Decisions (Living Will)	❏	❏	❏
❏ Medical Power of Attorney (MPOA)	❏	❏	❏
Name: _____			
Relationship: _____			
❏ Mental Healthcare Power of Attorney (MHPOA)	❏	❏	❏
Name: _____			
Relationship: _____			
❏ Combination Power of Attorney (that includes MPOA language)	❏	❏	❏
❏ Other: (specify)	❏	❏	❏

❏ Patient **HAS NOT** executed Advance Directive(s). (Check items below **ONLY** when talking with patient.)	**PATIENT Was Advised On** _____ . (date)
❏ **PATIENT** requests more information.	❏ of the *right to accept or refuse medical treatment.*
❏ Social Services notified.	❏ of the *right to formulate Advance Directives.*
❏ **PATIENT** chooses not to execute Advance Directives at this time.	❏ of the *right to receive medical treatment whether or not there is an Advance Directive.*

For Home Health/Hospice Use Only:

❏ Patient **HAS** EXECUTED Prehospital Medical Care (Arizona's Orange Card).

❏ Patient was advised of the *right to have Advance Directives followed by the health care facility and caregivers to the extent permitted by law.*

Signature of Facility Representative:	Department:	Date:

IF ADVANCED DIRECTIVE IS UNAVAILABLE, the patient indicates that the substance of the directive is as follows: *(see reverse for script)*

Living Will: _____

Medical Power of Attorney: _____

❏ Patient signature (legal representative if applicable): _____

❏ Witness signature (if patient physically unable to sign): _____ Reason: _____

Verification Upon Admit/Re-Admit or Transfer:

Verified with patient/legal representative that Advance Directives in medical record are current.	Verified with patient/legal representative that Advance Directives in medical record are current.	Verified with patient/legal representative that Advance Directives in medical record are current.
Signature:	Signature:	Signature:
Date:	Date:	Date:

PATIENT IDENTIFICATION

FIGURE 8–10 ▲ Advance directive checklist.

Directions for Completing the Advance Directive Checklist

A. Complete the first section as follows:

1. Write patient's name in the designated area and place patient label in lower right corner.
2. Offer a brochure. Check the appropriate box.
3. Indicate from whom the information was obtained: Patient or Other.
   If "Other", indicate the relationship to the patient.

B. Information for the second section may come from someone other than the patient.

1. Ask which (if any) advance directives the patient has executed and verify currency. Check all boxes that apply.
2. If a copy is provided check the box in the "Copy Received, This Admit" column across from the specific advance directive. If a copy was provided prior to this visit, check the appropriate box in the "Copy Received, Prior Admit" column. If neither, ask for a copy and check the "Copy Requested" column.

C. Information for the third section must be obtained from the patient.

1. If the patient has not executed advance directives, ask if the patient would like more information (in which case, Social Services should be notified), or if the patient chooses not to execute advance directives at this time. Check the corresponding box.
2. Advise the patient of his/her rights as listed on the form, check each box as you read each right, and list the date in the space provided.

D. Fourth section to be completed by Home Health/Hospice admitting RN.

E. Sign the form, indicate your department and date of signing. <u>The patient, or if applicable, the patient's legal representative must sign the form. In the event the patient is mentally competent and able to communicate but physically unable to sign the form, a witness may sign the form. A reason must be indicated describing the physical ailment preventing the patient from signing.</u> The original form is kept in the medical record.

To determine substance of the document, it is best to query the patient in this way:

"Mr./Mrs. _____ , I understand you have a Living Will/MPOA.......Can you tell me what it says?" (If the patient is unable to indicate this, offer to have them execute new documents and refer to Social Services.)

F. The final section should be completed by any PHCT member receiving the patient upon admit/re-admit or transfer. Verify with patient/legal representative that Advance Directives in medical record are current. Signature and date required.

* **Refer to Advance Directives Policy, in the Patient Rights section of the Clinical Policy & Procedure Manual.**

FIGURE 8–10, cont'd ▲ Advanced directive checklist.

Date Ordered	
6-10-XX	Admitting diagnosis: acute exacerbation COPD, bronchitis, asthma, abd pain
	NKA
	VS q4h w/a
	I & O
	Reg NAS diet
	aminophylline 500 mg/500 cc D5W TKA 35 cc/hr
	O₂ 3L NP
	SMA, CBC, UA, EKG CXR
	Lasix 40 mg po now then 40mg po qam
	Theo level in am
	K-Dur ī lab BID
	Dr Hy Hopes

Authorization is given for dispensing non-proprietary name unless checked here. ☐

PHYSICIAN'S ORDERS

FIGURE 8–11 ▲ Physician's order form or doctor's order sheet.

to eliminate the need for carbon paper, or may be a single form. A duplicate of the original physician's order form may be sent to the pharmacy (commonly called the pharmacy copy) or the health unit coordinator may be required to fax a copy to the pharmacy to order the patient's medications. Sending a copy to the pharmacy helps to eliminate any drug errors that may occur in the transcription process. A copy (carbon or created on a fax machine) is also given to the appropriate nursing personnel.

2. Physician's Progress Record

The progress record is a form on which the physician records the patient's progress during the patient's hospitalization. The medical staff rules and regulations as well as the patient's condition dictate the interval allowed between notations (usually daily). The attending physician, residents, and consultants may write upon this form (Fig. 8–12).

3. The Nurse's Admission Record

The nurse's admission record (Fig. 8–13) usually precedes or leads into the nurse's notes. The patient upon his or her admission to the nursing unit answers printed questions on the form. A member of the nursing care team also compiles a short nursing history from the patient or family member regarding the patient's daily living activities, present illness, and medications the patient is taking. Also recorded on the nurse's admission history form are the patient's vital signs, height, weight, and any allergies to food

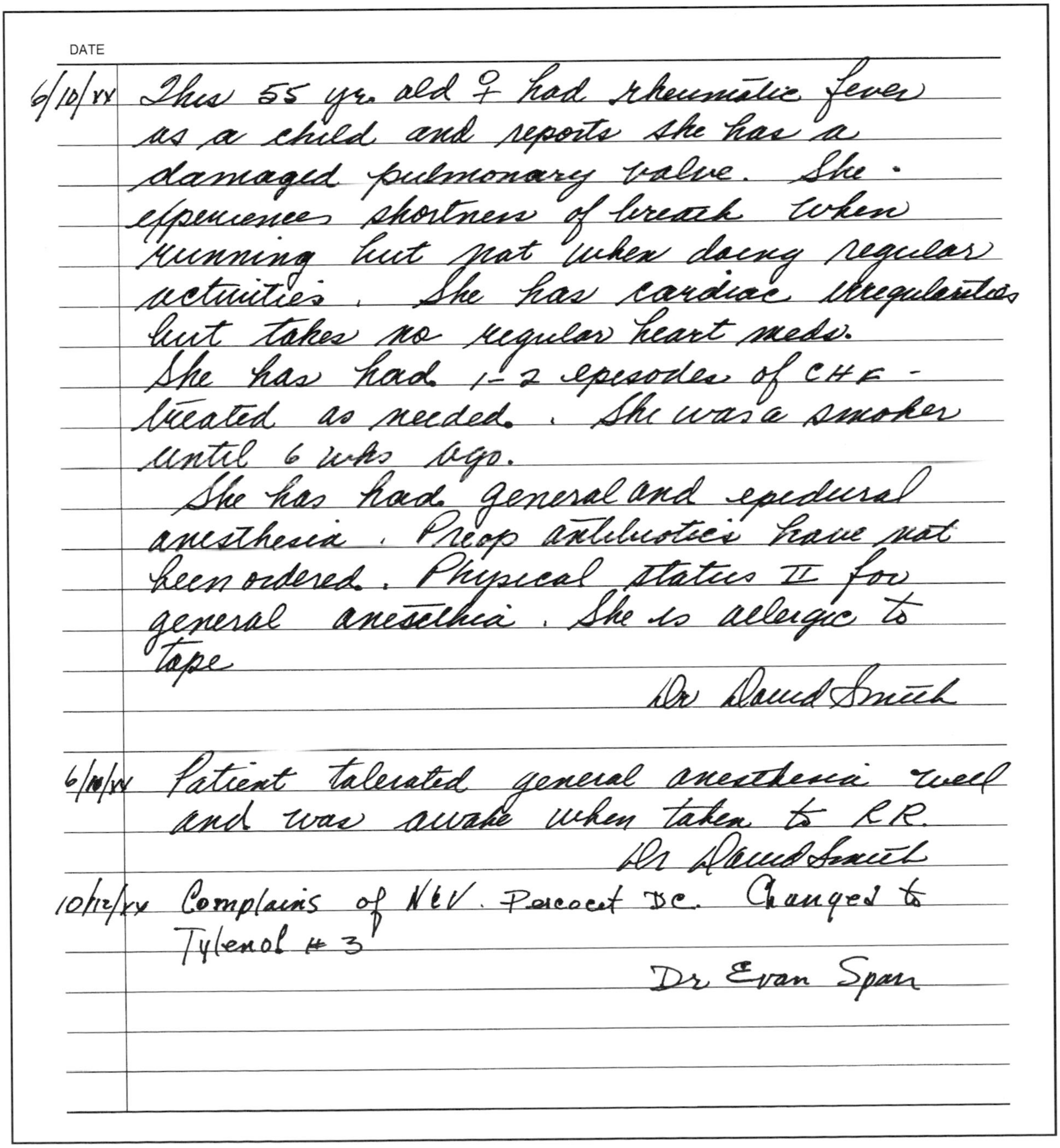

DATE

6/10/xx This 55 yr. old ♀ had rheumatic fever as a child and reports she has a damaged pulmonary valve. She experiences shortness of breath when running but not when doing regular activities. She has cardiac irregularities but takes no regular heart meds. She has had 1–2 episodes of CHF - treated as needed. She was a smoker until 6 wks ago.

She has had general and epidural anesthesia. Preop antibiotics have not been ordered. Physical status II for general anesthesia. She is allergic to tape

Dr David Smith

6/10/xx Patient tolerated general anesthesia well and was awake when taken to RR.

Dr David Smith

10/12/xx Complains of N&V. Percocet DC. Changed to Tylenol #3

Dr Evan Span

FIGURE 8–12 ▲ Physician's progress record.

SAINT, JOSEPH   MR 426-743
10/31/1939 M 57   963997
08/05/96 HOPES, HY

Admission Date _6/10/ XX_ Time _1200_ Room _T7_

Patient prefers to be called _Joe_

Primary Language Spoken _English_

MODE OF ADMISSION

☒ Ambulatory   Admitted from _home_   Patient oriented to room: ☒ Yes ☐ No

☐ Wheelchair   Valuables in safe: ☐ Yes ☐ No

☐ Stretcher   Identiband checked: ☐ Yes ☐ No

☐ _____

Vital signs: Temp _98.6_ Pulse _80_ Respirations _20_

Blood Pressure: Right _138/90_ Left _140/90_

Does patient smoke: ☒ Yes ☐ No Packs / day _one_

Does patient drink alcoholic beverages: ☒ Yes ☐ No Amount _1 drink/day_

Height _5'11'_ actual / stated Weight _210_ actual / stated Special diet / restriction _none_

Has patient experienced a change in weight in the last 6 months: ☐ Yes ☒ No Amount _____ ☐ Gained ☐ Lost

Signature _Barbara Smythe_ (R.N.) L.P.N., N.A. Date _6/10/XX_ Time _1250_

MEDICATION PROFILE: (PRESCRIPTION AND NON-PRESCRIPTION) Include eye drops, insulin, ointment, bowel care, etc.

DRUG NAME AND DOSE	HOW OFTEN	DATE / TIME OF LAST DOSE	SENT TO PHARMACY	LEFT AT BEDSIDE	AT HOME	SENT HOME
Dicumerol 100 mg	Tid	0900			✓	
Tagamet	Tid + hs	0900			✓	

Cortisone therapy: ☐ Yes ☒ No When _____ Therapy length _____

Injections _____ Oral _____

ALLERGIES

☐ None known   **Substance**   **Reaction**

Morphine   _nausea_

aspirin   _rash_

Tomatoes   _rash_

Patient's stated reason for admission and physical complaints: _Severe chest pain, shortness of breath coughing_

Physician notified at admission: _✓_

Attending _Dr Hy Hopes_ Date _6/10/XX_ Time _1220_

Resident _Dr Arthur Spence_ Date _6/10/XX_ Time _1225_

Emergency Contact _Jennie Saynt_ Phone Number _861 1902_

Signature _Barbara Smythe_ (R.N.) L.P.N. Date _6/10_ Time _1300_

MR-509-98 (9/91)

PATIENT ADMISSION

FIGURE 8–13 ▲ Nurse's admission record.

DIABETIC INFORMATION

Do you have diabetes? ☐ Yes ☒ No If yes, please complete the following questions:

Do you take insulin at home? ☐ Yes ☐ No

Do you check blood sugars at home? ☐ Yes ☐ No

Diabetes Educator notified? ☐ Yes ☐ No

Diet Office notified? ☐ Yes ☐ No

MEDICAL HISTORY (Pertinent / Current)

Illnesses (acute / chronic) _____

Recent hospitalizations _____

Recent surgeries _*Laparoscopic cholecystectomy*_

Injuries / accidents _*fractured left radius*_

Recent exposure to infections _*pneumonia approx 6 months ago*_

Current infections _*none*_

Pacemaker _*no*_

Do you have an Advanced Directive / Living Will? ☐ Yes ☒ No If yes, please submit copy.

Durable Power of Attorney for Health Care? ☐ Yes ☒ No If yes, please submit copy.

Are you a designated organ donor? ☐ Yes ☒ No

Name and relationship of person providing information if other than patient: _____

PROSTHESIS / APPLIANCES / VALUABLES

ITEM	YES	NO	TAKEN HOME	LOCKED IN SAFE	LEFT AT BEDSIDE
GLASSES					
CONTACT LENSES ☒ L ☒ R	✓				
HEARING AID ☐ L ☐ R					
DENTURES: FULL ☐ U ☐ L PARTIAL ☐ U ☐ L					
MOBILITY APPLIANCE					
OTHER (Identify):					
VALUABLES					

Signature _*Barbara Smythe*_ ®.N., L.P.N. Date _6/10/XX_ Time _1230_

PATIENT ADMISSION 2

FIGURE 8–13, cont'd ▲ Nurse's admission record.

or medications. The health unit coordinator enters this vital information, including height, weight, and allergies, into a patient profile screen on the computer. It is a responsibility of the health unit coordinator to label the front of the patient's chart with a red and white allergy sticker and to place a cardboard insert into a red plastic allergy bracelet for the patient to wear. It is standard practice in some facilities to use red ink to note the patient's allergies on chart forms. Some facilities also provide a separate allergy form that is included under the hard cover of the chart binder.

4. Nurse's Progress Notes

The nurse's progress notes is a standard chart form that is used to outline the patient's care and treatment and to record the treatment, progress, and activities of the patient. The form is often located on a nurse's clipboard, in a separate chart at the foot of the patient's bed or outside of the room in a Walla Roo. The nurse records his or her observations of the patient on the nurse's progress notes (Fig. 8–14). Entries must be signed by the nurse making the entry and usually includes the nurse's first name, last name, and professional status (RN, LPN). These notes relate to the patient's behavior and reaction to treatment and other care ordered by the physician. The form serves as the written communication between the doctor and the nursing staff. Nursing students as well as RNs, LPNs, and in some facilities, CNAs may record on this form. Black ink is preferred for all shifts because colored ink, especially red and green, does not photocopy or microfilm well. The form is used during patient care conferences to evaluate patient progress and to plan discharge and future care.

5. Graphic Record Form

The graphic record (Fig. 8–15) is a graphic representation of the patient's vital signs (temperature, pulse, respiration, and blood pressure) for a given number of days. Vital signs are ordered by the doctor, or taken according to the hospital routine.

It is the task of the health unit coordinator or nursing personnel to graph the vital signs on the graphic record form. (Temperature may be calibrated in degrees Fahrenheit or degrees Celsius.) Other items recorded on the graphic record form by nursing personnel include intake and output, weight, and bowel movements.

6. Medication Administration Record (MAR)

All medications given by nursing personnel are recorded on the medication administration record (MAR; Fig. 8–16). As the doctor orders new medications, the date, drug, dosage, administration route, and time frequency for administration of the medication are written on this form. This task is part of the transcription procedure and, therefore, is usually the responsibility of the health unit coordinator in many health care facilities. Some hospital pharmacies provide a computerized medication record for every patient each day; when a new medication is ordered, the nurse or health unit coordinator hand writes the medication with administration instructions on the computerized form.

7. Nurse's Discharge-Planning Form

The nurse's discharge-planning form (Fig. 8–17) is used to prepare the patient for discharge from the health care facility. The nurse usually records information about the patient's health status at the time of discharge and provides instructions for the patient to follow after discharge from the health care facility.

8. Physician's Discharge Summary

The physician's discharge summary (Fig. 8–18), which is used by the physician to summarize the treatment and diagnosis the patient received while hospitalized, includes discharge information. A coding summary or DRG sheet may either be part of the physician's discharge summary or a separate chart form.

Standard Patient Chart Form Initiated by the Physician

1. History and Physical Form

The history and physical form (H&P; Fig. 8–19) is a chart form that is usually dictated by the patient's doctor, hospitalist, or resident. A medical transcriptionist in the hospital health records department types the dictated report and sends it to the nursing unit to be placed in the patient's chart. Some doctors will send a completed copy of the patient's history and physical with the patient or send it to the hospital prior to the patient's admission. The H&P form is used to record the medical history and the present symptomatic history of the patient. A review of all body systems or physical assessment of the patient is also recorded (Fig. 8–20).

■ PREPARING THE PATIENT'S CHART

Each health care facility has specific standard forms that are placed in all patients' charts. These forms are preassembled, clipped together (by the health unit coordinator or by volunteers), and filed in a drawer or on shelves near the health unit coordinator area. These assembled forms are often referred to as the admission packet.

Upon a patient admission, the health unit coordinator will obtain an admission packet from the drawer or shelf and label each form with the patient's ID labels. The forms that need dates and days of the week are filled in (Fig. 8–21) and are then placed behind the proper chart divider in a chart binder.

Text continued on page 142

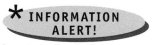

★ INFORMATION ALERT!

Twelve Standard Chart Forms

Initiated in the Admitting Department	Included in the Admission Packet
1. Face Sheet or Information Form	5. Physician's Order Form
2. Condition of Admission Form	6. Physician's Progress Record
3. Advance Directive Checklist	7. Nurse's Admission Record
	8. Nurse's Progress Notes
Initiated by the Physician	9. Graphic Record Form
4. History and Physical Form (H&P)	10. Medication Administration Record (MAR)
	11. Nurse's Discharge-Planning Form
	12. Physician's Discharge Summary

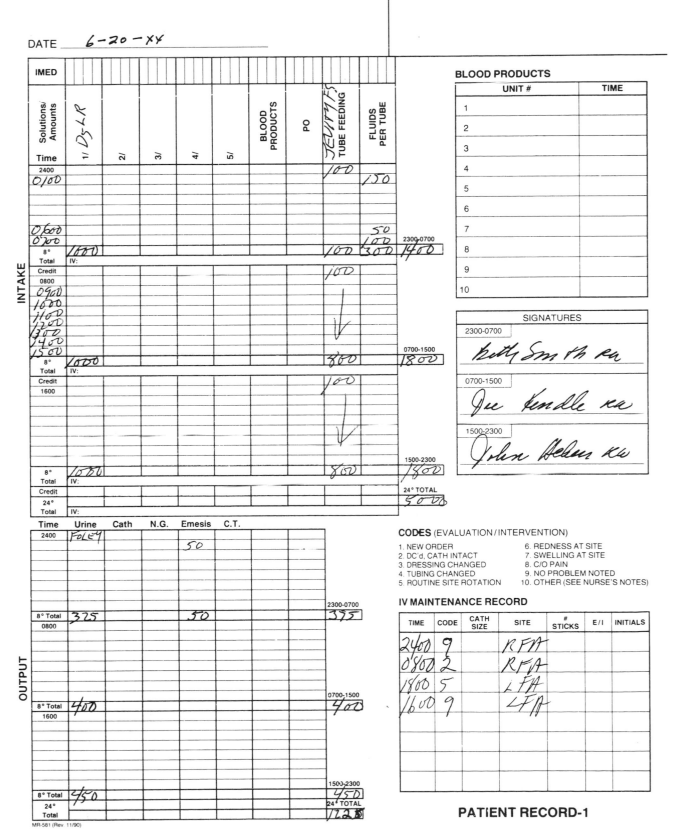

FIGURE 8–14 ▲ Nurse's progress notes.

Continued

DATE __6-20-XX__

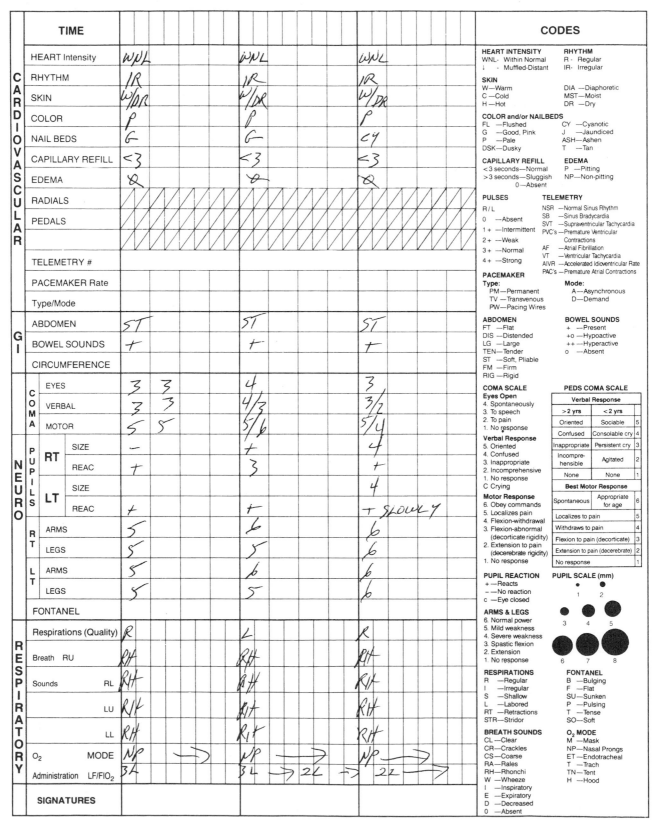

	TIME										CODES

CARDIOVASCULAR

HEART Intensity	WNL		WNL		WNL
RHYTHM	IR		IR		IR
SKIN	W/DR		W/DR		W/DR
COLOR	P		P		P
NAIL BEDS	G		G		CY
CAPILLARY REFILL	<3		<3		<3
EDEMA	Ø		Ø		Ø
RADIALS					
PEDALS					
TELEMETRY #					
PACEMAKER Rate					
Type/Mode					

CODES (Cardiovascular):

HEART INTENSITY
WNL- Within Normal
↓ - Muffled-Distant

RHYTHM
R - Regular
IR- Irregular

SKIN
W—Warm
C—Cold
H—Hot
DIA —Diaphoretic
MST—Moist
DR —Dry

COLOR and/or NAILBEDS
FL —Flushed
G —Good, Pink
P —Pale
DSK—Dusky
CY —Cyanotic
J —Jaundiced
ASH—Ashen
T —Tan

CAPILLARY REFILL
<3 seconds—Normal
>3 seconds—Sluggish
0—Absent

EDEMA
P —Pitting
NP—Non-pitting

PULSES
R / L
0 —Absent
1+ —Intermittent
2+ —Weak
3+ —Normal
4+ —Strong

TELEMETRY
NSR —Normal Sinus Rhythm
SB —Sinus Bradycardia
SVT —Supraventricular Tachycardia
PVC's—Premature Ventricular Contractions
AF —Atrial Fibrillation
VT —Ventricular Tachycardia
AIVR —Accelerated Idioventricular Rate
PAC's —Premature Atrial Contractions

PACEMAKER
Type:
PM—Permanent
TV —Transvenous
PW—Pacing Wires
Mode:
A—Asynchronous
D—Demand

GI

ABDOMEN	ST		ST		ST
BOWEL SOUNDS	+		+		+
CIRCUMFERENCE					

ABDOMEN
FT —Flat
DIS —Distended
LG —Large
TEN—Tender
ST —Soft, Pliable
FM —Firm
RIG —Rigid

BOWEL SOUNDS
+ —Present
+o —Hypoactive
++ —Hyperactive
o —Absent

NEURO

COMA
EYES	3	3	4		3
VERBAL	3	3	4/3		3/2
MOTOR	5	5	5/6		5/4

PUPILS
RT	SIZE	—		+		4
	REAC	+		3		+
LT	SIZE					4
	REAC	+		+		+ SLOWLY
RT	ARMS	5		6		6
	LEGS	5		5		6
LT	ARMS	5		6		6
	LEGS	5		5		6
FONTANEL						

COMA SCALE
Eyes Open
4. Spontaneously
3. To speech
2. To pain
1. No response

Verbal Response
5. Oriented
4. Confused
3. Inappropriate
2. Incomprehensive
1. No response
C Crying

Motor Response
6. Obey commands
5. Localizes pain
4. Flexion-withdrawal
3. Flexion-abnormal (decorticate rigidity)
2. Extension to pain (decerebrate rigidity)
1. No response

PUPIL REACTION
+ —Reacts
– —No reaction
c —Eye closed

ARMS & LEGS
6. Normal power
5. Mild weakness
4. Severe weakness
3. Spastic flexion
2. Extension
1. No response

PEDS COMA SCALE

Verbal Response		
>2 yrs	<2 yrs	
Oriented	Sociable	5
Confused	Consolable cry	4
Inappropriate	Persistent cry	3
Incomprehensible	Agitated	2
None	None	1

Best Motor Response		
Spontaneous	Appropriate for age	6
Localizes to pain		5
Withdraws to pain		4
Flexion to pain (decorticate)		3
Extension to pain (decerebrate)		2
No response		1

PUPIL SCALE (mm)
● ● ●
1 2
3 4 5
6 7 8

RESPIRATORY

Respirations (Quality)	R		L		R		
Breath RU	RH		RH		RH		
Sounds RL	RH		RH		RH		
LU	RH		RH		RH		
LL	RH		RH		RH		
O₂ MODE	NP →		NP →		NP →		
Administration LF/FIO₂	3L		3L → 2L		→ 2L		

RESPIRATIONS
R —Regular
I —Irregular
S —Shallow
L —Labored
RT —Retractions
STR—Stridor

FONTANEL
B —Bulging
F —Flat
SU—Sunken
P —Pulsing
T —Tense
SO—Soft

BREATH SOUNDS
CL —Clear
CR—Crackles
CS—Coarse
RA—Rales
RH—Rhonchi
W —Wheeze
I —Inspiratory
E —Expiratory
D —Decreased
0 —Absent

O₂ MODE
M —Mask
NP—Nasal Prongs
ET —Endotracheal
T —Trach
TN—Tent
H —Hood

SIGNATURES						

PATIENT RECORD - 2

FIGURE 8–14, cont'd ▲ Nurse's progress notes.

DATE ___6 – 20 x4___

PATIENT CARE		2400–0700	0800–1500	1600–2300	CODES
ISOLATION		BF ———→	BF ———→	BF ———→	**ISOLATION** AFB—Respiratory; BF—Blood & Body Fluids
TURN		c̄ ASSIST	c̄ assist	c̄ ASSIST	**TURN** R—Right; L—Left; B—Back
BATH			C BB		**BATH** C—Complete; P—Partial; PA—Partial/Assist; S—Shower; SA—Shower/Assist; SB—Self Bath; T—Tub Bath; TA—Tub Assist
ORAL/TRACH CARE			√		
PERI/FOLEY CARE			√		
ACTIVITY		B ———→	B C C B B B B →	C → B	**ACTIVITY** BRPA—; B—Bedrest; A—AROM; P—PROM; H—Held; PR—Playroom; BRP—Bathroom Privileges; BRPA—with assist; BSC—Bedside Commode; BSCA—with assist; C—Chair (Self); CA—with assist; DA—Dangle/Assist; W—Walking; WA—Walking/assist; S—Sleeping
BACK CARE					
LINEN CHANGE			√		
↑ SIDERAILS		↑↑	X2	↑X2	
DIET/APPETITE (% or cc's)		JEVITY FS	JEVITY FS	JEVITY FS	
EQUIPMENT		KANGAROO PUMP-TELE	K PUMP TELE	K PUMP-TELE	**RESTRAINTS** WRIST: left/right; ANKLE: left/right; BW—Both Wrists; BA—Both Ankles; P—Posey; CC—Cadillac Chair; CCA—with assist 2-3-4
GI TUBE	Placement Checked		√	√	
	Tube type/Suction	FLEX FLOW	Flexiflow	FLEXI FLOW	
	Hematest, Color, Char.				
STOOL	Method of Output				**DIET** FT—Fed Totally; FP—Fed Partially; TF—Tube Fed
	Amt Description		Lg gn solid	LG GN LIQ / SEMI SOLID	
	Hematest				
URINE	Catheter				**EQUIPMENT** IM—IMED; OX—Oximeter; KP—Kangaroo Pump; AM—Apnea Monitor; HO—Hypothermia Blanket; HP—Hyperthermia Blanket; A—Airshields Warmer; IS—Isolette; K—K-Pad
	Method of Output	FOLEY	foley	FOLEY	
	Specific Gravity Color, Char.	AMBER c̄ CLOTS	amber c̄ clots	AMBER c̄ CLOTS	
RESP	Rx Chest Pt.		SUN QID		
	Suctioned		X 2	X 2	**STOOL/METHOD** T—Toilet; D—Dilly; I—Incontinent
	Secretions (color, type, amt) ET / Oral	NON PROD LOOSE COUGH	occ prod cough	PROD COUGH	
TESTS/PROC	Specimen Sent			sputum sent	**URINE/METHOD** Catheter; Size/Date of insertion; D—Diaper; BP—Bedpan; I—Incontinent
	Procedures				
	Tests/X-rays		PORTABLE CHEST		**PERI/FOLEY CARE** P—Peri; F—Foley
DRAINS	Site Location				**DRAINAGE** CL—Clear; BL—Bloody; S—Serous; SS—Serosanguinous; T—Tan
	Dressing Change				
WOUND	Site: location/condition				
	Dressing Change				
	FLAPS/GRAFTS				
	SIGNATURES				

PATIENT RECORD - 3

FIGURE 8–14, cont'd ▲ Nurse's progress notes.

Continued

DATE 6-20 XX

NOTIFICATION	TIME	NURSING CONCERNS	RESPONSE TIME/ACTION TAKEN	INIT.

DISCHARGE/TEACHING INSTRUCTIONS

PATIENT BEHAVIORS/OBSERVATIONS/EVALUATION/INTERVENTIONS (NURSES' NOTES)

2406 PATIENT RESTING c̄ EYES CLOSED HOB ↑ VSS PULSE
130-150 TELE #21 AFIB c̄ FREQ PVC HEPLOCK PATENT
+ FLUSHED O₂ ON CONT. PT HAS LOOSE NO PRODUCTIVE
COUGH JEVITY FS THROUGH KANGAROO PUMP @ 100°
PT RECEIVED ALL MEDS THROUGH FT - TOLERATED WELL.
FOLEY IRRIGATED c̄ NS 50cc ↑ 50cc RETURN c̄ SOME
BLD CLOTS. FOLEY DRAINED 325cc OF DRK AMBER URINE
c̄ CLOTS RECOGNIZES RELATIVES - NEURO VS
INTACT UP IN CHAIR c̄ ASSIST. EMESIS - 50cc
0614 patient bathed turned freq - up in chair
Dr visit - alert @ times lg on stool -
foley patent. Jevity FS thru K pump @ 100/hr
tol well. occasional prod. cough pt.
resting @ intervals VSS - pulse reg
135 - 160 tele #21 Afib c̄ freq PVC
Heplock patent + flushed O₂ on cont.
good day. urine output - 400cc
1523 PT CONFUSED AT TIMES - UP IN CHAIR X1
FAMILY VISITED SHARED CONCERN OF PTS
CONFUSION. O₂ ON CONT. STOOL X1 FOLEY
PATENT JEVITY FS THRU K PUMP TOL WELL
HEPLOCK PATENT - FLUSHED TELE #21 AFIB OCC
PVC IV INFUSING PATIENT RESTING COMFORTABLY
NO COMPLAINTS OF PAIN OR NAUSEA URINE
OUTPUT - 450cc

PATIENT RECORD - 4

FIGURE 8-14, cont'd ▲ Nurse's progress notes.

GRAPHIC CHART (Fahrenheit)

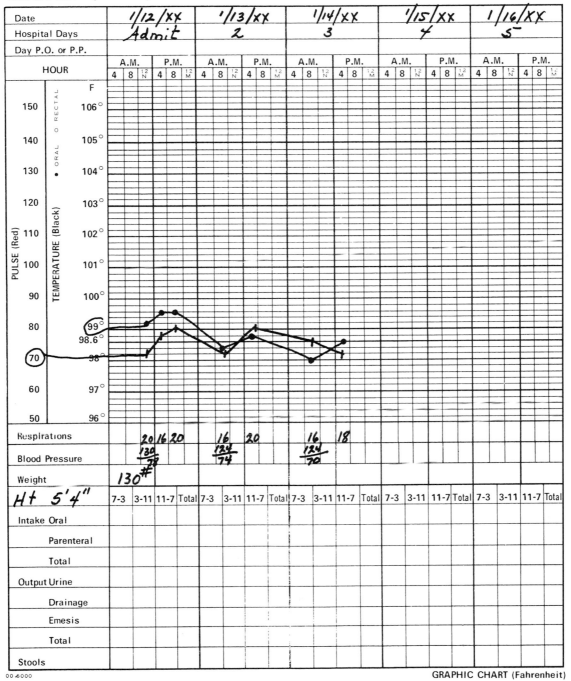

FIGURE 8–15 ▲ Graphic or clinical record. A, Fahrenheit.

Continued

967 896
MART TED
DR Y STOCKS
M 40 MED INS

GRAPHIC CHART (Centigrade)

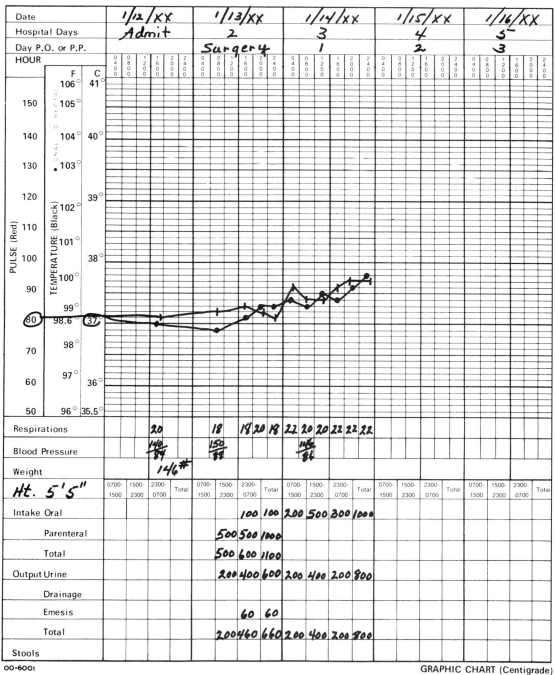

	1/12/XX	1/13/XX	1/14/XX	1/15/XX	1/16/XX
Date					
Hospital Days	Admit	2	3	4	5
Day P.O. or P.P.		Surgery	1	2	3

Respirations: 20 | 18 | 18 20 18 | 22 20 20 22 22 22

Blood Pressure: 140/84 | 150/88 | 146/86

Weight: 146#

Ht. 5'5"

	0700-1500	1500-2300	2300-0700	Total
Intake Oral	100	100	200	500 300 1000
Parenteral	500	500	1000	
Total	500	600	1100	
Output Urine	200	400	600	200 400 200 800
Drainage				
Emesis		60	60	
Total	200	460	660	200 400 200 800
Stools				

00-6001   GRAPHIC CHART (Centigrade)

B

FIGURE 8–15, cont'd ▲ Graphic or clinical record. *B*, Celsius (centigrade) with military time.

MEDICATION RECORD

SAINT, JOSEPH   MR 426-743
10/31/1939 M 57   963997
08/05/96 HOPES, HY

ROOM NO. 224-2			ROOM NO. 224-2			ROOM NO. 224-2		
LAST NAME Smyth			LAST NAME Smith			LAST NAME Smyth		
P.O. DAY			P.O. DAY			P.O. DAY		

	DATE	DRUG	DOSE	ROUTE	DATE DC	SCHEDULE	DATE 11-7	7-3	3-11	DATE 11-7	7-3	3-11	DATE 11-7	7-3	3-11
1	8/11	Dilantin	100mg	I.V. ⓟⓞ R. I.M.		tid	10	2	10						
2	8/11	Indocin	25mg	I.V. ⓟⓞ R. I.M.		bid	10		10						
3	8/11	Premarin	1.25mg	I.V. ⓟⓞ R. I.M.		qd	10								
4				I.V. P.O. R. I.M.											
5				I.V. P.O. R. I.M.											
6				I.V. P.O. R. I.M.											
7				I.V. P.O. R. I.M.											
8				I.V. P.O. R. I.M.											
9				I.V. P.O. R. I.M.											
10				I.V. P.O. R. I.M.											
11				I.V. P.O. R. I.M.											
12				I.V. P.O. R. I.M.											
13				I.V. P.O. R. I.M.											
14				I.V. P.O. R. I.M.											
15				I.V. P.O. R. I.M.											
16				I.V. P.O. R. I.M.											
17				I.V. P.O. R. I.M.											
18				I.V. P.O. R. I.M.											
19				I.V. P.O. R. I.M.											
20				I.V. P.O. R. I.M.											
21				I.V. P.O. R. I.M.											
22				I.V. P.O. R. I.M.											
23				I.V. P.O. R. I.M.											
24				I.V. P.O. R. I.M.											
25				I.V. P.O. R. I.M.											
26				I.V. P.O. R. I.M.											
27				I.V. P.O. R. I.M.											
28	8/13	Compazine	100mg	I.V. P.O. R. ⓘⓜ	8/16	q4h prn/iv	2³⁰ RT								
29	8/13	Ambien	5mg	I.V. P.O. R. I.M.	8/16	hs prn		10							
30	8/13	Demorol	50mg	I.V. P.O. R. ⓘⓜ	8/16	q4h prn	MN B³⁰ LT	MN	MN	MN	MN	MN	MN	MN	MN

CODES
LU - LUQ
RU - RUQ
OD - RT. EYE

O - NOT GIVEN
LT - LT. THIGH
RT - RT. THIGH
OS - LT. EYE

ABD - ABDOMEN
LA - LT. ARM
RA - RT. ARM
OU - BOTH EYES

IVPB - IV PIGGYBACK   SQ - SUBCUTANEOUS

IDIOSYNCRACIES
Morphine

DIAGNOSIS Cholecystitis

MR - 1012 REV. 12/84

MEDICATION RECORD

FIGURE 8–16 ▲ Medication administration record (MAR).

SAINT, JOSEPH   MR 426-743
10/31/1939 M 57   963997
08/05/96 HOPES, HY

Home Instructions

Name _Joseph Saint_

Attending Physician _Dr Hy Hopes_

Activity Guidelines (None indicated ☐)   **Room Checked For Patient Belongings** ☐

as tolerated

Diet/Nutrition (None indicated ☐) .

low fat diet
small meals

Treatments/Procedures/Dressings (None indicated ☐)

may shower.

Home Medications (None indicated ☐)   **Patients Own Medications Returned** ☐ **Yes** ☐ **No**

Name	Dose	Times	Special Considerations
Percodan	7	every 4 hours	For pain
Compazine	7	every 4 hours	For nausea

See General Information on Medication Use printed on the back of this form.
Food/Medication Instruction Sheet Provided ☒ Yes   ☐ None Indicated

Additional Information Provided (Handouts, Brochures) ☐ None Indicated
post op laparoscopic cholecystectomy instructions

Physician or Agency Referrals   Contact Person   Phone Number

I understand the guidelines for my care at home.

Joe Saint   _Mary Smit_   6/8
Responsible Person   LPN/RN/MD   Date

WHITE - Chart Copy; CANARY - Patient Copy; PINK - Physician Copy

09-9268 6/82 Rev. 9/94

FIGURE 8-17 ▲ Nurse's discharge planning form.

CODING SUMMARY

Attending Physician *Marietta Harris MD*   Other Attending *Pat Anderson MD*

Anesthesia *Philip Ellis MD*   Assistant Surgeon *Casey Hershfield MD*

Intern/Resident *Connie Estrella MD*

Consultant(s) *Richard Weber M.D.*   Date of Admission *11-6-XX*

Date of Discharge *11-21-XX*

Principal Diagnosis (Condition after study that occasioned the admission)	H.I.M.S. Codes
End Stage Renal Disease	403.9

Secondary Diagnosis (Including complications and co-morbidities if applicable)	H.I.M.S. Codes
Diabetes Mellitus	250.41
Blindness Secondary to Diabetic Retinopathy	250.51
Hypertension	369.00

Procedure(s) and Date(s) (List Principal Procedure first. Principal Procedure should be for definitive treatment.)		H.I.M.S. Codes
Kidney Transplant	11-8-XX	55.69
Excision of Tenckhoff catheter	11-8-XX	54.99

DISCHARGE STATUS:

☒ 1. Home   ☐ 5. Other Type Institute   ☐ 20. Expired
☐ 2. Other Acute Care   ☐ 6. Home Health Care   ☐ Autopsy
☐ 3. Skilled Nursing Facility   ☐ 7. Against Medical Advice   ☐ No Autopsy
☐ 4. Intermediate Care Facility   ☐ 8. Home with I.V. Therapy   ☐ Coroner's Case

ATTENDING PHYSICIAN OR CHIEF *Marietta Harris MD*   Date *11-21-XX*
(Signature Optional)

THIS SECTION TO BE UTILIZED BY HEALTH INFORMATION MANAGEMENT SERVICES

Coding *E MlC*

Hospital Service *Vascular Surgery* By *WK*   Analysis *WK*

00-0627 11/83 Rev. 10/95

Patient Label

FIGURE 8–18 ▲ Physician's discharge and coding summary sheet.

Physician: _____

Registration/Medical Record Number: _____

HISTORY

Present Illness: _____
_____
_____
_____
_____
_____

Past History: _____
_____
_____
_____
_____
_____

Present Medications: _____
_____
_____
_____
_____
_____

Allergies: _____
_____
_____
_____
_____

Diagnosis/Impression: _____
_____
_____
_____
_____

PHYSICAL EXAMINATION

General Appearance: Normal ☐   Abnormal ☐
_____

Head/ENT: Normal ☐   Abnormal ☐
_____

Heart: Normal ☐   Abnormal ☐
_____

Lungs: Normal ☐   Abnormal ☐
_____

Abdomen: Normal ☐   Abnormal ☐
_____

Genitalia: Normal ☐   Abnormal ☐
_____

Extremities: Normal ☐   Abnormal ☐
_____

Breast: Normal ☐   Abnormal ☐
_____

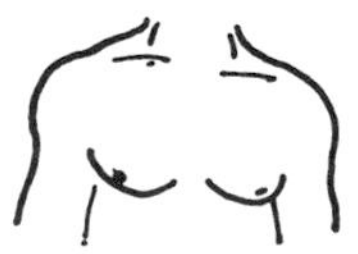

Focused Examination: _____
_____
_____
_____

Signature: _____ M.D.

FIGURE 8-19 ▲ History and physical (H&P) form.

Patient Number: 765 466
Patient Name Marcia Clerk
Physician Name   Joan Simone

HISTORY AND PHYSICAL EXAMINATION

Patient is a 56 year-old female admitted with the chief complaint of severe upper cervical spine pain The patient has rheumatoid spondylitis and has a fusion of most of the cervical spine, but the upper two vertebra still have motion in their joints, and the patient is experiencing considerable pain because of the progressive arthritis at this level.

PAST HISTORY: Reveals the patient to have some elevated blood pressure problems. She is currently taking Hygroton, aspirin and Indocin. Patient has had as appendectomy, hysterectomy and a bilateral salpingo-oophorectomy.

REVIEW OF SYSTEMS: No auditory or visual symptoms
CARDIORESPIRATORY: No orthopnea, dyspnea, hemoptysis.
G.I. TRACT: No weight gain, weight loss ., or change in bowel habits
G.U. TRACT: No pyuria, dysuria or frequency
NEUROMUSCULAR: See Present complaints.

PHYSICAL EXAMINATION: A somewhat frail female in no acute distress. Patient walks about room with neck flexed. She is unable to extend neck.

CHEST: Expansion is limited. The lungs are clear to auscultation. Heart tones are regular. No murmurs. No cardiomegaly.

ABDOMEN: Soft. LKS not palpable.

BACK: Marked limitations of lumbodorsal motion. No paraspinous muscle spasm noted.

EXTREMITY: The patient has limitations of right shoulder motion and active and passive motion causes her significant discomfort, and crepitation is noted. The neurovascular status of all extremities is intact.

Joan Simone, D. O.

FIGURE 8–20 ▲ Typewritten history and physical (H&P) form.

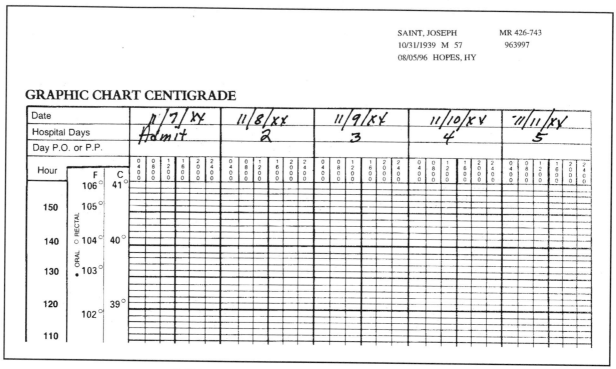

FIGURE 8–21 ▲ Graphic record with headings filled in.

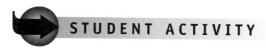

STUDENT ACTIVITY

To practice preparing a patient's chart, complete Activity 8–2 in the *Skills Practice Manual*.

■ SUPPLEMENTAL PATIENT CHART FORMS

Supplemental patient chart forms are additional to the standard chart forms and are added to the patient's chart according to his or her specific care and treatment. For example, if the patient is a diabetic and is receiving medication and being monitored, the supplemental form (diabetic record) will be added to the chart. This allows for information to be recorded separately from other data, making it easier for interpretation.

It is the responsibility of the health unit coordinator to obtain the needed forms, identify the form by using an ID label, and place the form behind the proper chart divider in the chart binder.

Clinical Pathway Record Form

Some hospitals utilize clinical pathway record forms for certain diagnoses or conditions, such as coronary artery bypass graft (CABG), or total hip or knee replacements. The clinical pathway record form is placed in the chart for those particular patients. The clinical pathway record form includes the surgeon's orders, a plan of care with treatment, and predicted outcomes (Fig. 8–22).

Anticoagulant Therapy Record

The anticoagulant record (Fig. 8–23) is used to maintain a record of blood test results and the anticoagulant medication received by the patient who is undergoing anticoagulant therapy. A flow sheet allows the doctor to make a comparison of the patient's blood test results and the medications prescribed over time.

Diabetic Record

The diabetic record (Fig. 8–24) is placed in the charts of patients who are receiving medication for diabetes. The results of the blood tests performed to monitor the effect of the diabetic medications are also recorded on the diabetic record.

Consultation Form

The patient's attending physician may wish to obtain the opinion of another doctor. In this event, he or she requests a consultation by writing it on the doctor's order sheet. Most doctors will dictate their report upon completing the consultation. The hospital medical transcription department personnel will type the dictated report and send it to the nursing unit to be filed in the patient's chart. Some doctors may prefer to write their findings on a consultation form. Additional information regarding consultations is found in Chapter 18.

Operating Room Records

The number of forms required to maintain a record of a patient's operation varies; those forms are usually assembled into a surgery packet. The records are utilized by operating room personnel, the anesthesiologist, and recovery room personnel (see Figs. 19–16, *A* and *B*). Additional responsibilities regarding the surgery chart are located in Chapter 19.

History: _____
IV: _____

Procedures: _____

Date _____

A = achieved · N = not achieved

	Pre-hospital	Day of Surgery	Post-op day 1	PO day 2	PO day 3	PO day 4 Discharge
Consult	Medical Clearance if necessary	PT consult in PM	PT therapy BID	PT BID Home Care and SS as appr	PT BID	PT
Tests	CXR, CBC, UA, PT, SMA20, EKG, Labs appropriate for age & health 72 hrs before	T & C 2 units (pre-op) (autologous when able) X-ray (in PACU)	H & H ☐ PT (if on coumadin) ☐	H & H ☐ PT ☐	H & H ☐ PT ☐	PT ☐
Mobility		dangle - stand prn	Knee exercises Chair BID (30 min) - up for dinner Stand/Amb	Cont exercises - Amb BID Chair BID (45 min) - up for lunch and dinner BRP	Continue mobility Chair (60 min) - up for all meals	Continue mobility Chair (60 min) - up for all meals
Treatments		Trapeze Drain IV therapy, incentive spir q2° DVT prophylaxes : (TED, foot compression device, coumadin, Lovenox) CPM 0 - 40° in PACU	Trapeze Drain Cap IV, incentive spir q2° DVT prophylaxes CPM 0 - 50°	Trapeze DC drain Cap IV, incentive spir q2° DVT proph Dressing change by physician CPM 0 - 60°	Trapeze Incentive spirometer DCIV DVT proph CPM 0 - 70°	CPM 0 - 80°
Meds		Pain Med (IV, IM) Pt states pain relief: A N Antibiotics ___	Pain Med (IV, IM) Pt states pain relief: A N DC Antibiotics	PO pain meds Pt states pain relief: A N	PO pain meds prn Pt states pain relief: A N	PO pain meds prn Pt states pain relief: A N
Nutrition Metabolic		DAT ___	DAT ___	DAT ___	DAT ___	DAT ___
Elimination		Catheter of choice prn st cath foley after 3rd time	DC foley	Eval. bowel function (BCOC)	Bowel movement: A N	Bowel movement: A N
Health /Home Management			Screen for Home Care & Social Service needs	Prescription for home equipment identified by PT Order equipment	Complete transfer form	☐ Home ☐ ECF
Health Perception	TKA pre-op teaching by Interdisciplinary Team	Review: ☐ TCDB, ☐ incentive spirometry, ☐ ankle pumps, ☐ ROM to arms, ☐ CPM, ☐ pain management	Instruct on: ☐ knee precautions	Instruct on: ☐ incisional care ☐ pain management	Discharge teaching: ☐ Medication ☐ review knee book	☐ Written discharge instructions to patient and family
Signature						
Signature						
Signature						

Outcomes		Date met/initials	Outcomes	Date met/initials
1. In-out of bed ☐ indep or with min assist	☐ mod - max assist		5. Evidence of wound healing, no drainage	
2. On-off commode or chair ☐ indep or with min assist	☐ mod - max assist		6. Performs total knee exercises without assistance	
3. Ambulates with assistive devices. ☐ 75 feet indep or with min asst	☐ 50 feet		7. Re-establish elimination pattern.	
4. AROM ☐ 0 - 70 - 90°	☐ 0 - 60°		8. Utilizes oral analgesics for pain control.	

FIGURE 8–22 ▲ Clinical pathway for total knee arthroscopy.

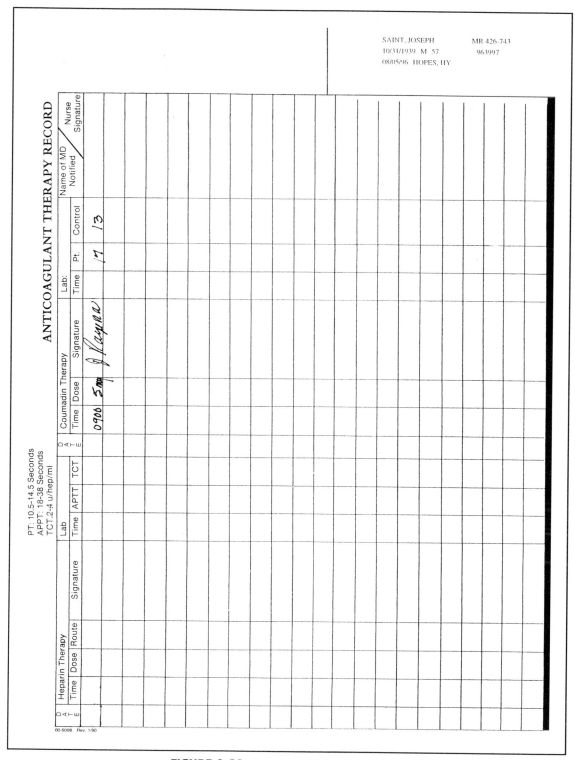

FIGURE 8–23 ▲ Anticoagulant therapy record.

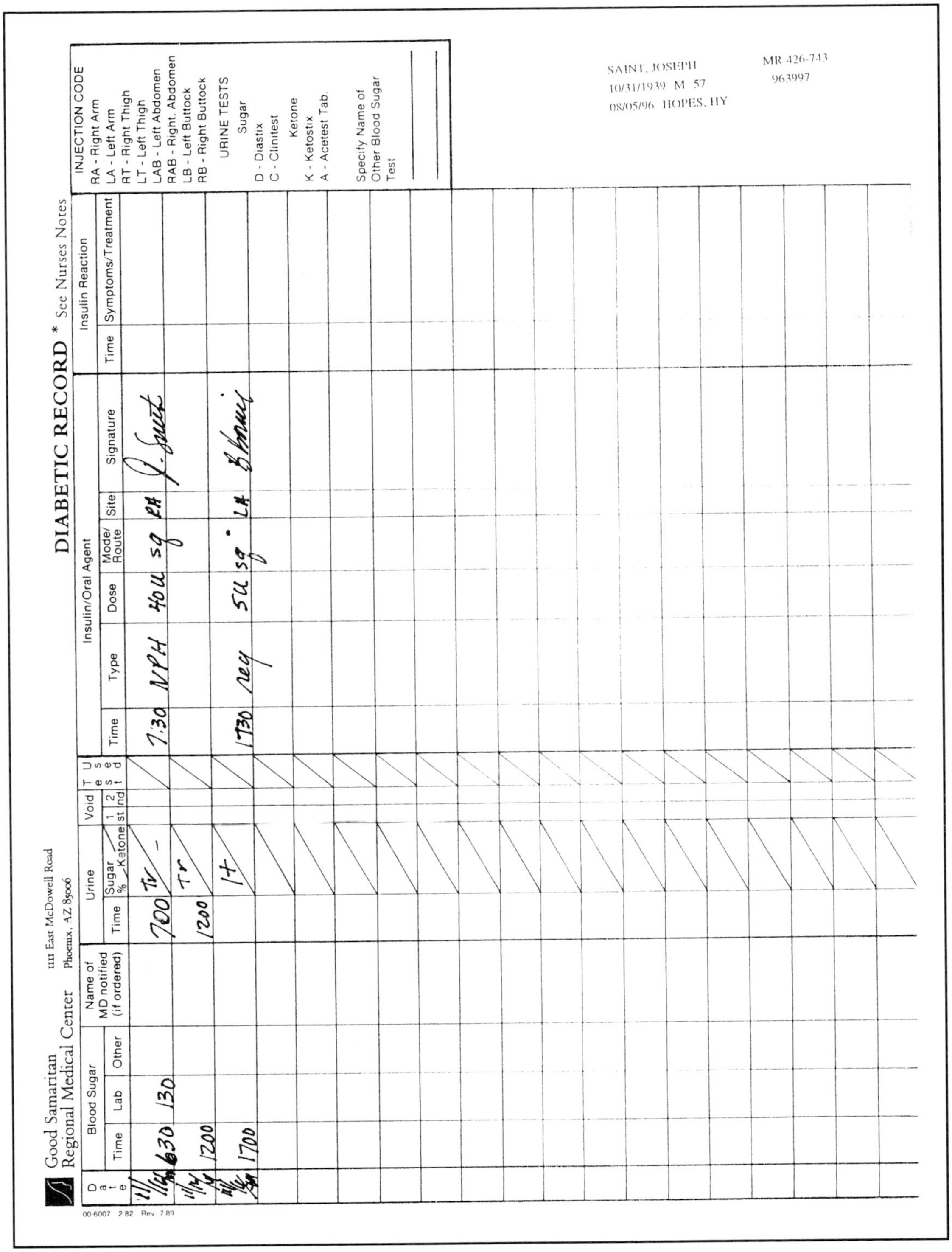

FIGURE 8–24 ▲ Diabetic record.

```
INSTITUTE OF REHABILITATION MEDICINE          967 896
         PROGRESS NOTES                        MART TED
Home Care, Orientation & Mobility, Occupational DR Y STOCKS
  Therapy, Physical Therapy, Speech Pathology   M 40 MED INS
              & Orthotics
```

DATE & SERVICE	
	P.T.
11/12/xx	Patient seen bid in a.m. for exercise in supine position. Ambulated 25' c̄ arm support + minimal assistance for balance. In p.m. pt seen for ambulation 25'. C/o light headache so returned to bed.
	R. Wentcomb, RPT
11/13/xx	In a.m arm ROM 5-10 reps in all planes. Pt. cooperated c̄ program. Transferred to chair for 10 min.
	R. Wentcomb, RPT.

FIGURE 8–25 ▲ Therapy records. *A*, Physical therapy progress notes. *Illustration continued on opposite page.*

Therapy Records

Health care facilities use individual record sheets for recording treatments. It is possible to have record sheets for physical therapy, occupational therapy, respiratory care, diet therapy, radiation therapy, and others. These departments are discussed elsewhere in Section 3 (Fig. 8–25).

Parenteral Fluid or Infusion Record

A patient who receives an intravenous infusion may have a parenteral fluid record (Fig. 8–26) placed in his or her chart. This form, when completed, is a written record of types and amounts of intravenous fluids administered to the patient. If bedside charting is in use, the parenteral fluid record or vital signs record may be initiated when the information is entered into the computer.

Frequent Vital Signs Record

The frequent vital signs record (Fig. 8–27) is used when vital signs are taken more often than every 4 hours.

■ CONSENT FORMS

Surgery or Procedure Consent Form

There are a number of conditions that require the patient or a responsible party to sign a special form granting permission for surgery or other invasive procedures to be performed upon the patient (Fig. 8–28).

The patient who is hospitalized for surgery is required to sign a form permitting his or her doctor to perform the surgery named on the consent form. The form should not be signed until the physician has explained the surgery or procedure and its risks, alternatives, and likely outcomes (informed consent). After receiving an explanation, a competent patient can give informed consent.

Other procedures requiring consent forms to be signed by the patient or a responsible party are covered in chapters related to the specific procedures.

The health unit coordinator may prepare the consent form for the physician or nurse to take to the patient for the patient's signature. If the surgery should be cancelled, the surgery permit is still valid unless the doctor or the surgical procedure has been changed.

Consent forms for surgery and certain other procedures are legal agreements between the patient and the physician. In some health care facilities it may be the physician's responsibility to write the name of the doctor who is to perform the surgery or procedure, and to write the name of the procedure to be done.

Procedure for Preparing Consent Forms

In most facilities, the health unit coordinator prepares the consent form for the nurse or doctor to present to the patient for signature. The following steps will assist you in preparing the consent form.

1. Affix the patient's ID label to the consent form.
2. Write in black ink the first and last names of the doctor who is to perform the surgery or procedure.

DEPARTMENT OF RESPIRATORY CARE

TREATMENT RECORD

967 901
SAAKE PETE
DR B GOOD
M 46 MED INS

DATE	
11/19/XX	SVN Rx given c̄ 0.2 cc Alupent + 2 cc N.S via N/P c̄ C/A at 5 L/M ×10 min. Pulse 104 and stable. Breath sounds essentially clear. Pt. tolerated Rx well. Productive cough c̄ sm. amt. thin white sputum
Bonnie Flowers RT.

B

DIETETIC PROGRESS NOTES

967 900
CIDER IDA
DR C BARRELL
F 58 SURG INS

DATE	
2/1/XX	Appetite poor × 4 mo. 150# → 124# States Dr. told her to avoid all fruits and juices and also no red meat. Pt does not tolerate milk products except cheese. Does not tolerate Ensure and Sustacal (diarrhea) Takes Vit. C + E. at home. Pt is 58 yr. old female c̄ lung cancer and mass in abdomen. Also dehydrated. Has med. visceral protein loss. Diet: Soft c̄ Sustacal supplement.
Doris Kay, R.D.

C

FIGURE 8–25, cont'd ▲ *B,* Respiratory treatment record. *C,* Dietetic therapy progress notes.

967 896
MART TED
DR Y STOCKS
M 40 MED INS

PARENTERAL FLUID SHEET

DATE	TIME STARTED	TYPE OF SOLUTION, RATE, SITE MODE OF ADMINISTRATION SIZE & KIND-NEEDLE/CANNULA	STARTED BY	MEDICATION ADDED BY	AMT. INF.	TIME DISC. BY	REMARKS
9/26/xx	1100	1000 cc D₅W @125 cc/h Lt hand c̄ #21 Butterfly	H. Jones		1000 cc	1900	No redness or edema at site

FIGURE 8–26 ▲ Parenteral fluid or infusion record.

967 896
MART TED
DR Y STOCKS
M 40 MED INS

VITAL SIGNS RECORD

DATE 11/6/XX

Time	BP	T	P	R	Oral	N/G	IV	Blood	Misc.	Urine	N/G	Stool	Emesis	Misc.	Spec. Grav.	CVP
						INTAKE						OUTPUT				
0900	110/50	98	60	16			100 cc						50 cc			
1000	112/54	98⁴	64	16	60 cc		100 cc			100 cc						
1100	112/57	98⁴	60	18	60 cc		100 cc					ṫ				
1200	110/56	98⁸	68	18	60 cc		100 cc			150 cc			100 cc			

FIGURE 8–27 ▲ Frequent vital signs record.

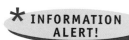
★ INFORMATION ALERT!

Some physicians may have preprinted consent forms for certain procedures or surgeries.

3. Write in black ink the surgery or procedure to be performed exactly as the physician wrote it on the physician's order sheet, except that abbreviations must be spelled out. For instance, if the procedure is the "amputation rt index finger," the consent form should read "amputation of the right index finger."

4. Spell correctly and write all information legibly.

5. Do not record the date and time. The person obtaining the patient's signature will complete this.

CONSENT FORM

1. I authorize and direct_____*Roderick Currten*_____, ("Physician"), and/or such associates and assistants as the Physician chooses, to perform upon_____*Darina Parker*_____ ("Patient"), the following procedure(s):
   _____*bilateral salpingo-oophorectomy*_____
   _____
   _____

2. I also authorize the Physician to perform any other procedures that, in the Physician's judgment, are reasonable and necessary for the Patient's well-being, including, but not limited to, the administration of anesthesia and the performance of pathology and radiology services.

3. For purposes of medical education, I authorize the Physician to admit observers to the operating room.

4. The Physician has explained to me the nature, purpose, and possible consequences, risks, and complications of the procedure, as well as alternative methods of treatment. I understand that the explanation I have received is not exhaustive and that other, more remote risks and consequences may occur. I understand that a more detailed and complete explanation of any of the foregoing matters will be given to me if I so desire. No warranty or guarantee has been made to me regarding the results or cure that may be obtained.

5. I understand that my private attending Physician and any anesthesiologists, radiologists, pathologists, or other private physicians who may be involved in the Patient's care are not employees or agents of this hospital, nor are they controlled by this hospital. Rather, they are independent contractors who act on the Patient's behalf using independent medical judgment. The only exceptions are employees of the hospital who provide these services.

6. I authorize the hospital pathologist to dispose of any severed tissue, body part, or explant as the pathologist best sees fit, except (specify desired disposal):
   _____
   _____

BY SIGNING THIS FORM, I HEREBY CERTIFY THAT I HAVE READ AND UNDERSTAND THIS CONSENT FORM IN ITS ENTIRETY, THAT ALL STATEMENTS MADE HEREIN ARE TRUE, AND THAT I CONSENT TO ALL TERMS STATED HEREIN.

_____*Darina Parker*_____   _____*8/10/XX*_____
Signature of Patient or Authorized Decision-Maker* (Specify Relationship)   Date & Time

_____*Bertha Graham*_____   _____*8/10/XX*_____
Signature of Witness/Two Witnesses Required for Telephone Consent   Date & Time

*If not signed by Patient, specify reason:
_____ Patient is a minor;
_____ Patient is unable to sign because:_____

CONSENT FORM

MR-10-303 (2/94)

FIGURE 8–28 ▲ Surgery consent form.

The patient may be required to sign other permit or release forms during his or her hospitalization. The following are examples of situations that usually require a signature by the patient or the patient's representative.

1. Release of side rails (Fig. 8–29)
2. Refusal to permit blood transfusion (Fig. 8–30)
3. Consent form for human immunodeficiency virus (HIV) testing (Fig. 8–31)
4. Consent to receive blood transfusion (Fig. 8–32)

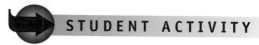

STUDENT ACTIVITY

To practice preparing a consent form for surgery, complete Activity 8–3 in the *Skills Practice Manual*.

Most health care facilities require that only licensed personnel witness the signing of consent forms. However, in some health care settings the health unit coordinator may be asked to witness

---

RELEASE OF SIDE RAILS

Having been informed by Good Samaritan Hospital that protective side rails should be placed on my bed and raised for my personal protection, I hereby instruct the hospital and its employees not to place or raise protective side rails on my bed and hereby assume all risks in connection therewith and fully release the said hospital, its employees and my physician from any and all liability for any injury or damage to me by reason of its failure to place or raise protective side rails on my bed.

Signature_____

Room No._____

Witness_____

Witness_____

Date_____Hour_____.M.

51–98

Release of Side Rails

FIGURE 8–29 ▲ Release of side rails form.

PATIENT LABEL

Refusal To Permit Blood Transfusion

1. I request that no blood derivatives be administered to _Richard Kramer_
   during this hospitalization.

   (patient name)

2. I hereby release the hospital, its personnel and the attending physician from any responsibility whatever for unfavorable reactions or any untoward results due to my refusal to permit the use of blood or its derivatives.

3. I fully understand the possible consequences of such refusal on my part.

Rich Kramer	_9/10/xx_	_1200_
Patient's Signature	Date	Time

Signature of parent, legally appointed guardian or responsible person
(for patients who cannot sign)

Alan Carlof	_9/10/xx_	_1200_
Witness	Date	Time
Donna Small	_9/10/xx_	_1200_
Witness	Date	Time

00-0038 6/90

REFUSAL TO PERMIT BLOOD TRANSFUSION

FIGURE 8–30 ▲ Form for refusal to permit blood transfusion.

CONSENT FOR HIV TESTING

1. My physician, _____, has recommended that I (my child) receive a blood test to detect the presence of antibodies to Human Immunodeficiency Virus (HIV), the virus that causes Acquired Immune Deficiency Syndrome (AIDS). I consent to this testing.

   It has been explained to me that in some cases the tests may be positive when I have (my child has) not been infected with HIV. This is a false positive.

   If the screening is positive, a second confirming test is done.

   I understand that a negative result usually means that I have (my child has) not been exposed to HIV. However, there is a possibility of a false-negative result, especially in the time period immediately after exposure to the virus.

2. I have been advised by my physician and I understand the following:

   ● Positive test results could mean that I have (my child has) been exposed to the HIV; this would not necesarily mean that I have (my child has) AIDS, or will develop AIDS.

   ● That if I am (my child is) HIV positive, I (my child) can transmit the virus to other individuals by sexual contact, by sharing needles, or by the donation of organs, blood, and blood products.

   ● That if I am (my child is) HIV positive, I (my child) should not donate blood or blood products, or body organs because the virus can be transmitted to the recipient.

3. I understand that Arizona State Law and Regulations require the reporting of HIV cases to the Department of Health Services and that if my (my child's) test results are positive, they will be submitted to the Arizona Department of Health Services, and others whose authority is established by law, regulation, or court order.

4. I also understand that my request for the test and the test results will be part of my (my child's) Hospital medical record and may therefore be requested by others, including insurers, third party payors or other individuals as outlined in the Conditions of Admission.

   I have been given the opportunity to ask quesitons, I understand what is involved in HIV testing, and I freely consent to it.

   _____   _____
   DATE   SIGNATURE

   _____   _____
   LEGAL GUARDIAN   WITNESS SIGNATURE
   (If patient cannot sign or under age)

FIGURE 8–31 ▲ Consent form for human immunodeficiency virus (HIV) testing.

the signing. Personnel must follow the following general rules when asking patients to sign consent forms.

1. The patient must not be under the influence of any "mind-clouding" medications.
2. The patient must be of legal age (18 years in most states).
3. The patient must be mentally competent.

■ METHODS OF ERROR CORRECTION

Since the chart is considered a legal document, information recorded on a chart form must not be erased or obliterated by pen, by pasting over, or by liquid correction fluid. Only certain methods of correcting errors recorded on the chart are permitted.

Chart forms that are affixed with the wrong or incorrect ID label may be shredded if no notations have been made on them. If the chart form has notations on it, the chart form cannot be shredded. Draw an X with a black ink pen through the incorrect label and write "mistaken entry" with the date, time, your first initial, last name, and status above the incorrect label. Affix the correct patient ID label on the form next to the incorrect label (do not place correct label over incorrect label). It is also permissible to hand print the patient information in black ink next to the incorrect label that you have drawn an X through (Fig. 8–33).

To correct an error of a written entry made on a chart form, draw (in black ink) one single line through the error. Record "mistaken entry" with the date, time, your first initial, last name, and status in a blank area near (directly above or next to) the error (Fig. 8–34). Follow your facility policy for correction of erroneous computer entries. The procedure for correcting an error on the graphic sheet is covered in Chapter 21.

CONSENT FOR TRANSFUSION

OF BLOOD OR BLOOD PRODUCTS

1.   My physician has informed me that I need, or may need during treatment, a transfusion of blood and/or one of its products in the interest of my health and proper medical care.

2.   My physician has explained to me the nature, purpose and possible consequences of the procedures relating to transfusion, as well as significant risks involved, possible complications of and alternatives to transfusion and possible options of obtaining blood and blood products. I understand that transfusion involves some risks to the patient even though precautions are taken. I also understand that despite the exercise of due care, the transfusion of blood and blood products may transmit infectious diseases such as hepatitis or HIV (AIDS) or may result in an allergic reaction of the patient.

3.   The alternatives to transfusion, including the risks and consequences of not receiving this therapy, have been explained to me.

4.   I have had the opportunity to ask questions.

5.   I consent to transfusion(s) as ordered by my physician(s) during my hospitalization.

_____   _____   _____
Signature of Patient   Date   Time

_____   _____   _____
Signature of Parent/Guardian or   Date   Time
Responsible Person (for minors or
patients who are unable to sign)

_____   _____   _____
Witness   Date   Time

MR-2320 (8/91)

FIGURE 8–32 ▲ Consent form for receiving blood transfusion.

11/7/XX mistaken entry W. Andrew CHUC

967-811 MR 243-687 ~~967-801   MR-243-687~~
Kay, JoAnn ~~Kay, JoAnn~~
A. Heart ~~A. Hart~~

NURSES NOTES

F 39 Ortho CHAMPUS ~~F 39 Ortho CHAMPUS~~

DATE TIME	

FIGURE 8–33 ▲ Method for correcting labeling error.

MEDICATION RECORD

Routine Medications

◯ - CIRCLE ALL DOSES NOT GIVEN - STATE REASON IN NURSES NOTES

DATE			11/6/XX	11/7/XX	11/8/XX	11/9/XX	11/10/XX
DAY OF WEEK			Sun.	Mon.	Tues.	Wed.	Thurs.
MEDICATION *11/6/84 mistaken entry* ~~prednisalone~~ *A. Hay. Chuc*			11-7				
			7-3				
DOSE *5 mg*	ROUTE	FREQUENCY	3-11				
MEDICATION *Prednisone*			11-7				
			7-3				
DOSE *5 mg*	ROUTE *p.o.*	FREQUENCY *Bid.*	3-11				
MEDICATION			11-7				
			7-3				
DOSE	ROUTE	FREQUENCY	3-11				
MEDICATION			11-7				
			7-3				
DOSE	ROUTE	FREQUENCY	3-11				
MEDICATION			11-7				
			7-3				
DOSE	ROUTE	FREQUENCY	3-11				
~ICATION			11-7				
	ROUTE	FREQUENCY					

FIGURE 8–34 ▲ Method for correcting a written error on the chart.

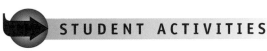

To practice correcting labeling and written errors on a chart form, complete Activities 8–4 and 8–5 in the *Skills Practice Manual.*

■ MAINTAINING THE PATIENT'S CHART

As the person in charge of the clerical duties on the nursing unit, you are responsible for maintaining the patient's chart. The following is a list of duties that will assist you in the maintenance of the patient's chart.

1. Place all charts in proper sequence (usually according to room number) in the chart rack when they are not in use.
2. Place new chart forms in each patient's chart before the immediate need arises. In many health care facilities, this is referred to as "stuffing the chart." Label each chart form with the patient's ID label before placing it in the chart. New chart forms are placed on top of old chart forms for easy access. The new forms may be folded in half to show the old form has not been completely used.
3. Place diagnostic reports in the correct patient's chart behind the correct divider. Match the patient's name on the report with the patient's name on the front of the chart. (Don't depend on room numbers because patients are often transferred to another room.)
4. Review the patient's charts frequently for new orders (always check each chart for new orders prior to returning them to the chart rack).
5. Properly label the patient's chart so that it can easily be located at all times.
6. Check each chart to be sure all the forms are labeled with the correct patient's name. Chart forms should be in the proper sequence.
7. Check the chart frequently for patient information forms or face sheets. Usually five copies are maintained in the chart. Physicians may remove copies for billing purposes. The health unit coordinator may print additional copies of the face sheet from the computer or may order them from admitting.
8. Assist physicians or other professionals in locating the patient's chart.

Splitting or Thinning a Patient's Chart

The chart of a patient who remains in the health care facility for a long time becomes very full and eventually becomes unmanageable. When this occurs, the health unit coordinator may "thin"

or "split" the chart. A doctor's order is not required to thin a patient's chart. To thin the chart, certain categories of chart forms may be removed and placed in an envelope for safekeeping on the unit. The following guidelines will assist you in thinning a patient's chart.

1. Remove older graphic records, nurse's notes, medication forms, and other forms that are no longer needed in the chart binder. (Check the hospital policy and procedure manual to verify forms that may and may not be removed.)
2. Place the removed forms in an envelope.
3. Place the patient's ID label on the outside of the envelope.
4. Write "thinned chart" and record the date with your first initial and last name on the outside of the envelope.
5. Place a label stating that the chart was thinned, along with the date, your first initial, and last name on the front of the patient's chart.

If the patient is transferred to another unit, transfer the thinned-out forms with the patient's chart.

When the patient is discharged, send all the thinned-out forms with the patient's chart to health records.

Reproduction of Chart Forms Containing Patient Information

There are occasions that necessitate the use of a copier to reproduce portions of a patient's chart. For example, when a patient is discharged to another health care facility, to ensure the continuity of care the attending physician requests that specific information on the patient's chart be reproduced. Depending on hospital policy, either the health unit coordinator has the responsibility of copying the chart forms or the patient's chart will be sent to the health records department to be copied. After the forms are reproduced on the copier, the original forms are replaced in the patient's chart and the copied records are sent to the receiving facility.

■ SUMMARY

The chart is a record of care rendered and the patient's response to care during hospitalization. The nursing unit to which the patient is assigned adds forms to the chart. The record is a legal document and should be maintained as such. Standard forms are placed on all patients' charts; supplemental forms may be added according to the need dictated by each patient's treatment and care. The purpose of the forms is the same for each hospital, but the sequence of forms in the chart and the placement of blank forms that are added may differ from hospital to hospital. The information contained in the patient's chart must always be regarded as confidential.

REVIEW QUESTIONS

1. A patient who has been admitted to the health care facility for at least 24 hours for treatment and care is called a/an:

   _____

2. List six duties that will assist the health unit coordinator to properly maintain a patient's chart.

   a. _____

   b. _____

   c. _____

   d. _____

   e. _____

   f. _____

3. State the purpose of the following:

   a. physician's order form:

      _____

   b. graphic record form:

      _____

   c. physician's progress record:

      _____

   d. history and physical form:

      _____

   e. nurse's progress notes:

      _____

   f. medication administration record:

      _____

4. List three standard patient chart forms that are initiated in the admitting department and describe the purpose of each.

   a. _____

   b. _____

   c. _____

5. Define what is meant by a supplemental patient chart form and give two examples of supplemental forms.

   a. definition:

   _____

   b. 1st example:

   _____

   c. 2nd example:

   _____

6. List six reasons for keeping a chart on each patient.

   a. _____

   b. _____

   c. _____

   d. _____

   e. _____

   f. _____

7. A patient receiving care by a health care facility for less than 24 hours is referred to as a/an:

   _____

8. A group of patient chart forms preassembled to be used for new patients is usually called a(n):

   _____

9. Describe how to correct the following errors on a chart form:

   a. a written entry error:

   _____

   b. a labeling error:

   _____

10. 3:30 PM in military time is _____.

11. 2345 military time in standard time is _____.

12. Define the following terms:

   a. stuffing charts:

   _____

   b. "split" or thinned chart:

   _____

   c. patient identification labels:

   _____

   d. name alert:

   _____

   e. allergy labels:

   _____

   f. old record:

   _____

   g. Walla Roo:

   _____

13. List five guidelines for preparing consent forms:

   a. _____

   b. _____

   c. _____

   d. _____

   e. _____

14. List four types of permit or release forms that a patient may be required to sign during his or her hospital stay.

   a. _____

   b. _____

   c. _____

   d. _____

TOPICS FOR DISCUSSION

1. Discuss possible consequences of allowing a stranger access to a patient's chart.

2. Discuss possible consequences of leaving a patient's side rails down without having him or her sign a release.

3. Discuss possible consequences of a patient signing a consent form after he or she has been sedated or adding an additional procedure or changing the wording of a procedure after a patient has signed it.

4. Discuss what would happen if surgery personnel came to pick up the patient for surgery and it was discovered that the wording on the consent form was not exactly the same as the doctor's order.

Transcription of Doctors' Orders

Chapter Objectives

Upon completion of this chapter, you will be able to:

1. Define the terms in the vocabulary list.

2. Describe the health unit coordinator's role in executing doctors' orders.

3. Name two criteria the health unit coordinator can use to recognize a new set of doctors' orders that need transcription.

4. List the four categories of doctors' orders and explain the characteristics of each.

5. Describe the purpose of and process for kardexing.

6. List five areas commonly found on the Kardex form.

7. Describe the purpose of and process for ordering doctors' orders.

8. Name the symbols used in transcribing doctors' orders, and describe the purpose of and process for using each.

9. Describe the purpose of and process for signing-off doctors' orders.

10. Explain why all entries on the doctor's order sheet are recorded in ink.

11. List in order the 10 steps of transcription.

12. Discuss why accuracy is important in the transcription procedure.

13. Discuss the types of errors that may occur during the transcription procedure and the methods of avoidance that may be used.

14. List seven guidelines for recording telephoned doctors' orders.

Vocabulary

Flagging ▲ A method used by the doctor to notify the nursing staff that she or he has written a new set of orders

Kardex File ▲ A portable file that contains and organizes by room number the Kardex forms for each patient on the nursing unit

Kardex Form ▲ A form on which the health unit coordinator records doctors' orders to be used by the nursing staff for a quick reference of the patient's current orders

Kardexing ▲ The process of recording and updating doctors' orders on the Kardex form (many hospitals have eliminated the paper Kardex form in favor of entering all patient orders into the computer)

One-Time or Short-Series Order ▲ A doctor's order that is executed according to the qualifying phrase, and then is automatically discontinued

Ordering ▲ The process of ordering diagnostic procedures, treatments, or supplies from hospital departments other than nursing

Requisition ▲ The form used to order diagnostic procedures, treatments, or supplies from hospital departments other than nursing when the computer is down (also called a downtime requisition)

Set of Doctor's Orders ▲ An entry of doctors' orders made at one time on the doctor's order sheet, dated, notated for time, and signed by the doctor; may include one or more orders

Signing-Off ▲ A process of recording data (date, time, name, and status) on the doctor's order sheet to indicate the completion of transcription of a set of doctor's orders

Standing Order ▲ A doctor's order that remains in effect and is executed as ordered until the doctor discontinues or changes it

Standing PRN Order ▲ Same as a standing order, except that it is executed according to the patient's needs

Stat Order ▲ A doctor's order that is to be executed immediately, then automatically discontinued

Symbols ▲ Notations written in black or red ink on the doctor's order sheet to indicate completion of a step of the transcription procedure

Telephoned Orders ▲ Orders for a patient telephoned to a health care facility by the doctor

■ DOCTORS' ORDERS

During the patient's stay in a health care facility, the doctor's orders for a patient's care are expressed in handwriting or preprinted on the doctor's order sheet. In some hospitals, doctors enter their orders into a computer. These orders include such things as diagnostic procedures, medications, surgical treatment, diet, patient activities, discharge, and so forth. As you will recall from Chapter 8, written doctors' orders are legal documents and become a permanent record of the patient's chart.

The doctor writes all of the orders in ink, writes the date and time, and signs each entry. The doctor may write one order or a series of orders; this is referred to as a *set of doctor's orders*. The doctor indicates to the nursing staff that he or she has written a new set of orders by *flagging* the chart. Flagging techniques vary among health care facilities. New orders can also be identified by absence of symbols, and absence of sign-off information. See Figure 9–1 for an example of a set of written doctor's orders. Sometimes the doctor may write new orders and forget to flag the chart. Always check for new orders before returning a chart from the counter into the chart rack.

If the new orders are recorded at the top of the doctor's order sheet, check the previous sheet to see if the orders are continued. When orders are recorded near the bottom of the doctor's order sheet, make diagonal lines across the remaining space so new orders will not be recorded there, and then continue on the following page. When this happens it is easy to miss the orders at the bottom of the first page (Fig. 9–2).

Recording Telephoned Doctors' Orders

Many health care facilities have a policy that states only the registered nurses can record telephoned doctors' orders. However, policies vary and some hospitals may allow the health unit coordinator to record telephoned doctors' orders. Since you may have the responsibility of recording doctors' or-

Physician's Order Sheet

	Joint, Jane	MR: 168495
	Acct#: 428975	DOB: 04-16-42
	DOA: 09-16-03	Dr.: T. Arthro
	Serv: Med Fe	Rm: 318-2

Date Ordered	Physician's Orders
6-4-00	CBR (Complete bed rest*)
10:45 AM	CBC (Complete blood count, laboratory tests*)
	consultation with Dr. F.L. Payne
	please call
	Dr J. Arthro

FIGURE 9–1 ▲ Example of a set of written doctor's orders. *Note:* The typed interpretations of the abbreviations shown with an asterisk here and in subsequent figures are included for your information only and would not be seen on a typical set of orders. These abbreviations will be covered in succeeding chapters.

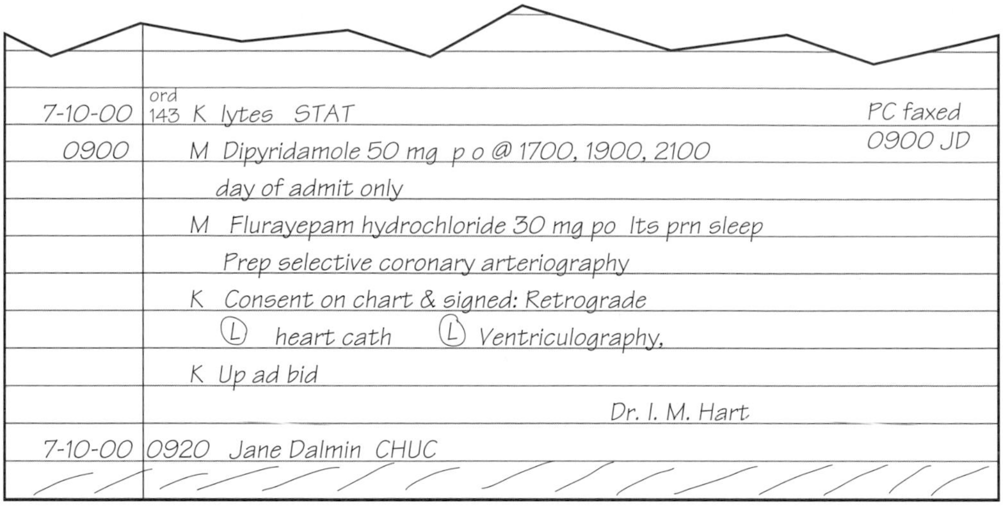

7-10-00	ord 143 K lytes STAT	PC faxed
0900	M Dipyridamole 50 mg p o @ 1700, 1900, 2100	0900 JD
	day of admit only	
	M Flurayepam hydrochloride 30 mg po lts prn sleep	
	Prep selective coronary arteriography	
	K Consent on chart & signed: Retrograde	
	Ⓛ heart cath Ⓛ Ventriculography,	
	K Up ad bid	
	Dr. I. M. Hart	
7-10-00	0920 Jane Dalmin CHUC	

Physician's Orders

FIGURE 9–2 ▲ Diagonal lines drawn at the bottom of a nearly filled doctor's order sheet.

ders, we are including guidelines and exercises for the practice of those guidelines. The activities in the Skills Practice Manual will also assist you in reading and understanding doctors' orders.

Recording of doctors' orders is a serious matter; error could cause harm to the patient. Accuracy is an absolute must. Use the following guidelines to ensure accuracy in recording the orders.

Guidelines for Recording Doctors' Orders

1. Make sure you have the correct chart. Check both the chart spine and the patient ID label on the doctor's order sheet.

2. Begin recording the orders directly below the last entry on the doctor's order sheet (sign-off of last set of orders). In other words, do not leave a space between your entry and the last entry.

3. Record the orders in ink.

4. Record the date and time.

5. Record each order as the doctor states it. Do not hesitate to ask questions if you do not understand what is being said.

6. Read the entire set of orders back to the doctor. *Do not skip any part of this step.*

7. Sign the orders as shown in Figure 9–3.

The doctor is expected to cosign the orders within 24 hours.

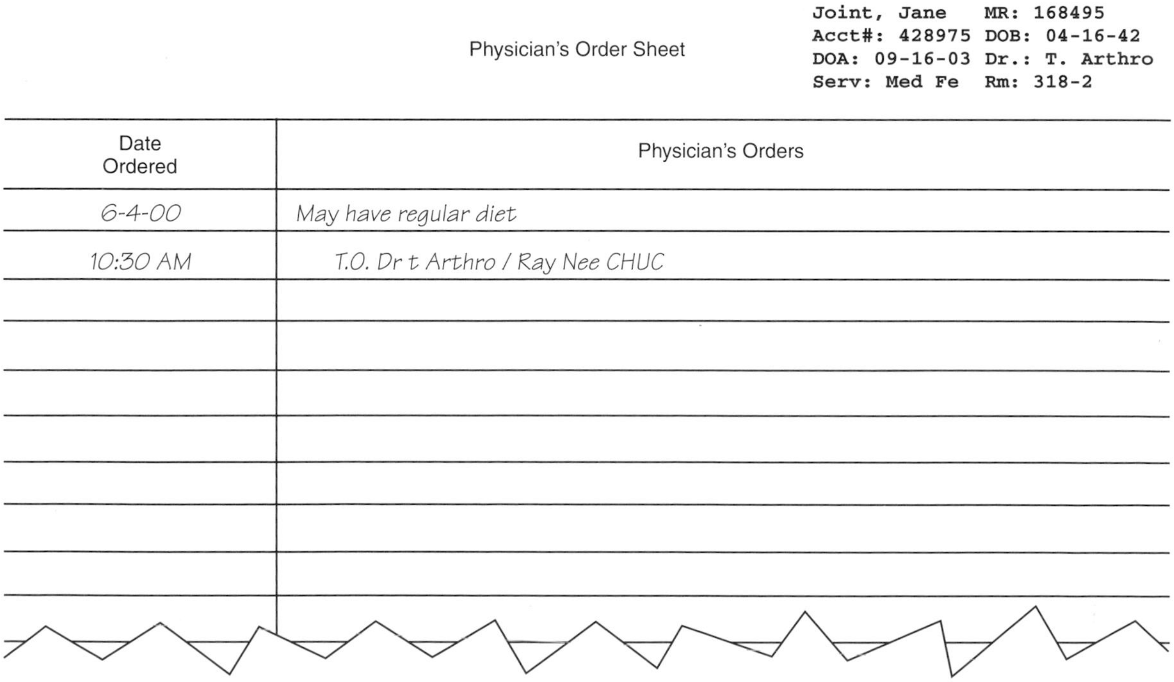

Physician's Order Sheet

```
Joint, Jane    MR: 168495
Acct#: 428975 DOB: 04-16-42
DOA: 09-16-03 Dr.: T. Arthro
Serv: Med Fe  Rm: 318-2
```

Date Ordered	Physician's Orders
6-4-00	May have regular diet
10:30 AM	T.O. Dr t Arthro / Ray Nee CHUC

FIGURE 9–3 ▲ Example of a telephoned doctor's order recorded by a certified health unit coordinator.

Categories of Doctors' Orders

Doctors' orders may be categorized according to when they are carried out and the length of time they are in effect. The transcription procedure varies according to the category of the order; therefore, it is necessary for you to be able to recognize each category. The four categories are: (1) standing, or continuing, orders, (2) standing, or continuing, PRN orders, (3) one-time, or short-series orders, and (4) stat orders.

Standing (Continuing) Orders

The majority of doctors' orders fall into this group. Standing orders are in effect and executed routinely as ordered until they are discontinued or changed by a written doctor's order. For example, in the order:

- *BP lying, sitting, and standing tid*

the doctor has ordered the patient's blood pressure (BP) to be taken with the patient lying, sitting, and standing and recorded three times a day (tid). A time sequence such as 0800, 1400, and 2000 is set up for the blood pressure to be taken daily. This routine continues until changed or discontinued by the doctor. Another example of a standing order:

- *Regular diet*

This order means that the patient receives a regular diet each day of his or her hospital stay unless the order is changed or discontinued by the doctor.

Standing (Continuing) PRN Orders

The Latin words *pro re nata,* meaning "as circumstances may require," are abbreviated as *prn* and are used by the doctor in a written order to indicate that the order is to be executed as needed. Standing prn orders, like standing orders, are in effect until changed or discontinued by the doctor. They differ from standing orders in that they are executed according to the patient's needs. For example, in the order:

- *Acetaminophen 325 mg $\bar{1}$ or $\bar{11}$ PO q 4h prn headache*

the nurse may give 325-mg $\bar{1}$ or $\bar{11}$ capsules as often as every 4 hours (q 4h) as needed by the patient to relieve a headache. This does not mean the patient necessarily receives the medication every 4 hours, because he or she may not have a headache at those times; therefore, it is impossible to set up a time sequence as we discussed with the standing order.

In the order:

- *Compazine 10 mg IM q 6h for nausea or vomiting*

the doctor uses a qualifying phrase, *for nausea or vomiting,* to indicate it is a prn order.

Remember: A prn order may be recognized either by the abbreviation prn or by the content of a qualifying phrase and is in effect until changed or discontinued by the doctor.

One-Time or Short-Series Order

The doctor may want a treatment or medication carried out once only or for a short series. This is indicated by a qualifying phrase, such as *give at 2:00 PM* or *give tonight and in AM.* Upon comple-

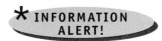

tion of the one time or short series, the order is automatically discontinued. For example, in the order:

- *Give patient Fleets enema this PM*

this PM makes it a one-time order—thus, the order is discontinued after the enema is given.

Here is another example; in the order:

- *Blood pressure q 2h until awake*

until awake makes it a short-series order.

Remember: A one-time or short-series order may be recognized by the content of the qualifying phrase and is automatically discontinued after completion.

Stat Orders

Stat is the abbreviation for the Latin word *statim,* which means "at once." When included in a doctor's order it indicates that the order is to be carried out immediately. Stat orders are usually written during an emergency or for patients who are critically ill. Because of the urgency of stat orders, they are communicated to the nurse and/or department personnel responsible for carrying out the order immediately. Stat orders are transcribed first when included in a set of orders. Stat orders are recognized by the word *stat* included in the order, for example:

- *CBC stat*

In the orders:

- *CBC now (or CBC immediately)*

the words *now* and *immediately* are usually considered to indicate stat orders that should receive urgent attention.

The Kardex File and Kardex Form

Each nursing unit may maintain a portable file, often referred to as the Kardex. The Kardex file contains the Kardex forms, one for each patient on the unit. Approximately 15 to 20 individual patient Kardex forms are contained in one Kardex file; large nursing units of 30 or more patients may maintain two Kardex files. Patient information such as room number, name, doctor's name, and diagnosis is recorded at the bottom of the Kardex form, so that, when filed in the Kardex file, this information remains visible for each location of each patient's Kardex form (Fig. 9–4).

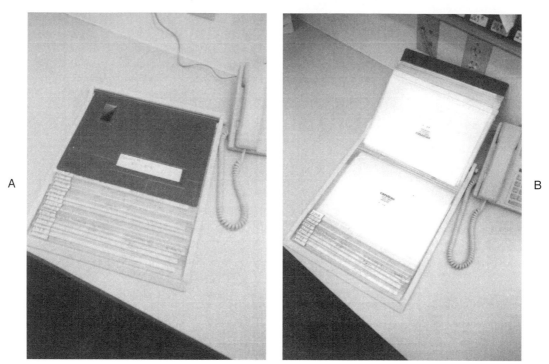

FIGURE 9–4 ▲ A portable file (a Kardex) as it appears closed, *A*, and open, *B*.

Kardex Form

Activity	Date Ord	Treatments	Date Ord	Laboratory	Date Ord	Allergies	
						Diagnostic Imaging	Date to
Diet							be Done
Vital signs							
Weight							
IV		Respiratory Care		Pre OP Orders		Diagnostic Studies	
				Daily Lab			
I & O							
Retention Cath (Foley)		Physical Medicine					
☐ Health Records _____							
Adm. Date		Consultations:		Surgery: Date:			
Name	Doctor	Age		Diagnosis		Date of admission	

FIGURE 9–5 ▲ A Kardex form.

Five main areas common to most Kardex forms are listed below.

1. Activity
2. Diet
3. Vital sign frequency
4. Treatment
5. Diagnostic studies

Other areas, such as intravenous therapy, intake and output, and weight, are also usually included on the form.

The Kardex form may also include an area for a patient care plan. The nursing staff completes this area. The purpose of the Kardex is to maintain a current profile of a patient's information, his or her doctor's orders, and the patient's nursing needs. It provides a quick reference for the nursing staff, and it is also used for planning and designating patient care and for reporting patient information to the oncoming shift. The design of the Kardex form varies according to hospital and nursing unit needs. However, the basic concept remains constant. See Figure 9–5 for a typical Kardex form.

Note: Many hospitals are using a computerized kardexing system, eliminating the need for the Kardex form and the Kardex file.

Kardexing

Kardexing is the process of recording all new doctor's orders onto each patient's Kardex form. The purpose of kardexing all the doctors' orders is to communicate new orders to the nursing staff and to update the patient's profile on the Kardex form. Kardexing is usually done in pencil, since new doctors' orders may involve

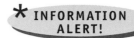

★ INFORMATION ALERT!

Many hospitals have eliminated the paper Kardex form in favor of entering all patient orders into the computer. A summary sheet may then be printed for each patient, showing current and active orders.

changing or discontinuing an existing order. However, information not subject to change, such as the patient's name, is usually recorded in black ink and allergies are always recorded in red ink.

Accuracy in kardexing is absolutely essential. An error could result in the patient receiving the wrong, and perhaps harmful, treatment. The patient's Kardex form is usually not considered a legal document and in the past it was usually discarded when the patient was discharged from the hospital. However, the present trend is toward filing the nursing care plan portion of the Kardex form with the patient's chart in the health records department.

Ordering

Ordering is the process of inputting the doctor's orders into the computer or of copying the doctor's order onto a requisition (Fig. 9–6). Whichever method is used, the purpose of ordering is to forward the doctor's orders to the various hospital departments that will execute the orders.

Doctor Ordering_____ □ Stat
Today's Date_____ □ T/Stat
Draw @ Date_____Time_____ □ Routine
Collected Date_____ _Time_____
Collected by_____
Request by_____

Hematology	**Serology**	**Urinalysis/Urine Chemistry**
□ Bleeding Time, Ivy	□ ANA	□ Routine Ua
□ CBC c̄ Diff	□ ASO Titer	□ Amylase (2hr)
□ CBC c̄ Manual Diff	□ CEA	□ Bilirubin
□ Factor VIII	□ CMV	□ Calcium
□ Fibrinogen	□ IgG	□ Chloride
□ HCT	□ IgM	□ Creatinine Clearance
□ HGB	□ Cocci Screen	□ Glucose Tolerance
□ H & H	□ EBV Panel	□ Nitrogen
□ Eosinophil Ct Absolute	□ Enterovirus Ab Panel 1	□ Occult Blood
□ Eosinophil Smear	□ Enterovirus Ab Panel 2	□ Osmolality
□ ESR	□ HbsAb	□ Phosphorus
□ LE Cell Prep	□ HbsAg	□ Potassium
□ Platelet Ct	□ HIV	□ Pregnancy
□ PT	□ Monospot	□ Protein
□ PTT (APTT)	□ PSA Screen	□ Sodium
□ RBC	□ Ra Factor	□ Sp Gravity
□ RBC Indicies	□ RPR	□ Uric Acid
□ Reticulocyte Ct	□ RSV	□ Other_____
□ Sickle Cell Prep	□ Rubella Screen	
□ WBC	□ Streptozyme	
□ Other_____	□ VDRL	
	□ Other_____	

Write in Orders:_____

_____

Revised 11/26/02

FIGURE 9–6 ▲ Example of a laboratory ordering screen.

Doctors' orders that involve diagnostic procedures, treatment, or supplies other than nursing usually require the ordering step. Ordering by computer requires the health unit coordinator to select the patient's name from a computer screen and follow the steps to input the ordering information (according to the hospital computer program used). Ordering by requisition requires the health unit coordinator first to affix that patient's ID label on the requisition and, second, to copy or fill in all the pertinent data from the doctor's orders.

Symbols

As the health unit coordinator completes a part of the transcription procedure, he or she places a *symbol* on the doctor's order sheet to indicate completion of the task. The symbol is written in black or red ink, depending on hospital policy, in front of the doctor's order (Fig. 9–7).

By using symbols, the health unit coordinator has a written record of the steps completed and reduces the possibility of omitting or forgetting to complete a part of the transcription procedure. There are constant interruptions, which would make it easy to forget where you left off when returning to transcribing a set of orders. Omission can cause delay in treatment, which may slow down or be harmful to the patient's recovery.

The following list of symbols will be used in this textbook; however, symbols vary among hospitals. Your instructor, therefore, may wish you to become familiar with a different set of symbols commonly used in hospitals in your area.

PC sent or faxed: Indicates that the pharmacy copy of the doctor's order sheet was forwarded to the pharmacy. Record the time the copy was sent and your initials.

Ord: Indicates diagnostic tests, treatments, or supplies have been ordered by either computer or requisition. When using the computer method, record the computer order number above each ordered item.

K: Indicates the order has been transcribed on the patient's Kardex form. It is also used to indicate that a discontinued order has been erased from the Kardex. Each order kardexed requires the date and its own line on the Kardex.

M: Indicates transcription of a medication order on the medication administration record form (MAR).

Called (name and time): Indicates completion of a telephone call necessary to complete the doctor's order. Document the time of call, the name of the person you spoke to, and your initials above the order on the doctor's order sheet.

Notified (name and time): Indicates that the appropriate health care team member has been notified of a *stat* order. Document the time of notification, the name of the person you spoke to, and your initials above the order on the doctor's order sheet.

Signing Off Doctors' Orders

Signing off is the process used to indicate completion of the transcription procedure of a set of a doctor's orders. To sign off, the health unit coordinator records the date, time, and his or her full name and status (may use the abbreviation *SHUC* if a student HUC or *CHUC* if certified) on the line directly below the doctor's signature, as shown in Figure 9–8. Once again, this is done in black or red ink, because the doctor's order sheet is a legal document. In some hospitals a registered nurse is required to cosign the transcribed orders. Some hospitals use the *independent transcription method*, meaning that the registered nurse does not

Physician's Order Sheet	Joint, Jane MR: 168495 Acct#: 428975 DOB: 04-16-42 DOA: 09-16-03 Dr.: T. Arthro Serv: Med Fe Rm: 318-2

Date Ordered	Physician's Orders
6-4-00 10am K	CBR (Complete bed rest*)
#254 ord K	CBC (Complete blood count, laboratory test*)
K	Consultation with Dr. TL Payne
Called Pat 1005	please call
Mary Smith	Dr. T. Arthro

FIGURE 9–7 ▲ Example of a doctor's order sheet with the transcription symbols recorded.

	Physician's Order Sheet	Joint, Jane	MR: 168495
		Acct#: 428975	DOB: 04-16-42
		DOA: 09-16-03	Dr.: T. Arthro
		Serv: Med Fe	Rm: 318-2

Date Ordered	Physician's Orders
6-4-00 10am K	CBR (Complete bed rest*)
#254 ord K	CBC (Complete blood count, laboratory test*)
K	Consultation with Dr. TL Payne
Called Pat 1005	please call
Mary Smith	Dr. T. Arthro
6-4-00	1005 Ella Bow/CHUC

FIGURE 9–8 ▲ Example of a transcribed set of doctor's orders, showing HUC's sign-off data.

cosign the doctor's orders. He or she may sign the orders to indicate he or she has read them. All hospitals require the registered nurses to perform 24-hour chart checks in which they will sign off on their assigned patients.

The sign-off procedure varies among health care facilities. For example, some health care facilities use black ink for the sign-off procedure. Some hospitals use red ink to distinguish the sign-off information from the written doctor's orders, and some require the health unit coordinator to draw a line to box off the orders when signing off.

■ TRANSCRIPTION OF DOCTORS' ORDERS

Transcription of doctors' orders is a written process used to communicate doctors' orders to the nursing staff and other hospital departments. The transcription procedure includes kardexing, ordering, using symbols, the signing-off process, and sometimes other steps. How the health unit coordinator goes about performing this procedure varies among health care facilities and from individual to individual.

Ten Steps for Transcription of Doctors' Orders

For learning purposes we have outlined 10 steps that make up the transcription procedure. It is important to note that each type of doctors' orders may require some or all of the steps to complete the transcription procedure. Always compare each order with the 10 steps of transcription when choosing the steps that

are required for complete transcription of each order. Using this procedure allows for the simplest yet most efficient method for transcribing doctors' orders.

The following 10 steps of transcription will assist you in transcribing doctors' orders efficiently and accurately.

1. Read the complete set of doctors' orders.
2. Order medications by sending or faxing the pharmacy copy of the doctor's order sheet to the pharmacy department.
3. Complete all stat orders.
4. Place telephone calls as necessary to complete the doctor's orders.
5. Select the patient's name from the census on the computer screen or collect all necessary forms.
6. Order diagnostic tests, treatments, and supplies.
7. Kardex all the doctor's orders except medication orders.
8. Complete medication orders by writing them on the MAR.
9. Recheck your performance of each step for accuracy and thoroughness.
10. Sign-off the completed set of the doctor's orders.

Procedure 9–1 describes carrying out the 10 steps of transcription.

Avoiding Transcription Errors

Throughout this chapter we have mentioned the importance of accuracy during the transcription procedure, so errors that may cause serious harm to the patient can be avoided. Consider, for example, the consequences of the health unit coordinator, during the transcription procedure, overlooking a doctor's order for the patient to have a stat medication, or the consequences of a

Text continued on page 172

Procedure 9–1: TRANSCRIPTION OF DOCTORS' ORDERS

STEP TASK	NOTES
1. Read the complete set of doctor's orders.	**1.** *Reading the complete set of orders gives an overview of the task at hand. Accurate reading and interpretation of each word of the doctor's orders are vital, since each word or abbreviation carries a specific meaning.*

2. Order medications.
  a. Remove and send the pharmacy copy of the doctor's order sheet or fax original copy of doctor's order sheet to the pharmacy.
  b. Write PC sent or faxed, time, and your initials on the doctor's order sheet (Fig. 9–9, *B*).
	2. *Sending a copy or faxing a copy of the original doctor's order to the pharmacy helps avoid medication errors because no rewriting is involved. Completing this step first allows for the patient to receive the medication as soon as possible.*

3. Complete all stat orders.	**3.** *Stat orders are always transcribed first.*
4. Place telephone calls as necessary to complete the doctor's orders. Upon completing this task, write the symbol *called* and the time called (be sure to include AM or PM or use military time) and the name of the person receiving the call in ink in front of the doctor's order on the doctor's order sheet (Fig. 9–10).	**4.** *Doctors' orders may require you to place a telephone call to another department or health agency to schedule appointments, procedures, etc. Recording the person's name receiving the call is helpful if a follow-up is necessary.*
5. Select the patient's name from the census on the computer screen and collect all necessary forms.	**5.** *This varies according to the type of doctors' orders included in the set. Collecting all forms at once saves time.*

6. Order all diagnostic tests, treatments, and supplies.
Computer method: (see Figure 9–9)
  a. Select patient's name from the census on the view screen.
	6. *This step includes ordering diagnostic procedures, and treatments and ordering supplies form hospital departments other than the nursing department.*
	   Check both the patient's name and hospital number with the same information on the chart back label.

b. Select the department from the department menu on the viewing screen.	
c. Select the test, treatment, or supply from the menu on the viewing screen.	
d. Fill in required information.	
e. Order test, treatments, or supplies.	
f. Write the symbol *ord* or computer number in ink in front of the doctor's order on the doctor's order sheet.	
Requisition Method	
a. Affix the patient's ID label to the requisition	*Selection of the correct patient's label is absolutely essential. The wrong selection could easily cause a patient to receive a diagnostic test or treatment intended for another patient. Always compare the name and patient's hospital number you have labeled on the requisition form with the same information on the chart back label. Remember: There may be more than one patient on the unit with the same last name. Label all requisitions at the same time.*

Procedure 9-1: TRANSCRIPTION OF DOCTORS' ORDERS—cont'd

STEP	TASK	NOTES

b. Place a checkmark on the requisition to indicate the test, treatment, or supply being requisitioned.

c. Fill in today's date and the date the test or treatment is to be done in the appropriate spaces.

d. Write in pertinent data, such as, "patient blind" or "isolation."

e. Sign your name and status in the appropriate space on the requisition form.

f. Write the symbol *ord* in ink in front of the doctor's order on the doctor's order sheet. (see Fig. 9–9, *B*)

7. Kardex all the doctors' orders. Begin with the first order, then proceed to the next until all the orders are completed (Fig. 9–11, *A*). Complete kardexing by:

a. Writing the date followed by the order in pencil under the correct column of the Kardex form. Carefully read what is already written in the column to evaluate whether the new order cancels an existing order. If this occurs, erase the existing order. If an order is discontinued, erase it from the Kardex.

b. Write the symbol *K* in ink in front of the doctor's order on the doctors' order sheet (Fig. 9–11, *B*)

8. Complete medication orders by:

a. Writing the medication order on the medication administration record.

b. Placing the symbol *M* in ink in front of the doctor's order on the doctors' order sheet.

9. Recheck your performance of each task for accuracy and thoroughness.

10. Sign off the completed set of orders by writing the following in ink on the line directly below the doctor's signature:

a. Date

b. Time

c. Full signature

d. Status

Figure 9-12 provides an example of this step.

NOTES

7. *Nursing orders that need to be implemented during the shift are often recorded on a clipboard in order to bring them to the immediate attention of the nurse.*

Remember: All doctors' orders are kardexed. Make sure you have selected the right patient's Kardex forms; many patients' Kardex forms are filed in one Kardex file. To ensure accurate selection, check the names of the patient and doctor on the Kardex form with the labeled information on the chart back label.

Remember: There may be more than one patient on the unit with the same last name.

Note: Many hospitals are using a computerized Kardexing system.

8. *This procedure is covered in more detail in Chapter 13.*

10. *It is important that you have completed all the tasks of transcription before signing off.*

A

Doctor Ordering ___T. Arthro___   □ Stat
Today's Date ___6/4/00___   □ T/Stat
Draw @ Date _____ Time_____   ☒ Routine
Collected Date ___6/4/00___ Time ___1430___
Collected by ___J. Jackson___
Request by ___E. Bow___

Joint, Jane   MR: 168495
Acct#: 428975   DOA: 09-16-03   Dr.: T. Arthro
Serv: Med Fe   Rm: 318-2

Hematology	Serology	Urinalysis/Urine Chemistry
□ Bleeding Time, Ivy	□ ANA	□ Routine Ua
☒ CBC c̄ Diff	□ ASO Titer	□ Amylase (2hr)
□ CBC c̄ Manual Diff	□ CEA	□ Bilirubin
□ Factor VIII	□ CMV	□ Calcium
□ Fibrinogen	□ IgG	□ Chloride
□ HCT	□ IgM	□ Creatinine Clearance
□ HGB	□ Cocci Screen	□ Glucose Tolerance
□ H & H	□ EBV Panel	□ Nitrogen
□ Eosinophil Ct Absolute	□ Enterovirus Ab Panel 1	□ Occult Blood
□ Eosinophil Smear	□ Enterovirus Ab Panel 2	□ Osmolality
□ ESR	□ HbsAb	□ Phosphorus
□ LE Cell Prep	□ HbsAg	□ Potassium
□ Platelet Ct	□ HIV	□ Pregnancy
□ PT	□ Monospot	□ Protein
□ PTT (APTT)	□ PSA Screen	□ Sodium
□ RBC	□ Ra Factor	□ Sp Gravity
□ RBC Indicies	□ RPR	□ Uric Acid
□ Reticulocyte Ct	□ RSV	□ Other_____
□ Sickle Cell Prep	□ Rubella Screen	
□ WBC	□ Streptozyme	
□ Other_____	□ VDRL	
	□ Other_____	

Write in Orders: _____

_____

Revised 11/26/02

B

Physician's Order Sheet

Joint, Jane   MR: 168495
Acct#: 428975   DOB: 04-16-42
DOA: 09-16-03   Dr.: T. Arthro
Serv: Med Fe   Rm: 318-2

Date Ordered	Physician's Orders	PC Faxed
6-4-00 2 PM	CBR (Complete bed rest*)	1410 EB
#254 ord	CBC (Complete blood count, laboratory test*)	
Called Pat 1405	consultation with Dr. TL Payne. Please call	
Mary Smith	Fowler's position	
	wt daily (wt: weight*)	
	rectal temp. q4h (q4h: every 4 hours*)	
	intake and output	
	Compazine 10 mg IM q4h nausea or vomiting	
	Dr. T. Arthro	

FIGURE 9–9 ▲ Example of using the symbol to indicate that the pharmacy copy has been faxed (step 2 of the transcription procedure), and example of requisitioning (step 6 of the transcription procedure). A, Completed laboratory ordering screen. B, Symbols recorded on the doctor's order sheet to show completion of step 6.

Physician's Order Sheet

Joint, Jane   MR: 168495
Acct#: 428975   DOB: 04-16-42
DOA: 09-16-03   Dr.: T. Arthro
Serv: Med Fe   Rm: 318-2

Date Ordered	Physician's Orders	PC Faxed
6-4-00 2 PM	CBR (Complete bed rest*)	1410 EB
#251 ord	CBC (Complete blood count, laboratory test*)	
Called Pat 1405	consultation with Dr. TL Payne, please call	
Mary Smith	Fowler's position	
	wt daily (wt: weight*)	
	rectal temp q4h (q4h: every 4 hours*)	
	intake and output	
	Compazine 10 mg. IM q4h nausea or vomiting	
	Dr. T. Arthro	

FIGURE 9–10 ▲ Example of using the symbol for placing a telephone call, step 4 of the transcription procedure.

Kardex Form

Activity 6-4-00	Date Ord	Treatments	Date Ord	Laboratory	Date Ord	Allergies	
CBR			6-4	CBC			
Fowler's position							
						Diagnostic Imaging	To be
Diet							Done
Vital signs 6-4-00							
®temp q4h							
Weight							
6-4-00 daily							
IV		Respiratory Care		Pre OP Orders		Diagnostic Studies	
				Daily Lab			
I & O							
6-4-00							
Retention Cath (Foley) ☐ Health Records ___		Physical Medicine					
Adm. Date 6-4-00		Consultations: 6-4-00 Dr. T. L. Payne		Surgery: Date:			

Name Joint, Jane L.   Doctor T. Arthro   Age 25   Diagnosis Arthritis   Date of admission

A

Physician's Order Sheet

Joint, Jane   MR: 168495
Acct#: 428975   DOB: 04-16-42
DOA: 09-16-03   Dr.: T. Arthro
Serv: Med Fe   Rm: 318-2

Date Ordered		Physician's Orders	PC Faxed
6-4-00 2 PM K	CBR	(Complete bed rest*)	1410 FB
#251 ord K	CBC (Complete blood count, laboratory test*)		
Called Pat 1410 K	consultation with Dr. TL Payne, please call		
Mary Smith K	Fowler's position		
K	wt daily (wt: weight*)		
K	rectal temp q4h (q4h: every 4 hours*)		
K	intake and output		
M	Compazine 10 mg. IM q4h nausea or vomiting		
	Dr. T. Arthro		

B

FIGURE 9–11 ▲ An example of kardexing, step 7 of the transcription procedure. A, The doctor's orders are recorded in pencil on the Kardex form. B, The symbols recorded on the doctor's order sheet to show completion of step 7.

Physician's Order Sheet

Joint, Jane   MR: 168495
Acct#: 428975   DOB: 04-16-42
DOA: 09-16-03   Dr.: T. Arthro
Serv: Med Fe   Rm: 318-2

Date Ordered		Physician's Orders	PC Faxed
6-4-00 2 PM K	CBR	(Complete bed rest*)	1410 EB
#25.7 ord K	CBC (Complete blood count, laboratory test*)		
Called Pat 1410 K	consultation with Dr. TL Payne, please call		
Mary Smith K	Fowler's position		
K	wt daily (wt: weight*)		
K	rectal temp q4h (q4h: every 4 hours*)		
K	intake and output		
M	Compazine 10 mg. IM q4h nausea or vomiting		
	Dr. T. Arthro		
6-4-00	1420 Ella Bow CHUC		

FIGURE 9–12 ▲ Example of a transcribed set of doctor's orders, showing step 10 of the transcription procedure, the signing-off of a doctor's orders.

TABLE 9–1	Avoiding Transcription Errors	
Type of Error	**Method of Avoidance**	
Errors of Omission	1. Read and understand each word of doctors' orders. If in doubt, check with a patient's nurse or the doctor.	
	2. Use symbols. It is especially important for you to write the symbol after you have completed each step of transcription.	
	3. When new orders are recorded at the top of the doctors' order sheet, check the previous order sheet to see if these orders are continued from the previous page.	
	4. If the set of orders finishes near the bottom of the doctors' order sheet, cross through the remaining space with diagonal lines. This is done so that newly written orders will begin at the top of the new doctors' order form. When orders are recorded at the bottom of one page and continued on the next, it is easy to miss transcribing those recorded on the first page.	
	5. Record the signing off information on the line directly below the doctor's signature to avoid leaving space in which future orders could be written and missed.	
	6. Check for new orders before returning a chart from the counter or elsewhere to the chart rack.	
Errors of Interpretation	1. When in doubt about the correct interpretation of doctors' orders, always check with the registered nurse or the doctor.	
Errors in the Selection of the Patient's ID label or Errors in Selection of the Patient's name on the Computer Screen	1. Compare the patient's name and the hospital number on the patient's ID you have placed on the order requisition form or selected on the computer screen with the same information on the patient's chart cover. Never select computer labels by the patient's room number only. *Note:* Many people on the nursing staff use the computer to retrieve information and may change screens while you are transcribing orders. Always double-check the name on the screen when entering orders into the computer.	
Errors in the Selection of the Patient's Kardex Form	1. Compare the patient's name and the doctor's name on the Kardex form with the same information on the label on the patient's chart cover. Do not use the information on the doctors' order sheet. It may have the wrong information on it. Never select by using room number alone. If the patient has been transferred, the room number imprinted on chart forms may no longer be correct. *Note:* Many people on the nursing staff use the Kardex for a quick reference and may flip to another patient's Kardex form while you are transcribing orders. Remove the Kardex form from the holder when transcribing orders and return it to its proper place in the Kardex holder when you are finished.	
Errors in Reading the Doctor's Poor Handwriting	1. When you cannot read an order because of the doctor's handwriting, refer to the progress record form in the patient's chart. The orders are often recorded on this form also, and using this information may assist you in interpreting the orders on the physicians' order form. If the order remains unclear, ask the doctor who wrote it for clarification. Don't waste time asking others. They may be guessing also. If a doctor has a reputation for poor handwriting, ask him or her to wait while you read the orders so he or she can clarify orders that you can't read.	

How to Avoid Errors of Transcription

- Ask the doctor or nurse for assistance if you cannot read or understand a doctor's order.
- Use patient information from the chart cover to select the computer screen or patient ID label.
- Record the sign-off information on the line directly below the doctor's signature.
- Check the previous page for orders when the orders begin at the top of the page.
- Void space if three or more lines are left at the bottom of the doctor's order sheet.

health unit coordinator ordering a diet for a patient who has been ordered by the doctor to have nothing by mouth for a pending surgery or procedure.

Table 9–1 outlines the types of errors that may occur during the transcription procedure and methods you may use to avoid making these errors.

■ SUMMARY

Transcription of doctors' orders is the single most responsible task you perform as a health unit coordinator. An error may result in a patient being harmed or his or her recovery time being extended. You owe it both to the patient and the health care facility to complete the transcription procedure promptly, accurately, and thoroughly.

REVIEW QUESTIONS

1. Why are symbols used as a part of the transcription procedure?

   _____

2. Demonstrate how you as the health unit coordinator would sign-off a set of a doctor's orders.

   _____

   _____

3. List *in order* the 10 steps of transcription.

   a. _____

   b. _____

   c. _____

   d. _____

   e. _____

   f. _____

   g. _____

   h. _____

   i. _____

   j. _____

4. Explain why doctors' orders, symbols, and sign-offs are recorded in ink on each doctor's order sheet.

   _____

   _____

5. Symbols are recorded on the doctor's order sheet (circle one):

   a. after the step of transcription is completed

   b. before the step of transcription is completed

   c. at any time, as long as they are recorded accurately

   d. after the patient's nurse has verified that the step of transcription is complete

6. List two ways that the health unit coordinator would recognize newly written doctors' orders that need transcription.

   a. _____

   b. _____

7. Why are doctors' orders recorded on the Kardex form?

   _____

8. Why are doctors' orders written on the Kardex form in pencil?

   _____

9. Define the following terms:

   a. ordering: _____

   b. kardexing: _____

   c. requisition: _____

   d. flagging: _____

10. Regarding the doctor's order sheet:

    a. Which line of the doctor's order sheet is used for the signing-off procedure?

    _____

    b. Why?

    _____

11. Why is accuracy necessary in the transcription procedure?

    _____

12. Write in the symbol used to indicate completion of the following:

    a. ordering   _____

    b. writing of a medication order on the MAR   _____

    c. kardexing   _____

    d. telephone call   _____

    e. pharmacy copy sent or faxed   _____

    f. notification to appropriate person of a stat order _____

13. When is it necessary to use the ordering step when transcribing doctors' orders?

    _____

14. List five areas commonly found on a Kardex form.

    a. _____

    b. _____

c. _____

d. _____

e. _____

15. List the four categories of doctors' orders and write a brief description of each.

a. _____

b. _____

c. _____

d. _____

16. Identify each type (category) of order written below.

a. blood pressure q 3h until alert _____

b. morphine 8–12 mg IM q 3–4h prn pain _____

c. diazepam 10 mg PO now _____

d. Premarin 1.25 mg PO daily _____

e. regular diet _____

f. Fleets enema this PM and repeat in AM _____

17. How would a stat order be identified?

_____

18. Describe precautions you would take to avoid making the following transcription errors:

a. errors of omission (missing written doctors' orders):

_____

b. errors of interpretation (not understanding the written doctors' orders):

_____

c. errors in the selection of the patient's ID label or errors in the selection of the patient's name on the computer screen:

_____

d. errors in the selection of the patient's Kardex form:

_____

e. errors in reading the doctor's poor handwriting:

_____

19. List the seven guidelines for recording telephoned doctors' orders.

a. _____

b. _____

c. _____

d. _____

e. _____

f. _____

g. _____

TOPICS FOR DISCUSSION

1. Discuss the possible consequences of a medication being written on the wrong patient's medication administration record.

2. While transcribing a set of a doctor's orders, you place an "ord" symbol above an order for a chest x-ray prior to actually entering the order into the computer. A doctor asks you to help her find a chart and someone borrows the chart you have been working on before you have an opportunity to complete the orders. Discuss what could happen when the chart is returned and you finish transcribing the orders.

Patient Activity, Patient Positioning, and Nursing Observation Orders

Chapter Objectives

Upon completion of this chapter, you will be able to:

1. Define the terms in the vocabulary list.
2. Write the meaning of each abbreviation and write the abbreviation for each term in the abbreviation list.
3. Interpret patient activity, patient positioning, and nursing observation orders.

Vocabulary

Activity Order ▲ A doctor's order that defines the type and amount of activity a hospitalized patient may have

Afebrile ▲ Without fever

Apical Rate ▲ Heart rate obtained from the apex of the heart

Axillary Temperature ▲ The temperature reading obtained by placing the thermometer in the patient's axilla (armpit)

Bedside Commode ▲ A chair or wheelchair with an open seat, used at the bedside by the patient for the passage of urine and stool

Blood Pressure ▲ The measurement of the pressure of blood against the walls of the blood vessels

Febrile ▲ Elevated body temperature (fever)

Fowler's Position ▲ A semi-sitting position

Intake and Output ▲ The measurement of the patient's fluid intake and output

Neurologic Vital Signs (Neurochecks) ▲ The measurement of the function of the body's neurologic system; includes checking pupils of the eyes, verbal response, and so forth

Nursing Observation Order ▲ A doctor's order that requests the nursing staff to observe and record certain patient signs and symptoms

Oral Temperature ▲ The temperature reading obtained by placing the thermometer in the patient's mouth under the tongue

Pedal Pulse ▲ The pulse rate obtained on the top of the foot

Positioning Order ▲ A doctor's order that requests that the patient be placed in a specified body position

Pulse Oximetry ▲ A noninvasive method to measure the oxygen saturation of arterial blood

Pulse Rate ▲ The number of times per minute the heartbeat is felt through the walls of the artery

Radial Pulse ▲ Pulse rate obtained on the wrist

Rectal Temperature ▲ The temperature reading obtained by placing the thermometer in the patient's rectum

Respiration Rate ▲ The number of times a patient breathes per minute

Temperature ▲ The quantity of body heat, measured in degrees—either Fahrenheit or Celsius

Tympanic Membrane Temperature ▲ The temperature reading obtained by placing an aural (ear) thermometer in the patient's ear

Vital Signs ▲ Measurements of body functions, including temperature, pulse, respiration, and blood pressure

Abbreviations

Abbreviation	Meaning	Example of Order
A & O	alert and oriented	D/C to home when A & O
ABR	absolute bedrest	ABR × 12 hr
ad-lib	as desired	up ad-lib
amb	ambulate	amb c̄ help
as tol	as tolerated	up as tol
ax	axilla or axillary	ax temp tid
bid	two times per day	up in chair 20 min bid
BP	blood pressure	BP tid standing & lying
BR	bedrest	BR until A & O
BRP	bathroom privileges	BRP only
BSC	bedside commode	may use BSC
c̄	with	up c̄ help
CBR	complete bed rest	CBR today
CMS	circulation, motion, and sensation	check CMS fingers rt hand
CVP	central venous pressure	measure CVP q 4h
D/C *or* DC	discontinue *or* discharge	D/C BSC *or* DC to home today
HOB	head of bed	↑ HOB
h, hr, hrs	hour, hours	flat in bed for 8 h
I & O	intake and output	Strict I & O
lt, Ⓛ	left	↑ lt arm on pillow
min	minutes	up in chair for 5 min today
NVS or neuro ✓s	neurologic vital signs or checks	NVS q 4h & record
°	degree or hour	elevate head of bed 30°
OOB	out of bed	OOB ad lib
P	pulse	BP & P q 4h
prn	as necessary	up prn
q	every	wt q day
qd	every day or daily	wt qd
qid	four times a day	VS qid
qod	every other day	wt qod
qh *or* q _h	every hour *or* every (fill in number) hour	check VS q 2h
R	rectal	R temp
RR	respiratory rate	monitor RR q 1h
rt, Ⓡ	right	↑ rt arm on pillow
Rout	routine	rout VS
SOB	shortness of breath	evaluate for SOB & notify physician
temp	temperature	rectal temp
tid	three times a day	up in chair tid
TPR	temperature, pulse, respiration	TPR & BP q 4h
VS	vital signs	VS q 4h
wt	weight	wt daily
↑	increase, above, or elevate	↑ arm on 2 pillows
↓	decrease, below, or lower	if BP ↓ 100/60 call me

EXERCISE 1

Write the abbreviation for the following terms.

1. complete bed rest _____

2. with _____

3. alert and oriented _____

4. four times a day _____

5. degree or hour _____

6. blood pressure _____

7. every _____

8. ambulatory _____

9. absolute bed rest _____

10. increase or elevate _____

11. bathroom privileges _____

12. respiratory rate _____

13. as desired _____

14. every other day _____

15. two times a day _____

16. every day _____

17. three times a day _____

18. every hour _____

19. temperature _____

20. as tolerated _____

21. right _____

22. left _____

23. discontinue or discharge _____

24. vital signs _____

25. intake and output _____

26. out of bed _____

27. minutes _____

28. weight _____

29. bed rest _____

30. rectal _____

31. axilla or axillary _____

32. temperature, pulse, respiration _____

33. pulse _____

34. hour or hours _____

35. as necessary _____

36. neurologic vital signs or neurologic checks _____

37. decrease, below, or lower _____

38. head of bed _____

39. bedside commode _____

40. every 4 hours _____

41. circulation, motion, and sensation _____

42. shortness of breath _____

43. central venous pressure _____

44. routine _____

EXERCISE 2

Write the meaning of each abbreviation.

1. lt or Ⓛ _____

2. rt or Ⓡ _____

3. D/C or DC _____

4. VS _____

5. BP _____

6. tid _____

7. CBR _____

8. c̄ _____

9. TPR _____

10. BR _____

11. min _____

12. BRP _____

13. ad lib _____

14. ↑ _____

15. *OOB*

_____

16. *A & O*

_____

17. *wt*

_____

18. *amb*

_____

19. *qod*

_____

20. *qd*

_____

21. *bid*

_____

22. *qid*

_____

23. *qh*

_____

24. *ABR*

_____

25. *temp*

_____

26. *as tol*

_____

27. *I & O*

_____

28. *q*

_____

29. *P*

_____

30. *ax*

_____

31. *R*

_____

32. *prn*

_____

33. *RR*

_____

34. *q 4h*

_____

35. *h, hr, or hrs*

_____

36. *NVS or neuro ✓s*

_____

37. ↓

_____

38. *rt*

_____

39. *SOB*

_____

40. *HOB*

_____

41. BSC

_____

42. CMS

_____

43. CVP

_____

44. rout

_____

■ PATIENT ACTIVITY ORDERS

Background Information

Patient activity refers to the amount of walking, sitting, and other motions that the patient may do in a given period during his or her hospital stay. The prescribed activity changes to coincide with the patient's stage of recovery. For example, following some major surgery the doctor may want the patient to remain in bed; as the patient recovers, the doctor increases the activity accordingly. The doctor indicates the degree of activity the patient should have by writing an activity order on the doctor's order sheet. Common activity orders are listed here with interpretations.

☑ Doctors' Orders for Patient Activities

CBR
The patient is to remain in bed at all times.

BR c̄ BRP
The patient may use the bathroom for the elimination of urine and stool, but otherwise must remain in bed.

Dangle Tonight
The patient may sit and dangle his feet over the edge of the bed. The doctor may specify the number of times per day the patient should dangle, such as *Dangle bid*, or he or she may specify a period of time, such as *Dangle 5 min tid*.

Use Bedside Commode or **Use BSC**
The patient may use a portable commode at the bedside.

Up c̄ Help
The patient may be out of bed when assisted by a member of the nursing staff.

Up in Chair
The patient may sit in a chair. The doctor may specify the length of time and/or number of times per day, especially if he or she orders this activity following CBR. Example: *Up in chair 5 min tid*.

BRP When A & O
The patient may use the bathroom as desired when alert and oriented.

Up in Hall
The patient may walk in the hall.

Up as Tol
The patient may be out of bed as much as he or she can physically tolerate.

Up Ad Lib
The patient has no restriction on activity.

OOB
The patient may be out of bed. The doctor may qualify this order with another statement, such as *OOB bid*.

Amb
This is another way of saying the patient may be up as desired.

May Shower
The patient may have a shower. A doctor's order is necessary for a hospitalized patient to have a shower or tub bath.

These orders are written in abbreviated form as the doctor would write them on the doctor's order sheet, *with one exception*: they are not written in a doctor's handwriting. Reading doctors' handwriting can be a difficult task. However, the repetitive reading of doctors' handwritten orders soon prepares you to become an expert in this area. For assistance with abbreviations, refer to the abbreviation list at the beginning of the chapter.

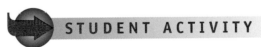

STUDENT ACTIVITY

To practice transcribing an activity order, complete Activity 10–1 in the *Skills Practice Manual.*

■ PATIENT POSITIONING ORDERS

Background Information

Patient positioning is often determined by the nursing staff; however, the doctor may want the patient to remain in a special body position to maintain body alignment, promote comfort, and fa-

Communication and Implementation of Patient Activity, Patient Positioning, and Nursing Observation Orders

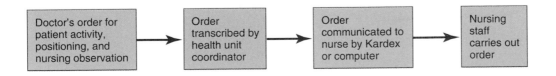

cilitate body functions. For example, the doctor may order the head of the bed to be elevated to ease the patient's breathing, or he or she may want the nurse to turn the patient to the unaffected side to promote healing. The doctor indicates a special position by writing the order on the doctor's order sheet. Since it would be impossible to discuss all patient positioning orders, only those that are most typical are described here. The following positioning orders are written in the same terms as you will find on a doctor's order sheet. Refer to the abbreviation list at the beginning of the chapter for assistance.

☑ DOCTORS' ORDERS FOR PATIENT POSITIONING

Elevate Head of Bed 30° or ↑ HOB 30°
The head of the bed is to be elevated 30 degrees. (The degree of elevation may vary according to the purpose of the order; for example, the doctor may write ↑ *head of bed 20°*.)

Elevate Lt Arm on Two Pillows
The left arm is to be elevated on two pillows. Variations of this order include the degree of elevation and also include other limbs; for example, *Elevate rt foot on pillow*.

Fowler's Position
The patient is placed in a semi-sitting position by elevating the head of the bed approximately 18–20 inches, or 45 degrees, with a slight elevation of the knees. The semi-Fowler's position is the same as Fowler's, but with the head of the bed elevated 30° (Fig. 10–1).

Log Roll
The patient is turned from side to side or side to back while keeping the back straight like a log, with a pillow between the knees.

Turn to Unaffected Side
The doctor wishes the patient to lie on the side that is free of injury.

Flat in Bed for 8 h No Pillow
The patient is to remain flat in bed for 8 hours, after which the standing activity order is resumed.

Turn q 2h
The patient's position is changed every 2 hours to prevent skin breakdown (bedsores).

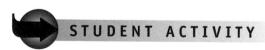

STUDENT ACTIVITY

To practice transcribing a patient positioning order, complete Activity 10–2 in the Skills Practice Manual.

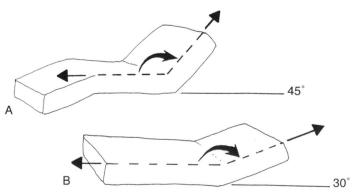

FIGURE 10–1 ▲ *A,* Fowler's position, *B,* Semi-Fowler's position.

■ NURSING OBSERVATION ORDERS

Background Information

The doctor may wish to have the nursing staff make periodic observations of the patient's condition; these observations are referred to as *signs and symptoms*. Some doctors may write "call orders" indicating he or she is to be called in the event of certain circumstances. For example, call if P ↑ 110, R ↓ 10, T ↑ 101°, B/P systolic ↑ 160, diastolic ↑ 90. The doctor may need this information to assist in diagnosing the patient's illness or interpreting the patient's progress. The doctor writes an order to request the information wanted. It is difficult to record all doctors' orders that you will encounter in this area; however, we have outlined some of the more common ones for you, written as you may find them on the doctor's order sheet. For assistance with the interpretation of the abbreviations, refer to the abbreviation list at the beginning of the chapter.

☑ DOCTORS' ORDERS FOR NURSING OBSERVATION

VS q 4h
The patient's vital signs are to be taken and recorded every 4 hours. Vital signs include *temperature* (Fig. 10–2), *pulse rate, respiration rate,* and *blood pressure reading*. The temperature may be taken using an aural, oral, or rectal thermometer. Oral and rectal thermometers may be glass or electric (Fig. 10–2). The results of the temperature will indicate whether the patient is febrile or afebrile. The pulse is obtained from the radial artery in the wrist, unless otherwise indicated. Variations of this type of order may include other time sequences and can read, for example, *VS q 1h, VS q 2h,* or may include a qualifying phrase, such as *VS q 1h until stable then q 4h.*

BP q h × 4
The blood pressure is to be taken and recorded every hour for 4 hours. Variations to this order may involve other time sequences, such as *BP q 4h, BP tid,* and so forth, or a qualifying phrase, such as *BP q 3h while awake* or *BP q 4h if ↓ 100/60 call me.*

Observe for SOB and Notify Physician
The patient will be observed for shortness of breath and, if severe, the nurse will notify the physician of the patient's condition.

Apical Rate
The patient's heart rate is to be taken at the apex of the heart with a stethoscope.

Check Pedal Pulse R foot q 2h
The pulses are obtained from an artery (dorsalis pedis) on top of the foot.

Neuro √s q 2h
The patient's neurologic vital signs are taken and recorded every 2 hours.

I & O
The patient's fluid intake and output is measured and recorded at the completion of each shift. It is then calculated for 24-hour periods. See Figure 10–3, a typical intake and output form used by the nursing staff to calculate the patient's intake and output for an 8-hour shift.

Wt Daily
The patient is to be weighed daily and the weight recorded. A variation of this order may be *wt qd.*

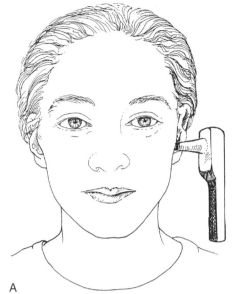
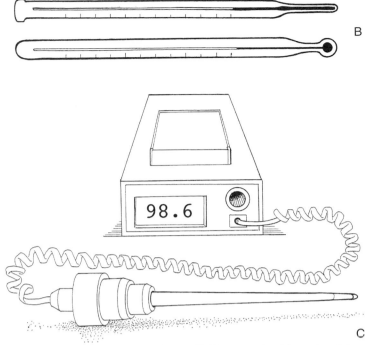

FIGURE 10–2 ▲ Types of thermometers. *A*, Aural— used to take tympanic membrane temperature in the ear. *B*, Glass—used to take oral, rectal, and axillary temperatures. *C*, Electric—used to take oral and rectal temperatures.

FIGURE 10–3 ▲ An intake and output form.

24 Hour Intake and Output

Name _Mary Ryan_
Room _403A_
Date _9/10/00_

Shift	Fluid Intake			Fluid Output		Other	Stools
	Oral	I.V.	Piggy Back	Urine	Emesis	Suction ☐	
0700-1500	08³⁰ 100cc 10⁰⁰ 30cc 12⁰⁰ 320cc 15⁰⁰ 500cc 210	Credit _300_ Add _1000_ Add _____	50	07³⁰ 200cc 11⁰⁰ 300cc 13⁰⁰ 175cc	200cc		x1 lg amt
8 hr.	1160		50	675			
1500-2300		Credit _500_ Add _____ Add _____					
8 hr.							
2300-0700		Credit ____ Add _____ Add _____					
8 hr.							
24 hr.							

Iced Tea - 6 oz. (180 cc)
Water Glass - 6 oz. (180 cc)
Milk (carton) - 8 oz. (240 cc)
Fruit Juice - 4 oz. (120 cc)
Soup - 4 oz. (120 cc)
Ice Cream - 3 oz. (90 cc)
Jello - 3.5 oz. (105 cc)

Cup of Coffee or Tea - 7 oz. (210 cc)
Styrofoam Cup - 150 cc
Paper Cup - 150 cc
Coffee Creamer - .5 oz. (15 cc)
Cereal Creamer - 2 oz. (60 cc)
Coca Cola and Sprite - 12 oz. (360 cc)
H_2O Pitcher - 30 oz. (900 cc)

Tympanic Membrane Temp q 4h

The temperature is to be measured every 4 hours, using the aural thermometer (see Fig. 10–2) as opposed to the oral method. A third method of measuring the body temperature is the axillary method. The doctor's order for this method may read, *axillary temp q 4h*. A fourth is the rectal method. The doctor's order will read, *rectal temp q 4h*.

CVP q 2h

A catheter is inserted, usually through the right or left subclavian vein, and threaded through the vein until the tip reaches the right atrium of the heart (see Fig. 11–11). The catheter is inserted by the doctor; the pressure readings are done by the nurse.

Pulse Oximetry q 4h

The oxygen saturation of arterial blood is to be measured every 4 hours. A portable pulse oximeter with a special sensor is used. The nursing staff or respiratory therapist may perform pulse oximetry. The sensor may be left in place for continuous monitoring.

Check CMS Fingers Rt Hand

The circulation, motion, and sensation of the patient's right-hand fingers are to be checked as often as the nurse determines it to be necessary. This type of order specifies observation of the patient's signs and symptoms relative to the patient's diagnosis and treatment. For example, this order was written following the application of a cast to the patient's right arm and hand.

vsq shift

Vital signs are measured to detect changes in the patient's condition, assess response to treatment, and recognize life-threatening situations. Accurate recording of vital signs is essential. Vital signs consist of:

Blood pressure	Temperature	Pulse	Respiration rate
	Oral	Apical	
	Tympanic membrane	Radial	
	Axillary	Pedal	
	Rectal	Femoral	
		Carotid	
		Popliteal	
		Brachial	

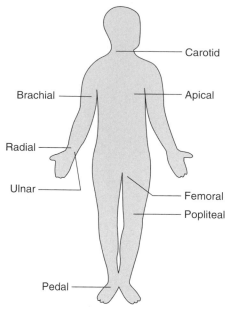

FIGURE 10–4 ▲ Location of the pulse points on the body.

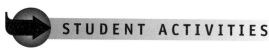

STUDENT ACTIVITIES

- To practice transcribing a nursing observation order, complete Activity 10–3 in the *Skills Practice Manual*.
- To practice transcribing, automatically canceling, and discontinuing doctors' orders, complete Activity 10–4.
- To practice transcribing a review set of doctors' orders, complete Activity 10–5.
- To practice recording telephoned doctors' orders and to practice recording telephoned messages, complete Activities 10–6 and 10–7.

■ SUMMARY

Transcription of doctors' orders is a major responsibility in health unit coordinating. This chapter introduced you to doctors' orders for patient activity, patient positioning, and nursing observation. Refer back to this chapter as needed.

REVIEW QUESTIONS

1. Define the following terms.

   a. nursing observation orders

   _____

   b. activity order

   _____

   c. positioning order

   _____

d. vital signs

_____

e. temperature

_____

   i. oral

   _____

   ii. rectal

   _____

   iii. axillary

   _____

   iv. tympanic membrane

   _____

f. pulse oximetry

_____

g. febrile

_____

h. afebrile

_____

2. Write out each doctor's order in the space provided.

   a. CBR

   _____

   b. BR c̄ BRP when A & O

   _____

   c. wt qod

   _____

   d. VS qid

   _____

   e. TPR & BP tid

   _____

   f. HOB 20°

   _____

g. check dressing prn

_____

h. temp R or ax only

_____

i. neuro ✓s q 2h

_____

j. I & O q shift

_____

k. OOB ad lib

_____

l. up as tol

_____

m. TPR & BP q 4h

_____

n. amb today

_____

o. DC VS

_____

p. ↑ HOB 30°

_____

q. may use BSC

_____

r. log roll q 2h

_____

s. check CMS toes lt foot

_____

t. CVP q 3h

_____

u. call me if pt SOB

_____

TOPICS FOR DISCUSSION

1. Discuss errors that could occur because of misinterpretation of abbreviations.

2. Discuss possible consequences of a positioning or activity order being recorded incorrectly.

3. Discuss possible consequences of an order for NVS being overlooked or not carried out.

Nursing Treatment Orders

Chapter Objectives

Upon completion of this chapter, you will be able to:

1. Define the terms in the vocabulary list.
2. Write the meaning of the abbreviations in the abbreviations list.

3. Describe the function of the central service department with regard to nursing treatment orders.
4. Explain why reusable equipment should be returned to the central service department as quickly as possible.
5. List the types of items stored in the central service department stock supply closet (C-locker or cart) on the nursing units.
6. List the types of items stored in the central service department.
7. List the types of enemas.
8. State the two types of urinary catheterization procedures.
9. State two methods of administering intravenous therapy.
10. List three parts of an intravenous therapy order.
11. List two types of commercially prepared intravenous solutions.
12. Explain the importance of correct labeling of a blood specimen being sent for a type and crossmatch.
13. Explain the health unit coordinator's role in obtaining blood from the blood bank and the correct storage of blood.
14. List the various suction devices and explain the use of each.
15. List the devices used for heat therapy.
16. List the devices used for cold therapy.
17. Review the procedure for obtaining blood glucose levels.
18. Explain other health unit coordinator tasks that may be necessary when transcribing intravenous infusion orders.

Vocabulary

Autologous Blood ▲ The patient's own blood donated previously for transfusion as needed by the patient; also called autotransfusion

Binder ▲ A cloth or elastic bandage usually used for abdominal or chest support

Catheterization ▲ Insertion of a catheter into a body cavity or organ to inject or remove fluid

Central Venous Catheter ▲ A catheter is threaded through to the superior vena cava or right atrium used for the administration of intravenous therapy

Donor-Specific or Donor-Directed Blood ▲ Blood donated by relatives or friends of the patient to be used for transfusion as needed

Egg-Crate Mattress ▲ A foam rubber mattress

Enema ▲ The introduction of fluid and/or medication into the rectum and sigmoid colon

Foley Catheter ▲ A type of indwelling retention catheter

Gastric Suction ▲ Used to remove gastric contents

Harris Flush or Return Flow Enema ▲ A mild colonic irrigation that helps expel flatus

Hemovac ▲ A disposable suction device (evacuator unit) that is connected to a drain inserted into or close to a surgical wound

Heparin Lock ▲ A vascular access device (also called intermittent infusion device) placed on a peripheral intravenous catheter when used intermittently

Incontinence ▲ Inability of the body to control the elimination of urine and/or feces

Indwelling (Retention) Catheter ▲ A catheter that remains in the bladder for a longer period until a patient is able to void completely and voluntarily or as long as hourly accurate measurements are needed.

Infusion Pump ▲ A device used to regulate flow or rate of intravenous fluid. It is commonly called an IV pump

Intermittent (Straight) Catheter ▲ A single-use catheter that is introduced long enough to drain the bladder (5 to 10 minutes) and then removed

Intravenous Infusion ▲ The administration of fluid through a vein

Irrigation ▲ Washing out of a body cavity, organ, or wound

Jackson-Pratt (JP) ▲ A disposable suction device (evacuator unit) that is connected to a drain inserted into or close to a surgical wound

K-Pad ▲ An electric device used for heat application (also called a K-thermia pad, aquathermia pad, or aquamatic pad)

Nasogastric Tube (NG Tube) ▲ A tube that is inserted through the nose into the stomach

Orthostatic Vital Signs ▲ The measurement of blood pressure and pulse rate first in supine (lying), then in sitting, and finally in standing positions.

Patency ▲ A term indicating that there are no clots at the tip of the needle or catheter and that the needle tip or catheter is not against the vein wall (open)

Penrose Drain ▲ A drain that that is inserted into or close to a surgical wound and may lie under a dressing, extend through a dressing, or be connected to a drainage bag or a suction device

Peripheral Intravenous Catheter ▲ A catheter that begins and ends in the extremities of the body; used for the administration of intravenous therapy

Pneumatic Hose ▲ Stockings that promote circulation by sequentially compressing the legs from ankle upward, promoting venous return (also called sequential compression devices)

Rectal Tube ▲ A plastic or rubber tube designed for insertion into the rectum; when written as a doctor's order, *rectal tube* means the insertion of a rectal tube into the rectum to remove gas and relieve distention

Restraints ▲ Devices used to control patients exhibiting dangerous behavior or to protect the patient

Sheepskin ▲ A pad made out of lamb's wool or synthetic material; used to prevent pressure sores (used primarily in long-term care)

Sitz Bath ▲ Application of warm water to the pelvic area

Ted Hose ▲ A brand name for antiembolism (A-E) hose

Urinary Catheter ▲ A tube used for removing urine or injecting fluids into the bladder

Urine Residual ▲ The amount of urine left in the bladder after voiding

Venipuncture ▲ Needle puncture of a vein

Void ▲ To empty, especially the urinary bladder

▶ Abbreviations

Abbreviation	Meaning	Example of Usage on a Doctor's Order Sheet
@	at	Run @ 100 cc/hr
abd	abdominal	Up c̄ abd binder
ac	before meals	Accu-Chek ac and hs
ASAP	as soon as possible	Start IV ASAP
B/L	bilateral (both sides)	B/L Teds
cath	catheterize	Cath q 8 hr prn
CBI	continuous bladder irrigation	CBI c̄ NS 50 cc/hr
cc	cubic centimeter (equivalent to milliliter [mL])	IV 1000 cc 5% D/W 125 cc/hr
cm	centimeter	Chest tube 20 cm neg pressure
con't	continue, continuous	Foley cath to con't drainage
CVC	central venous catheter	Blood draws through CVC
D/LR	dextrose in lactated Ringer's	IV 1000 cc 5% D/LR at 125 cc/hr
D_5W	5% dextrose in water	1000 mL D_5W @ 125 mL/hr
$D_{10}W$	10% dextrose in water	1000 cc $D_{10}W$ @ 100 cc/hr
DW	distilled water	Irrig cath prn c̄ DW
ETS	elevated toilet seat	Order ETS for home use
gtt(s)	drop(s)	IV @ 60 gtts/min
HL or hep lock	heparin lock	convert IV to Hep lock

H_2O_2	hydrogen peroxide	Irrigate wound $\bar{c}$ H_2O_2 & NS equal strength
hs	bedtime, hour of sleep	Give TWE @ hs
irrig	irrigate	Irrig cath $\bar{c}$ NS prn
IV	intravenous	Con't IVs as ordered
IVF	intravenous fluids	DC IVF at 1000 today
KO	keep open	KO IV $\bar{c}$ 1000 cc 5% D/W
LR	lactated Ringer's	1000 mL LR 125 mL/h
min, m	minute	Run @ 30 gtts/min
mL	milliliter	1000 D_5W @ 100 mL/hr
MR	may repeat	SSE now MR × 1
nec	necessary	SSE now MR if nec
NG	nasogastric	Insert NG tube
NS	normal saline	Give NS enema now
ORE	oil-retention enema	ORE today
$\bar{p}$	after	Up $\bar{p}$ breakfast
PICC	peripherally inserted central catheter	Insert PICC, follow protocol
SCD	sequential compression device	apply SCD when in bed
sol'n	solution	irrig cath $\bar{c}$ NS sol'n
SSE	soap suds enema	SSE now
st	straight	retention cath to st drain
TCDB	turn, cough, and deep breathe	TCDB q 2h
TKO	to keep open	1000 cc D_5W TKO
TWE	tap-water enema	give TWE
VAD	vascular access device	use VAD for blood draws
Δ	change	Δ catheter daily
/	per, by	run IV @ 150 cc/hr

EXERCISE ❶

Write the abbreviation for each term.

1. soap suds enema _____

2. keep open _____

3. may repeat _____

4. solution _____

5. necessary _____

6. centimeter _____

7. tap-water enema _____

8. nasogastric _____

9. normal saline _____

10. dextrose in lactated Ringer's _____

11. bedtime _____

12. distilled water _____

13. at _____

14. oil-retention enema _____

15. irrigate _____

16. intravenous _____

17. catheterize _____

18. lactated Ringer's _____

19. straight _____

20. cubic centimeter _____

21. after _____

22. abdominal _____

23. turn, cough, and deep breathe _____

24. minute _____

25. drops _____

26. change _____

27. as soon as possible _____

28. per _____

29. hydrogen peroxide _____

30. before meals _____

31. continue _____

32. continuous bladder irrigation _____

33. to keep open _____

34. milliliter _____

35. intravenous fluids _____

36. elevated toilet seat _____

37. peripherally inserted central catheter _____

38. vascular access device _____

39. central venous catheter _____

40. 5% dextrose in water _____

41. 10% dextrose in water _____

42. bilateral _____

43. heparin lock _____

44. sequential compression
    device _____

EXERCISE 2

Write out each doctor's order in the space provided.

1. *1000 mL LR @ 125cc/hr, then DC*

   _____

2. *SSE HS MR × 1*

   _____

3. *Give ORE follow c̄ TWE if nec*

   _____

4. *Irrig cath tid c̄ NS sol'n*

   _____

5. *1000 cc D_5W 0.9 NS @ TKO*

   _____

6. *Insert NG tube*

   _____

7. *TCDB q 2h*

   _____

8. *Δ IV tubing ASAP*

   _____

9. *Please obtain ETS for patient*

   _____

10. *Start IVF of $D_{10}W$ @ 120 cc/hr*

    _____

11. *Insert HL*

    _____

12. *Shave B/L inguinal groin area*

    _____

13. *Apply SCD when in bed*

    _____

▆ COMMUNICATION WITH THE CENTRAL SERVICE DEPARTMENT

The central service department (CSD) distributes the supplies used for nursing procedures. Central processing department (CPD), products and materials (PAM), and supplies, processing, and distribution (SPD) are other names used for the central service department. Although CSD supplies are frequently used without being a part of the doctor's orders, obtaining these supplies for the nursing staff may be a step of the transcription procedure for nursing treatment orders. For example, in the order *footboard to bed*, the health unit coordinator would order the footboard from the CSD. It is therefore necessary for you to be familiar with frequently used CSD items and to learn your hospital's system for obtaining them.

The system for obtaining central service supplies varies among hospitals; thus, it is impossible to outline one procedure to cover all hospital systems. Disposable or frequently used items are stored on each nursing unit (items will vary depending on the specialty of the nursing unit). That storage space is often referred to as the CSD closet or C-locker. Usually a central service technician will take a daily inventory of the items stored in the closet or C-locker. He or she then replaces the used items, and collects the patient's CSD current charge cards. Some hospitals have an exchange cart system. The carts are supplied with frequently used items and exchanged every 24 hours. The unit receives another completely supplied cart while CSD replenishes the used cart. Reusable or infrequently used items are stored in the CSD. Refer to Table 11–1 for a comparison of items commonly stored on the nursing units and items often stored in the central service department (note that items in each category could vary among hospitals).

The health unit coordinator, when transcribing a treatment order, orders only those items stored in the central service department, since the nursing staff can quickly obtain the items needed from the CSD stock supply. Items from CSD are ordered

TABLE 11–1	Items Obtained from the Central Service Department

Items that May Be Stored on the Nursing Unit CSD Closet or C-Locker	Items that May Be Stored in the Central Service Department
Fleet enema	Alternating pressure pad
Rectal tube	Egg-crate mattress
Irrigation trays	Ted hose
Urinary catheter trays	Pneumatic hose
IV solutions*	Colostomy kit
IV catheters and needles	Stomal bags
IV tubing	Elastic abdominal binder
Suction catheters and tubing	Footboard
Sterile gloves	Foot cradle
Exam gloves	Feeding pump and tubing
Masks	IV infusion pump
Syringes and needles	Hypothermia machine
Disposable suture removal kits	K-pad
Dressings	Restraints
Abdominal pads	Adult disposable diapers
Telfa pads	Sitz bath, disposable
Gauze pads in various sizes	Sterile trays
Kling	Tracheostomy
Vaseline gauze	Bone marrow
Tape (various types)	Paracentesis
Alcohol pads	Lumbar puncture (spinal tap)
Glycerin swabs	Thoracentesis
Irrigation solutions, etc.	Central line, etc.

*IV solutions are obtained from the pharmacy in some hospitals.

by computer or by completing a requisition. It is important to remember that supplies used from the nursing unit supply closet or C-locker are also charged to the patient. The charging process is done by removing a bar-code label from the item and placing it on the patient's CSD charge card (Fig. 11–1). The person removing the supplies is responsible for placing the bar-code label on the patient's CSD card. Figure 11–2 is an example of central department ordering computer screen.

Many items used for nursing treatments, such as enema bags or urinary catheterization trays, are *disposable.* This means that once the item has been used for the patient, it is either discarded or given to the patient for future use. The patient is charged for the disposable equipment.

Other items are *reusable.* They are cleaned or sterilized, if necessary, after use by a patient. Those items are then available for another patient. The patient usually pays a fee for the use of these items. Reusable items are numbered and are tracked to the appropriate patient for charging or discontinuing charge. When a reusable item, such as an IV infusion pump, is discontinued, it is placed in the dirty utility room. A central service technician will pick up the item and return it to CSD. If there is a rental charge, it is terminated and the equipment is readied for use by other patients.

Equipment is discussed and illustrated throughout this chapter as it relates to nursing treatment orders. Although you will not use the equipment yourself, recognizing frequently used items will assist you in the ordering step of the transcription procedure.

Learn which items are stored on the unit and those stored in CSD. If size and/or weight is required when ordering an item, check with the patient's nurse and enter the information when ordering the item (example: Ted hose).

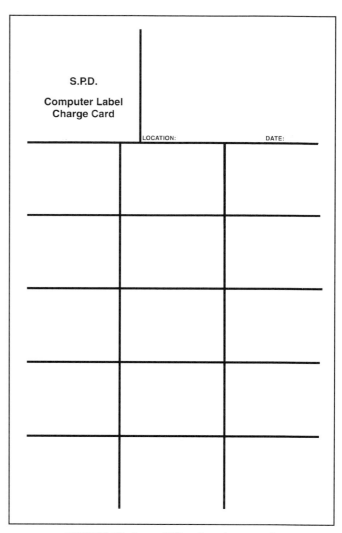

S.P.D.

Computer Label
Charge Card

LOCATION: DATE:

FIGURE 11–1 ▲ CSD patient charge card.

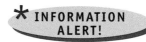

✱ INFORMATION ALERT!

As a health unit coordinator, you can best assist the nursing staff when transcribing nursing treatment orders by learning about the equipment and supplies on the unit where you work so you can have the items needed by the staff to carry out the treatments.

▪ INTESTINAL ELIMINATION ORDERS

Background Information

Enemas, rectal tubes, and colostomy irrigations are treatments used to remove stool and/or flatus (gas) from the large intestine.

An enema is the introduction of fluid into the rectum and sigmoid colon for the purpose of relieving distention (trapped gas) or constipation, or to prepare the patient for surgery or diagnostic tests. A doctor may order a "*high*" or "*low*" cleansing enema. The terms *high* and *low* refer to the height from which the

Doctor Ordering_____ ☐ Stat
Today's Date_____ ☐ Routine
Requested by_____

CSD (Central Service Department)

☐ Adult disposable diapers
☐ Alternating pressure pad
☐ Colostomy kit
☐ Colostomy irrigation bag
☐ Egg-crate mattress
☐ Elastic abdominal binder   size_____
☐ Footboard
☐ Feeding pump with bag and tubing
☐ Feeding bag and tubing
☐ Footboard
☐ Foot cradle
☐ Hypothermia machine
☐ Isolation pack
☐ IV infusion pump with tubing
☐ K-pad with motor
☐ Nasal gastric tube   type_____ size_____
☐ Pleur-evac
☐ Pneumatic hose
☐ Restraints   type_____
☐ Sitz bath, disposable
☐ Stomal bags   type_____ size_____
☐ Suction canister and tubing
☐ Suction catheter   type_____ size_____
☐ Ted hose   size_____
☐ Vaginal irrigation kit

Sterile Trays:

☐ Bone marrow
☐ Central line
☐ Lumbar puncture (spinal tap)
☐ Paracentesis
☐ Thoracentesis
☐ Tracheostomy

☐ Write in item _____

FIGURE 11–2 ▲ An example of CSD requisition.

enema container is held, which determines the pressure with which the fluid is delivered. High enemas are given to cleanse the entire colon, while low enemas cleanse only the rectum and sigmoid colon. Common types of enemas are:

1. Oil retention
2. Soap suds
3. Tap water
4. Normal saline

Figure 11–3 is an example of a disposable enema bag used to administer these types of enemas.

Fleet enema is a disposable, commercially prepackaged sodium phosphate enema that is frequently used (Fig. 11–4).

The order for a *rectal tube* means the insertion of a disposable plastic, latex-free, or rubber tube into the rectum for the purpose of relieving distention or draining feces. The rectal tube may be attached to a bag that captures the flatus and/or feces (Fig. 11–5).

Harris flush is a return-flow enema and is used to relieve distention. A disposable enema bag is used to inject fluid into the rectum. The fluid is allowed to return into the bag. The process is repeated several times.

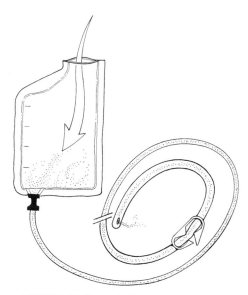

FIGURE 11–3 ▲ A disposable enema bag.

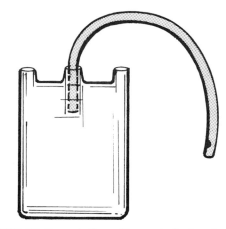

FIGURE 11–5 ▲ A disposable rectal tube in a flatus bag.

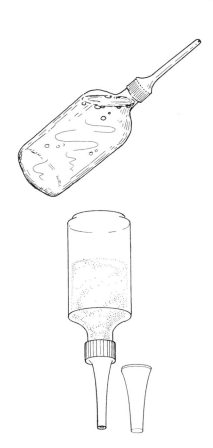

FIGURE 11–4 ▲ Commercially prepackaged enema.

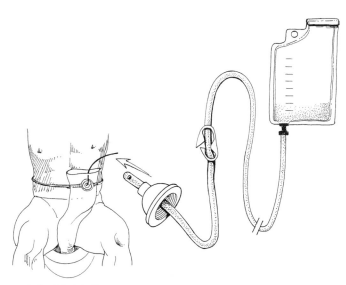

FIGURE 11–6 ▲ A disposable colostomy irrigation apparatus.

Colostomy (an artificial opening in the colon for passage of stool) irrigation (the flushing of fluid) resembles an enema and is used to regulate the discharge of stool. Figure 11–6 shows a disposable colostomy irrigation bag used for this treatment.

A doctor's order is required for the administration of an enema, rectal tube, or Harris flush. The order contains the name of

the treatment, the type (when pertinent), and the frequency. If the frequency is not indicated (such as in the order, *tap-water enema*), it is considered a one-time order.

Examples of intestinal elimination orders are listed below as they are usually written on the doctor's order sheet. Refer to the abbreviations list at the beginning of the chapter for interpretation of the abbreviations.

☑ DOCTORS' ORDERS FOR INTESTINAL ELIMINATION

- *TWE now MR × 1 prn*
- *Give ORE followed by NS enemas this AM*
- *Harris flush for abdominal distention*
- *NS enemas until clear*
- *Give Fleet enema qd prn constipation*
- *Rectal tube prn for distention*

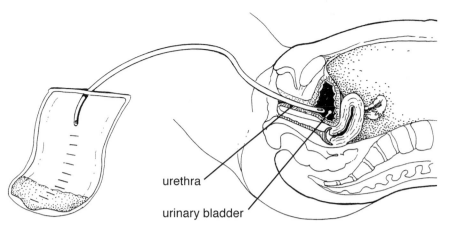

FIGURE 11–7 ▲ An intermittent (straight) catheter in place.

urethra

urinary bladder

■ URINARY CATHETERIZATION ORDERS

Background Information

Urinary catheterization is the insertion of a latex-free tube called a catheter through the urethral meatus into the bladder for the purpose of removing urine. The tube is usually made of plastic, and it varies in size. The doctor may order two types of catheterization procedures: retention and nonretention. Disposable sterile catheterization trays are used. Because different equipment is needed for each procedure, two types of catheter trays are available. One is used for the insertion of the retention catheter and the other is used for the insertion of the nonretention catheter. Each tray is marked with the size and type of catheter it contains.

An intermittent nonretention catheter, sometimes referred to as a *straight catheter*, is used to empty the bladder, to collect a sterile urine specimen, or to check residual. *Residual* is the amount of urine remaining in the bladder after voiding. The in-

termittent catheter is removed from the bladder after completion of the procedure (5 to 10 minutes) (Fig. 11–7).

An indwelling retention catheter (also called a Foley catheter) remains in the bladder and is usually connected to a drainage system that allows for continuous flow of urine from the bladder to the container. Doctors refer to this type of drainage system as a straight drain (Fig. 11–8).

The doctor may order the indwelling catheter to be irrigated on an intermittent or continuous basis to maintain patency (to keep the catheter open). This is referred to as a closed system (Fig. 11–9) and is usually used for those who have had surgery involving the urinary or reproductive systems. The open irrigation system is used for irrigating the catheter at specific intervals. The open system requires the nurse to open a closed drainage system and insert an irrigation solution. A disposable irrigation tray is used for this procedure. The doctor indicates the solution to be used (normal saline, acetic acid, distilled water). For continuous and intermittent irrigation, special set-ups are used (Fig. 11–9).

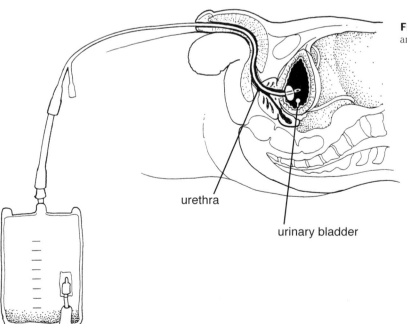

FIGURE 11–8 ▲ An indwelling (Foley) catheter in place and connected to a drainage bag (called *straight drainage*).

urethra

urinary bladder

Communication and Implementation of Nursing Treatment Orders

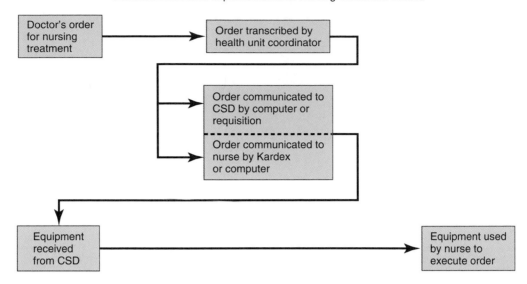

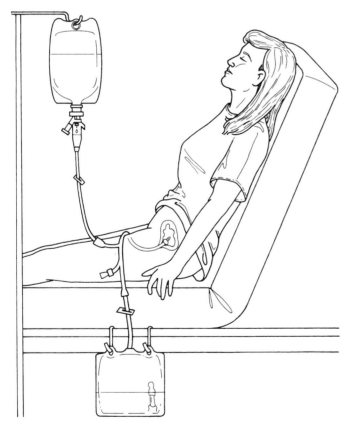

FIGURE 11-9 ▲ A set-up used for intermittent or continuous bladder irrigation.

☑ *DOCTORS' ORDERS FOR CATHETERIZATION*

Intermittent (Straight) Catheter
- *May cath q 8h prn*
- *Straight cath prn*
- *Cath in 8 hr if unable to void*
- *Cath for residual*
- *Stand to void p̄ 4 PM—cath if nec*

Indwelling (Retention) Catheter
- *Insert Foley*
- *Indwelling cath to st drain*
- *Insert Foley cath for residual; if over 200 mL, leave in*
- *DC cath in AM; if unable to void in 6 hr reinsert*
- *DC cath this AM*
- *Clamp cath 4 hr then drain*

Catheter Irrigation
- *CBI; use NS @ 50 mL/hr*
- *Irrig Foley c̄ NS bid*
- *Irrig cath prn patency*
- *Intermittent CBI q 4h × 6*

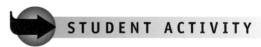

STUDENT ACTIVITY

To practice transcribing intestinal elimination and urinary catheterization orders, complete Activity 11–1 in the *Skills Practice Manual.*

■ INTRAVENOUS THERAPY ORDERS

Background Information

Several types of typical doctor's orders related to urinary catheterizations are listed in the text that follows, recorded in abbreviated form as they would appear on the doctor's order sheet. Refer to the abbreviations list at the beginning of the chapter for assistance with abbreviations.

Until 1949 intravenous therapy consisted of the administration of simple solutions, such as water and normal saline, through peripheral veins. Equipment was a glass bottle, rubber tube, and a needle. Today, intravenous therapy is the parenteral administration of fluids, medications, nutritional substances, and blood transfusions through peripheral veins and through central veins. The availability of sophisticated equipment allows intravenous therapy to be administered to the patient at home as well as in the hospital. Fluids can be administered continuously or intermittently and intravenous administration is done by the nurse, by the patient, or by the patient's family. The purpose of the intravenous therapy is to:

■ Administer nutritional support such as total parenteral nutrition (TPN) (covered in Chapters 12 and 13)
■ Provide for intermittent or continuous administration of medication
■ Transfuse blood or blood products
■ Maintain or replace fluids and electrolytes

Intravenous Therapy Catheters and Devices

Peripheral Intravenous Therapy

In peripheral intravenous therapy, peripheral refers to the blood flow in the extremities of the body. To administer therapy, the cannula is inserted into a vein in the arm, hand, or on rare occasion in the foot (adult). A vein in the scalp or foot is often used when administering peripheral intravenous therapy to infants. The cannula is short, less than 2 inches, so that it ends in the extremity. It is not threaded to the larger veins or the heart as in central venous therapy (Fig. 11–10). Peripheral intravenous therapy is:

■ Usually initiated by the nurse at the bedside
■ Usually started in a vein in the arm by a venipuncture
■ Used for short-term IV therapy, a week or less
■ Basic and easiest to initiate

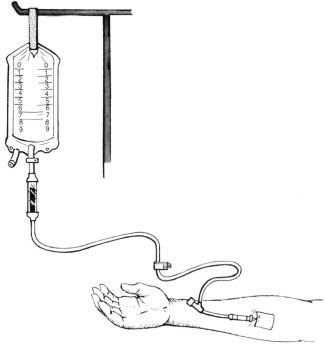

FIGURE 11–10 ▲ Peripheral intravenous therapy (venipuncture).

■ Commonly used in hospitals
■ Sometimes given through a vascular access device (VAD)

Central Intravenous Therapy

In central intravenous therapy, *central* refers to the blood flow in the center of the body. To administer therapy the catheter is inserted into the jugular or subclavian vein or a large vein in the arm and threaded to the superior vena cava or right atrium of the heart. A central venous catheter (CVC) is used. It is commonly referred to as a central venous line or a subclavian line. (Fig. 11–11). The health unit coordinator orders a central line tray and an infusion pump from the central service department and prepares a consent form.

Types of Central Venous Catheters

A peripherally inserted central catheter (PICC or PIC) is:

■ Initiated by the doctor or by a nurse certified in the procedure at the bedside, and requires a consent form
■ Inserted in the arm and advanced until the tip lies in the superior vena cava
■ X-rayed to verify placement
■ Used when therapy is needed longer than 7 days
■ Used for antibiotic therapy, total parenteral nutrition, chemotherapy, cardiac drugs, or other drugs that are potentially harmful to peripheral veins
■ Sometimes used for blood draws

A percutaneous central venous catheter is:

■ Sometimes referred to as a subclavian line
■ Initiated by the doctor at the bedside and requires a consent form
■ Inserted through the skin directly into the subclavian (most common) or jugular vein and advanced until the tip lies in the superior vena cava or right atrium of the heart
■ X-rayed to verify placement
■ Used for short-term therapy, 7 days to several weeks
■ Used for antibiotic therapy, TPN, or chemotherapy,
■ Sometimes used for blood draws

A tunneled catheter is:

■ Initiated by the doctor, is considered a surgical procedure, and requires a consent form
■ Inserted through a small incision made near the subclavian vein
  ■ A catheter is inserted and advanced to the superior vena cava
  ■ A device called a tunneler is used to exit the catheter low in the patient's chest
  ■ This allows for the patient to administer his or her own therapy, and the tips can be placed under clothing
  ■ Hickman, Raaf, Groshong, and Broviac are types of tunneling catheters
■ Inserted for long-term IV therapy, longer than a month
■ Used for home care, in long-term care facilities, and for self-administration
■ Sometimes used for blood draws

An implanted port is:

■ A surgical procedure, performed by the doctor in a surgical setting

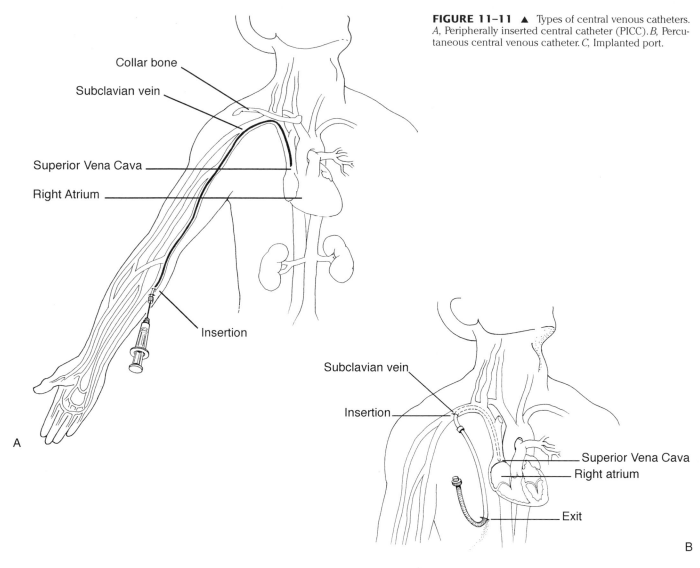

FIGURE 11–11 ▲ Types of central venous catheters. *A*, Peripherally inserted central catheter (PICC). *B*, Percutaneous central venous catheter. *C*, Implanted port.

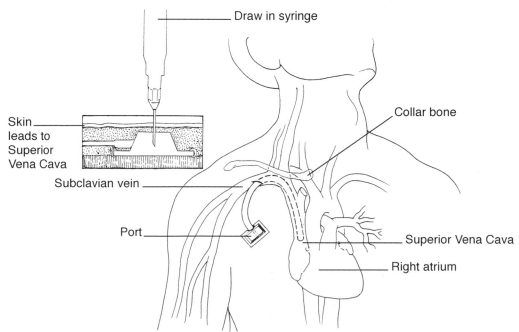

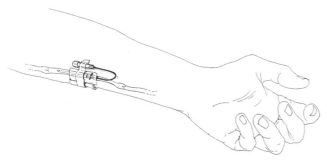

FIGURE 11–12 ▲ Intermittent infusion device (heparin lock).

- Inserted into the subclavian or jugular vein
  - A port (container) is implanted under the skin in the chest wall
  - The incision is closed and the device cannot be seen but can be identified by a bulge
  - Implanted ports differ from other long-term catheters in that there are no external parts, they are located under the skin, and do not require daily care
  - A special needle is inserted into the port to administer the therapy
  - Port-A-Cath and Med-I-Port and Infus-A-Port are types of implanted ports
- Used for long-term and or intermittent use; often used for chemotherapy administration

Heparin Lock (Heplock)

A heparin lock or Heplock is a venous access device (also called an *intermittent infusion device*) placed on a peripheral intravenous catheter when used intermittently. The Heplock is used to establish an intermittent line when IV fluids are no longer needed but IV entry is still required. It is commonly used for the administration of medication. It consists of a plastic needle with an attached injection cap. The device is kept patent by heparin or saline flushes administered at specific intervals (flushes require a doctor's order) (Fig. 11–12).

Intravenous Infusion Pump

An intravenous infusion pump is an electrical device used in the administration of intravenous fluid. It is used to measure a precise amount of fluid (regulates drips per hour) to be infused for a stated amount of time. The pump is ordered from CSD and is manufactured under several brand names (Fig. 11–13).

▋ FLUIDS AND ELECTROLYTES

The doctor orders the type, the amount, and the flow rate of the solutions to be given. For example, in the IV order:

1000 mL D₅W @ 125 mL/hr

D₅W is the type of solution. There is a large variety of solutions on the market, and the doctor must select the one that best meets the patient's needs.

Continuing this example, 1000 mL is the amount of solution the doctor wants the patient to have. Solutions are most commonly packaged in amounts of 1000 mL; however, 250 mL or 500 mL may also be ordered.

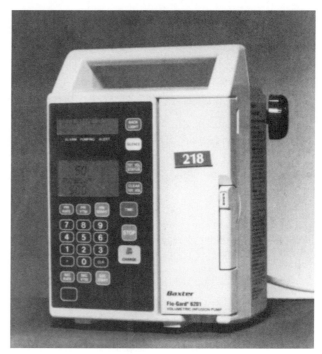

FIGURE 11–13 ▲ Infusion pump. (From Ignatavicius DD, Workman ML, Mishler MA: Medical-Surgical Nursing: A Nursing Process Approach, 2nd ed. Philadelphia: W. B. Saunders, 1995.

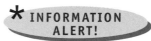
✱ INFORMATION ALERT!

To determine the amount of time it will take for IV infusion, divide the number of milliliters in the IV bag by the rate of flow. In the doctor's order: 1000 mL 5% D/W @ 125 mL/h, divide 1000 by 125. The answer is 8. The IV will run for 8 hours. Use this information to order the number of 1000-mL IV bags needed for a given amount of time.

The notation 125 mL/hr indicates the rate of flow per hour of the solution into the vein. Other examples of phrases used in stating the rate of flow are 60 gtts per min, to run for 8 hr; or to keep open (usually 50 to 60 mL/hr).

Frequently, the health unit coordinator is required to order IV solutions at specific intervals; therefore, it is necessary to know the length of time it takes the IV to infuse. An IV of 1000 mL running at 125 mL/h runs for 8 hours (1000 mL / 125 mL = 8 hours). How many hours will an IV running at 100 mL/h take to infuse?

Several one-time, continuous, and discontinuation IV orders, written in abbreviated form as commonly seen on the doctor's order sheet, follow. Use the abbreviations list at the beginning of the chapter for assistance in interpreting these, if necessary.

☑ DOCTORS' ORDERS FOR INTRAVENOUS THERAPY

- *1000 mL LR 125 mL/h then DC*
- *Con't IVs alternate 1000 cc/RL c̄ 1000 cc D₅W each to run for 8 h via CVC*

COMMON COMMERCIALLY PREPARED IV SOLUTIONS

- Sodium chloride 0.45% (NaCl 0.45%, or half-strength NaCl)
- Sodium chloride 0.9% (NaCl 0.9%, or normal saline)
- 5% dextrose in water (5% D/W, or D_5W)
- 10% dextrose in water (10% D/W, or $D_{10}W$)
- 5% dextrose in 0.2% sodium chloride (5% D/0.2% NaCl)
- 5% dextrose in 0.45% sodium chloride (5% D/0.45% NaCl)
- 5% dextrose in 0.9% sodium chloride (5% D/0.9% NaCl)
- Lactated Ringer's solution with 5% dextrose (LR/5%D)
- 5% dextrose in 0.2% normal saline
- 5% dextrose in 0.45% normal saline
- Lactated Ringer's solution

There are other IV solutions containing essential body elements that are sold under trade names. For example, McGaw, a manufacturer of parenteral fluids, markets an IV solution with electrolytes as Isolyte M. The same formula is sold by Abbott Laboratories as Ionosol T. Your instructor will give you the trade names used in your hospital.

- *KVO IV rate 30 cc/h c̄D_5W*
- *DC IV when present bottle is finished*
- *D_5LR 100 cc/h follow c̄1000 cc 5% Isolyte M at same rate*
- *Alternate the following Ivs*
  - *1000 mL D_{10}LR via Groshong cath*
  - *1000 cc 5% D/W plus 20 mEq KCl to run at 125 cc/h*
  - *1000 cc D_5 0.9 NS @ 100 cc/h if pt not tol fluids*
- *DC IV fluids, convert to hep lock c̄ rout saline flushes*
- *Have IV team insert PICC*
- *Use Port-A-Cath for blood draws*

▌ TRANSFUSION OF BLOOD, BLOOD COMPONENTS, AND PLASMA SUBSTITUTES

Background Information

An intravenous infusion of blood is called a *blood transfusion*. It is usually ordered for patients who have lost blood because of hemorrhage from trauma or surgery. Before the administration of blood and blood products, the patient must sign a specific consent form. A refusal form must be signed if the patient refuses to have a blood transfusion Refer to Chapter 8, page 151 to see a blood transfusion.

The use of whole blood for transfusion is gradually lessening, and only parts or components of blood are being used. You will find the following in transfusion orders:

1. Packed cells (red blood cells) (frequently used)
2. Plasma
3. Platelet concentrate
4. Washed cells
5. Fresh frozen plasma (FFP)
6. Cryoprecipitates
7. Gamma globulins
8. Albumin
9. Factor VIII

Transcribing Doctors' Orders for Blood Transfusions

A type and crossmatch is a laboratory study performed to determine the type and compatibility of the blood and is done before the patient receives blood or certain blood components. A type and crossmatch is performed in the blood bank division of the hospital laboratory. It is essential that the health unit coordinator match the patient's name and information on the patient ID label affixed to the blood specimen to the patient name and information on the 'doctor's order sheet, and to the name and information on the computer order screen. The specimen will be discarded if the specimen patient ID label and the patient name on the requisition are not the same. The patient will then need to have his or her blood redrawn, causing additional discomfort and delaying their treatment.

The equipment used for infusion of blood is similar to that used for the infusion of intravenous solutions. Blood is packaged in plastic containers and ordered by the unit. The intravenous tubing used for blood contains a filter. Normal saline solution is generally used, along with the administration of blood. All equipment items must be disposed of after the blood is transfused.

The transfusion of blood is a potentially dangerous procedure. Special precautions are taken by the nursing staff to ensure the correct administration of blood. Proper storage of blood is also essential to ensure safe administration. Blood is stored in the blood bank, in a special refrigerator designed to maintain constant temperature for safe storage of the blood. It is often the health unit coordinator's responsibility to pick up the blood from the blood bank and bring it to the nursing unit. If blood for two different patients is to be obtained from the blood bank at the same time, two different health care personnel should pick up the blood. It is important for the health unit coordinator to know that if the blood is not used immediately it must be returned to the blood bank for storage. Blood should only be stored in refrigerators designated for blood storage.

Planning for blood transfusions is becoming common practice because it greatly reduces the risk of acquiring bloodborne infections such as human immunodeficiency virus (HIV) or hepatitis B. Patients, family, or friends may donate blood for a patient in advance. The patient's own blood transfusion is called autologous or autotransfusion; blood of relatives or friends is called donor-directed, or donor-specific. Blood may also be collected from the patient during surgery from the surgery site. This blood is then transfused back to the patient. The blood is collected in a device called a cell-saver, or autotransfusion system.

Plasma extenders or plasma substitutes are ordered by the doctor to increase the level of circulating fluid in the body. They are obtained from the pharmacy.

☑ DOCTORS' ORDERS FOR TRANSFUSION OF BLOOD, BLOOD COMPONENTS, AND PLASMA SUBSTITUTES

The nurse carries out the following orders for the administration of blood, blood components, and plasma substitutes; however, the transcription procedure requires the ordering step of tran-

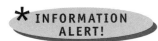

*INFORMATION ALERT!

Ordering and Obtaining Blood

A mistake in labeling a blood specimen sent to the laboratory for a type and cross-match will be discarded and the patient will have to have his or her blood drawn again. Avoid errors in labeling, which cause the patient additional discomfort and a delay in their treatment by:

- Matching the patient's name and information on the ID label affixed to the blood specimen to the patient name and information on the 'doctor's order sheet and the name and information on the computer order screen.

  If two units of blood need to be picked up from the blood bank for two different patients on your nursing unit, avoid an error in identifying the units of blood by:

- Having another person go with you to the blood bank to pick up the second unit

  or

- Making two trips to pick up one unit at a time

  When blood is brought to the unit and cannot be given immediately, return the blood to the blood bank for storage, where the storage temperature will ensure the safety of the blood.

scription. Blood bank ordering is described in Chapter 14,"Laboratory Orders."

- *Give 2 units of whole blood now*
- *T & X-match 2 units PC & hold for surgery*
- *Give 1 unit of packed cells tonight and one in the* AM
- *Give 2 units of plasma stat*
- *Give 1 unit PC now, draw stat H & H₂O p̄ completion of transfusion*
- *Give 2 units PCs c̄ 20 mg Lasix p̄ 1st unit*
- *Transfuse 1 unit of autologous blood today*
- *Autotransfusion per protocol*

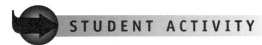

STUDENT ACTIVITY

To practice transcribing intravenous therapy orders, complete Activity 11–2 in *the Skills Practice Manual*.

Doctors' orders for total parenteral nutrition and for intravenous medication are covered in Chapter 13.

■ SUCTION ORDERS

Background Information

Suction may be ordered by the doctor to remove fluid or air from the body cavities and surgical wounds. Suction may be ordered intermittently or continuously and may be accomplished manually or mechanically. The doctor sets up some types of suction ap-

paratuses during surgery, and the nursing staff may initiate some, such as gastric suction. The doctor may write orders for the establishment, maintenance, or discontinuance of suction. Wall suction is installed at each patient's bedside. Usually tubing and suction catheters used with wall suction are stored on the nursing unit supply closet or C-locker. The unit coordinator may be asked by the nurse to order additional tubing or a specific type and/or size of catheter for a patient.

Following are doctors' orders relating to suctioning, with a brief interpretation. Refer to the abbreviations list at the beginning of the chapter for assistance, if necessary.

✓ DOCTORS' ORDERS FOR SUCTIONING

- *Suction throat prn to clear airway*

When a patient is unable to clear respiratory tract secretions by coughing, the doctor may order manual (bulb suction device) or mechanical (wall suction) suctioning to clear the airways (Fig 11–14). Three ways of suctioning respiratory tract secretions are through the nose, through the mouth, or through an artificial airway using tubing connected to the wall suction.

- *Suction tracheostomy prn*

A tracheostomy is an artificial opening into the trachea (windpipe), performed to facilitate breathing. When the patient is unable to cough, suctioning is necessary to remove secretions. Usually small catheters and tubing connected to a wall suction are used to remove secretions (Fig. 11–15).

- *Assess character of penrose drainage*

Patients often return from surgery with a drain inserted into or close to their surgical wound if a large amount of drainage is expected. A drain such as a penrose may lie under a dressing, extend through a dressing (Fig. 11–16), or be connected to a drainage bag or a disposable wound-suction device (also called evacuator units).

- *Keep Hemovac compressed*

- *Empty and record J-P drainage q shift*

Hemovac (Fig. 11–17, *A*) and Jackson-Pratt (J-P) (Fig. 11–17, *B*) are names of disposable wound-suction devices (evacuator units) that are attached to an incisional drain during surgery. These devices exert a constant low pressure as long as the suction device is fully compressed.

- *Insert NG tube, connect to intermittent low gastric suction*

The nurse or doctor inserts a nasogastric tube through the nose or mouth into the stomach (an x-ray is usually ordered to check tube placement). The tube is then connected to a wall-mounted suction unit (Fig. 11–18). The suction unit provides an intermittent removal of gastric contents and is usually set on low. (A high-pressure setting is never used without specific orders.) Gastric suction is often ordered following gastrointestinal or other abdominal surgery, to prevent vomiting or for various other reasons. Levin and Salem sumps are examples of tubes that may be used for gastric suction (Fig. 11–19).

- *Irrig NG per rout*

The nurse irrigates the nasogastric tube per facility policy. An irrigation tray, usually disposable, is used for this procedure.

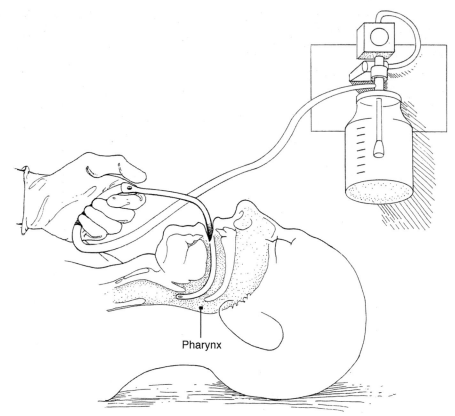

Pharynx

FIGURE 11–14 ▲ Throat-suctioning apparatus.

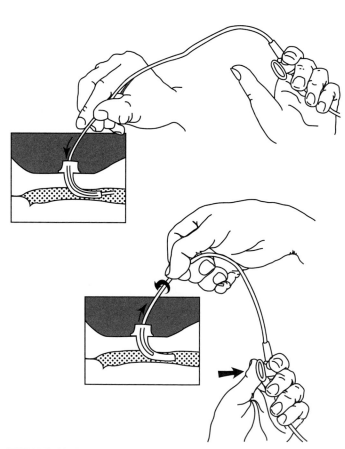

FIGURE 11–15 ▲ Suctioning of a tracheostomy using a small catheter and tubing attached to wall suction.

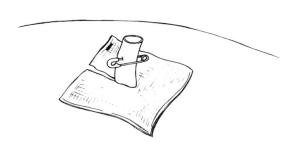

FIGURE 11–16 ▲ A penrose drain. (From Potter PA, Perry AG: Fundamentals of Nursing, 5th ed. St. Louis: Mosby, 2001.)

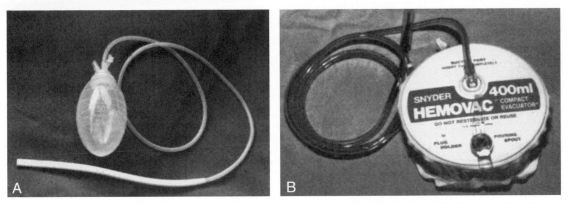

FIGURE 11-17 ▲ *A*, Jackson-Pratt. *B*, Hemovac, a disposal wound-suction apparatus. (From Ignatavicius DD, Workman ML, Mishler MA: Medical-Surgical Nursing: A Nursing Process Approach, 2nd ed. Philadelphia: W. B. Saunders, 1995.)

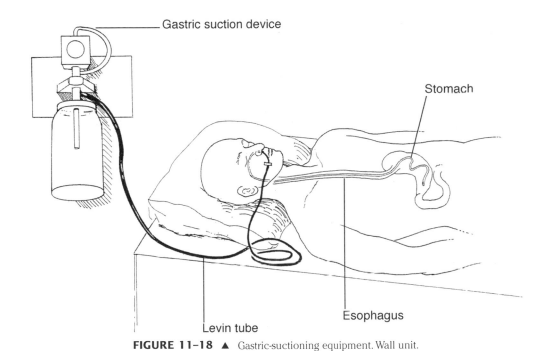

Gastric suction device

Stomach

Esophagus

Levin tube

FIGURE 11-18 ▲ Gastric-suctioning equipment. Wall unit.

Markings indicate tube placement

Small lumen (air vent)

SALEM SUMP TUBE

LEVIN TUBE

FIGURE 11-19 ▲ Two types of nasogastric tubes. (From Ignatavicius DD, Workman ML, Mishler MA: Medical-Surgical Nursing: A Nursing Process Approach, 2nd ed. Philadelphia: W. B. Saunders, 1995.)

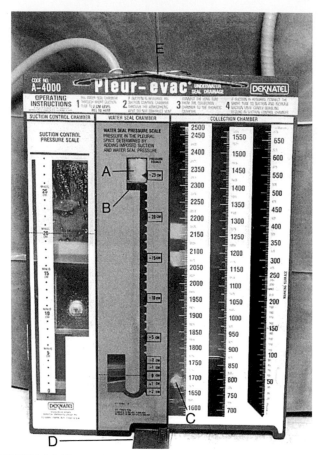

FIGURE 11–20 ▲ Pleur-evac—one of many available brands of chest-draining systems.

■ *Clamp NG tube intermittently q 1h*
A clamp is applied to the NG tube or a plug is inserted in the distal end of the tube at 1-hour intervals and then reconnected to the suction machine for 1-hour intervals.

■ *Remove NG tube and gastric suction*
This is a typical example of an order to discontinue the gastric suction.

■ *Chest tube 20 cm neg pressure*
A chest tube is a catheter that is inserted through the thorax (chest) to reexpand the lungs by removing air or fluids that collect in the pleural cavity. Chest tubes are used after chest surgery and chest trauma. The chest tube is connected to a closed chest-drainage system, such as Pleur-evac or Thora-Sene III, that is connected to wall suction. The drainage system and chest tubes are disposable items (Fig. 11–20).

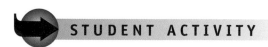

STUDENT ACTIVITY

To practice transcribing suction orders, complete Activity 11–3 in the *Skills Practice Manual*.

■ HEAT AND COLD APPLICATION ORDERS

Background Information

Heat and cold treatments are ordered for the patient by the doctor. Heat treatment is used to promote comfort, relaxation, and healing; to reduce pain and swelling; and to promote circulation. Cold treatment may be used to relieve pain, reduce inflammation, control hemorrhage, and decrease circulation.

Various methods for application of heat and cold are used, and thus there are a variety of doctors' orders to prescribe the methods intended. Typical doctors' orders for the common procedures used for heat and cold applications follow, with an explanation.

☑ DOCTORS' ORDERS FOR HEAT APPLICATIONS

■ *K-pad to lower lt arm 20 min qid*
An aquamatic K-pad is a device in which the water is electrically heated in a container and circulated through a network of tubes in a pad. K-pads are used for the application of continuous dry heat to various parts of the body. The temperature for the water in the K-pad is preset in CSD. A doctor's order for a temperature setting higher than one approved by the hospital must be communicated to CSD, since the CSD personnel can make the setting change. The K-pad is a reusable item (Fig. 11–21).

■ *Hot compresses to abscess on lt ankle 10 min qh*
Hot compresses are warm, wet gauze applied to a body part. They are used to treat small areas of the body. Usually, disposable items are used for this procedure.

■ *Soak rt hand 20 min in warm NS solution q 4h while awake*
A soak is usually ordered to facilitate healing. For this order the right hand is placed in a container of the prescribed solution to soak for 20 minutes every 4 hours while the patient is awake.

■ *Sitz bath 30 min tid*
A sitz bath is used for the application of warm water to the pelvic area. Special tubs may be used for this procedure or a disposable sitz bath that fits under a toilet seat may be ordered from CSD (Fig. 11–22). Obstetric units have sitz baths included in patient bathrooms.

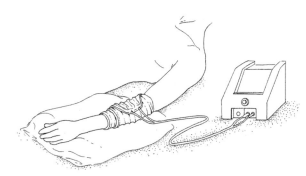

FIGURE 11–21 ▲ Aquamatic K-pad.

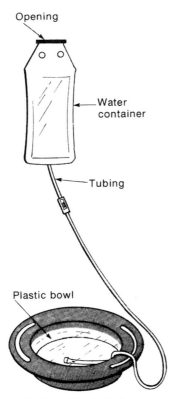

FIGURE 11-22 ▲ A disposable sitz bath apparatus. (Courtesy of Baxter Travenol Laboratories, Inc.)

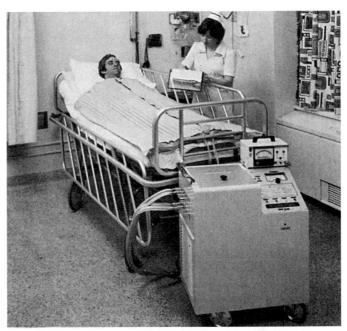

FIGURE 11-23 ▲ A hypothermia machine. (Courtesy of Cincinnati Sub-zero Products.)

☑ DOCTORS' ORDERS FOR COLD APPLICATIONS

▪ *Alcohol sponge for temp over 102°*
Alcohol sponge is the bathing of a patient with a solution of alcohol and water for the purpose of reducing the patient's temperature

▪ *Ice bag to scrotum as tolerated for 24 hr*
An ice bag may be a plastic or rubber container or sometimes a rubber glove filled with ice. It is a reusable item that is usually stored on the nursing unit supply closet or C-locker. Commercially prepared disposable ice bags are also used.

▪ *Hypothermia machine PRN if temp ↑ 104°*
The hypothermia machine circulates fluid through a network of tubing in a mattress-sized pad. It is used for prolonged cooling and to reduce body surface temperature (Fig. 11–23). This is a reusable item and is returned to the CSD when discontinued by the doctor.

■ COMFORT, SAFETY, AND HEALING ORDERS

Background Information

The nursing staff determines and performs many tasks to promote the comfort, safety, and healing of the patient. However, you will encounter doctors' orders relating to these areas also. Because such orders are so varied, only typical examples with the interpretation of each are listed.

☑ DOCTORS' ORDERS FOR PATIENT COMFORT, SAFETY, AND HEALING

▪ *Air therapy bed*
The air therapy bed is a low-air-loss therapy bed. Types include Respair, Flexicare, and Kinair. The health unit coordinator must include the patient's height and weight when ordering the bed from CSD.

A variety of specialty beds are available to reduce the hazards of immobility to the skin and musculoskeletal system. Other types of specialty beds that may be used include BioDyne, Pulmonair-40, Rescue, RotoRest, Tilt and Turn, and Clinitron.

▪ *Egg-crate mattress*
The Egg-crate mattress is a foam rubber pad resembling an egg crate or carton, used to distribute body weight more evenly (Fig. 11–24). It is a disposable item, and is used most often in long-term care.

Other mattresses used to reduce the hazards of immobility to the skin and musculoskeletal system include Lotus Water Flotation Mattress, Bio Flote (an alternating air mattress), static air mattress, and foam mattress.

▪ *Sheepskin on bed*
A sheepskin is made either of lamb's wool or of a synthetic material. It measures approximately three quarters of the length and the same width as the bed. The sheepskin is placed directly below the patient and is used to relieve pressure and prevent bedsores (decubitus ulcers). A sheepskin is usually considered a disposable item, and is mostly used in long-term care.

▪ *Footboard on bed*
A footboard is placed at or near the foot of the bed so that the patient's feet, when placed against it, are at a right angle to the bed. It is used to prevent footdrop of patients who are in bed for

FIGURE 11–24 ▲ An egg-crate mattress.

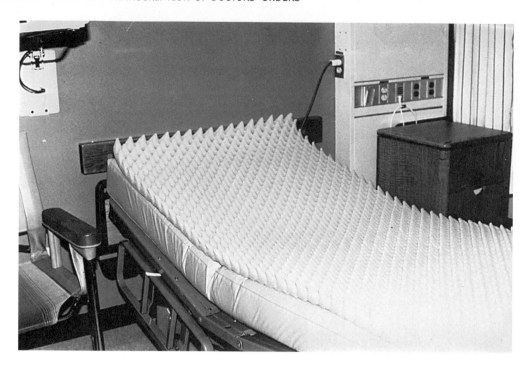

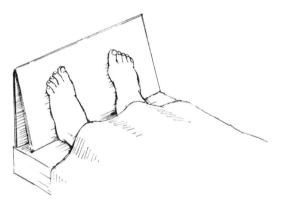

FIGURE 11–25 ▲ A footboard.

long periods (Fig. 11–25). A footboard is a reusable item and would be ordered from CSD.

▪ *Foot cradle to bed*

A foot cradle is a metal frame placed on the bed to prevent the top sheet from touching a specified part of the body. A foot cradle is a reusable item and would be ordered from CSD.

▪ *Immobilizer to lt knee 20° flexion*

Immobilizers are used to keep a limb or body part in alignment (Fig. 11–26). Immobilizers are reusable. Immobilizers would be stored on the CSD closet or C-locker on an ortho unit, but would need to be ordered from CSD if ordered for a patient on another unit.

FIGURE 11–26 ▲ Immobilizer.

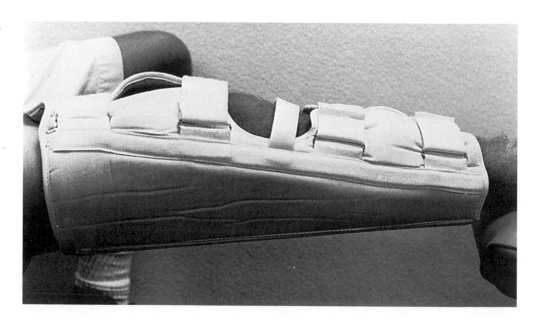

• *Sand bags to immobilize lt leg*

Sand bags are placed on both sides of the leg to immobilize the leg. Sand bags are stored on the CSD closet or C-locker on ortho units, but would need to be ordered from CSD on other units.

• *OOB with elastic abd binder*

An elastic abdominal binder is often ordered following surgery for patient support (Fig. 11–27). It is a disposable item. It is usually necessary to include the measurement of the patient's waist and hips on the requisition to obtain the correctly sized binder. The doctor may also order an elastic binder for the chest following chest surgery.

• *Sling to rt arm when up*

A sling is a disposable bandage used to support an arm (Fig. 11–28). Slings would be stored on the CSD closet or C-locker on an ortho unit, but would need to be ordered from CSD if ordered for a patient on another unit.

• *Thigh-high Teds to both legs*

Teds is a brand name for antiembolism hose (AE hose) and are made in various sizes and may be ordered as thigh high or knee high. Teds are ordered to promote circulation to the lower extremities and therefore prevent blood clots or emboli. The patient takes the stockings home with him or her. The health unit coordinator will need to obtain the size prior to ordering them from the nurse after the nurse measures the patient's leg (Fig. 11–29).

• *Soft wrist restraints for agitation and patient safety*

When they are absolutely necessary for patient safety, restraints are ordered by the doctor. There are various methods of restraint, and several types of commercial equipment available. The patient's mental and physical status must be assessed at close and regular intervals as prescribed by law and the agency's policies. Careful nursing documentation is essential when restraints are applied. The health unit coordinator may need to place a restraint documentation form in the patient's chart (Fig. 11–30).

• *May shampoo hair*

A doctor's order is necessary for the hospitalized patient to have a shampoo. The appropriate equipment is usually requisitioned from CSD and is reusable. Some hospitals have a beauty shop located on the campus, for ambulatory patients.

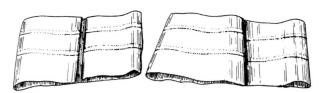

FIGURE 11–27 ▲ An elastic binder.

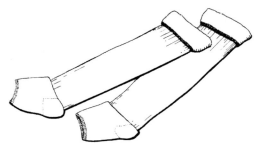

FIGURE 11–29 ▲ Ted hose (antiembolism stockings).

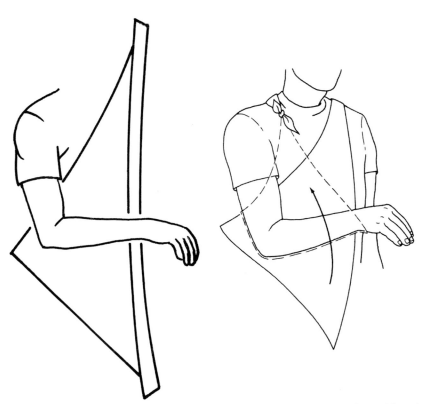

FIGURE 11–28 ▲ A sling used to support a patient's arm. (From deWit SC: Rambo's Nursing Skills for Clinical Practice, 4th ed. Philadelphia: W. B. Saunders, 1994.)

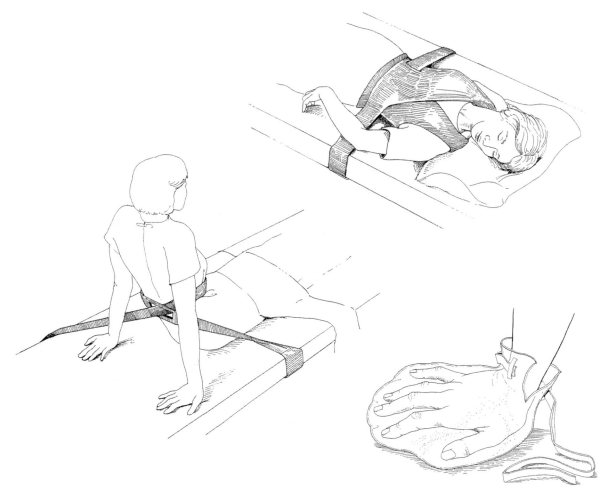

FIGURE 11–30 ▲ Types of restraints.

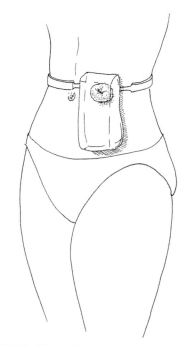

FIGURE 11–31 ▲ Stomal bag covering a colostomy.

- *Change surgical dressings bid*
A bandage or other application over an external wound is called a dressing. Items used for this treatment are disposable and usually stored on the nursing unit supply closet or C-locker.

- *Pneumatic hose to left leg*
An electrical pump with a pneumatic hose (also called sequential compression devices) is used to provide alternating pressure and thereby prevent clots from forming in the legs from inactivity. The stockings are disposable; the pump is reusable.

- *TCDB q 2h*
The nursing staff turns the patient to a different position (right side, left side, back) every 2 hours and encourages him or her to take deep breaths and cough. TCDB is frequently ordered following surgery.

- *ET nurse referral*
ET is the abbreviation for enterostomal therapist. The term is now outdated but is used to refer to the nurse who is trained to care for ostomy patients. The ET nurse is notified and will perform the care needed or will provide ostomy training to the patient. Figure 11–31 displays a stomal bag used for ostomy care.

- *Give warm water vaginal irrigation (douche) in* AM
- *Change surgical dressing and record observations bid*

To practice transcribing heat and cold applications, comfort, safety and healing orders, complete Activity 11–4 in the *Skills Practice Manual*.

■ BLOOD GLUCOSE MONITORING ORDERS

Blood glucose monitoring is routinely performed by the nursing staff (referred to as point-of-care testing, POCT) for diabetic patients or patients who are receiving nutritional support (total parenteral nutrition). There are different kinds of blood glucose monitoring devices used to obtain capillary blood, usually from the patient's finger. One type of monitor is the Accu-Chek Advantage (referred to as Accu-Chek), in which a drop of blood is placed on a chemically treated strip. The strip is placed in a blood glucose monitor and the patient's blood glucose results are displayed in numbers. The monitor is turned off by pressing the "O" button. Another type of blood glucose monitor is the One Touch, which can be used on the patient's arm rather than the finger. The nurse uses the results of the blood glucose level to administer or adjust insulin dosage according to the doctor's orders (see Chapter 13). The order for blood glucose monitoring is usually written on the Kardex form during the transcription procedures. The doctor may use the trade name of the device when ordering blood glucose monitoring, such as Accu-Chek or One Touch (Fig. 11–32)

Note: Other POCT will be discussed in Chapter 14.

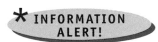 **DOCTORS' ORDERS FOR BLOOD TESTING FOR GLUCOSE**

▪ *Accu-Chek ac and hs*
Accu-Chek is a type of commercial blood glucose monitor used to check the glucose level of blood. The doctor has ordered the test to be done four times a day (the order may be written as qid, which would be performed ac and hs).

✱ INFORMATION ALERT!

Types of Nursing Treatment Orders

Intestinal elimination orders
Urinary catheterization orders
Intravenous therapy orders
Blood transfusion orders
Suction orders
Heat and cold application orders
Comfort, safety, and healing orders
Blood glucose monitoring orders

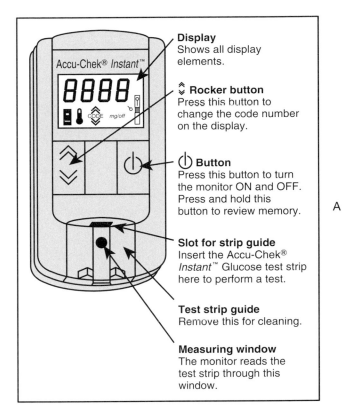

Display
Shows all display elements.

⌃⌄ Rocker button
Press this button to change the code number on the display.

⏻ Button
Press this button to turn the monitor ON and OFF. Press and hold this button to review memory.

Slot for strip guide
Insert the Accu-Chek® *Instant*™ Glucose test strip here to perform a test.

Test strip guide
Remove this for cleaning.

Measuring window
The monitor reads the test strip through this window.

A

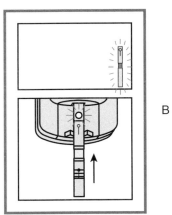

B

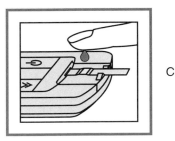

C

FIGURE 11–32 ▲ *A*, Example of a blood glucose monitor. *B*, The strip is placed on the monitor. *C*, Blood glucose results are displayed in numbers; the monitor is turned off by pressing the "O" button. (From Stepp CA, Woods MA: Laboratory Procedures for Medical Office Personnel. Philadelphia: W.B. Saunders, 1998.)

STUDENT ACTIVITIES

To practice transcribing a blood glucose monitor order, complete Activity 11–5 in the *Skills Practice Manual*. To practice transcribing a review set of a doctor's orders, complete Activity 11–6.

supplies and/or equipment delays the treatment, but probably would not harm the patient. When in doubt about the supplies or equipment needed, check with the nurse or with the CSD. The health unit coordinator who is able to recognize supplies and equipment and their uses and effectively uses the central service department system plays an invaluable role in helping the nursing staff to practice quality patient care.

■ SUMMARY

The transcription procedure for nursing treatment orders is fairly simple once you become familiar with the supplies and equipment necessary to implement each order. Ordering the wrong

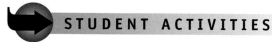

STUDENT ACTIVITIES

To practice recording telephoned doctors' orders, complete Activity 11–7 in *the Skills Practice Manual*. To practice recording telephone messages, complete Activity 11–8.

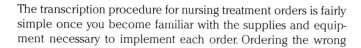

REVIEW QUESTIONS

1. List five nursing treatment items that would be located on the nursing unit supply closet or C-locker.

    a. _____

    b. _____

    c. _____

    d. _____

    e. _____

2. List five nursing treatment items that would be stored in the central service department.

    a. _____

    b. _____

    c. _____

    d. _____

    e. _____

3. List three types of enemas a doctor may order.

    a. _____

    b. _____

    c. _____

4. List two types of urinary catheters and describe the function of each.

    a. _____

    b. _____

5. List three parts of an IV order.

    a. _____

    b. _____

    c. _____

6. List two types of suction devices that could be inserted in surgery.

    a. _____

    b. _____

7. State two methods of administering IV therapy.

    a. _____

    b. _____

8. List two types of IV solutions commonly used.

    a. _____

    b. _____

9. Explain what would happen if a patient's blood specimen sent for a type and crossmatch was labeled incorrectly (the patient's name on the ID label does not match the patient's name on the order requisition).

    _____

    _____

10. List two devices used for heat application.

    a. _____

    b. _____

11. List two devices used for cold application.

    a. _____

    b. _____

12. Define the following terms.

    a. Heplock

    _____

    b. Hemovac

    _____

  c. Jackson-Pratt (J-P) _____

  _____

  d. autologous blood _____

  _____

  e. donor-specific blood _____

  _____

  f. catheterization _____

  _____

  g. penrose drain _____

  _____

  h. central venous catheter _____

  _____

  i. Accu-Chek _____

  _____

13. Define "urine residual."

  _____

14. Rental equipment should be promptly returned to the central service department because:

  a. _____

  b. _____

15. The patient's nurse asked you to pick up a unit of packed cells from the blood bank. When you return to the nursing unit with the packed cells, the nurse tells you she is not able to start the transfusion for an hour. Explain what you would do with the packed cells until the nurse can start the transfusion.

  _____

  _____

16. You are asked to pick up two units of packed cells from the blood bank for two separate patients on your unit. Explain what you would do.

  _____

  _____

17. Briefly describe the function of the CSD as it relates to nursing treatment orders.

_____

_____

18. True or False

   a. _____ A consent is required for the insertion of a PICC.

   b. _____ A consent is required for a peripheral intravenous catheter.

   c. _____ A consent is required for the insertion of a Heplock.

   d. _____ A Hemovac is connected to a drain in or near the surgical site and is inserted in surgery.

   e. _____ A central line tray would need to be ordered for insertion of a PICC.

19. Rewrite the following doctors' orders using abbreviations.

   a. Have the intravenous team insert a peripherally inserted central catheter.

   _____

   b. Continuous intravenous fluids; alternate one thousand cubic centimeters of lactated Ringer's with one thousand cubic centimeters of five percent dextrose in water at one hundred twenty-five cubic centimeters per hour via central venous catheter.

   _____

   c. Insert nasal gastric tube and connect to low gastric suction.

   _____

TOPICS FOR DISCUSSION

1. Discuss what your greatest fears might be if you were a hospital patient.

2. Discuss what patients have the right to expect of the nursing staff, including the health unit coordinator.

3. Discuss how the health unit coordinator can have a direct impact on the delivery of patient care.

4. Discuss why communication and teamwork between the health unit coordinator and the nursing staff are important.

WEB SITES OF INTEREST

www.Accu-Chek.com
www.lifescan.com
www.cdc.gov/hiv/pubs/saq15.htm
www.niddk.nih.gov

Dietary Orders

Chapter Objectives

Upon completion of this chapter, you will be able to:

1. Define the terms listed in the vocabulary list.
2. Write the meaning of the abbreviations in the abbreviations list.
3. Interpret the dietary orders included in this chapter.
4. Explain the importance of communicating patient food allergies to the dietary department.
5. List the diets that provide change in the consistency of food.
6. Identify five therapeutic diets.
7. List four diets that may be selected for the patient who is on *diet as tolerated*.
8. List three types of formula or preparations used for tube feeding.
9. List three methods of administering tube feedings.
10. List three items a health unit coordinator may need to order when transcribing an order for tube feeding.

Vocabulary

Calorie ▲ A measurement of energy generated in the body by the heat produced after food is eaten

Diet Manual ▲ Hospitals are required to have an up-to-date diet manual available in the dietary office and on all nursing units that has been jointly approved by the medical and dietary staffs

Diet Order ▲ A doctor's order that states the type and amount of food and liquids the patient may receive

Enteral Feeding Set ▲ Equipment needed to infuse tube feeding; includes plastic bag for feeding solution and may be ordered with or without pump

Enteral Nutrition ▲ The provision of liquid formulas into the GI tract by tube or orally

Food Allergy ▲ A negative physical reaction to a particular food involving the immune system (people with food allergies must avoid the offending foods)

Food Intolerance ▲ A more common problem than food allergies, involving digestion (people with food intolerances can eat some of the offending food without suffering symptoms)

Gastrostomy Feeding ▲ Feeding by means of a tube inserted into the stomach through an artificial opening in the abdominal wall

Gavage ▲ Feeding by means of a tube inserted into the stomach, duodenum, or jejunum through the nose or an opening in the abdominal wall; also called *tube feeding*

Ingestion ▲ The taking in of food by mouth

Kangaroo Pump ▲ A brand name of a feeding pump used to administer tube feeding

Nutrients ▲ Substances derived from food, which are utilized by body cells; for example, carbohydrates, fats, proteins, vitamins, minerals, and water

Percutaneous Endoscopic Gastrostomy (PEG) ▲ Insertion of a tube through the abdominal wall into the stomach using endoscopic guidance

Registered Dietitian (RD) ▲ One who has completed an educational program, served an internship, and passed an examination sponsored by the American Dietetic Association

Regular Diet ▲ A diet that consists of all foods, designed to provide good nutrition

Therapeutic Diet ▲ A regular diet with modifications or restrictions (also called a *special diet*)

Total Parenteral Nutrition (TPN) ▲ The provision of all necessary nutrients via veins (discussed in detail in Chapter 13)

Tube Feeding ▲ Administration of liquids into the stomach, duodenum, or jejunum, through a tube

Abbreviations

Abbreviation	Meaning	Example of Usage on a Doctor's Order Sheet
ADA	American Diabetic Association	1200 cal ADA diet
cal	calorie	1800 cal diet
CHO	carbohydrate	high protein, low CHO diet
chol	cholesterol	low chol diet
cl	clear	cl liq diet
DAT	diet as tolerated	advance DAT
FF	force fluids	soft diet FF
FS	full strength	Δ Jevity FS @ 50 mL/h
K or K+	potassium	high K+
liq	liquid	full liq diet
MN	midnight	NPO MN
Na or Na+	sodium	4000 mg Na diet (4000 mg4 g)
NAS	no added salt	reg diet, NAS
NPO	nothing by mouth	NPO after midnight
NSA	no salt added (same as NAS)	
PEG	percutaneous endoscopic gastrostomy	PEG in AM
RD	registered dietitian	RD consult requested
reg	regular	reg diet

EXERCISE 1

Write the abbreviation for each term.

1. sodium _____
2. midnight _____
3. nothing by mouth _____
4. regular _____
5. clear _____
6. calorie _____
7. American Diabetic Association _____

8. liquid _____
9. cholesterol _____
10. diet as tolerated _____
11. force fluids _____
12. carbohydrate _____
13. no salt added _____
14. full strength _____
15. percutaneous endoscopic gastrostomy _____
16. no added salt _____
17. registered dietitian _____
18. potassium _____

EXERCISE 2

Write the meaning of each abbreviation listed below.

1. *Na or Na+* _____
2. *NPO* _____
3. *reg* _____
4. *MN* _____
5. *liq* _____
6. *cal* _____
7. *NSA* _____

8. ADA

_____

9. DAT

_____

10. cl

_____

11. chol

_____

12. CHO

_____

13. FF

_____

14. FS

_____

15. PEG

_____

16. NAS

_____

17. RD

_____

18. K or K+

_____

■ COMMUNICATION WITH THE DIETARY DEPARTMENT

The procedure for ordering a new diet or a change/modification to an existing diet requires the health unit coordinator to communicate the order by computer to the dietary department. The health unit coordinator chooses the correct patient from the unit census screen on the computer, selects dietary department from the department ordering screen, then checks the box to order the specific diet from the options on the dietary screen along with other items that apply (e.g., dietitian consult) (Fig. 12–1). The patient's food allergies and intolerances must be communicated to the dietary department (noted on the order). Some food aller-

FIGURE 12–1 ▲ A computer screen for ordering from the dietary department.

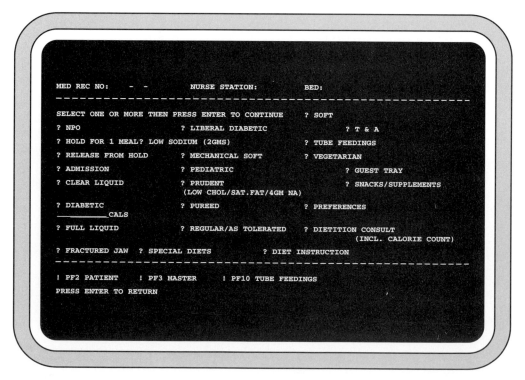

```
MED REC NO:     - -          NURSE STATION:          BED:
-----------------------------------------------------------------------

SELECT ONE OR MORE THEN PRESS ENTER TO CONTINUE    ? SOFT

? NPO                        ? LIBERAL DIABETIC              ? T & A

? HOLD FOR 1 MEAL? LOW SODIUM (2GMS)        ? TUBE FEEDINGS

? RELEASE FROM HOLD          ? MECHANICAL SOFT    ? VEGETARIAN

? ADMISSION                  ? PEDIATRIC              ? GUEST TRAY

? CLEAR LIQUID               ? PRUDENT            ? SNACKS/SUPPLEMENTS
                             (LOW CHOL/SAT.FAT/4GM NA)

? DIABETIC                   ? PUREED             ? PREFERENCES
          CALS
? FULL LIQUID                ? REGULAR/AS TOLERATED   ? DIETITION CONSULT
                                                         (INCL. CALORIE COUNT)

? FRACTURED JAW  ? SPECIAL DIETS          ? DIET INSTRUCTION
-----------------------------------------------------------------------

! PF2 PATIENT    ! PF3 MASTER    ! PF10 TUBE FEEDINGS
PRESS ENTER TO RETURN
```

gies and intolerances cause minor discomforts such as hives or upset stomach. True food allergies such as allergies to tree nuts, fish, shellfish, and peanuts can produce life-threatening changes in circulation and bronchioles called anaphylactic shock. NKFA indicates that the patient has no known food allergies.

There is also a "write-in" option for additional comments. The diet order would be sent to the dietary department by pressing "enter" on the computer keyboard.

If the computer is shut down, order the diet from the dietary department by telephone or written requisition. The diet order is later entered into the computer to maintain a record (Fig. 12–2).

Most health care facilities provide each patient with the next day's menu of items that are allowed for the particular diet the doctor has ordered for the patient. The patient checks what foods he or she would like from the menu. The menu is then sent to the dietary department. Many facilities have initiated a system to better serve the patient as well as save the cost of printing the menus. This involves the diet aide or technician interviewing each patient upon admission to obtain and record his or her food preferences and allergies. The diet aide may use a laptop computer to record the information. The doctor, nurse, diet aide, or diet technician may request the dietitian to consult with the patient. Many patients have food preferences or restrictions based on their culture or religion or religious holidays. This information is used to prepare food for those patients.

All dietary information must be sent to the dietary department, including orders for nothing by mouth, tube feedings, allergies, limit fluids, force fluids, and calorie count, so the necessary adjustments will be made when preparing the patient's trays. The dietitian also maintains a record (usually on computer) on each patient, which will be updated with each order received (Fig. 12–3).

Background Information

During hospitalization, the doctor orders the type of diet the patient is to receive. The food is prepared by the dietary department and is designed to attain or maintain the health of the patient. Di-

---

✱ INFORMATION ALERT!

Patients' food allergies and intolerances must be communicated to the dietary department (noted on the order). Some food allergies and intolerances cause minor discomforts such as hives or upset stomach. True food allergies such as allergies to tree nuts, fish, shellfish, and peanuts can produce life-threatening changes in circulation and bronchioles called anaphylactic shock. NKFA indicates that the patient has no known food allergies.

✱ INFORMATION ALERT!

It is essential that all dietary information be sent to the dietary department, including orders for nothing by mouth, tube feedings, allergies, limit fluids, force fluids, and calorie count, so the necessary adjustments will be made when preparing the patient's tray. All admitted patients require a diet order.

FIGURE 12–2 ▲ A diet requisition.

Doctor Ordering _____ ☐ Routine
Today's Date _____ ☐ Stat
Requested by _____

Dietary Department

☐ Bland	☐ Kosher	☐ Restrict fluids to_____
☐ _____Calorie ADA	☐ Low cholesterol	☐ Snacks/supplements
☐ Calorie count	☐ Low sodium	☐ _____Sodium
_____Calorie	☐ Mechanical soft	☐ Soft
☐ Clear liquid	☐ Modified fat_____	☐ Vegetarian
☐ Dietitian consult	☐ NPO	
☐ Early tray	☐ Pediatric	
☐ Finger food	☐ Protein modified_____g	
☐ Force fluids	☐ Prudent cardiac	
☐ Full liquid	☐ Pureed	
☐ Guest tray	☐ Regular	
☐ Gluten free	☐ Release from hold	
☐ Hold tray_____	☐ Renal	

☐ Other_____

Food allergies_____
Preferences_____
Comments_____

| Room number_____ Patient name_____ Doctor_____ |
| Patient age_____ Height_____ Weight_____ Comments_____ |
| _____ |
| Date admitted_____ Food allergies_____ |

Date	Dietary orders	Diagnosis and notes	Food preferences

FIGURE 12–3 ▲ A sample of a dietary record maintained by the dietitian.

ets for the hospitalized patient can be divided into three groups: standard diets, therapeutic diets, and tube feedings (Table 12–1).

■ STANDARD DIETS

Standard hospital diets consist of a regular diet and diets that vary in consistency or texture (clear liquid–solid) of foods. A regular diet, also called general, house, routine, and full, is planned to provide good nutrition and consists of all items in the four basic food groups. This diet is ordered for hospitalized patients who do not require restrictions or modifications of their diets. Clear liquid, full liquid, soft, mechanical soft, and bland are types of diets that vary in food texture or consistency. Modifications may be added to these diets (e.g., Reg, 2.5 g Na).

☑ DOCTORS' ORDERS FOR STANDARD DIETS

- *Regular diet*
This diet is nutritionally adequate and includes all the foods a healthy person should eat.

- *Soft diet*
This diet is often used in the progression from a full liquid diet to a regular diet. It consists of nonirritating, easily digestible foods and modified fiber content, such as broiled chicken and boiled vegetables. It may be ordered postoperatively, for acute infections, or for gastrointestinal disorders.

- *Full liquid diet*
A full liquid diet is often ordered as a transitional step between a clear liquid diet and a soft diet. Some of the foods included in this diet are milk, creamed soup, custards, ice cream, and fruit and vegetable juices. It is often ordered for patients who have dif-

ficulty chewing or swallowing, who are acutely ill, or who have just had surgery.

- *Clear liquid diet*
This diet is used for patients who cannot tolerate solid foods, such as those suffering an acute illness or who have just had surgery. It includes clear liquids only, such as tea, coffee, soda, broth, water, Jello, and clear juices.

- *Mechanical soft diet*
This is a regular diet that is prepared to meet the needs of patients who have difficulty chewing. The meat is ground and vegetables are diced or chopped. Variations may include mechanical soft, ground, or pureed depending on a patient's ability to chew food.

- *Diet as tolerated (DAT)*
When the doctor writes this order, the nurse selects a clear liquid, full liquid, soft, or regular diet for the patient, according to his or her tolerance of food. For example, immediately following surgery the nurse may select a clear liquid diet for the patient. Normally, the patient is advanced to full liquid, soft, and then regular diet, according to the stage of recovery.

- *Bland diet*
A bland diet is considered a transitional diet used during severe inflammation and to determine food intolerances. It is designed to avoid chemical, thermal, and mechanical irritations of the GI tract and to decrease peristalsis.

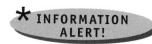
★ INFORMATION ALERT!

An order sent to dietary for a liquid diet must indicate *clear* or *full* or the dietary personnel will not know what to send to the patient.

TABLE 12-1	Description and Purpose of Common Hospital Diets		
Type	**Description**	**Purpose**	**Tray Condiments**
Bland diet	May be used for patients who experience stomach irritation. Spicy foods containing black or red pepper and chili powder are omitted. Beverages that contain caffeine, cola, coffee, cocoa, and tea are omitted. Chocolate is also omitted. Any foods known to cause discomfort are omitted.	For patients with ulcers and other problems.	Salt, sugar
Prudent—low-cholesterol/ reduced sodium	Controls the type of fat in the diet. Limits saturated fat and cholesterol found in foods from animal sources like eggs, dairy products, meat, and fish. Limits salt added to foods and on tray.	For patients who have high levels of blood cholesterol.	Pepper, sugar, salt substitute or herbal seasoning mix.
Sodium-controlled diet	Controls the amount of sodium in the diet. Salt and foods containing salt are high in sodium and are limited. The sodium-controlled diet will vary according to the amount of sodium allowed.	For patients with heart disease, high blood pressure, kidney disease, or who are using certain drugs.	Sugar, pepper, salt substitute, if ordered.
Diabetic diet	Total amount of food (calories) is carefully planned. Diabetics cannot receive too much or too little food; therefore, portion sizes must be followed. Concentrated sweets, like syrup, jelly, sweet desserts, and sugar are omitted. Snacks may be planned in between meals to keep blood sugar levels balanced.	For patients who cannot produce enough insulin. Insulin is a substance important in helping sugar enter body cells. When there is not enough insulin made, sugar will build up in the blood.	Salt, pepper, sugar substitute
Renal	Based on individual needs, diet is controlled in one or more of the following: protein, sodium, potassium, total fluid, phosphorous.	For patients with renal disease.	Sugar, pepper No salt substitutes
Neutropenic—no fresh fruits/vegetables low bacteria	No fresh fruits or vegetables allowed.	Reduce the number of bacteria entering the stomach for patients on chemotherapy or those with immune deficiency diseases.	Sugar No pepper or salt
Lactose controlled	Limits intake of milk and milk products.	For patients who experience stomach disturbances after drinking/eating milk-containing foods.	Salt, pepper, sugar
NPO—nothing by mouth	Patient cannot receive fluids or solid foods.	Presurgery, procedures, test, or as Indicated.	None
Clear liquid	Foods that are liquid or become liquid at room or body temperatures. Includes foods like tea, coffee, clear broth, gelatin, carbonated beverages. Foods you can see through (e.g., apple, cranberry, grape juice).	For patients who are very sick and cannot eat anything else. For patients before or after surgery.	Sugar
Full-liquid diet	Includes food from the clear-liquid diet, with the addition of juices with pulp, such as orange. Includes milk, ice cream, puddings, refined cooked cereals, strained cream soups, and egg nog.	For patients who cannot eat solid foods. For patients after surgery, following the clear-liquid diet.	Salt, pepper, sugar
Regular diet/DAT	All foods and beverages are allowed.	For patients who have no dietary restrictions.	Salt, pepper, sugar
GI soft diet	Limits raw, highly seasoned, and fried foods.	For patients with nausea and distention in the postsurgical patient.	Salt, pepper, sugar
Mechanical soft diet	Any diet made soft with ground meats, soft canned fruits, and well-cooked vegetables.	For patients who have trouble chewing or swallowing.	Salt, pepper, sugar
Puree	Mechanically altered foods and full liquids allowed.	For patients with problems in chewing and swallowing.	Salt, pepper, sugar
No thin liquids/thick liquids only	No milk (except milk shakes), juice (except nectars), broth soups (only cream soups), no coffee, tea, or soda pop.	To prevent choking.	Salt, pepper, sugar

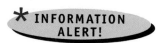

INFORMATION ALERT!

When the doctor writes an order to advance diet as tolerated (DAT), he or she usually orders the initial diet. The nurse may then select from the standard (consistency) diets such as clear liquid, full liquid, soft, or regular to advance the diet. Variations may include mechanical soft, ground, or pureed depending on the patient's ability to chew. The health unit coordinator needs to ask the patient's nurse for the diet selection then send this information to the dietary department. The dietary department cannot make the evaluation of what the patient can tolerate.

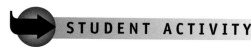

STUDENT ACTIVITY

To practice transcribing a standard hospital diet order, complete Activity 12–1 in the *Skills Practice Manual.*

■ THERAPEUTIC DIET ORDERS

Therapeutic diets must be ordered by a doctor, and differ from the regular diet in that the foods served are modified to vary in caloric content, level of one or more nutrients, bulk, or flavor. The following list contains common therapeutic diets named according to the modification.

Low-cholesterol diet
Low-cholesterol, sugar-free diet
Prudent cardiac diet
Low-fat diet
High-carbohydrate diet
Hypoglycemic diet

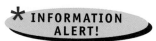

INFORMATION ALERT!

An order modifying a nutrient or number of calories would not change the consistency of a patient's diet.

Example: If a patient is on a "soft diet" and the doctor then wrote an order for "low fat," the patient's diet would be "soft, low fat."

Renal diet
Sodium-restricted diets:
    Regular, no salt added diet
    2.5 g Na diet (mild restrictions)
    1.0 g Na diet (moderate restrictions)
    500 mg Na diet (severe restrictions); may also be called *low Na+ diet*
High-fiber diet
Potassium-modified diets:
    Potassium-restricted diet
    High-potassium diet
High-protein, moderate-carbohydrate diet
Low-triglyceride diet
Diabetic diet (ADA)
Liberal diabetic diet
Calorie-restricted diets:
    1200-calorie diet
    1400-calorie diet
Vegetarian diet (usually a patient request)
Kosher diet (usually a patient request)

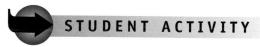

STUDENT ACTIVITY

To practice transcribing a therapeutic diet order, complete Activity 12–2 in the *Skills Practice Manual.*

Communication and Implementation of Dietary Orders

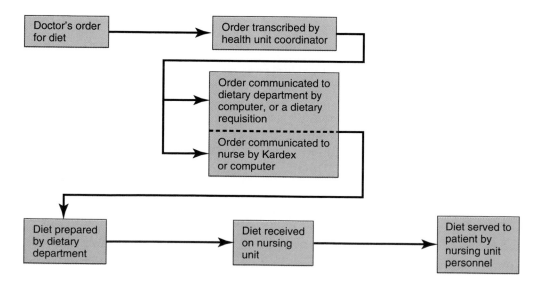

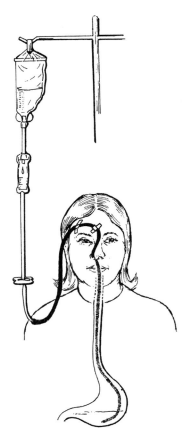

FIGURE 12–4 ▲ Feeding tube. (Courtesy of Baxter Travenol Laboratories, Inc.)

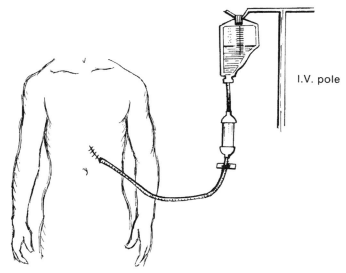

FIGURE 12–5 ▲ Gastrostomy feeding.

I.V. pole

■ TUBE FEEDINGS

Tube feeding, also called gavage, is the administration of liquefied nutrients into the stomach, duodenum, or jejunum through a tube inserted either through the nose (a nasogastric or nasoenteral tube; see Fig. 12–4) or through an opening in the abdominal wall (gastrostomy, duodenostomy, or jejunostomy; see Fig. 12–5). Tube feedings are ordered for patients who have difficulty swallowing, are unable to eat sufficient nutrients, or who cannot absorb the nutrients from the food they eat.

Administration of tube feedings may be by bolus, continuous, or cyclic:

- Bolus—infusing 300 to 400 mL of formula over a short period of time (10 minutes) with a syringe, or 300 to 400 mL every 3 to 6 hours over a 30- to 60-minute period using an enteral feeding bag.
- Continuous—administered by using a mechanical feeding infusion pump (called enteral feeding pump or Kangaroo pump) to control the rate of infusion (Fig. 12–6).
- Cyclic—infused over 8 to 16 hours either during the day or night. Nighttime feedings allow for more freedom during the day. Daytime feedings are recommended for patients who have a greater chance of aspiration or tube dislodgment.

Types of nasogastric or nasoenteral tubes used for feedings include Entron, Dobbhoff, and Levin. Some of the commercially prepared formulas, including Isocal HN, Deliver 2.0, Ultracal HN

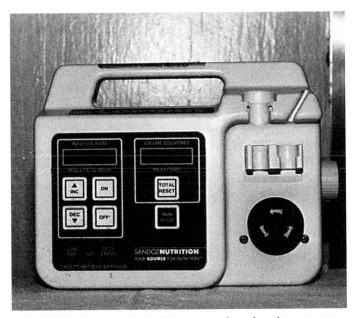

FIGURE 12–6 ▲ Feeding infusion pump, also referred to as an enteral feeding pump or Kangaroo pump.

Plus, Pulmocare, Jevity, Boost High Nitrogen, Boost Plus, Respalor, or Megnacal, may be ordered for tube feedings. To transcribe a tube-feeding order, the health unit coordinator may need to order a nasogastric tube, formula, and a feeding infusion pump.

☑ DOCTORS' ORDERS FOR TUBE FEEDING

Several types of formulas and preparations are available to meet nutritional needs for different disease states. There are more than 50 medical food products available and changes are constantly made as a result of new knowledge. Examples of a typical doctor's order for tube feeding are written below.

- *Insert NG feeding tube, verify placement, and begin feeding of Isocal HN (1 cal/cc) @ FS 40 cc/hr. Progress by 10 cc/hr q 2 hrs as tolerated to final rate of 90 cc/hr.*
The nurse may verify the tube placement by withdrawing a small amount of stomach contents or by injecting air with a syringe through the tube and listening with a stethoscope as air enters the stomach. The doctor has ordered that the prepared formula be started at full strength and the amount increased every 2 hours as tolerated to a final rate.

- *Tube feeding of Boost Plus (1.5 cal/cc) FS bolus by syringe 45 cc q 6 hrs given over 20 min. Flush tube c̄ 5 cc H₂O q 2 hrs.*
The doctor is ordering the formula to be given full strength by bolus using a syringe every 6 hours and to be given over 20 minutes. The nurse will flush the tube with water as ordered.

- *Megnacal FS @ 40 cc/hr through gastrostomy tube*

- *Insert jejunostomy tube. X-ray for placement. When in proper position, begin via pump to deliver 2.0 (2 cal/cc) @ 30 cc/hr for 8 hrs, then 40 cc/hr for 8 hrs, then increase to final rate of 50 cc/hr.*
In this order for tube feedings, the doctor is requesting an x-ray to determine the correct placement of the tube before the administration of the formula.

 STUDENT ACTIVITY

To practice transcribing a tube-feeding order, complete Activity 12–3 in the *Skills Practice Manual*.

✓ DOCTORS' ORDERS: OTHER DIETARY ORDERS

The following orders pertain to the patient's intake of foods and liquids but are not orders for a type of diet.

- *Force fluids*
This order is probably written in addition to the patient's dietary order. The doctor wants the patient to drink more fluids. The health unit coordinator would send this order to the dietary department so more fluids could be included on the patient's trays.

- *Limit fluids to 1000 cc per day*
This order is also written in addition to the diet order. The patient's fluid intake is to be restricted to 1000 cc per day. A restriction of fluids is usually ordered for patients who are retaining fluids (a condition known as edema) because of a disease process. The dietary department should be notified of this order so fluids would be limited on the patient's trays and the dietitian would also become involved.

- *NPO*
This order means the patient is to have nothing by mouth. This is usually ordered following major surgery, or during a critical illness. This information is sent to the dietary department to update the patient's dietary record so a tray would not be prepared for the patient.

- *NPO midnight*
The patient is to have nothing by mouth after midnight. This is ordered to prepare a patient for surgery, treatment, or a diagnostic procedure. The dietary department is notified so that a tray would not be sent to the patient.

- *Sips and chips*
The patient may have only sips of water and ice chips. This order would also be sent to the dietary department to update the patient's dietary record.

- *Have dietitian see patient*
The doctor is requesting the dietitian to discuss the diet with the patient or teach the patient about his or her diet. This order may require a phone call in addition to sending a requisition to the dietary department.

- *Calorie count today and tomorrow*
This is usually ordered to document amount and types of food consumed by the patient for further nutritional evaluation by the dietitian. Send this information to the dietary department and notify the nurse caring for the patient. You may be required to prepare a form to record the patient's caloric intake.

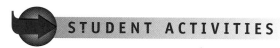 **STUDENT ACTIVITIES**

To practice transcribing a review set of doctors' orders, complete Activity 12–4 in the *Skills Practice Manual*.
To practice recording telephoned doctors' orders and telephone messages, complete Activities 12–5 and 12–6 in the *Skills Practice Manual*.

■ SUMMARY

Accuracy is essential in the transcription of dietary orders, because an error could result in serious consequences. Imagine, for example, a patient who is NPO for surgery receiving breakfast, or a severely diabetic patient receiving a regular diet.

Hospitalized patients are dependent upon the hospital personnel to meet their dietary preferences and needs. The diet ordered by the doctor for the patient may be an integral part of the treatment plan, or it may be ordered to maintain health. In either case, mealtime is an important time for many patients, and for some it may be the most positive experience of the day. The health unit coordinator is responsible for ordering late trays when a patient has missed a meal because of a test or procedure. It is important that the tray is ordered and delivered to the patient promptly. The dietary and nursing departments must work closely together to provide the patient with proper and pleasant meals. Thorough and prompt communication by the health unit coordinator facilitates this tremendously.

REVIEW QUESTIONS

1. Rewrite the following doctors' orders using symbols and/or abbreviations. Or, to practice writing doctors' orders, have someone read the orders to you while you record them. Again, practice using symbols and abbreviations while you do this.

   a. nothing by mouth after midnight

   _____

   b. clear liquid breakfast, then nothing by mouth

   _____

   c. one-thousand-calorie American Diabetic Association diet

   _____

   d. low-cholesterol diet

   _____

   e. diet as tolerated

   _____

   f. regular diet

   _____

   g. low-sodium diet

   _____

   h. no salt added

   _____

2. Define the terms listed below.

   a. therapeutic, or special, diet

   _____

   b. regular diet

   _____

   c. tube feeding

   _____

   d. nothing by mouth

   _____

3. List three methods of administering tube feedings.

   a. _____

   b. _____

   c. _____

4. Below is a list of diets the doctor may order for the patient. Identify each diet as standard or therapeutic.

   a. soft diet _____

   b. potassium-restricted diet _____

   c. 1200-cal diet _____

   d. full liquid diet _____

   e. 500-mg Na diet _____

   f. mechanical soft diet _____

   g. hypoglycemic diet _____

   h. low-triglyceride diet _____

5. For the doctor's order advance *diet as tolerated* (DAT), list four diets that may be selected by the nurse for the patient.

   a. _____

   b. _____

   c. _____

   d. _____

6. Explain why a doctor's order for DAT requires the health unit coordinator to ask the nurse what diet to order from the dietary department.

   _____

   _____

7. List two reasons why a doctor would order the patient NPO MN.

   a. _____

   b. _____

8. List three commercially prepared formulas or preparations that may be ordered for tube feedings.

   a. _____

   b. _____

   c. _____

9. Would a doctor's order for 2.5 g Na change a patient's previous order for a soft diet?

_____

10. Would a doctor's order for limit fluids to 1200 cc/day change a patient's previous order for a regular diet?

_____

11. Would an order for a patient to have sips and chips need to be sent to dietary?

_____

12. Why is it important to notify dietary of a patient's food allergy?

_____

_____

▼ **TOPICS FOR**
DISCUSSION

1. Discuss the possible consequences of a patient's food allergy not being communicated to the dietary department.

2. Discuss the importance of ordering a patient's diet as soon as possible when he or she returns to the nursing unit after undergoing a procedure and is cleared to eat.

Medication Orders

Chapter Objectives

Upon completion of this chapter, you will be able to:

1. Define the terms in the vocabulary list.

2. Write the meaning of each abbreviation in the abbreviations list.

3. Define *standing, standing prn, stat, one-time,* and *short-series* medication orders.

4. List the five components of a medication order.

5. List four groups of drugs that usually have automatic "stop dates."

6. Name two reference books for medications.

7. List four routes by which medications are administered.

8. Demonstrate the procedure for using the *Physicians' Desk Reference* (PDR).

9. Describe the general purpose for selected drug groups.

10. Name the skin test for TB.

11. Identify the most commonly used drugs, which are listed in italics in the "Drug Groups" section of the chapter, and name the drug group to which each belongs.

Vocabulary

Admixture ▲ The result of adding a medication to a container of intravenous solution

Ampoule (Ampule) ▲ Small glass vial sealed to keep contents sterile; used for subcutaneous, intramuscular, and intravenous medications

Apothecary System ▲ Ancient system of weight and volume measurements used to measure drugs and solutions

Automatic Stop Date ▲ Date on which specific categories of medications must be discontinued unless renewed by the physician

Bolus ▲ Concentrated dose of medication or fluid, frequently given intravenously

Capsule ▲ Gelatinous, single-dose container in which a drug is enclosed to prevent the patient from tasting the drug

Central Line Catheter or Central Venous Catheter (CVC) ▲ Large catheter that provides access to the veins and/or to the heart to measure pressures

Extravasation ▲ Leakage of fluid into tissue surrounding a vein

Hypnotics ▲ Drugs that reduce pain or induce sleep; can include sedatives, analgesics, and anesthetics

Infiltrate ▲ To strain through or pass into a substance or space

Intramuscular (IM) Injection ▲ Injection of a medication into a muscle

Intravenous (IV) ▲ Administered directly into a vein

Intravenous Hyperalimentation or Total Parenteral Nutrition (TPN) ▲ Method used to administer calories, proteins, vitamins, and other nutrients into the bloodstream of a patient who is unable to eat. Must be infused into the superior vena cava through a central line catheter—not given through a peripheral IV catheter

IV Push (IVP) ▲ Method of giving concentrated doses of medication directly into the vein

Lozenge ▲ Medicated tablet or disk that dissolves in the mouth

Medication Administration Record (MAR) ▲ List of medications that each individual patient is currently taking; it is used by the nurse to administer the medications

Medication Nurse ▲ Registered nurse or licensed practical nurse who administers medications to patients

Metric System ▲ A system of weights and measures based on multiples of 10

Narcotic ▲ Controlled drug that relieves pain or produces sleep

Oral ▲ By mouth

Parenteral Routes ▲ Methods other than oral for giving fluids or medications (i.e., injections or intravenously)

Patient-Controlled Analgesia (PCA) ▲ Medications administered intravenously by means of a special infusion pump controlled by the patient within order ranges written by the physician

Piggyback ▲ A method by which drugs are usually administered intravenously in 50 to 100 mL of fluid

Skin Tests ▲ Tests in which the reactive materials are placed on the skin or just beneath the skin to determine the presence of certain antibodies within the body

Subcutaneous (SQ) Injection ▲ Injection of a small amount of a medication under the skin into fatty or connective tissue

Suppository ▲ Medicated substance mixed in a solid base that melts when placed in a body opening; suppositories are commonly used in the rectum, vagina, or urethra

Suspension ▲ Fine-particle drug suspended in liquid

Tablet ▲ Solid dosage of a drug in a disk form

Topical ▲ Direct application of medication to the skin, eye, ear, or other parts of the body

Abbreviations

Abbreviation	Meaning	Order Example
ac	ante cibum (before meals)	Sliding scale insulin ac
amp	ampoule	Add 1 amp multivitamins to TPN bag q 24h
ASA	acetylsalicylic acid (aspirin)	ASA 325 mg × 2 PO q 4h prn
cap	capsule	ampicillin 1 cap 500 mg q 6h
cc	cubic centimeter (same as mL)	Give NS @ 75 cc/h
dr or ʒ	dram	elixir of phenobarb ʒ ī PO tid
G, gm, or g	gram	Cefadyl 1 g IVPB q 6h
gr	grain	chloral hydrate gr XV PO hs prn
IM	intramuscular	vitamin B_{12} 1000 μg deep IM tomorrow
IVP	intravenous push	Versed 2 mg IVP now
IVPB	intravenous piggyback	Keflin 0.5 g IVPB q 8h
KCl	potassium chloride	Add 40 mEq KCl to each IV
L	liter	1 L 5% D/W to run @ 125 mL/h
LOC	laxative of choice	LOC prn constipation
μg or mcg	microgram	vitamin B_{12} 1000 mcg IM
mEq	milliequivalent	Give 20 mEq KCl per open heart protocol
mg	milligram	Achromycin 250 mg PO qid
mL	milliliter (same as cc)	1000 mL 5% D/W @ KO rate
MOM	milk of magnesia	MOM 30 cc hs prn
MS or MSO_4	morphine sulfate	MS 10 mg IM q 4h prn pain

noc	night	LOC q noc
NTG	nitroglycerin	May leave NTG tablets @ bedside
N/V	nausea & vomiting	Compazine 10 mg IM q 6h prn N/V
OD	oculus dexter (right eye)	Timoptic XE 0.25% 1gtt OD bid
OS	oculus sinister (left eye)	Garamycin ophth sol gtt OS tid
OU	oculus unitas (both eyes)	Neosporin ophth sol gtts OU bid
oz	ounce	Add 8 oz of juice to Metamucil packet
pc	post cibum (after meals)	Maalox 15 cc tid pc
PCA	patient-controlled analgesia	PCA MS 2 mg q 15 min
PCN	penicillin	PCN 250 mg PO q 6h
PO	per os (by mouth)	Librium 5 mg PO tid
pr	per rectum	Dulcolax supp 10 mg now pr
prn	pro re nata (as needed)	Maalox 30 cc prn GI discomfort
SC, sq, or sub-q	subcutaneous	heparin 5000 U SC qd
stat	immediately	Valium 10 mg IVP stat
subling, SL	sublingual (under tongue)	nitroglycerin tab SL prn anginal pain
supp	suppository	acetaminophen supp prn for temp ↑ 100°(R)
syr	syrup	ipecac syr dr ĪĪ now
tab	tablet	prednisone 25 mg PO tab bid
tinct or tr	tincture	tinct belladonna gtts ac
TPN	total parenteral nutrition	↑ TPN to 100 cc/h
U	unit	heparin gtt @ 100 U/h
ung	unguent (ointment)	Neosporin ung tid to (R) elbow
WA	while awake	Hycodan 5 cc PO q 4h WA

EXERCISE 1

Write the abbreviation for each term.

1. liter _____
2. aspirin _____
3. immediately _____
4. capsule _____
5. tablet _____
6. milk of magnesia _____
7. unit _____

8. right eye _____
9. milligram _____
10. potassium chloride _____
11. gram _____
12. both eyes _____
13. milliliter _____
14. milliequivalent _____
15. after meals _____
16. ointment _____
17. while awake _____
18. nausea and vomiting _____
19. grain _____
20. intramuscular _____
21. sublingual _____
22. tincture _____
23. by mouth _____
24. ounce _____
25. left eye _____
26. ampoule _____
27. dram _____
28. suppository _____
29. nitroglycerin _____
30. subcutaneous _____
31. microgram _____
32. night _____
33. syrup _____
34. intravenous piggyback _____
35. before meals _____
36. penicillin _____
37. per rectum _____
38. total parenteral nutrition _____

39. patient-controlled analgesia _____

40. cubic centimeter _____

41. intravenous push _____

42. laxative of choice _____

43. morphine sulfate _____

44. pro re nata (as needed) _____

EXERCISE 2

Write the meaning of each abbreviation.

1. KCl

_____

2. OS

_____

3. amp

_____

4. syr

_____

5. dr or ʒ

_____

6. noc

_____

7. μg, mcg

_____

8. oz

_____

9. SC, sq, or sub-q

_____

10. stat

_____

11. ac

_____

12. mEq

_____

13. pc

_____

14. ung

_____

15. mL

_____

16. PO

_____

17. tinct

_____

18. IM

_____

19. gr

_____

20. mg

_____

21. supp

_____

22. G, gm, or g

_____

23. *OU*

_____

24. *N/V*

_____

25. *WA*

_____

26. *NTG*

_____

27. *ASA*

_____

28. *cap*

_____

29. *tab*

_____

30. *MOM*

_____

31. *L*

_____

32. *U*

_____

33. *OD*

_____

34. *subling, SL*

_____

35. *IVPB*

_____

36. *PCN*

_____

37. *TPN*

_____

38. *PCA*

_____

39. *pr*

_____

40. *cc*

_____

41. *prn*

_____

42. *LOC*

_____

43. *IVP*

_____

44. *MS or MSO₄*

_____

EXERCISE 3

The following is a list of medication orders typical of those you may see on the patient's chart. Write the meanings of the underlined abbreviations in the space provided.

1. *MS 14 mg IM q 3h prn severe pain*

_____

2. *Keflin 0.5 g IVPB q 8h*

_____

3. *Librium 10 <u>mg</u> <u>PO</u> qid*

_____

4. *Neosporin ophthalmic <u>gtts</u> <u>OU</u> bid*

_____

5. *Nitroglycerin 0.4 <u>mg</u> <u>subling</u> <u>prn</u> chest pain*

_____

6. *<u>MOM</u> 30 <u>cc</u> hs <u>prn</u> constipation*

_____

7. *NPH insulin 25 <u>U</u> qd*

_____

8. *<u>ASA</u> 325 <u>mg</u> <u>PO</u> q 4h prn for fever > than 101 <u>pr</u>*

_____

9. *Run <u>TPN</u> @ 50 <u>cc</u>/h x 2 hrs, then 125 <u>cc</u>/h*

_____

10. *Check blood sugar <u>ac</u>*

_____

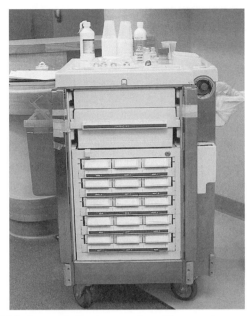

FIGURE 13–1 ▲ Medication cart (from Pharmacology and the Nursing Process, 3rd ed., Lilley & Aucker, Mosby, p. 86).

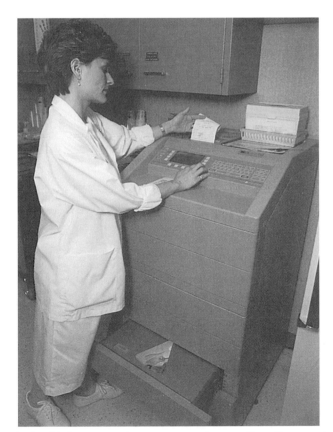

FIGURE 13–2 ▲ Computerized medication cart (from Pharmacology and the Nursing Process, 3rd ed., Lilley & Aucker, Mosby p. 86).

■ BACKGROUND INFORMATION

Communicating with the Pharmacy

The physician, nurse practitioner, or physician assistant commonly orders medications. An important part of the transcription procedure for medication orders is to communicate the order to the pharmacy. This is done by faxing or sending the pharmacy copy of the doctors' orders to the pharmacy. The pharmacist fills the medication orders by reading the copy of the doctor's order sheet, thus reducing the possibility of error.

The pharmacist labels the medication with the patient's name, room number, and bed number, and the name, dosage, and frequency of administration. The medication is then sent back to the nursing unit, where it is placed in a medicine room (med room), medication cart, or individual patient medication drawer.

The medicine cart is a vehicle in which the patient's medications are stored in separate drawers or bins that are labeled for each patient. The medication cart can be wheeled to the patient's bedside for the administration of the medication (Fig. 13–1.) Some facilities now use a computerized medication cart that requires the

user to enter a confidential user ID and password to unlock the cart. The medication cart computer asks the user to verify the name of the medication, the dose, and the patient's name before removing the medication. The computerized medication carts remain in the medication room and are not taken room to room (Fig. 13–2).

Filling Out the Medication Administration Record (MAR)

Transcribing medication orders may require the health unit coordinator to write the order on a medication administration record (MAR) and/or enter the medications on the patient's medication profile in the computer. A registered nurse or a licensed practical nurse is assigned to give the medications. The "med nurse" (as he or she is called) uses the MAR as a reference while preparing the medications for administration and also while giving the medications. Accuracy in copying the order from the order sheet onto the MAR and entering it into the computer is absolutely essential.

In hospitals where the MAR is used, the health unit coordinator initiates the record on the patient's admission. The record varies in the number of days that medications may be entered. When the last date of the dated period on the MAR is reached, a new record with new dates is prepared and all medications still in use are copied onto the new form. The MAR is a part of the patient's chart and is a legal document that is written in ink. To discontinue medications on the MAR, indicate "DC" on the correct day and time and draw a line through the days that medication will not be used (Fig. 13–3). A yellow highlight is usually then drawn over the medication entry that is discontinued.

Facilities utilizing computerized charting for patient care require the nurse to document medication administration in the computer rather than a written MAR. The updated, computerized MARs for each individual patient will be sent to the nursing units each morning for the nurses to check against current chart orders. When the patient is discharged, an MAR with all computer entries is printed and placed on the patient's chart.

Medication Reference Books

Reference books usually kept on nursing units that are most helpful to doctors, nurses, and allied health personnel are *The American Hospital Formulary* (published by the American Society of Hospital Pharmacists), the *Physicians' Desk Reference* (PDR; published yearly by Medical Economics, Inc.). Various nursing drug handbooks are also frequently used on nursing units.

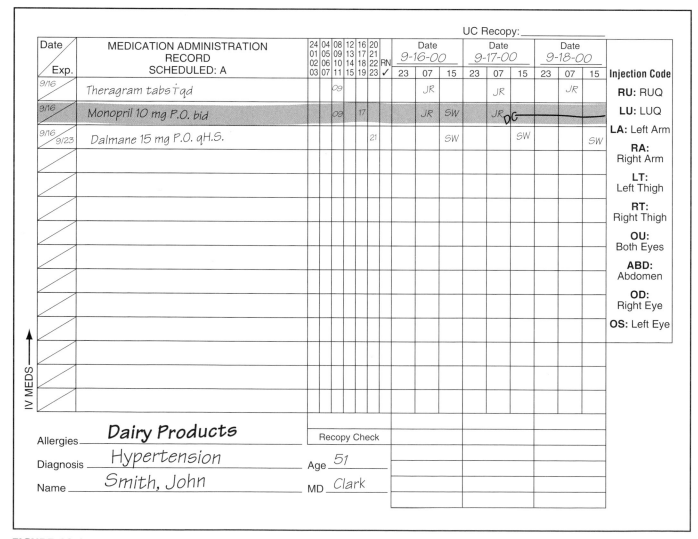

FIGURE 13–3 ▲ A medication administration record (side A) showing a method of discontinuing a standing medication. Illustration continued on following page.

The individual hospital pharmacy frequently supplies each nursing unit with a listing of medications and dosage forms available in that particular pharmacy. The listing is the specific formulary compiled for that health care facility. Other reference books for medications are frequently available on the nursing units.

The PDR has different sections listed under the table of contents. Each section is printed on a different color paper. The "Product Name" and the "Generic and Chemical Name Index" are the two sections that are most useful to the health unit coordinator.

Use of the PDR

The following exercises will introduce you to the use of the PDR. Your instructor will assist you, if necessary. It is recommended that during transcription of medication orders you use the PDR for spelling, drug category names, or other information you may need to know in order to transcribe the order accurately.

EXERCISE 4

Using the PDR, in the section titled "Product Name Index," locate the following drugs in the "Product Information Section," and briefly state the purpose of each. (Read the paragraph titled "Indications and Usage" under the drug name to locate the purpose. Ignore entries listed in the "Product Identification" section. This section shows pictures of the drugs and dosages only.)

Example: *Amesec—given for asthma*

_____

1. *Soma compound w/codeine*

_____

2. *Kay Ciel oral solution*

_____

3. *Indocin SR capsules*

_____

4. *Senokot tablets*

_____

PATIENT _Smith, John_   ALLERGIES _**Dairy Products**_

Date / Exp.	MEDICATION ADMINISTRATION RECORD PRN-ONE TIME & STAT: B	RN ✓	Date 9-16-00 23	07	15	Date 9-17-00 23	07	15	Date 9-18-00 23	07	15

PRN → ONE-TIME ↑

FIGURE 13–3 ▲ Continued; side B of a medication administration record

5. *Decadron elixir*

_____

Using the "Generic and Chemical Names Index," locate the following and state the purpose of each.

6. *furosemide*

_____

7. *meperidine hydrochloride*

_____

Naming Medications

Most medications have several names. They are:

1. *Official name:* This is the name under which the drug is listed in official government publications of drug standards. This name may be followed by the initials U.S.P. (United States Pharmacopeia) or N.F. (National Formulary). These are the two official volumes in which drug standards are published.
2. *Chemical name:* This name describes the chemical composition of the drug.
3. *Generic name:* This is a shortened name given to the drug by the developer so that the longer chemical name does not have to be used. Many states require the pharmacist to use the generic name on the label. Generic names are not capitalized.

4. *Brand name, trade name, or proprietary name:* This is the name given to and registered by the manufacturer. The general public often knows the drug best by this name. *The brand name is always capitalized and may have a trademark symbol (™ or ®).* Each company that manufactures a drug of the same chemical composition may assign it a brand name. For example, Tylenol, the brand name under which McNeil Laboratories manufactures acetaminophen (its generic name) is named Datril by Bristol Laboratories. *A drug has only one generic name but may have many trade names, depending on how many companies manufacture it.*

Some hospitals have a substitution rule. Under this rule the pharmacist may substitute a different brand from the one that is prescribed or the pharmacist may substitute the generic equivalent. It is good practice for the pharmacist to put an "equivalent" label on the container to decrease confusion on the nursing unit.

■ COMPONENTS OF A MEDICATION ORDER

Each medication order is written using specific components that include directions for the person giving the drug. You may see them written in slightly different order, but the components remain the same.

Example:

Tylenol	325 mg	PO	q4h	WA
1	2	3	4	5

The numbered portions of this drug order are:

1. Name of drug   Tylenol
2. Dose of drug (amount)   325 mg

COMMUNICATION AND IMPLEMENTATION OF MEDICATION ORDERS

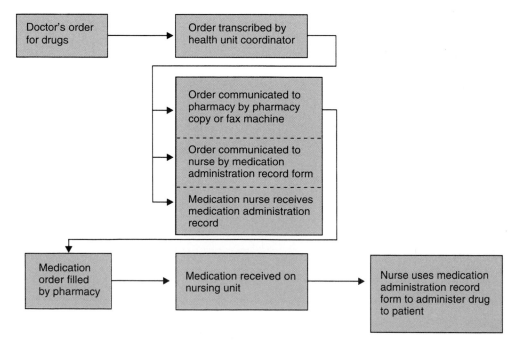

3. Route of administration   PO (by mouth)
4. Time of administration (frequency)   q 4h (every 4 hours)
5. Qualifying phrase   WA (while awake)

Component 1: Name of the Drug

It is impossible for you to learn the names of all the drugs on the market, therefore, as a beginning or new health unit coordinator you may wish to keep a small notebook with an alphabetical index to jot down names of drugs that you encounter frequently. Periodic reviewing will help you to become more familiar with medication names.

Many medications are prepared in different forms, depending on their use. The form is often included with the name of the drug, such as Neosporin *ointment* (see the Box *Examples of Doctors' Medication Orders That Indicate a Specific Form of Medication*). For example, ointments are used on the skin or the mucous membranes of the body. Other medications may include a letter, as shown in Components 2 and 3.

Component 2: Dosage

The apothecary system and the metric system are the two methods of weights and measures in present-day hospital use. The metric system, which is based on multiples of 10, is the system of choice in scientific fields and is gradually replacing the apothecary system. However, until the apothecary system is completely phased out, the health unit coordinator must continue to be knowledgeable about both systems.

Apothecary System

The apothecary system for weighing and measuring drugs and solutions is an ancient system that was brought to the United States from England during the colonial period. Only those terms still used frequently today are listed.

Terms Relating to Weight (Solid or Powder)

Grain (gr)
Dram (dr or ʒ)
Ounce (oz or ℥)

> ### EXAMPLES OF DOCTORS' MEDICATION ORDERS THAT INDICATE A SPECIFIC FORM OF MEDICATION
>
> - *Neosporin ung ophthalmic OD bid*
>   *Ophthalmic* indicates that this ointment is to be used in the eye only.
>
> - *aspirin EC tab ī q 3h prn*
>   The *enteric-coated* (EC) aspirin dissolves only in the small intestine.
>
> - *aspirin T-R 650 mg PO q hs*
>   *Time-released* (T-R) aspirin has a longer-lasting effect.
>
> - *aspirin supp 325 mg q 3h for temp 101 (R)*
>   Aspirin is contained in *suppository* (supp) form for insertion into the rectum.

Terms Relating to Volume (Liquid)

Fluid dram (fl dr or ʒ)
Fluid ounce (fl oz or ℥)

The abbreviation fl is not frequently used.

Measurements in this system are written in lowercase Roman numerals. These numerals have a line over them and may be dotted to avoid confusion with similar-appearing letters or numerals. Also the unit of measure precedes the numeral.

> **Examples:** one grain—gr ī
>   five grains—gr v̄

A medication dosage that is less than 1 is written as a fraction.

> **Example:** one-sixth grain—gr $\frac{1}{6}$.

Metric System

The metric system is used everywhere except in the United States. The weight, volume, and measurement units are used in other hospital departments as well as in the pharmacy. These basic units are:

Weight = gram (g)
Volume = liter (L)
Length = meter (M)

Smaller and larger units in the metric system can be indicated by attaching prefixes to the basic units. This text will not cover all the prefixes used in the metric system because not all are used in doctors' orders.

To enlarge the basic unit 1000 times, the prefix *kilo* is added.

> **Example:** kilogram (kg) = 1000 g.

To diminish the basic unit by 100, the prefix *centi* is added. The prefix *milli* diminishes the basic unit by 1000. A milligram (mg), milliliter (mL), and millimeter (mm) represent 1/1000 of the basic unit. The symbol μ represents the prefix *micro*.

> **Example:** 1 μ = 1 micrometer or 0.001 millimeter.

The terms *milliliter* (mL) and *cubic centimeter* (cc) are used interchangeably.

> **Example:** 1 L = 1000 cc or 1000 mL.

The metric system uses the Arabic numerals that we all know—1, 2, 3, and so forth. Abbreviations are placed after the number, as in 50 mg or 500 mL.

Quantities less than 1 and fractions are written in decimal form (for example: 0.25 mg, 1.25 mg, and 1.5 g).

Abbreviations used in medication dosages that *do not fall* within the apothecary or metric systems are: gtt (drop), mEq (milliequivalent), and U (unit). Examples of their usage in doctors' orders are:

Pilocarpine 1% gtts OU tid
Add 40 mEq KCl to each IV
Bicillin 600,000 U bid × 3 days

EXERCISE ❺

Write the following doses in the correct form using the proper abbreviations. (Do not convert to different systems.)
1. Two grains   _____

2. Five cubic centimeters   _____

3. Four drams   _____

4. One-half gram   _____

5. One and one-half grains   _____

6. Five hundred milligrams   _____

7. Fifteen grains   _____

8. One liter   _____

9. One thousand grams   _____

10. One-sixth grain   _____

11. One one-hundred-fiftieth grain   _____

Component 3: Routes of Administration

Medications may be administered to patients using different routes of administration. Also, any one medication may be given by several different methods. The route of administration should always be included in a medication order; however, when in doubt, the route of administration should always be clarified. The following list contains the routes most frequently used in medication administration, with an example of each. (Fig. 13–4)

- **Oral** (mouth or PO)

The patient swallows the medication, which may be in the form of a capsule, pill, tablet, or liquid.

> **Example:** Librium 10 mg PO tid.

- **Sublingual**

The tablet is placed under the tongue, where it is slowly absorbed.

> **Example:** Nitroglycerin gr 1/150 subling prn anginal pain.

- **Inhalation**

Liquid medications are most commonly administered by the respiratory care department as part of their treatment procedure.

> **Examples:** SVN c̄ UD (unit dose) ventolin tid
> 1PPB c̄ 3cc saline qid

- **Topical**

Applied to skin or mucous membrane. Medications in this category may be in the form of lotions, liniments, ointments, powders, sprays, solutions, suppositories, or transdermal preparations.

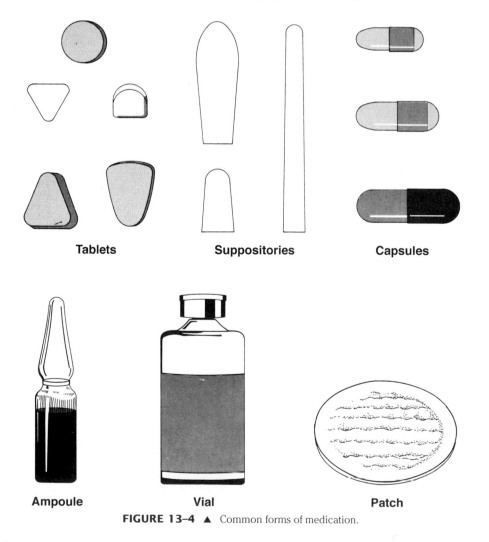

Tablets   Suppositories   Capsules

Ampoule   Vial   Patch

FIGURE 13–4 ▲ Common forms of medication.

FIGURE 13–5 ▲ Angle of needle insertion for parenteral injections.

a. Applied to skin

Example 1: Apply Neosporin ointment to rt leg ulcer bid.
Example 2: Transderm-Nitro qd. (The medication is part of a flat disk that is applied to the body, usually the chest; the medication is released over a specified period.)

b. Spraying onto skin or mucous membrane

Example 1: Spray lt ankle wound with Neosporin aerosol tid.
Example 2: Chloraseptic throat spray q 3h prn for throat irritation.

c. Instillation
These liquids are dropped into the eye, ear, or nose.

Example: Instill 2 gtts q 6h into rt ear.

d. Insertions of drugs into body openings—suppositories

Example 1: Compazine supp 5 mg q 4h prn N/V.
Example 2: Mycostatin vag supp q AM.

■ **Parenteral**
Fluids or medications given by injection or intravenously.
a. Intradermal: Injected between two skin layers. These injections are principally for diagnostic testing.

Example: PPD intermediate today. PPD (purified protein derivative) is a tuberculin skin test order. The word "intermediate" indicates the strength of the drug.

b. Subcutaneous (SC or SQ): The medication is injected with a syringe under the skin into the fat or connective tissue.

Example: heparin 5000 U SQ stat

c. Intramuscular (IM): The medication is injected directly into the muscle (Fig. 13–5).

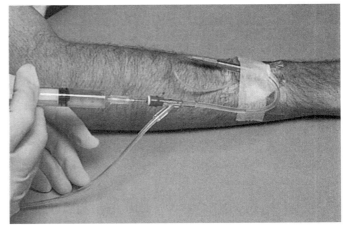

FIGURE 13–6 ▲ Intravenous push (IV push) (from Pharmacology and the Nursing Process, 2nd ed., Lilley & Aucker, Mosby, p. 72).

d. Intravenous push (IV push or IVP): A method of infusing a concentrated dose of medication over 1 to 5 minutes (Fig. 13–6).

e. Intravenous piggyback (IVPB): IVPB is a method of intermittent infusion of medication that has been diluted in 50 to 100 cc of a commercially prepared solution and infused over 30 to 60 minutes through an established IV line (Fig. 13–7). The medication concentration in the IVPB is lower than the medication concentration in the IV push and is administered over a longer period of time.

f. Heparin lock: A device used for intermittent intravenous infusion of medication, also used to maintain patent venous access for the infusion of medications in an emergency (Fig. 13–8).

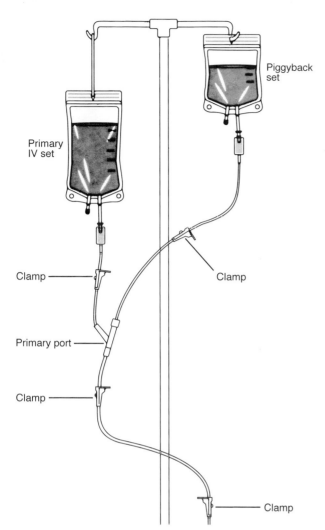

FIGURE 13–7 ▲ An intravenous set with piggyback bags.

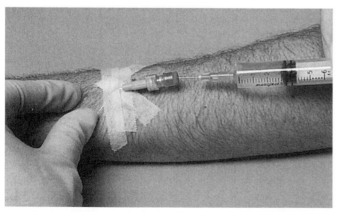

FIGURE 13–8 ▲ Heparin lock (from Pharmacology and the Nursing Process, 2nd ed., Lilley & Aucker, Mosby p. 73).

Total Parenteral Nutrition (TPN)

Total parenteral nutrition (TPN) or intravenous hyperalimentation is the process of intravenously infusing carbohydrates, proteins, fats, water, electrolytes, vitamins, and minerals. These nutrients are infused through a catheter that is placed directly into a large central vein and advanced into the superior vena cava. The veins most often used are the jugular and the subclavian veins. It is common procedure for providing nutrients to patients who are unable to receive food via the digestive tract. Some diseases that require TPN intervention are ileitis, bowel obstructions, massive burns, and severe anorexia. Patients receiving TPN require frequent (daily) blood tests for electrolyte and lipid levels.

Total parenteral nutrition is usually a long-term therapy and is administered through central venous catheters that are designed for long-term use. Some common types of long-term central venous catheters are Hickman, Boviac, Groshong, and Port-A-Cath. The type of catheter used is dependent on the length of treatment. Insertion of a central catheter requires an informed consent and is surgically inserted under local anesthesia and sterile conditions.

The complex composition of TPN solution requires a written doctor's order and is prepared by the pharmacist under sterile conditions using a laminar flow hood. The solution is kept refrigerated until 30 to 40 minutes before infusion. The infusion rate is controlled by an infusion pump (Fig. 13–9). The infusion of TPN is closely monitored by the nurse, since fluid overload is a serious complication for the patient receiving fluids via central venous access. Other complications that may develop are infections, phlebitis, thrombosis, electrolyte imbalance, and hyperglycemia. The nurse will assess the patient for change in status and he or she will use strict aseptic technique when changing dressings and when handling the administration equipment and solutions.

The order for TPN is a preprinted form that is filled in by the doctor (Fig. 13–10). This form takes the place of the regular doctor's order form and a copy is sent to the pharmacy. Because of the length and complexity of the TPN order, many hospitals transcribe only the date, TPN with rate, and check chart on the medication administration record. When the TPN solution is delivered from the pharmacy, the registered nurse will check it against the doctor's order on the preprinted form. Many times the doctor will use the regular doctor's order form to make small changes in the compo-

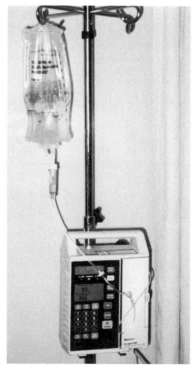

FIGURE 13–9 ▲ Example of an intravenous infusion pump (from Foundations of Nursing, 4th ed., Christensen & Kockrow, Mosby, p. 606).

ADULT TPN ORDER FORM

	Custom	Standard Central	Standard Peripheral
BASE SOLUTION	☐	☐	☐
gm AA (60-120/d : 4 cal/gm : 10 gm/100 ml)	_____gm	50gm/L	30gm/L
gm Dextrose (200-700/d : 3.4 cal/gm : 70 gm/100 ml)	_____gm	200gm/L	75gm/L
gm Lipid (0-100/d : 9 cal/gm : 20 gm/100 ml).................	_____gm		40gm/L
ADDITIVES			
meq NaCl (60-150/d)	_____/bag	35/L or ____/L	35/L or ____/L
meq NaAcetate	_____/bag	____/L	____/L
meq KCl (30-100/d)	_____/bag	____/L	____/L
meq KAcetate	_____/bag	20/L or ____/L	20/L or ____/L
meq KPO4 (15-40/d)......................................	_____/bag	15/L or ____/L	15/L or ____/L
meq NaPO4	_____/bag	____/L	____/L
meq CaGluconate (9-18/d)................................	_____/bag	4.5/L or ____/L	4.5/L or ____/L
meq MgSO4 (5-15/d)	_____/bag	5/L or ____/L	5/L or ____/L
mg ZnSO4	_____/bag	____/L	____/L
Multivitamin-12	_____/bag	Standard	Standard
Trace Elements (Zn, Cu, Mn, Cr).........................	_____/bag	Standard	Standard
Human Insulin R	_____/bag	____/L	____/L
Other: _____	_____	____/L	____/L
Other: _____	_____	____/L	____/L
Other: _____	_____	____/L	____/L
FINAL VOLUME to be infused over 24 hours	_____	_____	_____
RATE ml/hr..	_____	_____	_____

_____ ml Iron Dextran/wk (0.5 ml = 25 mg Fe+ + q wk; incompatible with lipid-containing solutions. Lipids will be omitted from
solution on the day iron is administered.)
_____ mg Vitamin K/wk (5 mg q wk)

IVPB Lipids _____ ml _____% Lipid q _____ . Run over _____ hrs.

LABORATORY
Daily: _____ Electrolytes _____ BUN _____ Creat _____ Glucose _____ CBC
Q Mon & Thurs: _____ SMA-20 _____ Mg+ + _____ CBC
Q Week: _____ Protime _____ Platelets
Other: _____
Other: _____
Other: _____

_____ Fingerstick glucose q _____ hrs.   Weight q _____

SLIDING SCALE:

Glucose	Sub Q Human Insulin R
Less than 80 mg%	Call M.D.
80 - 150 mg%	_____ units
151 - 200 mg%	_____ units
201 - 250 mg%	_____ units
251 - 300 mg%	_____ units
301 - 350 mg%	_____ units
Greater than 350 mg%	Call M.D.

Sign. _____

Date _____ Time _____

Phone or pager _____

IV Pharmacy Phone: X4557

ADULT TPN ORDER FORM

FIGURE 13-10 ▲ Total parenteral nutrition order form.

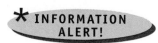

Any change in the TPN order must be immediately sent to the pharmacy. The TPN solution is very expensive and is wasted if there is any change in the formula after it has been prepared.

sition of the original order. You must discontinue the original order on the MAR and rewrite the order by again noting as above.

Peripheral Parenteral Nutrition (PPN)

Peripheral Parenteral Nutrition (PPN) is one route of administration for nutrition that is used for short-term therapy that is usually less than 2 weeks in length. A peripheral catheter is usually inserted into a large vein in the arm, and the nurse must be alert to the most adverse effect of PPN, which is phlebitis. Phlebitis is a severe inflammation of a vein. PPN is used for patients who need temporary nutritional supplements and who can tolerate a higher fluid infusion amount. The dextrose or sugar content of the formula is lower than parenteral nutrition that is given through the central veins.

Component 4: Frequency of Administration

Each hospital maintains a schedule of hours for administration of medications. These schedules are set up by the hospital nursing service, and you are required to learn the hours that are standard for your hospital.

Table 13–1 lists examples of time frequencies used to administer medication. Remember that this varies among hospitals.

Also, military time may be used in place of standard time. If the schedule does not coincide with the schedule at your hospital, write in the times you will be using.

Note: Standard prn orders are never assigned a time, because the drugs are administered as they are needed by the patient.

Component 5: Qualifying Phrases

There are times when the doctor may wish the drug to be administered only for specific conditions. He or she then includes a phrase to this effect as the fifth part of the medication order. Not all orders contain qualifying phrases; however, when included, they are an important part of the order. Some phrases you may see commonly used are:

For severe pain
For stomach spasms
For N/V
While awake
For insomnia

Examples of Doctors' Orders with a Qualifying Phrase

- *Demerol 75 mg IM q 3h prn <u>severe pain</u>*
- *Compazine supp q 4h <u>for NV</u>*
- *May give Maalox 30 cc <u>for upset stomach</u>*

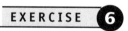

EXERCISE 6

It is necessary for the health unit coordinator to identify the parts of a medication order quickly in order to recognize whether the order is complete and to transcribe it correctly. The following exercise provides you with practice for this task.

TABLE 13–1	Medication Time Schedule		
Time Symbols	**Meaning**	**Time Schedule**	**Military Time**
qd	Once a day	9:00 AM	0900
		(5:00 PM [daily] for anticoagulants—to allow for results of prothrombin time)	1700
		(7:30 AM [daily] for insulin, which must be administered before breakfast)	0730
bid	Two times a day during waking hours	9:00 AM and 5:00 PM (9-5)	0900—1700
tid	Three times a day during waking hours	9:00 AM—1:00 PM—5:00 PM (9-1-5)	0900—1300—1700
qid	Four times a day during waking hours	9:00 AM—1:00 PM—5:00 PM—9:00 PM (9-1-5-9)	0900—1300—1700—2100
ac	One-half hour before meals. This varies according to when food cart arrives on unit.		
pc	One-half hour after meals. This varies according to when food cart arrives on unit.		
q3h	Every 3 hours	9:00 AM—12:00 Noon—3:00 PM—6:00 PM—9:00 PM—12:00 Mid—3:00 AM—6:00 AM (9-12-3-6-9-12-3-6)	0900—1200—1500—1800—2100—2400—0300—0600
q4h	Every 4 hours	9:00 AM—1:00 PM 5:00 PM 9:00 PM—1:00 PM—5:00 AM (9-1-5-9-1-5)	0900—1300—1700—2100—0100—0500
q6h	Every 6 hours	9:00 AM—3:00 PM—9:00 PM—3:00 AM (9-3-9-3)	0900—1500—2100—0300
q8h	Every 8 hours	9:00 AM—5:00 PM—9:00 AM (9-5-1)	0900—1700—0100
q12h	Every 12 hours	9:00 AM—9:00 PM (9-9)	0900—2100

Following the example below and using the numbers to indicate each part of a medication order, complete the following exercise.

Example:

<u>Demerol</u>	<u>50 mg</u>	<u>IM</u>	<u>q 4h prn</u>	<u>for severe pain</u>
1	2	3	4	5

1. List the five parts of a medication order in consecutive order as used in the example above.

   a. _____

   b. _____

   c. _____

   d. _____

   e. _____

2. Identify each component of the medication orders below by writing the number of the component below the component part, as shown in the preceding example.

   a. Compazine 10 mg IM stat

   b. Ativan .05 mg IV q 6h prn anxiety

   c. Xanax .05 mg po qid

   d. Ambien 5 mg po hs prn

   e. Lomotil Ī caps po after each loose stool

   f. Percodan Tabs 1–2 po q 4h prn severe pain

   g. Lente Insulin 25 U sq qd

   h. Amoxicillin 500 mg po q 8h

   i. Compazine 5 mg IM q 6h prn N/V

   j. Tigan supp 100 mg pr now

EXERCISE 7

Test your knowledge of material covered thus far by completing the following exercise. You will find a list of doctors' orders for medications written, as they would be spoken. Rewrite the orders as they would be written, using abbreviations where needed, and use the correct form for the apothecary and metric systems.

Example: Demerol fifty milligrams intramuscularly every four hours whenever necessary for severe pain.

Answer: Demerol 50 mg IM q 4h prn severe pain.

1. *Tylenol five hundred milligrams every four hours by mouth for pain.*

   _____

2. *Ampicillin two hundred fifty milligrams by mouth four times a day.*

   _____

3. *Penicillin one million six hundred thousand units intramuscularly every twelve hours.*

   _____

4. *Donnatal elixir five milliliters by mouth three times a day before meals.*

   _____

5. *Neo-Synephrine ophthalmic 10% drops two in right eye twice a day.*

   _____

6. *Benadryl fifty milligrams by mouth immediately.*

   _____

7. *Equanil four hundred milligrams by mouth twice a day and at bedtime.*

   _____

8. *Coumadin five milligrams by mouth daily.*

   _____

■ THE FIVE RIGHTS OF MEDICATION ADMINISTRATION

It is vital that the health unit coordinator is accurate when reading and transcribing medication orders. Use the five rights listed below as a guide when transcribing medications.

1. *Right Drug:* It is important that close attention be paid to the drug order when transcribing medications. Many drugs have similar names and spellings.
2. *Right Dose:* Once again, accuracy in transcribing the medication dose is vital to patient safety.
3. *Right Time:* Pay special attention to stat or one-time orders and let the nurse know if a stat or now medication is ordered.
4. *Right Route:* Never assume the route for a medication; always check if the order is not clear.
5. *Right Patient:* It is critical that medication orders are transcribed on the correct patient's chart or medication administration record. Always double-check the name on the chart as you transcribe medication orders. If an error is made, make the correction immediately and notify the nurse of the correction.

■ CATEGORIES OF DOCTORS' ORDERS RELATED TO MEDICATION ORDERS

Categories of doctors' orders are especially relevant to medication orders. For example, a standing medication order must have times assigned on the medication administration record or medication Kardex form, whereas the standing prn order does not have times assigned. To review, read "Categories of Doctors' Orders," Chapter 9, then read and complete the following unit.

Standing Orders

Fill in the definition below.

A standing order is: _____

_____

Examples of Standing Medication Orders

Lente Insulin U 40 qd
This medication is administered one time each day, such as 0800, until discontinued.

Penicillin 600,000 U IM q 6h
This medication is administered every 6 hours, such as 0900, 1500, 2100, 0300, until discontinued.

Vitamin B$_{12}$ 1000 mcg IM twice a week
This medication is to be administered twice a week, such as Monday and Thursday at 0900, until discontinued.

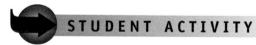
STUDENT ACTIVITY

To practice transcribing standing medication orders, complete Activity 13–1 in the *Skills Practice Manual.*

Standing PRN Orders

Fill in the definition below.

A PRN order is: _____

_____

Examples of Standing PRN Orders

MS 10 mg IM q 4h prn severe pain
The morphine sulfate may not be given to the patient more often than every 4 hours and then only if needed. In a prn order it is impossible to set up a time sequence.

MOM 30 mL hs prn constipation
Milk of magnesia, a laxative, is given as needed, usually when the patient communicates to the nurse that he or she is constipated. This order is in effect until discontinued by the doctor. Laxatives are usually administered at bedtime.

Vistaril 25 mg IM q 3h prn restlessness
Vistaril may not be given more often than every 3 hours, and only if the patient exhibits restlessness.

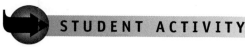
STUDENT ACTIVITY

To practice transcribing standing prn medication orders, complete Activity 13-2 in the *Skills Practice Manual.*

One-Time or Short-Series Orders

Fill in the definition below.

A one-time or short-series order is: _____

_____

Examples of One-Time or Short-Series Order Medication Orders

Penicillin 600,000 U IM @ 6 PM today and 6 AM tomorrow
This medication is given at the two times ordered and then discontinued.

Compazine 10 mg IM to be given 1 h before therapy tomorrow
This medication is to be administered 1 hour before the patient is sent for therapy tomorrow and then the order is discontinued.

Give Dulcolax supp tonight
This medication is to be administered the evening the order was written; then it is discontinued.

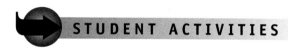
STUDENT ACTIVITIES

To practice transcribing one-time medication orders, complete Activity 13–3 in the *Skills Practice Manual.* To practice transcribing short-series order medication orders, complete Activity 13–4.

Stat Orders

Fill in the definition below.

A stat order is: _____

_____

Examples of Stat Orders

Heparin 20,000 U IV push stat
This order indicates that the heparin should be given immediately. The order then is to be discontinued.

Achromycin 500 mg PO now and then q 6h
This medication order is in two parts. The first part calls for the antibiotic Achromycin to be given immediately. Part 2 of this order contains a standing order for the medication to be given four times a day, such as 0900, 1500, 2100, 0300. The standing order remains in effect until the doctor discontinues it.

Communication of Stat Medication Orders

The medication must be ordered immediately from the pharmacy via phone, fax, or pharmacy copy. Immediately communicate the medication order to the nurse verbally. The nurse giving the medication must then review the order directly from the doctor's order sheet.

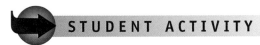

STUDENT ACTIVITY

To practice transcribing and communicating stat medication orders, complete Activity 13–5 in the *Skills Practice Manual.*

■ CONTROLLED SUBSTANCES

In 1971, the Controlled Substances Act updated previous laws that regulated the manufacture, sale, and dispensing of narcotics and drugs having potential for abuse. These drugs are referred to as *controlled drugs* or *controlled substances*. Controlled substances are divided into five classes, or schedules. Each of these classes differs according to its potential for abuse and therefore each is controlled to a different degree. The U.S. attorney general has the authority to reschedule the class in which a drug is placed, remove a substance from the controlled list, or assign an unscheduled drug to a controlled category. Therefore, the drugs in particular classes are subject to change. Examples of scheduled drugs follow.

Schedule I

This group has such a high potential for abuse that they usually are nonexistent in a health care setting except for specific, approved research. Examples are heroin and marijuana.

Schedule II

This group has a high potential for abuse and may lead to severe physical or psychological dependence. Examples are Percodan, morphine, meperidine (Demerol), amphetamines, and codeine.

Schedule III

There is moderate or low potential for abuse in this group. Examples are Tylenol with codeine, Phenaphen with codeine, Doriden, and Fiorinal.

Schedule IV

The potential for abuse is lower in this class than for drugs in schedule III. Examples are Talwin, Valium, meprobamate, Equagesic, and Centrax.

Schedule V

The abuse potential of these drugs is limited. Examples are Actified with codeine, Lomotil, Phenergan with codeine, and Triaminic Expectorant with codeine.

As dispensers of controlled substances for medicinal purposes, hospital pharmacies are required to be registered with the Drug Enforcement Administration, which mandates that records be maintained on certain drugs (Fig. 13–11).

Controlled drugs must be kept in a locked cupboard, medication cart, or computerized medication dispensing system on the nursing unit. This is because of the potential for theft and because the law requires it. A nurse carries the key to the locked cupboard or medication cart. If the medications are kept in a computerized medication system, an ID and password and/or fingerprint identification may be utilized to access the medication drawers.

Each time a medication from the locked cupboard or cart is given, the nurse who administers the medication is responsible for writing the required information on the disposition sheet. Each drug and each dosage of the drug requires the use of a separate disposition sheet. When the disposition sheet is completed, it is returned to the pharmacy. If a computerized system is used, the nurse must verify the count of the medications left in the drawer after removal of the drug. The count is then maintained on a computerized log.

Replacement of the drugs in the cupboard or cart is usually under the direction and supervision of pharmacy personnel who deliver the drugs in person to the nursing unit and in return receive a signed delivery slip from the nurse who accepts the drugs. The computerized cart keeps track of the number of medications given, to whom they were given, and the name of the nurse removing the drug.

The computerized medicine cart allows controlled, regularly scheduled, and prn medications to be computer dispensed. The pharmacist receives the medication orders by one of the three methods of ordering from the pharmacy department. Using the medication orders the pharmacist will then load the computer system with that patient's medication, usually for a 24-hour period.

Each nurse has a password that will allow him or her to access the system. The nurse must input the patient's name, and the drug along with the dosage. The patient's medical record number may also be used. Dispensing medication by the computer method significantly decreases medication errors because the system will not dispense the drug if there is a discrepancy in the patient's orders and the drug requisitioned by the nurse.

Two advantages of using the computer-dispensing method are a decreased number of errors in medication administration and an increased accuracy in accounting and billing. One disadvantage to the computerized system is that all new and changed medication orders written after the system has been loaded will have to be handled in the regular fashion. The computer system works best on nursing units where changes in orders are infrequent.

Medications that fall in the category of controlled drugs have an automatic stop date. An automatic stop date means that after a certain period, for example 72 hours, the drug may no longer be given to the patient unless renewed by a written order. Controlled substances usually have a 72-hour limit. Each health care facility develops its own list of drugs that have automatic stop dates.

Although other types of drugs are included under the heading "controlled substances," narcotics and hypnotics are the most frequently used.

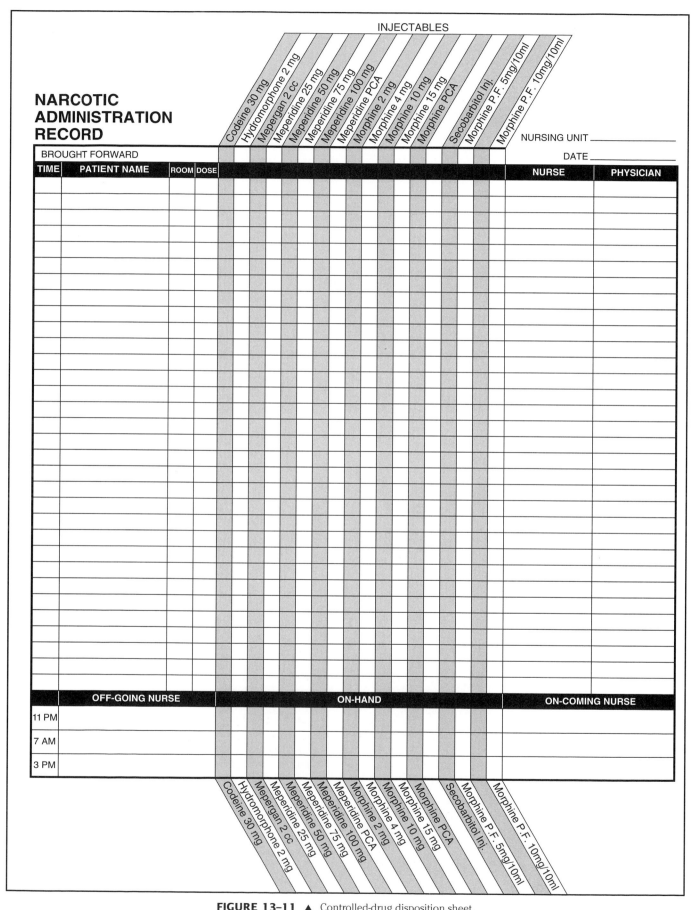

FIGURE 13–11 ▲ Controlled-drug disposition sheet.

■ DRUG GROUPS

Drugs are categorized into specific groups according to function or use, and are listed here by their trade names. There are many more drug groups than can be addressed in this brief introduction to drug categories. The following identifies the major groups of drugs and a description of each. Drugs listed in italics are the most commonly used drugs. Be able to identify the italicized drugs in order to meet Chapter Objective #11. Trade names of drugs are listed first and are capitalized. Generic names for drugs are not capitalized, and appear in parentheses.

Drugs that Affect the Nervous System

Narcotics or Opioids, Analgesics with Narcotics, and Nonnarcotic Analgesics

Narcotics or opioids, analgesics with narcotics, and nonnarcotic analgesics are all drugs that are ordered to relieve pain and may also be called painkillers. Narcotics and analgesics with narcotics are usually ordered to relieve moderate to severe pain, have an automatic stop date, and are commonly administered orally, intramuscularly, or intravenously (Fig. 13–12).

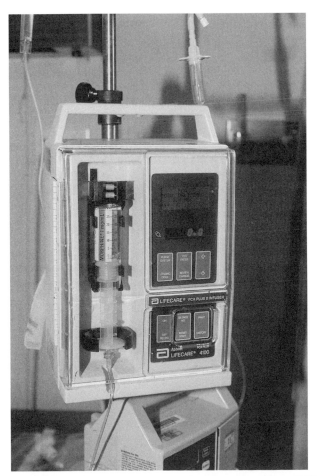

FIGURE 13–12 ▲ Example of a patient-controlled analgesia (PCA) pump (from Foundations of Nursing, 4th ed., Christensen & Kockrow, Mosby, p. 606).

Examples of Narcotics and Analgesics with Narcotic

Narcotics
- *Codeine*
- *Demerol* (meperidine)
- (methadone)
- *Morphine* (morphine sulfate)

Analgesics with narcotic
- (aspirin) *with Codeine #1, #2, #3,* or *#4*
- *Percocet* (oxycodone with acetaminophen)
- *Percodan* (oxycodone with aspirin)
- *Tylenol* (acetaminophen) *with codeine #1, #2, #3, or #4*

Examples of Nonnarcotic Analgesics

- Ascriptin
- Bufferin
- *Ecotrin* (enteric-coated aspirin)
- Excedrin (aspirin)
- *Motrin* (ibuprofen)
- *Tylenol* (acetaminophen)

Patient-Controlled Analgesia

Patient-controlled analgesia (PCA) allows the patient to self-administer small doses of narcotics intravenously. A special IV infusion pump is used. The physician orders the amount of individual doses, the frequency of delivery, and the total dose permitted within certain time periods called lockout intervals. The nurse receives the narcotic from the pharmacy either in a syringe form or a small cassette that fits into the PCA (see Fig. 13–12).

An internal system within the PCA unit is programmed and does not permit the patient to overdose or self-administer the medication too frequently. The most common narcotics used in PCA systems are meperidine and morphine. Some conditions for patients using PCAs are severe postoperative pain or the chronic pain of a terminal illness.

Sedatives and Hypnotics

Sedatives are drugs that cause relaxation and reduce restlessness without causing sleep. A sedative given in higher doses may also be called a hypnotic. A hypnotic is stronger than a sedative and

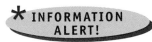

✱ INFORMATION ALERT!

Numbers that are assigned to analgesics containing codeine differentiate the amount of codeine found in the medications. The numbers mean:

\# 1 contains gr $\frac{1}{8}$ (8 mg) codeine
\# 2 contains gr $\frac{1}{4}$ (15 mg) codeine
\# 3 contains gr $\frac{1}{2}$ (30 mg) codeine
\# 4 contains gr 1 (60 mg) codeine

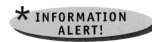

✱ INFORMATION ALERT!

There are too many nonnarcotic analgesics to list, but it is important to remember that nonnarcotic analgesics all relieve mild to moderate pain.

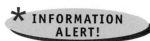

Drugs You Need to Identify to Meet Objective #11

Narcotics	Analgesics with Narcotics	Nonnarcotic Analgesics	Sedatives/ Hypnotics
Codeine	aspirin 1, 2, 3, or 4	Ecotrin	Ambien
Demerol	Percocet	Motrin	Dalmane
(meparidine)	Percodan	Tylenol	Nembutal
Methadone	Tylenol # 1,		Restoril
Morphine	2, 3, or 4		

is commonly used to induce sleep. There are also drugs that are classified as sedative-hypnotics and most have automatic stop dates. The side effects of these drugs include dizziness and excessive tiredness, so these patients must be closely watched following administration of sedatives and hypnotics.

Examples of Sedative-Hypnotics

- *Ambien*
- *Dalmane*
- Halcion
- *Nembutal*
- *Restoril*

STUDENT ACTIVITY

To practice transcribing orders for medications with automatic stop dates, complete Activity 13–6 in the *Skills Practice Manual.*

Psychotherapeutic Drugs

Psychotherapeutic drugs are used to treat anxiety, depression, emotional disorders, and mental illnesses. The drugs included in this broad category are among the most commonly prescribed medications in the United States.

Examples of Antianxiety and Antidepression Medications

Antianxiety Medications
- *Ativan* (lorazepam)
- *Valium* (diazepam)
- *Xanax* (alprazolam)

Drugs Used to Treat Depression
- Elavil (amitriptyline)
- Pamelor (nortriptyline)
- Zoloft (sertraline)

Anticonvulsants

Anticonvulsants are drugs that prevent or relieve convulsions caused by epilepsy or other disorders.

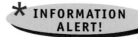

Drugs that are used to treat emotional and mental disorders vary according to the patient's diagnosis and may require that the patient try several to find the one that work's best for a specific condition.

Examples of Anticonvulsants

- Depakote (divalproex)
- *Dilantin* (phenytoin)
- Mysoline (primidone)
- *(phenobarbital)*
- *Tegretol* (carbamazepine)

Drugs that Affect the Respiratory System

Drugs affect the respiratory system by either assisting in drying secretions (antihistamines), relieving nasal stuffiness (decongestants), decreasing the cough reflex (antitussives), or assisting with increasing the flow of fluid in the respiratory tract, enabling secretions to be removed by the cough reflex (expectorants). Specific drugs given orally, via the IV route, or by inhalation are bronchodilators and are used to treat asthma and related conditions.

Examples of Antihistamines

- *Benadryl*
- Claritin

Nasal decongestants can be administered orally, through an inhaler, or topically.

Examples of Nasal Decongestants

- Afrin nasal spray (topical)
- Sudafed
- Vicks inhaler

Antitussives may or may not include a narcotic or opioid.

Examples of Antitussive Drugs in a Nonnarcotic Form

- Robitussin D-M
- Tessalon Perles
- Vicks Formula 44

Expectorants often contain a drug called *guaifenisin* and are found in medications such as Humibid and Robitussin.

Examples of Drugs Used to Treat Asthma and Related Conditions

- *(aminophylline)*
- *Bronkosol*
- Maxair inhaler
- *Proventil, Ventolin* (albuterol)
- *Theo-Dur* (theophylline)

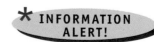

Codeine is frequently added to antitussive formulas, making them narcotic antitussive drugs, available by prescription only.

Drugs that Treat Infections

This is a huge category of medications used to treat a variety of infections that include antibiotic, antifungal, and antiviral drugs. Antibiotics are commonly prescribed for bacterial infections and it is important for the doctor to order the "right drug for the right bug" in order to give the patient the best treatment possible. That is why a culture of the wound or blood cultures are often drawn prior to beginning antibiotic therapy. There are many different classifications and combinations of antibiotics; penicillin is the oldest form of antibiotic. Antibiotics usually have automatic stop dates. (*Note:* Many antibiotic names end in *-cillin*, *-statin*, or *-mycin*; this makes identification easier.)

Examples of Antibiotics

- Amikin *(amikacin)*
- Polymax *(amoxicillin)*
- (bacitracin)
- Duricef (cefadroxil)
- *Ancef, Kefzol (cefazolin)*
- *Keflex (cefalexin)*
- *Keflin (Cephalothin)*
- *Cipro (ciprofloxacin)*
- (erythromycin base), (erythromycin ethylsuccinate, EES)
- Garamycin *(gentamycin* or *gentamicin)*
- *(penicillin)*
- *(vancomycin)*

Antifungals are drugs used to treat fungal infections. They are administered topically, orally, or through an intravenous piggyback (IVPB). Antifungals are also commonly used topically to treat oral fungal infections and vaginally to treat vaginal candidiasis.

Examples of Antifungals

- Amphotericin B
- (fluconazole)
- (nystatin)

Viral infections are difficult to treat because by the time the viral symptoms begin to appear, the virus has completed the replication process in the body. Antiviral drugs are only effective during the replication stage of the viral illness, so by the time the person knows that he or she is ill, it is often too late for the drugs to be effective. Antiviral drugs may be prescribed orally, intravenously, or as a nasal spray. Many new antiviral drugs are being tested to fight diseases such as acquired immunodeficiency syndrome (AIDS), human immunodeficiency virus (HIV), influenza A, cytomegalovirus (CMV), herpes simplex, and respiratory syncytial virus (RSV).

Examples of Antivirals

- (acyclovir)
- (ribavirin)
- (zidovudine)

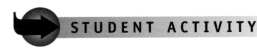

STUDENT ACTIVITY

To practice transcribing IV medication orders, complete Activity 13-7 in the *Skills Practice Manual*.

Drugs that Affect the Endocrine System

Drugs Used to Treat Diabetes: Antidiabetics

Antidiabetics are given to lower blood sugar and are ordered for the diabetic or hyperglycemic patient.

Standing Order for Insulin

A standing order for insulin to be administered once a day is commonly scheduled to be given 1/2 h a.c. breakfast. Also, if the doctor is normalizing the amount of insulin required by the patient, the doctor may order insulin to be given on a sliding scale.

Sliding-Scale Insulin Orders

The amount of sliding-scale insulin given is dependent upon the results obtained from blood glucose monitoring. This insulin may be given in addition to the daily insulin order the doctor has prescribed.

EXAMPLE

Sliding-Scale Order (using bedside blood glucose monitoring)	
Blood Sugar Level	**Dosage or Action**
200–249	5 U regular insulin
250–299	10 U regular insulin
300–349	15 U regular insulin
>350	Call doctor

Not all diabetic patients have sliding-scale orders or take insulin. Many diabetics control their illness with diet and exercise or use an oral medication to assist in controlling their blood glucose levels.

Examples of Oral Antidiabetic Drugs

- DiaBeta (glyburide)
- Glucophage (metformin)
- *Glucotrol* (glipizide)
- *Orinase* (tolbutamide)

Examples of Subcutaneous Insulin

- *Humalog*
- *Iletin, NPH*
- *insulin, regular*
- Novolin L
- Protamine Zinc & Iletin (PZI)

Hormones

Hormones are medications that either replace or regulate glandular secretions from glands such as the thyroid, pituitary, adrenals, and the male and female sexual organs. When these medications are ordered, the patient will be closely watched and the medication dosages may have to be changed several times to find the right level for each patient. Laboratory tests will also be done to determine blood levels.

Examples of Hormone Medications

- Decadron (Dexamethasone)
- Solu-Cortef (hydrocortisone)
- (prednisone)

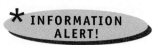

Drugs You Need to Identify to Meet Objective #11

Antianxiety Drugs	Anticonvulsants	Antihistamines
Ativan	Dilantin	Benadryl
Valium	phenobarbital	
Xanax	Tegretol	

Drugs Used to Treat Asthma and Related Conditions	Antibiotics	Antidiabetic Drugs
aminophylline	amikacin	Oral
Bronkosol	amoxicillin	Glucotrol
Proventil, Ventolin	Ancef, Kefzol	Orinase
Theo-Dur	(cefazolin)	Subcutaneous
	Keflex (cephalexin)	Insulin
	Keflin (cephalothin)	Humalog
	Cipro (ciprofloxacin)	Iletin, NPH
	gentamycin or	insulin, regular
	gentamicin	
	penicillin	
	vancomycin	

- Premarin (estrogen)
- Progesterone, Progestin
- Synthroid
- Tapazole
- (testosterone)

Drugs that Affect the Cardiovascular System

This is another large category of drugs that affect the heart and the vascular system in various ways. Many of these drugs also have effects on the kidneys or renal system. The subcategories of drugs in this section include antidysrhythmic agents, antianginal drugs, antihypertensive medications, diuretic drugs, potassium replacements, anticoagulant agents, antilipidemics, and other medications that affect the cardiovascular system.

Antidysrhythmic Agents

Antidysrhythmic medications correct abnormal cardiac beats by several functions. This group of drugs is divided into classes that are identified by how they affect the cardiac cells. You may hear these drugs called cardiotonics, beta-blockers, or calcium channel blockers depending on which drugs are ordered.

Examples of Antidysrhythmics

- quinidine
- *lidocaine*
- esmolol
- Inderal (propranolol)
- Isoptin (verapamil)

- amiodarone
- *Cardizem* (diltiazem)
- *Lanoxin (digoxin)*

Vasopressors

Vasopressors are medications given to treat shock, low blood pressure, and other related conditions. Vasopressors cause constriction of the smooth muscle of arteries and arterioles, which increases resistance to the flow of blood and thus elevates blood pressure.

Examples of Vasopressors

- *dopamine*
- *Levophed*

Antianginal Agents

The heart must pump blood to all of the organs and tissues of the body, 24 hours a day, 7 days a week—an enormous job! Antianginal drugs are medications that are used to treat pain that is caused when the heart muscle does not get enough oxygen and nutrients to meet this demand. When enough blood does not reach the heart muscle (myocardium), the chest pain that results from this is called angina pectoris. Lack of blood supply to the heart is called ischemic heart disease and is one of the primary causes of death in the United States.

Antianginal drugs include three primary categories of medications. These are nitrates or nitrites, and two categories that were just reviewed, beta-blockers and calcium channel blockers, both of which are commonly listed as antidysrhythmics and antianginals due to the effects that they have on the heart.

Examples of Antianginal Drugs in the Nitrate Category

- *Nitro-Bid (nitroglycerin)*
- *Nitrostat (nitroglycerin)*
- Isordil (isosorbide dinitrate)

It is common to see an order for "Nitroglycerin tabs to be left at bedside." If a patient begins to experience chest pain, the nurse then has the medication right at the bedside for the patient to place under his or her tongue.

Examples of Other Antianginal Medications

- Tenormin (atenolol)
- Inderal (propranolol)
- Lopressor (metoprolol)
- Procardia (nifedipine)
- Cardizem (diltiazem)

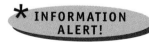

Antidysrhythmics that may be ordered *stat* for a patient in a cardiac emergency include amiodarone, bretylium, or possibly lidocaine. These would be transcribed as a stat, one-time order, or they might be included under the emergency standing orders for the patient. An example of this type of order would be:

Amiodarone 300 mg IV push now. May repeat once at 150 mg in 3-5 min.

Antihypertensive Agents

Antihypertensive drugs are the medications used to lower high blood pressure. It is not uncommon for patients to try several antihypertensive medications or combinations of various antihypertensives until finding what works best for them. It is important for patients to manage their hypertension because it is the number one risk factor for stroke, congestive heart failure, and peripheral vascular disease (PVD).

Antihypertensive medications also have several subcategories of drugs that all work in some way to lower blood pressure. These drugs may be ordered alone or in combination, depending on the needs of the patient. These categories are vasodilators, adrenergic agents, ganglionic blockers, angiotensin-converting enzyme (ACE) inhibitors, and calcium channel blockers.

Examples of Antihypertensives

- Catapres (clonidine)
- Minipress (prazosin)
- Vasotec (analapril)
- Apresoline (hydralazine)
- Nipride (sodium nitroprusside, most commonly used to manage a hypertensive crisis)

Diuretic Agents

These drugs are also sometimes called "water pills." Diuretics are among the first drugs that will often be prescribed to assist in the treatment of hypertension because they cause a quick decrease in circulating fluid volume, causing a decrease in pressure demand on the heart.

Examples of Diuretics

- *Lasix (furosemide)*
- Bumex (bumetanide)
- Edecrin (ethacrynic acid)
- Aldactone (spironolactone)
- *HydroDiuril (hydrochlorothiazide)*
- Osmitrol (mannitol)

Potassium Replacements

Potassium replacements replace potassium that has been lost because of the use of certain diuretics. Potassium may be given diluted in an IV medication, orally, or sprinkled on food or in fluid in granule form.

Examples of Potassium Replacements

- *Kaochlor, K-Lor, Micro K, Slow-K* (potassium chloride)
- *Klorvess Effervescent Granules*
- *Kaon*
- *K-Lyte* (potassium bicarbonate)

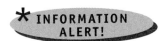

Diuretic orders may be written as a one-time order or a continuing order, but the dosages are frequently changed based on laboratory results and patient response.

Antilipidemics (Cholesterol-Lowering Drugs)

Many studies have demonstrated that lowering cholesterol can greatly reduce the risk of heart attack and death in people at high risk of a heart attack. Antilipidemic medications can lower cholesterol. They may be taken alone or used in combination.

Examples of Antilipidemics

- Questran (cholestyramine)
- Colestid (colestipol)
- Lopid (gemfibrozil)
- Tricor (fenofibrate)
- *Lipitor (atorvastatin)*
- *Mevacor (lovastatin)*
- *Zocor (simvastatin)*
- (niacin)

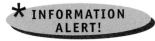

The antilipidemic drugs known as "statins" are indicated in italics above. It is important to note that a patient taking these medications should not eat grapefruit or drink grapefruit juice. Grapefruit interacts with statins, causing the blood level of the medications to rise, increasing the risk of side effects from the medications.

Anticoagulant Agents

Anticoagulants are drugs that thin the blood and prevent clots from forming in the blood.

Examples of Anticoagulants

- *Coumadin (warfarin)*
- Miradon (anisindione)
- *(heparin)*
- Fragmin (dalteparin) (a form of heparin)
- *Lovenox (enoxaparin)* (a form of heparin)

There are laboratory tests that are usually ordered if a patient is on anticoagulation therapy. These are the prothrombin time (PT) or the international normalized ratio (INR) if a patient is on Coumadin. If a patient is on heparin, different tests may be ordered, such as a PTT (activated partial thromboplastin time) or the activated clotting time (ACT). The timing of these tests is critical because the patient's next dose or immediate action that needs to be taken is dependent on the outcome of these tests.

Aspirin, ticlopidine (Ticlid), and dipyridamole (Persantine) are also considered a form of anticoagulant. These drugs actually work on the platelets in the blood to prevent them from sticking together and forming a clot.

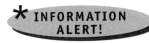

Oral Miradon and Coumadin are anticoagulants most frequently ordered for maintenance once patients have graduated from taking intravenous heparin, in the acute care setting.

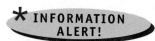

Drugs You Need to Identify to Meet Objective #11

Anticoagulants	Potassium Replacements	Antiemetics/Antinauseants
Coumadin (warfarin)	Kaochlor, K-Lor, Micro K	Compazine
heparin	Slow-K, Kaon, K-Lyte	Tigan
Lovenox	Klorvess Effervescent Granules	Vistaril

Cardiovascular Drugs

Antidysrhythmics	Antianginals	Diuretics	Vasopressors
Cardizem	Nitro-Bid (nitroglycerin)	HydroDiuril (hydrochlorothiazide)	dopamine hydrochloride
Lanoxin (digoxin)	Nitrostat (nitroglycerin)	Lasix (furosemide)	Levophed
lidocaine			

Drugs that Affect the Gastrointestinal System

Antacids

Too much acid in the stomach produces an often-painful condition called gastric hyperacidity. The category of both over-the-counter (OTC) and prescribed medications that are ordered for this condition is antacids. Many antacids are ordered as a prn order (e.g., May give Maalox 30 cc 3–4 x/d as needed for upset stomach).

Examples of Antacids

- Maalox
- Mylanta
- Tums
- Gaviscon

Antisecretory and Antiulcer Drugs

Antisecretory and antiulcer drugs decrease the acid production either by blocking the cells that help create acid or by inhibiting the proton pump, which pumps the acid.

Examples of Antisecretory Drugs

- Pepto-Bismol
- Zantac (ranitidine)
- Pepcid (famotidine)
- Tagamet (cimetidine)
- Prilosec (omeprazole)

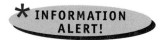

Carafate (sucralfate) is a common antiulcer drug. This drug is unique because it actually forms an inside "patch" over a stomach ulcer, protecting the stomach lining and allowing it to heal.

Antidiarrheals and Laxatives

Antidiarrheals are drugs that lessen or stop diarrhea. They include both OTC and prescription medications.

Examples of Antidiarrheals

- Kaopectate
- Imodium
- Lomotil
- Donnatal

Laxatives are the medications that are used to treat constipation. They can stimulate a bowel movement, soften the stool for easier passage, or may be a fiber supplement to increase and maintain normal bowel function. Laxatives are frequently ordered as a prn medication and may be given orally, as a suppository, or as an enema.

Examples of Laxatives

- Fiberall
- Dulcolax
- Senokot
- Fleet oral or enema preparation

Antiemetic or Antinausea Drugs

Nausea and vomiting need to be treated promptly because these can lead to serious complications for patients. Vomiting is also known as emesis; therefore, this category of drugs is often referred to as antiemetics. These drugs may be administered orally, intravenously, intramuscularly, or via suppository.

Examples of Antiemetics

- *Compazine* (prochlorperazine)
- Reglan (metoclopramide)
- *Vistaril* (hydroxyzine)
- *Tigan* (trimethobenzamide)

Drugs that Affect the Musculoskeletal System

Anti-Inflammatory Drugs

Anti-inflammatory drugs are used to reduce inflammation and relieve pain. They are most commonly used in arthritis and arthritis-like conditions. These drugs are divided into two groups, steroidal and nonsteroidal anti-inflammatory drugs (NSAID)

Examples of Steroidal Anti-Inflammatory Drugs

- Aristocort (triamcinolone)
- Cortef (hydrocortisone)
- Danocrine (danazol)
- Decadron (dexamethasone)
- Deltasone (prednisone)
- Pred Mild (prednisolone)

Note: Decadron, prednisone and hydrocortisone are also listed under hormones.

Examples of Nonsteroidal Anti-Inflammatory Drugs (NSAID)

- Acular
- Anaprox (naproxen)
- Ansaid (flurbiprofen)
- Arthropan
- Celebrex (celecoxib)
- Clinoril (sulindac)
- Disalcid (salsalate)
- Dolobid (diflunisal)
- Feldene (piroxicam)
- Motrin (ibuprofen)
- Tolectin (tolmetin)
- Voltaren (diclofenac)

Muscle Relaxants

Muscle relaxants reduce spasms in the muscles.

Examples of Muscle Relaxants

- Flexeril (cyclobenzaprine)
- Norflex (orphenadrine citrate)
- Soma (carisoprodol)

Antineoplastics (Chemotherapy)

Antineoplastic drugs are a large group of drugs that are used in the treatment of cancer. The uses and dosages vary widely depending on the type of cancer that the patient has. Some chemotherapy drugs require special handling of the drug itself, or the patient receiving the drugs may need special isolation precautions.

Examples of Antineoplastics

- Platinol–AQ (cisplatin)
- Cytoxan (cyclophosphamide)
- Adriamycin (doxorubicin)
- (interferon)
- (methotrexate)
- (tamoxifen)
- Oncovin (vincristine)

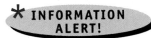

* INFORMATION ALERT!

Common Drug Dosages

The following list contains some frequently ordered medications and their usual adult dosages.

Codeine	15–60 mg
Coumadin	2–10 mg
Demerol	50–100 mg
heparin	5000 U
Lanoxin	0.125–0.25 mg
morphine sulfate	10–15 mg

Vitamins

Vitamins are organic substances found in food. Occasionally, the body becomes deficient in vitamins, especially during illness.

Examples of Vitamins:

- AquaMEPHYTON
- Berocca
- Multivitamin (MVI)
- Vitamin B-12

Topical Preparations

Topical preparations are frequently ordered for the eye or the ear or to be applied to the skin.

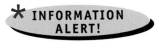

* INFORMATION ALERT!

Drugs You Need to Identify to Meet Objective #11

Antacids	Antisecretory Drugs	Antidiarrheals	Laxatives
Maalox	Tagamet	Imodium	Dulcolax
Mylanta		Lomotil	Fleets (oral & enema)

Antiemetics/ Antinauseants	Steroids	Nonsteroidal (NSAIDS)	Muscle Relaxants
Compazine	Aristocort	Anaprox—Naprosyn	Flexeril
Tigan	Cortef	Celebrex	Soma
Vistaril	Deltasone (prednisone)	Clinoril	
		Feldene	
		Motrin	

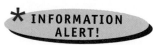

Drugs You Need to Identify to Meet Objective #11

Antineoplastics	Vitamins
Cytoxan	AquaMEPHYTON
Oncovin	Berocca
	Multivitamin (MVI)
	Vitamin B-12

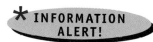

Many medications are spelled similarly, which increases the risk of making an error when interpreting doctors' handwriting. Below are some examples of similarly spelled medications.

Medication Order Written by Doctor	Medication that Could Cause Confusion
Quinine 200 mg PO	Quinidine 200 mg PO
Lamotrigine 150 mg	Lamivudine 150 mg PO
Sulfasalazine 500 mg qid	Sulfadiazine 500 mg qid
Indapamide 2.5 mg PO	Isradipine 2.5 mg PO
Norvasc TM 10 mg PO qd	Navane TM 10 mg PO qd
Hydroxyzine 25 mg PO	Hydralazine 25 mg PO
Losec TM 20 mg PO qd	Lasix TM 20 mg PO qd
Klonopin TM 0.5 mg PO	Clonidine 0.5 mg PO
Vinblastine	Vincristine
Platinol TM	Paraplatin TM

Examples of Ophthalmic Preparations (for the eye)

- Achromycin ophthalmic ointment
- Brinzolamide
- Cortisporin ophthalmic ointment and suspension
- Decadron phosphate ophthalmic ointment and solution
- Demulcents (artificial tears)
- Dorzolamide
- Garamycin ophthalmic ointment
- Neosporin ophthalmic ointment and solution
- Polysporin ophthalmic ointment
- Propine
- Silver nitrate solution
- Timoptic ophthalmic solution
- Tobrex

Examples of Otic Preparations (for the ear)

- Auralgan otic solution
- Cortisporin otic solution
- Cerumenex
- Vosol HC otic solution

Examples of Preparations for the Skin

- Aristocort
- Betadine spray
- Cortisporin ointment
- Cyclocort
- Furacin topical cream

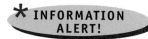

Drugs You Need to Identify to Meet Objective #11

Ophthalmic Preparations (eye)	Otic Preparations (ear)	Preparations for the Skin
Cortisporin ophthalmic ointment and suspension	Cerumenex	Betadine spray
Neosporin ophthalmic ointment and solution	Vosol HC otic solution	Hydrocortisone
Timoptic ophthalmic solution		Neosporin ointment

- Garamycin cream
- Hydrocortisone
- Lotrisone
- Mycolog cream and ointment
- Mycostatin cream and ointment
- Neosporin ointment
- Silvadene cream
- Topicort

EXERCISE 8

Briefly describe the general purpose for each of the following drug groups.

1. antidiabetics

_____

2. anticoagulants

_____

3. antiinfectives

_____

4. antisecretory or antiulcers

_____

5. antineoplastics

_____

6. sedatives

7. *hypnotics*

_____

8. *hormones*

_____

9. *potassium replacements*

_____

10. *narcotics or opioids, analgesics with narcotics, and nonnarcotic analgesics*

_____

11. *antihistamines*

_____

12. *antilipidemics*

_____

13. *antidysrhythmics*

_____

14. *antianginals*

_____

15. *antihypertensives*

_____

16. *diuretics*

_____

17. *laxatives*

_____

18. *antiemetics*

_____

19. *vasopressors*

_____

■ REAGENTS USED FOR DIAGNOSTIC TESTS

The following diagnostic procedures are performed by the nursing staff. The supplies used to perform the tests are requisitioned from the pharmacy during the transcription procedure.

Skin Tests

Skin tests are administered intradermally or subcutaneously for diagnostic purposes. Types and explanations of common skin tests follow.

☑ DOCTORS' ORDERS FOR SKIN TESTS

PPD today
This is a screening test for tuberculosis. The test agent that is administered to the patient is purified protein derivative (PPD). Inter (intermediate) is the dosage strength.

Cocci 1:100 now
This is a diagnostic test for coccidioidomycosis (valley fever). The ratio 1:100 refers to the dilution of the test material. It may also be administered in a 1:10 dilution.

Histoplasmin 0.1 mL today
This skin test is employed as an aid in diagnosing histoplasmosis, a fungal disease.

■ MEDICATION STOCK SUPPLY

Hospitals store a supply of medications on nursing units. This supply is often called the medication stock supply, and it includes such drugs as aspirin, acetaminophen, mineral oil, and milk of magnesia. When floor stock medicines are ordered from the pharmacy, they are charged to the unit budget.

■ RENEWAL MEDICATION ORDERS

Drugs such as narcotics, hypnotics, and other drugs controlled by federal or state laws have an automatic stop date. Hospital medical committees may also set automatic stop dates on anticoagulants and antibiotics. These drugs must be reordered before or when the stop date is reached. Your instructor or hospital pharmacist may provide you with a list of medications that have an automatic stop date in your hospital and the number of hours the drugs may be in effect before reordering is necessary.

A renewal stamp is used by some hospitals as a reminder of the automatic stop date (Fig. 13–13). This stamp is placed on the doctor's order sheet by nursing personnel shortly before the order is due to expire and when completed, it is regarded as a new order and is transcribed as such. Where permitted, this date may require only changing the dates on the medication Kardex form or medication administration record.

If the doctor wishes to discontinue the medication that is to be renewed, he or she may indicate this by writing "No" on the re-

DOCTOR, THE _____ *Narcotic* _____
HAS EXPIRED. DO YOU

WISH THE _____ *Demerol* _____
RENEWED? THANK YOU.

DR's. SIGNATURE _____ *Dr. Starr* _____

FIGURE 13-13 ▲ Drug renewal stamp.

newal stamp or by not signing the renewal stamp. This automatically discontinues the medication.

■ DISCONTINUING MEDICATION ORDERS

When a doctor discontinues a standing or standing prn order, he or she indicates this by writing an order on the doctor's order sheet: DC Achromycin 500 mg PO tid

 STUDENT ACTIVITIES

To practice renewing and discontinuing medication orders, complete Activities 13–8 and 13–9 in the *Skills Practice Manual.*

■ MEDICATION ORDER CHANGES

A patient's medication order may need to be changed for any number of reasons. The change may involve the dosage, route of administration, or frequency of a drug already ordered. Whenever this is done, it is considered a new order and should be written as such on the medication administration record. It is illegal to erase or cross out parts of an order or to write over an order on the MAR because this is a record of what medication has been administered to the patient. This may result in a serious medication error. The old order must be discontinued according to the policy and the new order written. (See also Fig. 13–2 for discontinuing medication on the MAR.)

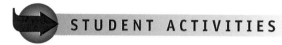 DOCTORS' ORDERS FOR MEDICATION ORDER CHANGES

- *Change Demerol 50 mg IM q 4h prn to Demerol 50 mg PO q 4h prn*
(change in route of administration)

- *Decrease ampicillin 500 mg PO qid to 250 mg PO qid*
(change in dosage)

- *Change Librium 5 mg PO tid to 5 mg PO qid*
(change in frequency of administration)

STUDENT ACTIVITIES

- To practice transcribing medication order changes, complete Activity 13–10 in the *Skills Practice Manual.*
- To test your skill in transcribing a review set of medication orders, complete Activity 13–11.
- To test your skill in transcribing a review set of doctor's orders, complete Activity 13–12.
- To practice locating medications in the *Physicians' Desk Reference,* complete Activity 13–13.
- To practice recording telephoned doctor's orders and to practice recording telephoned messages, complete Activities 13–14 and 13–15.

■ SUMMARY

Transcribing medication orders requires extreme accuracy. Errors may result in serious consequences to the patient and liability to the hospital and all involved personnel. The health unit coordinator must also be careful not to omit any orders from the several forms that he or she is responsible for during the transcription procedure. Each order must be transcribed exactly as written by the doctor. Write each order legibly so that it can be easily read by the nurse administering the medication.

An understanding of the type, form, and proper transcription procedure of medication orders should be acquired by all who work with drug orders. As you gain experience, you will learn the more commonly administered medications and the groupings to which they belong, such as laxatives, sedatives, and cardiac medications.

Whenever there is any doubt concerning a medication order or any order, always check with the nurse. Never hesitate to ask the nurse or to call the doctor whenever there is a possibility of misinterpreting the medication order or when the order cannot be read.

REVIEW QUESTIONS

1. Define the following:

   a. Standing medication order

   _____

   b. Standing prn medication order

   _____

   c. Stat medication order

   _____

   d. One-time medication order

   _____

   e. Short-series order for medication

   _____

   f. IV push

   _____

   g. Intramuscular injection

   _____

   h. Oral medication

   _____

   i. Automatic stop date

   _____

   j. Total parenteral nutrition

   _____

   k. Patient-controlled analgesia

   _____

   l. Intravenous

   _____

   m. Topical

   _____

   n. Peripheral parenteral nutrition

   _____

    o. Intravenous piggyback medication

    _____

2. Two reference books on medications that the health unit coordinator may refer to in the hospital are:

    a. _____

    b. _____

3. The five components of a medication order are:

    a. _____

    b. _____

    c. _____

    d. _____

    e. _____

4. Four routes by which medications may be administered are:

    a. _____

    b. _____

    c. _____

    d. _____

5. Two weights and measures systems used in the pharmacy are:

    a. _____

    b. _____

6. List the five rights of medication administration.

    a. _____

    b. _____

    c. _____

    d. _____

    e. _____

7. Identify the classification or group (use the list from Exercise 8) that the following medications would belong to:

a. Demerol _____

b. Tylenol _____

c. Motrin _____

d. Restoril _____

e. Codeine sulfate _____

f. Morphine _____

g. Tylenol # 3 _____

h. Percodan _____

i. Dalmane _____

j. Benadryl _____

k. Ativan _____

l. Insulin, regular _____

m. Penicillin _____

n. Cefazolin (Ancef, Kefzol) _____

o. Aminophylline _____

p. Xanax _____

q. Phenobarbital _____

r. Gentamycin _____

s. Coumadin (warfarin) _____

t. Lanoxin (digoxin) _____

u. K-Lyte _____

v. Tigan _____

w. Lasix _____

x. Nitostat (nitroglycerin) _____

y. heparin _____

z. K-Lor _____

8. Match the definition in the second column with the words in the first column by placing the correct letter in the space provided.

_____ 1. topical

a. an injection given under the skin into connective tissue

_____ 2. metric

b. by mouth

_____ 3. hypnotic

c. a gelatinous container enclosing a drug

_____ 4. parenteral

d. a drug that produces sleep

_____ 5. oral

e. a test to determine the presence of antibodies within the body

_____ 6. total parenteral nutrition

f. direct application of medication to the skin

_____ 7. narcotic

g. used to self-administer narcotics

_____ 8. skin test

h. also called intravenous hyperalimentation

_____ 9. patient-controlled analgesia

i. a weight and measure system

_____ 10. medication nurse

j. fluids or medications given by injection

_____ 11. subcutaneous injection

k. a drug that relieves pain

_____ 12. capsule

l. one who administers medications to a group of patients

TOPICS FOR DISCUSSION

1. A nurse asks you to change the medication dose that was listed on the physician's order sheet because he gave a different dose. Discuss what you would do and what you would say to the nurse.
2. The physician calls and starts to give you medication orders over the telephone, stating that she does not have time to wait for the nurse to take the order and these are "no big deal." It is hospital policy that telephone orders may only be given to a licensed nurse. Discuss what you would say to the doctor.
3. Discuss what you would do if you were not absolutely sure of the spelling of a medication when transcribing a doctor's order.

Laboratory Orders and Recording Telephoned Laboratory Results

Chapter Objectives

Upon completion of this chapter, you will be able to:

1. Define the terms in the vocabulary list.
2. Write the meaning of each abbreviation in the abbreviations list.
3. List the two general purposes of laboratory studies.
4. Name the three major laboratory divisions and briefly state the purpose of each.
5. Name six studies performed in each of the three major laboratory divisions.
6. List five specimens that may be studied in the laboratory.
7. Describe the health unit coordinator's responsibilities in sending specimens to the laboratory.
8. Name three methods of obtaining urine specimens.
9. List the four tests generally performed as part of electrolyte studies.
10. List five laboratory studies that may require a written consent form.
11. Describe the procedure for requisitioning stat blood tests from the laboratory.
12. Name the procedure that must be performed to order blood (packed cells) for transfusion.
13. Describe the health unit coordinator's responsibilities in an order for a 2 h PP.
14. Explain the difference between fasting and NPO.
15. Identify the laboratory department that would perform each of the tests that are marked with an asterisk.
16. Explain the procedure for ordering peak and trough drug levels.
17. Name three common urine chemistry tests (marked with an asterisk).
18. Describe how errors may be avoided in recording telephoned laboratory results.

Vocabulary

Amniocentesis ▲ A needle puncture into the uterine cavity to remove amniotic fluid, the liquid that surrounds the unborn baby

Antigen ▲ Any substance that induces an immune response

Antibody ▲ An immunoglobulin (protein) produced by the body that reacts with and neutralizes an antigen (usually a foreign substance)

Biopsy ▲ Tissue removed from a living body for examination

Clean Catch ▲ A method of obtaining a urine specimen using a special cleansing technique; also called a midstream urine

Culture and Sensitivity ▲ The growth of microorganisms in a special media (culture), followed by a test to determine the antibiotic to which they best respond (sensitivity)

Cytology ▲ The study of cells

Daily Laboratory Tests ▲ Tests that are ordered once by the doctor but are ordered every day until the doctor discontinues the order

Differential ▲ Identification of the types of white cells found in the blood

Dipstick Urine ▲ The visual examination of urine using a special chemically treated stick

Electrolytes ▲ A group of tests done in chemistry, which usually includes sodium, potassium, chloride, and CO_2

Erythrocyte ▲ A red blood cell

Fasting ▲ No solid foods by mouth and no fluids containing nourishment (e.g., sugar or milk)

Guaiac ▲ A method of testing stool and urine using guaiac as a reagent for hidden (occult) blood (may also be called a Hemoccult Slide Test)

Lumbar Puncture ▲ A procedure used to remove cerebrospinal fluid from the spinal canal

Occult Blood ▲ Blood that is undetectable to the eye

Pap Smear ▲ A test performed to detect cancerous cells in the female genital tract; the Pap staining method can also study body secretions, excretions, and tissue scrapings

Postprandial ▲ After eating

Paracentesis ▲ A surgical puncture and drainage of a body cavity

Pathology ▲ The study of body changes caused by disease

Plasma ▲ The fluid portion of the blood in which the cells are suspended; it contains a clotting factor called fibrinogen

Random Specimen ▲ A body fluid sample that can be collected at any time

Reference Range ▲ Range of normal values for a laboratory test result

Serology ▲ The study of blood serum or other body fluids for immune bodies, which are the body's defense when disease occurs

Serum ▲ Plasma from which fibrinogen, a clotting factor, has been removed

Sputum ▲ The mucous secretion from lungs, bronchi, or trachea

Sternal Puncture ▲ The procedure to remove bone marrow from the breastbone cavity for diagnostic purposes; also called a bone marrow biopsy

Thoracentesis ▲ A needle puncture into the pleural space in the chest cavity to remove pleural fluid for diagnostic or therapeutic reasons

Tissue Typing ▲ Identification of tissue types to predict acceptance or rejection of tissue and organ transplants

Titer ▲ The quantity of substance needed to react with a given amount of another substance—used to detect and quantify antibody levels

Type and Crossmatch ▲ The patient's blood is typed, then tested for compatibility with blood from a donor of the same blood type and Rh factor

Type and Screen ▲ The patient's blood type and Rh factor are determined, and a general antibody screen is performed

Urinalysis ▲ The physical, chemical, and microscopic examination of the urine

Urine Reflex ▲ Urine is tested; if certain parameters are met, a culture is performed

Abbreviations

Abbreviation	Meaning	Example of Usage on a Doctor's Order Sheet
Ab	antibody	Note: Many doctors' orders for laboratory tests are written on the doctors' order sheet as the abbreviation appears here; for example, CBC is the doctor's written order for complete blood count. Examples of doctors' orders are given only for those orders that require more than the abbreviation.
ADH	antidiuretic hormone (chemistry)	
AFB	acid-fast bacillus (microbiology)	
Ag	antigen	
ALP *or* alk phos	alkaline phosphatase (chemistry)	
ANA	antinuclear antibody (serology)	
BMP	basic metabolic panel (chemistry)	
BUN	blood urea nitrogen (chemistry)	
Bx	biopsy (cytology)	
Ca or Ca+	calcium (chemistry)	
CBC	complete blood count (hematology)	
CC, creat cl, or cr cl	creatinine clearance (chemistry)	
CEA	carcinoembryonic antigen (serology)	

Abbreviation	Meaning	Example of Usage on a Doctor's Order Sheet	Abbreviation	Meaning	Example of Usage on a Doctor's Order Sheet
Cl	chloride (chemistry)		LP	lumbar puncture (also called spinal tap)	LP in am
CMP	comprehensive metabolic panel (chemistry)		Lytes	electrolytes (chemistry)	
CMV	cytomegalovirus (microbiology, serology)		Mg or Mg+	magnesium (chemistry)	
CO_2	carbon dioxide (chemistry)		Na	sodium (chemistry)	
			NP	nasopharynx	NP smear for C&S
CPK or CK	creatine phosphoki-nase or creatine ki-nase (chemistry)		O&P	ova and parasites (parasitology)	Stool for O&P × 3
C&S	culture and sensitiv-ity (micro)	Sputum for C&S	PAP	prostatic acid phos-phatase (serology)	
CSF	cerebrospinal fluid (chemistry, hematology, microbiology)	CSF for serology	PC	packed cells (blood bank)	Give 2 U PC now
			PCV	packed-cell volume (hematology; same as hematocrit)	
Cx	culture (microbiology)		pH	hydrogen ion con-centration	
Diff	differential (hematology)		PKU	phenylketonuria (chemistry)	
EBV	Epstein-Barr virus (serology)		PO_2	partial pressure of oxygen	
ESR or sedrate	erythrocyte sedi-mentation rate (hematology)		PO_4 or phos	phosphorus (chemistry)	
FBS	fasting blood sugar (chemistry)		POCT or PCT	point-of-care testing (performed on the nursing unit)	
Fe	iron (chemistry)	Fe c̄ TIBC	PP	postprandial (chemistry)	2 h PP BS
FS	frozen section (cytology)		PSA	prostatic specific antigen (serology)	
GTT	glucose tolerance test (chemistry)		PT	prothrombin time (coagulation–hematology)	
HB_sAg	hepatitis B surface antigen (serology)		PTT or APTT	partial thromboplas-tin time or acti-vated partial thromboplastin time (coagulation–hematology)	
HCG	human chorionic go-nadotropin (test for pregnancy [chemistry])				
Hct	hematocrit (hematology)		RBC	red blood cell count (hematology)	
HDL	high-density lipopro-teins (chemistry)		RBS or BS	random blood sugar or blood sugar (chemistry)	
Hgb	hemoglobin (hematology)		RDW	red cell distribu-tion width (hematology)	
H&H	hemoglobin and hematocrit (hematology)		Retics	reticulocytes (hematology)	
$HIVB_{24}Ag$	human immunodefi-ciency virus screen (serology)		RSV	respiratory syncy-tial virus (microbiology)	
K	potassium (chemistry)		S&A	sugar and acetone (urinalysis)	
LDL	low-density lipo-proteins (chemistry)				

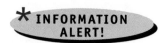

✱INFORMATION ALERT!

Most of the abbreviations listed on pp. 260 to 262 are for some commonly ordered laboratory tests. There are many more abbreviations for laboratory tests that will be covered throughout this chapter. The words in parentheses indicate in which division of the laboratory the test is performed.

Abbreviation	Meaning	Example of Usage on a Doctor's Order Sheet
T_3, T_4, T_7	thyroid tests (chemistry)	
T&X-match or T&C	type and cross-match (blood bank)	T&C for 2 U of packed red cells
TIBC	total iron-binding capacity (chemistry)	
T&S	type and screen (blood bank)	
TSH	thyroid-stimulating hormone (chemistry)	
T/Stat	timed stat (to be drawn stat at specified time)	
UA or U/A	(urinalysis)	
VDRL	Venereal Disease Research Laboratories (serology)	
WBC	white blood cell count (hematology)	
WNL	within normal limits	

EXERCISE 1

Write the abbreviation for each term listed below.

1. fasting blood sugar _____

2. ova and parasites _____

3. hemoglobin _____

4. erythrocyte sedimentation rate *or* sedimentation rate _____

5. potassium _____

6. acid-fast bacilli _____

7. red blood cell count _____

8. postprandial _____

9. cerebrospinal fluid _____

10. iron _____

11. culture and sensitivity _____

12. type and crossmatch _____

13. complete blood count _____

14. prostatic acid phosphatase _____

15. glucose tolerance test _____

16. packed cells _____

17. prothrombin time _____

18. urinalysis _____

19. alkaline phosphatase _____

20. hepatitis B surface antigen _____

21. frozen section _____

22. human immunodeficiency virus _____

23. magnesium _____

24. human chorionic gonadotropin _____

25. within normal limits _____

26. partial thromboplastin time *or* activated partial thromboplastin time _____

27. thyroid tests _____

28. thyroid-stimulating hormone _____

29. sugar and acetone _____

30. antigen _____

31. basic metabolic chemistry panel _____

32. cytomegalovirus _____

33. partial pressure of oxygen _____

34. type and screen _____

35. antibody _____

36. culture _____

37. respiratory syncytial virus _____

38. comprehensive metabolic panel _____

39. electrolytes _____

40. biopsy _____

41. point-of-care testing _____

42. packed-cell volume _____

43. random blood sugar *or* blood sugar _____

44. Venereal Disease Research Laboratories _____

45. reticulocytes _____

46. prostatic specific antigen _____

47. differential _____

48. white blood cell count _____

49. phosphorous _____

50. total iron-binding capacity _____

51. hematocrit _____

52. lumbar puncture _____

53. sodium _____

54. nasopharynx _____

55. hemoglobin and hematocrit _____

56. carbon dioxide _____

57. antinuclear antibody _____

58. high-density lipoproteins _____

59. blood urea nitrogen _____

60. calcium _____

61. creatinine clearance _____

62. chloride _____

63. carcinoembryonic antigen _____

64. timed stat _____

65. low-density lipoproteins _____

66. antidiuretic hormone _____

67. creatine phosphokinase or kinase _____

68. Epstein-Barr virus _____

69. hydrogen ion concentration _____

70. red cell distribution width _____

EXERCISE 2

Write the meaning of each abbreviation listed below.

1. *FBS*

_____

2. *O&P*

_____

3. *Hgb*

_____

4. *ESR* or *sedrate*

_____

5. *K*

_____

6. *AFB*

_____

7. *RBC*

_____

8. *PP*

_____

9. *CSF*

_____

10. *Fe*

_____

11. C&S

_____

12. T & X-match or T&C

_____

13. CBC

_____

14. PAP

_____

15. GTT

_____

16. PC

_____

17. PT

_____

18. Ua or U/A

_____

19. ALP or alk phos

_____

20. HB_5Ag

_____

21. FS

_____

22. $HIV B_{24}Ag$

_____

23. Mg or Mg+

_____

24. HCG

_____

25. WNL

_____

26. PTT or APTT

_____

27. $T_3T_4T_7$

_____

28. TSH

_____

29. S&A

_____

30. Ag

_____

31. BMP

_____

32. CMV

_____

33. PO_2

_____

34. T&S

_____

35. Ab

_____

36. Cx

_____

37. RSV

_____

38. CMP

_____

39. lytes

_____

40. Bx

_____

41. POCT or PCT

_____

42. PCV

_____

43. RBS

_____

44. VDRL

_____

45. retics

_____

46. PSA

_____

47. Diff

_____

48. WBC

_____

49. PO_4 or phos

_____

50. TIBC

_____

51. Hct

_____

52. LP

_____

53. Na

_____

54. NP

_____

55. H&H

_____

56. CO_2

_____

57. ANA

_____

58. HDL

_____

59. BUN

_____

60. Ca or Ca^+

_____

61. CC, creat cl, or cr cl

_____

62. Cl

_____

63. *CEA*

_____

64. *T/Stat*

_____

65. *LDL*

_____

66. *ADH*

_____

67. *CPK or CK*

_____

68. *EBV*

_____

69. *pH*

_____

70. *RDW*

_____

■ INTRODUCTION TO LABORATORY PROCEDURE

Tests performed by the laboratory are ordered for diagnostic purposes and for the evaluation of a prescribed treatment. See Appendix F for a comprehensive list of the studies that are performed in a laboratory.

Hospital size determines the number of divisions within the laboratory and the kinds of tests performed in each division. For example, a large hospital may have a microbiology division with subdivisions such as bacteriology, serology, parasitology, virology, and mycology. In smaller hospitals all the tests performed in the divisions mentioned above may be done in the microbiology division or sent to outside laboratories. (Figure 14–1 is a laboratory divisional chart.) Also, you may find in your hospital that the division and some test names vary from those used in this book.

In this chapter we will discuss three major laboratory divisions: hematology, chemistry, and microbiology; and five other divisions: toxicology, serology, pathology (including histology and cytology), blood bank, and urinalysis. The clinical laboratory may also perform tests related to nuclear medicine and gastroenterology when a hospital is not of sufficient size to maintain a separate nuclear medicine or gastroenterology department.

It is necessary for the health unit coordinator to interpret terms the doctor may use to write laboratory orders. The word *routine*, in a written laboratory order, would usually be performed within a 4-hour period, because there is no urgency for the test results. For example, the doctor may write the order *Routine CBC*, meaning that the blood specimen for the complete blood count may be drawn according to the hospital (laboratory) policy. Nursing personnel or laboratory personnel may draw blood specimens.

The doctor may also use the word *daily*, as in the order *daily Hgb*; this means that the test is ordered once by the doctor, but requisitioned every day or entered into the computer for multiple days in advance by the health unit coordinator until the order is discontinued. Some hospitals have a policy that requires the doctor to renew daily lab orders every 3 days or discontinue the orders.

The word *stat*, as you recall, means to be done immediately. Because of the urgency of a stat order, a different communication procedure is used. The procedure is to notify the laboratory by phone or verbally notify the appropriate nursing personnel on the unit. When calling the laboratory, supply the name of the patient, nursing unit, room number, and the test ordered. The order is entered into the computer immediately if a laboratory technician is to draw the blood. The order would be entered when the specimen is collected if collected by nursing personnel. When placing an order for a test that is to be drawn stat at a specified time such as drug levels or a 2 hr PP blood sugar, the term *T/Stat* (timed stat) is used.

Specimens

All laboratory tests require a specimen. Blood is the most common specimen used and is most often obtained by nursing or laboratory personnel through venipuncture (puncture into the vein), finger-stick (puncture into a capillary), or via peripheral arterial lines (Fig. 14–2).

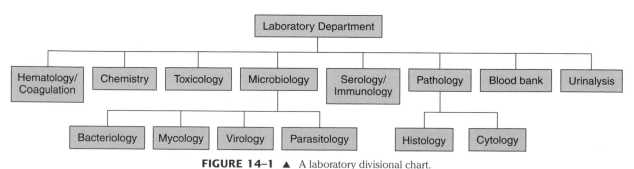

FIGURE 14–1 ▲ A laboratory divisional chart.

Blood specimens may need to be collected in different containers depending on the test ordered. For example, coagulation studies and chemistry studies must be in different tubes. Cultures performed on blood for different types of organisms (aerobic versus anaerobic bacteria) may also require different tubes. Clear and complete information on all tests to be collected reduces the need for the patient to be redrawn for additional blood specimens. When asked by a nurse to call the laboratory to inquire about amount or means of collecting a specimen; document what you are told and the name of the person giving you the information.

Some other specimens tested are urine, stool, sputum, sweat, wound drainage, discharge from body openings, and gastric washings (lavage). The nursing staff usually collects these specimens (Fig. 14–3, A-H).

The doctor usually obtains specimens by entering parts of the body or a body cavity. Types of specimens and the names of the procedures used to obtain them are listed below. Most hospitals have a policy that requires a written consent from the patient prior to performing these procedures, except for pelvic examination. (Review "Preparing a Consent Form," Chapter 8.) It may be your responsibility to order trays, such as a lumbar puncture tray, or other equipment from the CSD for the doctor to use to perform these procedures.

Specimen	Procedure Performed to Obtain Specimen
Spinal fluid	Lumbar puncture; also called spinal tap
Bone marrow	Sternal puncture; also called bone marrow biopsy
Abdominal cavity fluid	Abdominal paracentesis
Pleural fluid	Thoracentesis
Amniotic fluid	Amniocentesis
Biopsy specimen	Biopsy of a part of the body
Cervical smear	Pelvic examination

All specimens obtained by the nursing staff or doctor will usually be bagged and labeled (not always possible during an emergency) prior to handing them to the health unit coordinator. It is recommended that the health unit coordinator keep plastic gloves in her or his drawer to use when specimens are not bagged and wash his or her hands after handling specimens (even when placed in plastic bags). The label should have the date and time collected with initials of the person who collected the specimen.

Requisitions for laboratory tests of specimens obtained by the nursing staff or doctor are kept on the nursing unit until the specimen is collected or the order is entered into the computer when sending the specimen. The requisition or computer printout of the order is attached to the specimen bag, and then sent to the laboratory. It is essential that the health unit coordinator check the patient name on the specimen and computer order screen to compare to the doctor's order. Mislabeled specimens are usually discarded and the patient redrawn, causing a delay in diagnosis and treatment as well as causing the patient additional discomfort.

It is often your responsibility to take the specimen to the laboratory. This should be done as soon as possible. Some specimens (well wrapped) may be sent by the pneumatic tube system, especially when results are needed quickly (emergency department and surgery). Specimens that should *not* be sent by the pneumatic tube system are those that have been collected by an invasive procedure, such as cerebrospinal and amniotic flu-

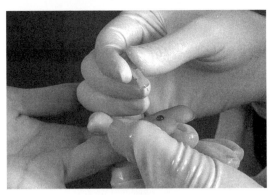

A

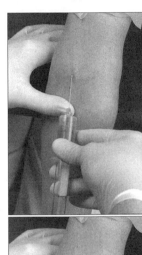

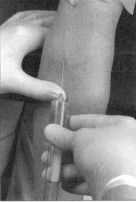

B

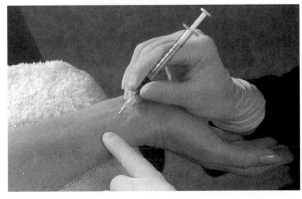

C

FIGURE 14–2 ▲ Methods of obtaining blood specimens: *A,* Finger stick. *B,* Venipuncture. *C,* Peripheral arterial draw. (From Sommer S. et al: Phlebotomy Worktext and Procedures Manual. St. Louis, Mosby, 2001.)

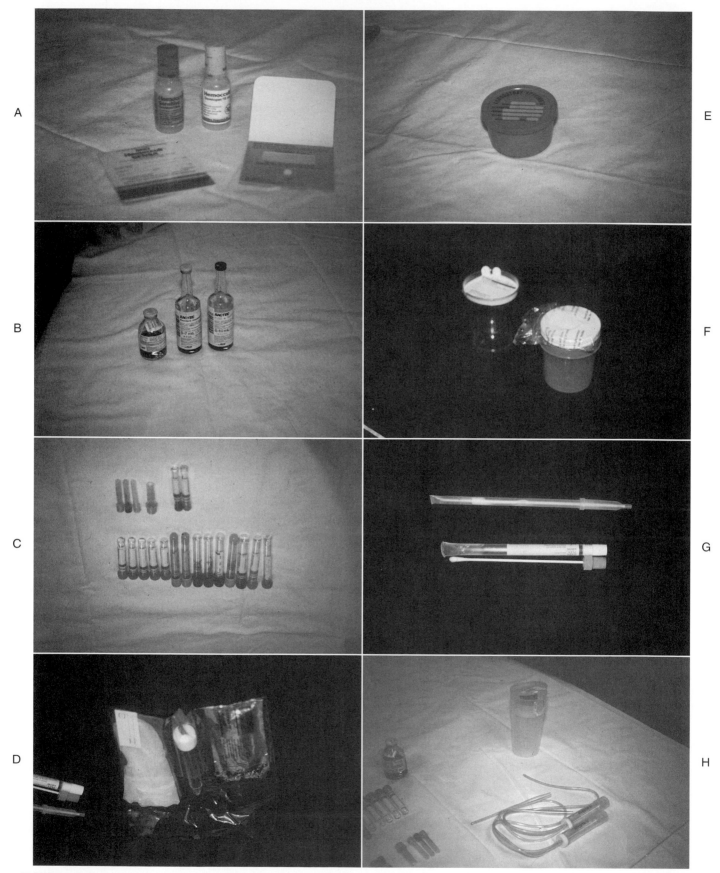

FIGURE 14–3 ▲ Specimen collection containers. *A,* Hemoccult slides for stool specimen. *B,* Containers for blood culture specimen. *C,* Various containers for blood specimen. *D,* Cath urine specimen container kit. *E,* Stool specimen container. *F,* Urine specimen containers: *left,* voided specimen; *right,* midstream specimen. *G,* Culturette and container for throat culture. *H,* Types of sputum collection containers.

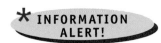

ids. When sending blood or urine by the pneumatic tube system, specimens must be well wrapped and cushioned. Some facilities may have a policy not to transport *any* specimens via the pneumatic tube system because of possible loss or spilling of the specimen.

Point-of-Care Testing

Many laboratory tests that were once only drawn and analyzed in the laboratory department may now be performed on the nursing unit. A laboratory test that is collected and analyzed on the hospital unit by nursing personnel is called a point-of-care lab test. Because of point-of-care testing, the procedure for ordering a test may change.

Results are obtained by utilizing several methods. These include analysis by portable automated analyzers, the use of reagents (chemicals), and microscopic visualization.

Portable automated analyzers may be used in departments that require immediate results, and they decrease the need for stat specimens to be sent to the laboratory. Some tests that may be done on the unit by this method are electrolytes, blood glucose, BUN, hemoglobin, and hematocrit. A pulmonary function test (see Chapter 16) or arterial blood gases (ABGs) may also be run on an automated analyzer on the unit.

Reagent-based tests may include a test for pregnancy or human chorionic gonadotropin (HCG), activated clotting time (ACT), and a test for *Helicobacter pylori* (CLO test), a bacterium that has been indicated in ulcers of the gastrointestinal system. The CLO test actually uses a biopsy specimen obtained in the endoscopy department (see Chapter 16) and may give positive results within 2 hours.

Some of the reagent-based tests that are considered point-of-care lab tests are those traditionally carried out by nursing personnel, and include blood and urine monitoring for the presence of ketones and the levels of glucose. These tests are discussed in Chapter 11. Guaiacs, gastroccults, or hemoccults, which use reagents to detect hidden blood in gastric and stool specimens, are also considered point-of-care tests in some health care facilities.

A test that uses both a reagent and microscopic visualization is the fern test, which is used to indicate the presence of amniotic fluid (due to the rupture of the amnion). The reagent portion utilizes a strip of paper that indicates acidity (pH paper), and the microscopic portion detects the characteristic fern pattern of crystallized amniotic sodium chloride (salt).

Communication with the Laboratory Department

All laboratory tests are communicated to the laboratory department by the ordering step of transcription.

■ DIVISIONS WITHIN THE LABORATORY

Hematology

The hematology division performs tests related to physical properties of the blood (including blood cells and their appearance), tests related to clotting and bleeding disorders, and coagulation (clotting) studies to monitor patients on anticoagulant therapy.

Specimen

The majority of these tests are done on a blood specimen. However, bone marrow and spinal fluid may also be studied in the hematology division.

Fasting

Fasting is generally not required for tests performed in the hematology division of the laboratory.

Communication with the Laboratory

Hematology studies are ordered by computer or by completing a requisition form (Fig. 14–4).

✔ DOCTORS' ORDERS FOR HEMATOLOGY STUDIES

It is impossible to list all doctors' orders relating to this division of the laboratory. However, we have listed the more common ones in their abbreviated forms with an interpretation for reference. Refer to the abbreviations list at the beginning of the chapter if necessary.

Note: All of the following tests are performed on blood specimens; therefore, as mentioned previously, nursing or laboratory personnel obtain the specimen or POCT performs them.

PT (prothrombin time)

A PT measures the clotting ability of blood. This test assists the doctor in determining the dosage of the drugs—usually Coumadin—prescribed in anticoagulant therapy. The health unit coordinator may be required to telephone the test results to the doctor. How the results are reported depends on the testing method used, such as patient/control in seconds (e.g., 17 sec/13 sec); or patient/% of prothrombin activity (e.g., 14 sec/70% activity).

In addition to the PT result, an additional result called the INR may be included. This is a calculation using the patient's PT result, the normal control result, and a coefficient factor that depends on the reagent used. The INR calculation is an attempt to standardize PT results.

APTT and PTT

An APTT (activated partial thromboplastin time) and a PTT (partial thromboplastin time) are coagulation studies. They are performed individually and are commonly used to monitor heparin dosage.

Bleeding time

Bleeding time is the measurement of the time it takes a standardized incision to cease bleeding. It differs from clotting time in that this test involves constriction of the smaller blood vessels. A standardized incision is an incision of specific length and depth. Several methods may be used, but the template bleeding time (TBT) is preferred, as the incision is standardized by the use of a cutting device called a template.

Doctor Ordering_____   ☐ Stat
Today's Date_____   ☐ Routine
Collection Date _____ Time _____
Collected by _____
Requested by_____

Hematology	**Serology**	**Urinalysis/Urine Chemistry**
☐ Bleeding Time, Ivy	☐ ANA	☐ Routine Ua
☐ CBC c̄ Diff	☐ ASO Titer	☐ Amylase (2hr)
☐ CBC c̄ Manual Diff	☐ CEA	☐ Bilirubin
☐ Factor VIII	☐ CMV	☐ Calcium
☐ Fibrinogen	☐ IgG	☐ Chloride
☐ HCT	☐ IgM	☐ Creatinine Clearance
☐ HGB	☐ Cocci Screen	☐ Glucose Tolerance
☐ H & H	☐ EBV Panel	☐ Nitrogen
☐ Eosinophil Ct Absolute	☐ Enterovirus Ab Panel 1	☐ Occult Blood
☐ Eosinophil Smear	☐ Enterovirus Ab Panel 2	☐ Osmolality
☐ ESR	☐ HbsAb	☐ Phosphorus
☐ LE Cell Prep	☐ HbsAg	☐ Potassium
☐ Platelet Ct	☐ HIV	☐ Pregnancy
☐ PT	☐ Monospot	☐ Protein
☐ PTT (APTT)	☐ PSA Screen	☐ Sodium
☐ RBC	☐ Ra Factor	☐ Sp Gravity
☐ RBC Indices	☐ RPR	☐ Uric Acid
☐ Reticulocyte Ct	☐ RSV	
☐ Sickle Cell Prep	☐ Rubella Screen	
☐ WBC	☐ Strptozyme	
	☐ VDRL	

Write in Orders: _____
_____

Revised 3/12/03

FIGURE 14–4 ▲ Computer ordering screen for hematology, serology, and urinalysis/urine chemistry.

Communication and Implementation of Laboratory Orders

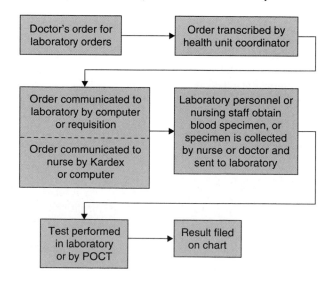

Clotting time
Clotting time is the determination of the time it takes blood to clot.

CBC (complete blood cell count) or Hemogram
A CBC or hemogram is composed of a number of tests, including RBC; Hgb; Hct; RBC indices; WBC; and Diff, blood smear, and platelet count. These tests may also be ordered separately. The number of tests included in a CBC may vary among hospitals.

RBC (red blood cell count)
RBC is the measurement of red blood cells (erythrocytes) per cubic millimeter of blood.

Hgb (hemoglobin)
HGB is the oxygen-carrying pigment of blood that gives it its red color. This test may determine the need for additional blood, or it may aid in diagnosing types of anemia.

Hct (hematocrit)
Hematocrit, also called PCV (packed-cell volume), is a measurement of the volume percentage of red blood cells in whole blood.

RBC (red blood cell) indices

Measurement of RBC indices is a method for determining the characteristics of red blood cells. The measurements are reported as MCH (content of hemoglobin in average individual red cell), MCHC (average hemoglobin concentration per 100 mL of packed red cells), and MCV (average volume of individual red cells).

WBC (white blood cell count)

A WBC (leukocyte count) is the count of the number of white blood cells that are present in the blood to fight disease-causing organisms. This test is often used in the diagnosis of infection.

Diff (differential)

A diff reports the various types of WBCs (or leukocytes) found in the blood specimen. Some of the types are lymphocytes (lymphs), monocytes (monos), neutrophils (neutros), eosinophils (eos), and basophils (basos). A diff is often included in a CBC.

Blood Smear

A blood smear is an examination using special stains of the peripheral blood and can provide a significant amount of information concerning drugs and disease that affect RBCs and WBCs.

Platelet Count (platelets)

Platelet count is the counting of clotting cells (platelets) essential for the coagulation process to take place.

RDW

The red cell distribution width is included on most instruments as part of a CBC. It measures the distribution of red cell volume.

ESR (erythrocyte sedimentation rate)

An erythrocyte sedimentation rate, also called sedrate, determines the rate at which RBCs settle out of the liquid portion of the blood. The test is used to determine the progress of inflammatory diseases.

Retics

The count of reticulocytes (immature red blood cells), determines bone marrow activity. It is often used in the diagnosis of anemia.

LE Cell Prep

LE cell prep is a diagnostic study for lupus erythematosus, an inflammatory disease

Refer to Appendix F for other tests performed in the hematology division.

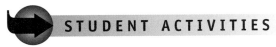

STUDENT ACTIVITIES

To practice transcribing hematology and coagulation orders, complete Activity 14–1 in the *Skills Practice Manual*. To practice transcribing daily laboratory orders, complete Activity 14–2 in the *Skills Practice Manual*.

Chemistry

The chemistry division performs tests related to the study of chemical reactions occurring in living organisms. When a disease process occurs, the chemicals within the body fluids vary from normal. Any variance permits a diagnosis or evaluation of the patient's health status to be made.

Specimens

Blood and urine are the specimens most commonly collected for study in this division of the laboratory. Whole blood, plasma, or serum may be used for chemistry tests. Many tests of the same name can be done on either blood or urine; therefore, often the doctor uses the word *serum* to indicate that the test is to be performed on blood and uses the term *urine* if the test is to be done on a urine specimen.

Specimens for urine chemistries may require the urine to be collected over a period of time, such as 24 hours. This is often referred to as a 24-hour urine specimen (Fig. 14–5). It may be the health unit coordinator's responsibility to obtain the receptacle from the laboratory to be used for the collection of the specimen. Some specimens that are to be kept for a period have a preservative added to the collection bottle before it is sent to the unit. Other 24-hour specimens may have to be iced in the patient's bathroom until the collection is completed (see the Box *Chemistry Tests That Require a 24-Hour Urine Specimen*).

Fasting

Many of the blood chemistry tests require the patient to fast or to be NPO. Fasting means that the patient has nothing to eat for 8 to 10 hours before the collection of the specimen to be tested; the patient may have water. NPO means nothing by mouth—food or fluid—after midnight. It may be your responsibility to notify the dietary department, or you may be asked to obtain bedside signs to be posted to remind personnel that the patient is being prepared for a test. Table 14–1 lists chemistry and other laboratory tests that require the patient to fast or be NPO. (Because some of these tests are not considered fasting by all laboratories, check with your instructor for their correct classification in your hospital.)

Communication with the Laboratory

Chemistry tests are requisitioned by using the computer or by completing a requisition form (see Fig. 14–4).

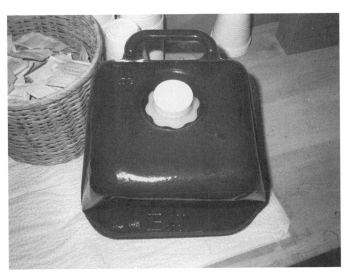

FIGURE 14–5 ▲ 24-hour urine specimen container.

CHEMISTRY TESTS THAT REQUIRE A 24-HOUR URINE SPECIMEN*

Epinephrine-norepinephrine	Homovanillic acid (HVA)
Albumin, quantitative & qualitative	17-Hydroxycorticosteroids
Aldosterone	5-Hydroxyindoleacetic acid, quantitative (5-HIAA)
Amino acids, quantitative-fractionated	17-Ketogenic steroids
Arsenic, quantitative	17-Ketosteroids
Calcium, quantitative	Lactose†
Catecholamines	Lead
Chlorides	Metanephrines
Chorionic gonadotropin (HCG)	Phosphorus
Coproporphyrin, qualitative & quantitative	Porphobilinogen, quantitative
	Potassium
Cortisol	Pregnanetriol
Creatine†	Protein, total
Creatinine	Sodium clearance
Epinephrine	Uric acid†
Estrogens, total	Uroporphyrins, qualitative & quantitative
FIGLU (N-formiminoglutamic acid)	Vanillylmandelic acid (VMA)†
Fluoride	Zinc
Follicle-stimulating hormone (FSH)	
Glucose, quantitative†	

*Note: Check with your laboratory concerning these tests. The methods used may vary from hospital to hospital.
†Common test.

Automated equipment permits many tests to be performed on a small sample of blood and in a short time. One requisition (or computer-entered laboratory request) is used to request a number of tests. Some of the automated instruments used are the Vitros, Paramax, Coulter, Astra, and Dacos. These automated multicomponent studies are called profiles, panels, or surveys.

✓ DOCTORS' ORDERS FOR BLOOD CHEMISTRY STUDIES

Listed below are frequently ordered blood chemistry tests, written in abbreviated form as the doctor would write them on the doctors' order sheet. The full name of each test is given in parentheses. Normal values for common blood chemistry studies are given on p. 273.

Note: Unless otherwise indicated, the specimen used for the following tests is serum, which is collected by either nursing or laboratory personnel.

Acid phos (acid phosphatase)
The level of acid phosphatase is used in diagnosing metastatic carcinomas of the prostate gland and breast, among other uses.

Alk phos (alkaline phosphatase)
The alkaline phosphatase level is used to evaluate bone and liver disease, among other uses.

Amylase (serum)
The level of amylase is elevated in acute pancreatitis, as well as some other illnesses.

TABLE 14-1	Fasting and/or NPO List for Laboratory Studies		
Procedure	**Fasting**	**NPO**	**Laboratory Division**
Bromsulphalein (BSP)	Yes	No	Chemistry
Cholesterol	Yes	No	Chemistry
Chromosomes	Yes	No	Blood bank
Deoxycorticosterone	Yes	No	Chemistry or nuclear medicine
D-Xylose (blood or urine)	Yes	Yes	Chemistry
Electrophoresis, lipids	Yes	No	Chemistry
Electrophoresis, lipoprotein	Yes	No	Chemistry
Factor VIII assay	Yes	Yes	Coagulation
Fasting blood sugar (FBS)	Yes	No	Chemistry
Gastrin (serum)	Yes	Yes	Chemistry or nuclear medicine
Glucose, fasting (FBS)	Yes	No	Chemistry
Glucose tolerance test (GTT)	Yes	Yes	Chemistry
Insulin tolerance test (ITT)	Yes	Yes	Chemistry
Iron (Fe)	Yes	Yes	Chemistry
Iron-binding capacity (IBC)	Yes	Yes	Chemistry
Lipids	Yes	Yes	Chemistry or GI lab
Neutral fat (lipid profile fractionization)	Yes	Yes	Chemistry or GI lab
Orinase tolerance test	Yes	Yes	Chemistry
Parathyroid hormone (PTH)	Yes	Yes	Chemistry or nuclear medicine
Phenolsulfonphthalein (PSP) urine	Yes	Yes	Chemistry
Phospholipids	Yes	Yes	Chemistry or GI lab
Plasma cortisol	Yes	Yes	Chemistry or nuclear medicine
Renin	Yes	Yes	Chemistry or nuclear medicine
Schilling test	No	Yes	Chemistry or nuclear medicine
Serum lipids	Yes	Yes	Chemistry or GI lab
SMA	Yes	Yes	Chemistry
Testosterone	Yes	Yes	Chemistry or nuclear medicine
Total iron-binding capacity (TIBC)	Yes	Yes	Chemistry
Triglycerides	Yes	Yes	Chemistry

AST (SGOT), CPK (CK), and LDH

AST, CPK, and LDH are known as cardiac enzymes. These tests are ordered when a myocardial infarction (heart attack) is suspected.

Bilirubin

This test measures liver function. Bilirubin is the result of red blood cells that have broken down and are excreted by the liver. In diseases in which a large number of red blood cells are destroyed (e.g., in liver disease and obstruction of the common bile duct), a high concentration of bilirubin is found in the blood serum. The doctor may order this test as total bilirubin, using the direct or indirect method of testing.

BMP (basic metabolic panel)

A BMP is a chemistry panel consisting of eight chemistry tests including glucose, BUN, Ca, creatine, Na, K, Cl, and CO_2.

BNP (beta natriuretic peptide)

Increased levels of BNP are released when ventricular diastolic pressure rises and may indicate congestive heart failure, or increased risk of congestive heart failure or mitral valvular disease.

BS (blood sugar) or Glucose

A BS or glucose test is used to determine the amount of sugar in the blood. It is usually ordered at a specific time, such as 4 PM BS, also called an *RBS*. The patient is not fasting when this test is performed.

BUN (blood urea nitrogen)

This test is useful in diagnosing diseases that affect kidney function.

Cholesterol

Cholesterol levels may be used to measure liver function. The patient is usually in a fasting state for this test. It is believed that cholesterol may sometimes be responsible for causing high blood pressure and hardening of the arteries (atherosclerosis). It is also important that the good cholesterol, or high-density lipoproteins (HDL), be measured in relation to total cholesterol.

CMP

A comprehensive metabolic panel consists of 14 chemistry tests including glucose, BUN, creatine, albumin, total bilirubin, Ca, Alk Phos, total protein, AST, Na, K, Cl, CO_2, and ALT.

CPK or CK (creatine phosphokinase or creatine kinase)

CPK or CK is an enzyme found in heart, brain, or skeletal muscle, which is released when there is damage from a disease process.

Creatinine clearance test

A creatinine clearance test is done to study kidney function. It requires testing the blood and urine.

Electrophoresis

An electrophoresis is a procedure performed to determine protein or fatty acid levels. The doctor may order any of three tests that result in a serum protein pattern. The tests are protein electrophoresis, lipoprotein electrophoresis, and immunoelectrophoresis.

FBS (fasting blood sugar)

An FBS, also called fasting glucose, determines the amount of sugar in the bloodstream after the patient has not eaten for 8 to 10 hours. This test is used in the diagnosis of and monitoring of diabetes treatment.

NORMAL VALUES FOR FREQUENTLY PERFORMED HEMATOLOGY—COAGULATION STUDIES AND BLOOD CHEMISTRY STUDIES

Hematocrit (Hct)
- *Male:* 45–50 vol/dL
- *Female:* 40–45 vol/dL

Hemoglobin (Hgb)
- *Male:* 14.5–16 g/dL
- *Female:* 13–15.5 g/dL

White blood cell count (WBC): 6000–9000/mm³
Prothrombin time (PT): 12–15 sec
Sodium (Na): 132–142 mEq/L
Potassium (K): 3.5–5.0 mEq/L
Fasting blood sugar (FBS): 70–120 mg/dL

GTT (glucose tolerance test)

A GTT is performed to determine abnormalities in glucose metabolism. The patient is in a fasting state. The test may be performed over several hours—usually three to six. The patient has an FBS drawn to establish baseline data and then is given a large amount of glucose solution to drink. Timed blood and urine specimens are taken. The urine specimens, collected by the nursing staff, must be carefully labeled with the time the urine was collected. At the completion of the test, all urine is sent to the laboratory. (The order has been communicated to the laboratory by requisition or computer to alert the laboratory personnel to perform a fasting blood sugar test before administering the sugar solution.)

HbA₁c, GHb, or GHB (glycosylated hemoglobin)

A HbA_{1c}, GHb, or GHB test is a reflection of the blood glucose on the red blood cells during the past 3 months. This test is used in monitoring patients with diabetes.

HDL (high-density lipoprotein)

An HDL "good" cholesterol level is thought to be important in the total cholesterol profile.

Isoenzymes (or isozymes)

Isoenzymes determine the source (body part enzymes) responsible for the elevation of enzymes such as LDH, CPK, or CK by determining the variations in these enzymes, such as CK-MB.

LDH (lactate dehydrogenase)

LDH is an enzyme released into the circulation after tissue damage to heart, liver, kidney, brain, or skeletal muscle.

Lytes (electrolytes)

Electrolytes consist of four tests: sodium (Na), potassium (K), chlorides (Cl), and carbon dioxide (CO_2). These four tests may be performed separately.

PAP (prostatic acid phosphatase)

A PAP is an enzyme produced by prostate tissue; it increases as prostate disease becomes more severe. PAP may be used to monitor patients with prostate cancer.

PSA (prostatic specific antigen)

A PSA measures the body's level of prostatic specific antigen. Increased PSA levels may indicate the presence of prostate cancer.

Serum creatinine

A serum creatinine test is performed to diagnose kidney diseases. It studies the creatinine level in the blood serum.

SGOT (serum glutamic-oxaloacetic transaminase)

Another name for SGOT is aspartate aminotransferase (AST). This enzyme is released into the circulation from destroyed skeletal or cardiac muscle, or the liver. The AST level is elevated in myocardial infarction, liver diseases, acute pancreatitis, acute renal diseases, and severe burns.

SGPT (serum glutamic-pyruvic transaminase)

Another name for SGPT is alanine aminotransferase (ALT). This enzyme is released into the circulation by destroyed liver cells.

TIBC (total iron-binding capacity)

A total iron-binding capacity test is useful in diagnosing anemia, some infections, and cirrhosis of the liver.

Troponin

Troponin is a test performed to diagnose acute myocardial infarction (AMI) from a few hours onset to as long as 120 hours. It is more sensitive in detecting unstable angina with minor myocardial cell damage than CK-MB.

2 h PP BS (2-hours postprandial blood sugar)

A 2-hours postprandial blood sugar test is performed to determine the patient's response to carbohydrate intake. It is the health unit coordinator's responsibility to notify the laboratory when the patient has finished eating. The blood for this test may be drawn 2 hours after any meal and if ordered for the laboratory to draw, is ordered T/Stat (timed stat) at the specified time.

Triglycerides

Triglycerides are the principal lipid (greasy organic substances) in the blood. The patient is in a fasting state for this study, which is important in diagnosing heart disease, hypertension, and diabetes.

Uric acid

Uric acid levels are used principally to diagnose gout.

Nuclear Chemistry Studies or Special Chemistry Studies

Many of the tests previously included in the nuclear chemistry division of the clinical laboratory or the nuclear medicine laboratory may now be performed using a non–radioisotope-based method, and may be included in the chemistry division as a special chemistry study. These tests are usually listed under the general heading of Chemistry on the computer order screen or on requisitions. The following studies are examples of tests that may be performed by these divisions (see Appendix F):

ACTH (adrenocorticotropic hormone)
Cortisol
Folate
FSH-urine (follicle-stimulating hormone)
LH (luteinizing hormone)
Schilling test
TBG (thyroxine-binding globulin)
  TSH (thyroid-simulating hormone)
  T_3 (triiodothyronine)
  T_4 (thyroxine)
  T_7 (free thyroxine index)

☑ DOCTORS' ORDERS FOR URINE CHEMISTRY STUDIES

Urine chemistry tests are listed below. Refer to the list presented earlier for the tests that require a 24-hour urine collection.

Urine glucose

Urine glucose is ordered in conjunction with the blood glucose for a glucose tolerance test. Determines the amount of glucose in the urine.

Urine creatinine

Urine creatinine is usually ordered in conjunction with the blood chemistry portion of the creatinine clearance test but may be ordered separately.

Urine protein

An elevated urine protein is found in inflammatory diseases of the urinary system and prostate gland.

Urine osmolality

Urine osmolality determines the diluting and concentrating ability of the kidneys.

Toxicology

Toxicology is the scientific study of poisons, their detection, their effects, and methods of treatment for conditions they produce. Tests for detecting drug abuse and for monitoring drug usage are also performed in toxicology. Special consents, handling, and labeling may be required.

Specimen

Specimens include blood and urine.

Communication with the Laboratory

Toxicology studies are ordered by computer or by completing a requisition form (Fig. 14–6).

☑ DOCTORS' ORDERS FOR TOXICOLOGY STUDIES

When the doctor wants to check levels of certain medications the patient is receiving, he or she orders peak-and-trough levels (Fig. 14–7). Sometimes, toxic blood levels accumulate instead of being excreted. Antibiotics such as amikacin, gentamicin, kanamycin, and tobramycin are examples of medications ordered for peak-and-trough levels. Other medication levels may include Dilantin (random), digoxin (random), and cyclosporine (trough level). For peak levels, the blood is usually collected 15 minutes after IV infusion and 30 to 60 minutes after IM injection. Trough levels usually require that blood be drawn 15 minutes before the next dose of the medication is given to the patient. For peak-and-trough orders, the health unit coordinator needs to work closely with the laboratory and nursing staff to assure proper scheduling of collections. When ordering peak-and-trough levels the health unit coordinator would order them T/Stat (timed stat), meaning that the blood should be drawn stat at the specified time.

▪ Gentamicin peak and trough around third dose

The health unit coordinator would need to check with the nurse to coordinate the times to order the gentamicin peak and trough and would order them T/Stat.

Doctor Ordering _____ ☐ Stat
Today's Date _____ ☐ T/Stat
Draw @ Date _____ Time _____ ☐ Routine
Drawn by _____
Requested by _____

Chemistry		**Toxicology**
☐ Acetone	☐ Cortisol	☐ Acetaminophen
☐ Acid phos.	☐ Electrolytes	☐ Peak
☐ ACE level	☐ Sodium	☐ Trough
☐ ACTH	☐ Potassium	☐ Aminophylline
☐ A/G ratio	☐ Chloride	☐ Peak
☐ Albumin	☐ Carbon Dioxide	☐ Trough
☐ Aldolase	☐ Folic Acid	☐ Digitoxin
☐ Alk Phos.	☐ Folate	☐ Peak
☐ Amylase	☐ FSH	☐ Trough
☐ ALT (SGPT)	☐ Glucose	☐ Digoxin
☐ Amino acid screen	☐ Glucose, _____ Hr PP	☐ Peak
☐ Bilirubin, total	☐ Glucose Tolerance _____ Hr	☐ Trough
☐ Direct	☐ Iron	☐ Drug Screen
☐ Indirect	☐ Lactic Acid	☐ Gentamycin
☐ BMP	☐ LDH Isoenzymes	☐ Peak
☐ BNP	☐ LH	☐ Trough
☐ BUN	☐ Lipase	☐ Kanamycin
☐ Calcium	☐ Magnesium	☐ Peak
☐ Cardiac Enzymes	☐ Osmolality	☐ Trough
☐ CK (CPK)	☐ Phosphorus	☐ Lidocaine
☐ LDH	☐ Protein	☐ Peak
☐ AST (SGOT)	☐ Protein Electrophoresis	☐ Trough
☐ Cltrate	☐ TBG	☐ Phenobarbital
☐ CKMB	☐ Triglycerides	☐ Peak
☐ CKMB Panel	☐ Troponin	☐ Trough
☐ Cholesterol	☐ TSH	☐ Vancomycin
☐ CMP	☐ T_3	☐ Peak
☐ C-reactive Protein	☐ T_4	☐ Trough
☐ Creatinine	☐ Uric Acid	
	☐ VMA	

Write in Orders: _____

Revised 2/4/03

FIGURE 14-6 ▲ Computer ordering screen for chemistry and toxicology.

STUDENT ACTIVITIES

For practice transcribing the following types of orders, please complete the following activities in the *Skills Practice Manual:*

- To practice transcribing blood chemistry orders, complete Activity 14–3.
- To practice transcribing stat laboratory orders, complete Activity 14–4.
- To practice transcribing fasting and NPO laboratory orders, complete Activity 14–5.
- To practice transcribing a review set of laboratory orders, including a toxicology order for peak and trough, complete Activity 14–6.

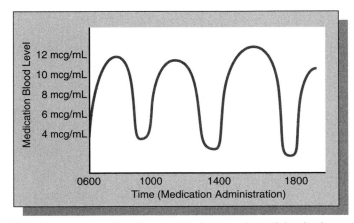

FIGURE 14-7 ▲ Graphic example of peak-and-trough levels of a medication.

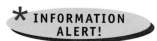

✳ **INFORMATION ALERT!**

Peak and trough, or random blood levels, are commonly drawn to check or monitor these medications:

amikacin
cyclosporine
digoxin
Dilantin
gentamicin
kanamycin
tobramycin
vancomycin

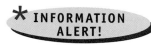

✳ **INFORMATION ALERT!**

Laboratory Divisions

- Hematology: Study of *physical properties* of blood, including blood cell studies and coagulation
- Chemistry: Study of *chemicals* of the blood and other body fluids
- Toxicology: Study of poisons, their detection, their effects and methods of treatment for conditions they produce.
- Monitoring of drug use and detection of drug abuse
- Microbiology: Study of the *organisms* that cause disease; includes bacteriology, mycology, virology, and parasitology
- Serology: Study of *immunologic* substances
- Pathology: Study of the nature and *cause of disease*, which involves changes in structure and function
- Histology: Study of the microscopic structure of tissue
- Cytology: Study of *cells* obtained from body tissues and fluid
- Blood Bank: *Blood typing* and crossmatching, storing blood and blood components for *transfusion*
- Urinalysis: Study of *urine*

Microbiology

The terms *microbiology* and *bacteriology* are sometimes used interchangeably. However, large laboratories may use the broader term microbiology as a division name within the hospital, with areas in that division designated for bacteriology, parasitology, mycology, and virology, to name a few.

Microbiology is the study of microorganisms that cause disease. Specimens are cultured, grown in a reproducing medium, identified using biochemical tests, and then tested for antibiotic sensitivity.

Parasites, organisms that live off other living organisms, are dealt with in parasitology. Fecal specimens are studied here for ova and parasites.

In mycology, cultures are set up to isolate and identify fungi. Because the plants must grow to produce spores, these cultures may take several weeks.

Virology is the study of viruses that cause disease. Identification of the exact virus or bacterium that is the causative organism of a specific disease is important, because isolation procedures are based on the methods by which organisms are spread.

Specimen

Almost any type of specimen may be studied in the microbiology division, including blood, urine, sputum, eye/ear drainage, and wound drainage.

Fasting

Fasting is not required for tests performed in the microbiology division of the laboratory.

Communication with the Laboratory

Microbiology tests are requisitioned by using the computer or by completing a requisition form (Fig. 14–8). The requisition form for the test remains on the unit until the specimen is obtained.

☑ DOCTORS' ORDERS FOR MICROBIOLOGY STUDIES

Frequently ordered tests performed in the microbiology division, with an interpretation relating to the health unit coordinator's role, are listed below. For assistance with abbreviations, check the abbreviations list at the beginning of the chapter.

Bacteriology

Culture and sensitivity: Can be ordered on blood, urine, stool, sputum, wound drainage, and nose and throat specimens. The specimen is placed on an appropriate medium for growth. If organisms grow, they are tested for antibiotic sensitivity, which determines those antibiotics that should be effective for treatment. The nursing staff is responsible for the collection of the specimen.

AFB culture (acid-fast bacilli): Performed to determine the presence of acid-fast bacilli such as *Mycobacterium tuberculosis,* which causes tuberculosis. The nursing staff is responsible for the collection of the specimen (usually sputum). A special stain may also be performed.

Urine for CC (colony count): Done to determine the number of bacteria present in a urine specimen.

Gram stain: Performed to classify bacteria into gram-negative or gram-positive groupings, thus allowing for differential diagnosis of the causative agent. Treatment can begin immediately, while awaiting the results of cultures.

Blood culture: Blood culture specimens may be collected as multiple specimens (different times or different sites) to ensure accurate isolation and identification of the causative organism.

Parasitology

Stool for O&P (ova and parasites): An order that is usually ordered times three, which requires three different stool specimens (three requisition forms must be prepared) to determine the presence of ova (eggs) or parasites in the stool. The nursing staff is responsible for the collection of the stool specimens.

Mycology

Mycology culture: A mycology culture is performed to determine the presence of fungi. It may be performed on blood or spinal fluid specimens. The results may take several weeks to determine. Studies may be performed to determine the presence of fungi such as *Histoplasma, Coccidioides,* and *Candida.*

Doctor Ordering _____   □ Stat
Today's Date _____   □ Routine
Collection Date _____ Time _____
Collected by _____
Requested by _____

Microbiology		**Fluids**	
Specimen Source	Test Requested	Specimen Source	Test Requested
□ Abscess	□ AFB Culture	□ Abdominal	□ Cell Count
	□ AFB Stain	□ Amniotic	[macron-c] Diff
_____	□ C & S	□ CSF	□ Glucose
□ Blood	□ C & S	□ Pericardial	□ LDH
□ Body Cavity	Anaerobic	□ Peritoneal	□ Occult Blood
_____	□ Fungal Culture	□ Pleural	□ Protein
□ CSF	□ GC Screen	□ Synovial	□ Sp Gravity
□ Ear Drainage	□ Strep Screen	□ Other	□ VDRL (CSF)
□ Right	□ Viral Culture		□ Other
□ Left	□ Other	# of Tubes _____	

Specimen Source (Microbiology)	Test Requested	**Cytology**	
□ Eye Drainage	_____	Specimen Source	Test Requested
□ Right		□ Amniotic	□ Pap
□ Left	□ Stool	□ Breast Bx	□ Fungal
□ Nasal Smear	□ Fat	□ Bronchial Asp	□ Buccal
□ Sputum	□ Fiber	□ Cervical Smear	□ Maturation
□ Stool	□ Occult Blood	□ Cervical Bx	Index
□ Throat	□ Ova & Parasites	□ Colon Bx	□ Other _____
□ Tissue	□ #1 of 3	□ CSF	
_____	□ #2 of 3	□ Gastric Fluid	
□ Urine	□ #3 of 3	□ Lung Asp	
□ Voided		□ Pleural	
□ Clean Catch		□ Pericardial	
□ St Cath		□ Peritoneal	
□ Foley Cath		□ Sputum	
□ Wound Drainage _____		□ Vaginal	
□ Other _____		□ Other _____	

Revised 3/11/03

FIGURE 14-8 ▲ Computer ordering screen for microbiology, fluids, and cytology.

Virology

Virus culture and virus serology: Virus cultures may be done on any specimen, and virus serology is done on a blood specimen to determine the presence of viruses or antibodies to viruses.

CMV (cytomegalovirus) cultures: Performed to detect cytomegalovirus infection, which is widespread and common. For culture specimens, a urine, sputum, or mouth swab is the specimen of choice. Fresh specimens are essential. The results may take about 3 to 7 days to complete.

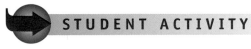

STUDENT ACTIVITY

To practice transcribing microbiology/bacteriology orders, complete Activity 14-7 in the *Skills Practice Manual*.

Serology

Serology is the study of antibodies and antigens useful in detecting the presence and intensity of a current infection. It may also be useful in identifying a previous infection or exposure to an organism. Autoimmune diseases may be studied, as well as pretransplant and posttransplant evaluations and treatment. Tests for syphilis, rheumatoid arthritis, HIV, some influenzae, and tissue typing are a few of the studies done in this area.

Immunology

The response of the body to a foreign substance may include mobilization of leukocytes (white blood cells) against the foreign substance as well as the production of certain proteins that neutralize the substance. These proteins are immunoglobulins (or more commonly antibodies) and circulate in the blood.

There are five main types of immunoglobulins: IgG, IgM, IgA, IgD, and IgE.

An important characteristic of antibodies is that much of the time they are produced specifically against a particular foreign substance, and are ordered in reference to that substance. Any substance that elicits an immune response is called an antigen. The measurement of the antibody level may be ordered as a titer. Many serologic tests are done to detect antibody levels, because the antibodies are usually in the serum portion of the blood. Serologic tests can also detect the presence of antigens.

Specimen

The majority of these tests are done on the serum portion of a blood specimen. However, other body fluids such as spinal fluid may be tested, as well as biopsy specimens and secretions from wounds.

Fasting

Fasting is not required for tests performed in the serology division of the laboratory.

Communication with the Laboratory

Serology studies are ordered by computer or by completing laboratory requisition form (see Fig. 14–4).

☑ DOCTORS' ORDERS FOR SEROLOGY

ANA (antinuclear antibody)
An ANA test determines the presence of certain autoimmune diseases such as SLE (systemic lupus erythematosus).

ASO titer (antistreptolysin O titer)
An elevated ASO titer usually indicates the presence of a streptococcal infection, such as acute rheumatic fever.

CEA (carcinoembryonic antigen)
An elevated level of CEA indicates liver, colon, or pancreatic cancer. It is also used to assess the treatment of these conditions.

CMV IgG (immunoglobulin G) and IgM (immunoglobulin M) antibodies
CMV IgG and IgM determines the levels of different types of antibodies (immunoglobulins) against cytomegalovirus. The presence of these antibodies may indicate exposure to or possible infection with cytomegalovirus.

Complement fixation titers
Complement fixation titers are done to detect various viral, fungal, and parasitic diseases.

EBV panel (Epstein-Barr virus)
An EBV panel determines various levels of antibodies (IgG and IgM) produced and directed against specific parts of the Epstein-Barr virus, such as viral capsid antigen (VCA) and Epstein-Barr virus nuclear antigen (EBNA). This can determine whether the patient has had a recent or previous EBV infection.

ELISA (enzyme-linked immunosorbent assay)
ELISA tests serum or plasma for antibodies and is widely used in the diagnosis of HIV and chlamydia.

FTA (fluorescent treponemal antibody)
FTA is a serology test for syphilis.

HB$_s$Ag (hepatitis B surface antigen)
HB$_s$Ag is a serum study to determine the presence of hepatitis B in the blood.

HIV-1 (human immunodeficiency virus) antibody test
HIV-1 antibody test uses oral mucosal transudate (OMT), a serum-derived fluid that enters saliva from the gingival crevice and across oral mucosal surfaces. The test is performed to diagnose HIV. A signed consent by the patient is required prior to HIV testing.

Heterophil agglutination test
An heterophil agglutination test is a diagnostic study for infectious mononucleosis.

RA (rheumatoid arthritis) factor
An RA factor is a specific test for rheumatoid arthritis.

VDRL (Venereal Disease Research Laboratory) or RPR (rapid plasma reagin) test
VDRL or RPR tests are performed on blood and are screening tests for syphilis.

Refer to Appendix F for other tests performed in the microbiology and serology divisions.

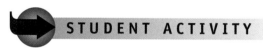

To practice transcribing serology orders, complete Activity 14–8 in the *Skills Practice Manual*.

Blood Bank

The blood bank, which is usually a part of the clinical laboratory, has the responsibilities of typing and crossmatching patient blood, obtaining blood for transfusions, storing blood and blood components, and keeping records of transfusions and blood donors.

Prior to the administration of whole blood, packed cells, and some other blood components, the patient must have a type and crossmatch done. This is a test that determines the patient's blood type and compatibility. *The four major blood groups are A, B, AB, and O.*

- Patients with type A blood may receive transfusions of types A and O.
- Patients with type B may receive types B and O.
- Patients with type AB may receive types A, B, AB, and O.
- Patients with type O may receive only type O blood transfusions.

This laboratory division also performs several other blood studies, including the Coombs' tests. The DAT (direct antiglobulin

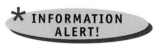

INFORMATION ALERT!

An order for transfusion of whole blood, packed red blood cells, and some other blood components automatically indicates that blood will be typed and crossmatched.

Doctor Ordering _____   ☐ Stat
Today's Date _____   ☐ Routine
Collection Date _____ Time _____
Collected by _____
Requested by _____

Blood Bank

☐ Routine   ☐ ASAP   ☐ Stat   ☐ For Hold

Date of Surgery _____   Date of Transfusion _____

Autologous Blood? yes ____ no ____   ☐ Whole Blood   # of Units ____
Donor Specific?   yes ____ no ____   ☐ Packed Cells   # of Units ____
☐ Type and X-match   ☐ Washed Cells   # of Units ____
☐ Type and Screen   ☐ Frozen Cells   # of Units ____
                                               ☐ Fresh Frozen Plasma   # of Units ____
☐ Coombs Test   ☐ Platelet Concentrate   # of Units ____
☐ Other _____   ☐ Cryoprecipitate   # of Units ____
                                               ☐ Other _____

Comments _____
_____
_____

Revised 3/11/03

FIGURE 14–9 ▲ Computer ordering screen for blood bank.

test) is a synonym for the Coombs' test. In a direct Coombs' test, a positive result is found in hemolytic disease of the newborn, hemolytic transfusion reactions, and acquired hemolytic anemia. The indirect Coombs' test detects the presence of antibodies to red blood cell antigens. This test is valuable in detecting the presence of anti-Rh antibodies in the serum of a pregnant woman before delivery.

Because the transfusion of blood and blood components is a treatment administered by nursing personnel, additional information on various types of blood transfusions (autologous, donor directed, and autotransfusion) is discussed in Chapter 11.

Specimen

A specimen of blood is used for type and crossmatch.

Fasting

Fasting is not required for this procedure.

Communication with the Laboratory

Blood bank orders are requisitioned by using the computer or by completing a requisition form (Fig. 14–9). The number of units to be given and the name of the blood components are items included on this requisition. A blood transfusion consent must be signed prior to administering blood or blood products. The patient may also sign a refusal of blood transfusion form.

☑ DOCTORS' ORDERS FOR BLOOD BANK

Listed below are examples of doctors' orders for blood component administration. Refer to Chapter 11 for examples of blood, blood components, and plasma substitutes.

- *T&C for 2 U packed cells*
- *Packed cells, 1 U (need type and crossmatching)*
- *Plasma, 3 U stat*
- *Give washed cells 1 U (need type and crossmatching)*
- *Cryoprecipitate 1 U*
- *Give 2 U of platelets (no crossmatching needed, but donor plasma and recipient RBCs should be ABO compatible)*
- *Normal serum albumin 5% (no crossmatching)*
- *T&C 6 U pc—hold for surgery in AM*

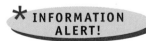
★ INFORMATION ALERT!

A blood transfusion consent must be signed prior to administering blood or blood products. The patient may also sign a refusal of blood transfusion form.

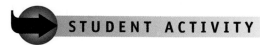

To practice transcribing blood bank orders, complete Activity 14–9 in the *Skills Practice Manual*.

Urinalysis

The urinalysis division of the laboratory studies urine specimens for color, clarity, pH (degree of acidity or alkalinity), specific gravity (degree of concentration), protein (albumin), glucose (sugar), blood, bilirubin, and urobilinogen. The sediment is viewed microscopically for organisms, intact cells, and crystals.

Specimen

Urine is the specimen used for this test; however, the doctor may indicate that the nursing staff should follow a special procedure to obtain the specimen.

Procedures for Obtaining Urine Specimens

- Voided urine specimen: The patient voids into a clean container.
- Clean catch, or midstream, urine specimen: The nursing staff uses a special cleansing technique to obtain this type of specimen.
- Catheterized urine specimen: This specimen is sterile and is obtained by catheterizing the patient. This procedure is usually done for culture and sensitivity testing, which is performed by microbiology.

Urine specimens that are collected at an unspecified time are called random specimens. However, the preferred collection time for a urine specimen is in the early morning upon rising.

Fasting

Fasting is not required for a urinalysis.

Communication with the Laboratory

Orders for urinalysis are entered into the computer or a requisition form (see Fig. 14–4) is used. Once again the requisition is held on the nursing unit until the specimen is collected or the order is entered when the specimen is obtained. The labeled specimen with the requisition or computer printout is sent to the laboratory.

☑ DOCTORS' ORDERS FOR URINALYSIS

Below are listed examples of doctors' orders for urinalysis.

- *Cath UA*
- *Clean catch UA*
- *Dipstick urine for ketones*
- *UA today*
- *Urine reflex (urine is tested in laboratory; if certain parameters are met, the specimen will be sent to microbiology to be cultured)*

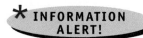

Points to Remember When Ordering Laboratory Studies:

- Determine whether the test ordered is a point-of-care test (POCT), or needs to be sent to the laboratory.
- All tests ordered require a specimen.
- Each specimen sent to the lab from the nursing unit requires a requisition and must be accurately labeled with patient ID label, with date, time, and initials of person who collected the specimen written on the label.
- Include date and time of collection on the requisition, as well as the name of the person collecting specimens.
- Order tests as efficiently as possible to avoid the necessity for the patient to be redrawn (e.g., routines with stats).
- Communicate stat laboratory tests immediately to the lab and/or nursing personnel, and include all pertinent information.

A urine specimen is sent to the laboratory. All regular urinalysis studies are performed, except the specimen is not examined microscopically.

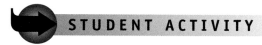

To practice transcribing urinalysis/urine chemistry orders, complete Activity 14–10 in the *Skills Practice Manual*.

The Following tests may be sent to several of the laboratory departments for testing.

Studies Performed on Pleural Fluid

Studies are performed on pleural fluid to determine the cause and nature of pleural effusion, including hypertension, CHF, cirrhosis, infections, and neoplasms.

Specimen

Pleural fluid is obtained when the doctor performs a thoracentesis. The patient must sign a consent form for this procedure.

Fasting

Fasting is not required for tests performed on pleural fluid.

Communication with the Laboratory

The doctor orders the tests to be done on the specimen and the health unit coordinator enters the orders into the computer or completes a requisition (see Fig. 14–8). As with any nonretrievable specimen obtained by invasive procedures it should be transported to the laboratory immediately, and should not be sent through a pneumatic tube system.

☑ DOCTORS' ORDERS FOR PLEURAL FLUID

Below are listed examples of doctors' orders performed on pleural fluid.

- *Thoracentesis, pleural fluid to lab for LDH, glucose, and amylase. CI: Cancer*
- *Pleural fluid for cell count, diff*
- *Pleural fluid for C&S*

Studies Performed on Cerebrospinal Fluid

Studies are performed on cerebrospinal fluid to determine various brain diseases or injuries.

Specimen

Cerebrospinal fluid (CSF) is obtained when the doctor performs a lumbar puncture. The patient must sign a consent form for this procedure.

Fasting

Fasting is not required for tests performed on CSF.

Communication with the Laboratory

The doctor orders the tests to be done on each specimen, of which there may be three or four. The health unit coordinator enters the respective tests into the computer or completes a requisition. The doctor will indicate in his or her orders the tube to be used for each test (usually three or four tubes). The health unit coordinator will enter this information into the computer or write it on the requisition. It is sometimes the health unit coordinator's responsibility to transport these specimens to the laboratory. It is important to transport CSF specimens to the laboratory immediately. Because they are difficult to obtain and would cause the patient further pain, never send the specimens via pneumatic tube.

☑ DOCTORS' ORDERS FOR CEREBROSPINAL FLUID

Below are listed examples of doctors' orders performed on cerebrospinal fluid (CSF).

- *Lumbar puncture, fluid to lab for cell count and diff*
- *CSF for serology*
- *CSF to lab for tube 1—cell count, protein, and glucose; tube 2—AFB and fungal culture; tube 3—Gram stain*

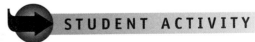
STUDENT ACTIVITY

To practice transcribing cerebrospinal fluid orders, complete Activity 14–11 in the *Skills Practice Manual*.

Pathology

Pathology is the study of the nature and cause of disease, which involve body changes. Histology and cytology are subdivisions of the pathology department. A pathologist is in charge of the pathology department.

Histology is the study of the microscopic structure of tissue. Cytology is the study of cells obtained from body tissues and fluid to determine cell type and to detect cancer or a precancerous condition.

Specimen

Organs, tissue, cells, and body fluids obtained from biopsies, centesis, sternal puncture, lumbar puncture, surgery, and autopsies are studied in the pathology department. A Pap smear is a staining method developed by Dr. George Nicolas Papanicolaou that can be performed on various types of specimens to determine the presence of cancer. However, cells from the cervix are the specimens most frequently studied (cervical smear). During a pelvic examination the doctor may remove tissue or cells from the cervix for study.

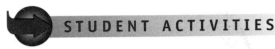
STUDENT ACTIVITIES

For practice transcribing the following types of orders, complete the following activities in the *Skills Practice Manual:*
- To practice transcribing a review set of laboratory orders, complete Activity 14–12.
- To practice transcribing a review set of doctors' orders, complete Activity 14–13.
- To practice recording telephoned doctors' orders, complete Activity 14–14.
- To practice recording telephoned messages, complete Activity 14–15.

■ RECORDING LABORATORY RESULTS

The results of laboratory tests are a valuable tool to the doctor in the diagnosis and treatment of patients; therefore, the test result values are often communicated to the doctor before the computer report can be placed on the patient's chart. Stat and/or abnormal laboratory test results are communicated verbally or by telephone to the doctor by the health unit coordinator or nurse. Also, the doctor may request on the doctor's order sheet that the laboratory test results be communicated to him or her by telephone immediately upon their completion.

To verbally communicate laboratory results, the laboratory personnel telephones the health unit coordinator on the nursing unit, who records the results on a telephone laboratory report sheet (Fig. 14–10). Laboratory results may also be sent to the unit via the computer printer. Also, results from an outside laboratory may be faxed to the nursing unit. The printed results also include the reference range, or range of normal values for each lab test (Fig. 14–11). The health unit coordinator should report the values to the patient's nurse who may request the results to be called to the doctor's office. Although the task may appear simple to perform, it is a very responsible task, because the doctor may prescribe treatment according to the laboratory values. Consider for a moment what the consequences could be should the value be recorded inaccurately. To avoid errors, always read the laboratory values you have recorded back to the person in the laboratory.

TELEPHONED LABORATORY RESULTS

Patient's Name _____ Report called by _____

Room Number _____ Report taken by _____

Date _____ Time _____

HEMATOLOGY

RBC _____
Hgb _____
Hct _____
WBC _____
   lymphs _____
   monos _____
   neutros _____
   eos _____
   basos _____
PLATELETS _____
RETICS _____
SED RATE _____
OTHER

CHEMISTRY

GLUCOSE
   Random _____
   FBS _____
E'LYTES
   Na _____
   K _____
   Cl _____
   CO_2 _____
CARDIAC ENZYMES
   SGOT _____
   LDH _____
   CPK _____
CALCIUM _____
PHOS _____
BUN _____
CREATININE _____
OTHER

URINE

COLOR _____
APPEARANCE _____
PH _____
SP. GRAVITY _____
ACETONE _____
GLUCOSE _____
BACTERIA _____
WBC _____
RBC _____
CASTS _____
OCCULT BLOOD _____
OTHER

COAGULATION

BLEEDING TIME _____
COAGULATION TIME _____
PROTIME _____
   Patient _____
   Control _____
   % _____
PT
   Patient _____
   Control _____
   INR _____
PTT _____

TELEPHONED BLOOD GAS REPORT

Patient's Name _____
Room Number _____
Date _____ Time _____
Report called by _____
Report taken by _____

O_2 CONCENTRATION _____
O_2 TENSION _____
CO_2 TENSION _____
PH _____
ACT BICARB _____
BASE EXCESS _____
O_2 SAT _____

FIGURE 14–10 ▲ Telephoned laboratory tests result form.

Always have the person you are communicating to in the doctor's office repeat his or her recorded values back to you. The written report should be placed on the patient's chart in a timely manner. Accuracy in the selection of the correct patient's chart as well as the appropriate location in the chart is very important.

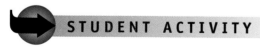

STUDENT ACTIVITY

To practice recording telephoned laboratory results, complete Activity 14–16 in the *Skills Practice Manual*.

■ SUMMARY

Laboratory studies are very useful diagnostic tools, and therefore they are frequently ordered. Accuracy in ordering is of utmost importance, because an error could result in the wrong test being performed or the wrong patient being tested. It is im-

perative that all specimens are properly labeled according to hospital policy and with the correct patient information. Prompt delivery of properly labeled specimens to the laboratory is also important.

One of your challenges as a health unit coordinator is to become familiar with the particular hospital's process of requisitioning laboratory orders. You should be able, after time, to process orders quickly and efficiently. Familiarize yourself with the various laboratory screens on the computer. Whether using the computer or a requisition, it is important to know from which laboratory department a particular test is requisitioned.

As diagnostic procedures from other departments are added to your medical knowledge, you may find that they may conflict with some laboratory tests, or vice versa. Coordinating laboratory studies with x-ray, nuclear medicine, or GI studies (to name a few) is one of the tasks you learn as you proceed with this program.

Most hospital units have a written laboratory procedure manual. If not, call the hospital laboratory help desk to get your questions answered.

```
                        COLLEGE HOSPITAL                      PAGE 1
                A. MELZER MD & D. RUDOLPH MD PATHOLOGISTS


                        *** RESULT INQUIRY ***
PATIENT NAME: WADSWORTH, JENNIFER          PATIENT #: 437592

LOC: 4W     AGE: 20    SEX: F     ADM PHY: PAYNE, IMA     ADM DATE: 10/9/04
---------------------------------------------------------------------------
CHEMISTRY PANEL           RESULT            UNITS      REFERENCE VALUES
---------------          -----------        -------    --------------------
SODIUM                 L   134              MMOL/L     (135-145     )
POTASSIUM              H   5.4              MMOL/L     (3.6-5.0     )
CHLORIDE                   96               MMOL/L     (96-110      )
CO2                        29               MMOL/L     (21-31       )
GLUCOSE                    103              MG/DL      (70-110      )
BUN                    H   33               MG/DL      (6-20        )
CREATININE                 1.2              MG/DL      (0.5-1.2     )
CALCIUM                    10.4             MG/DL      (8.5-10.5    )
URIC ACID                  4.8              MG/DL      (3.9-7.8     )
CHOLESTEROL                166              MG/DL      (140-200     )
T. BILIRUBIN               1.0              MG/DL      (0.0-1.2     )
T. PROTEIN                 6.9              GM/DL      (6.1-8.0     )
ALBUMIN                L   2.4              GM/DL      (3.5-4.8     )
ALK PHOS               H   132              U/L        (30-107      )
GGTP                   H   195              U/L        (8-69        )
ALT (SGPT)                 29               U/L        (0-55        )
LDH                    H   398              U/L        (94-172      )
AST (SGOT)                 29               U/L        (8-42        )
CPK                    L   27               U/L        (38-224      )
TRIGLYCERIDES              154              MG/DL      (30-64       )
PHOSPHORUS                 3.1              MG/DL      (2.4-4.3     )


COMPLETE BLOOD COUNT
--------------------
WHITE BLOOD CELL COUNT H   14.9             X10^3      (4.8-10.8    )
RED BLOOD CELL COUNT   L   4.29             X10^6      (4.7-6.10    )
HEMOGLOBIN             L   12.6             GM/DL      (14.0-18.0   )
HEMATOCRIT            L   37.3             %          (42.0-52.0   )
MCV                        87.0             U3         (80-94       )
MCH                        29.4             PG         (27-32       )
MCHC                       33.8             %          (33-37       )
RDW                    H   17.6             %          (11.5-14.5   )
POLYSEGMENTED NEUTROPHIL H 82               %          (50-70       )
BAND                       6                %          (0-10        )
LYMPHOCYTE             L   4                %          (20-40       )
MONOCYTE                   1                %          (0-10 ·      )
METAMYELOCYTE          H   6                %          (0           )
ATYPICAL LYMPHOCYTE    H   1                %          (0           )
PLATELET ESTIMATE          ADEQ
RBC MORPHOLOGY             SLT ANISO
                           SLT POLYC
PLATELET COUNT             220              X1000      (130-400     )
```

FIGURE 14-11 ▲ Computerized laboratory result sheet.

REVIEW QUESTIONS

1. List two general purposes of laboratory studies.

   a. _____

   b. _____

2. State the purpose of the following divisions of the laboratory:

   a. microbiology: _____

   b. chemistry: _____

   c. hematology: _____

3. Name three methods used by the nursing staff to collect urine specimens.

   a. _____

   b. _____

   c. _____

4. List five common types of specimens collected for laboratory study.

   a. _____

   b. _____

   c. _____

   d. _____

   e. _____

5. What is the procedure for ordering stat blood tests from the laboratory?

   _____

6. What are the health unit coordinator's responsibilities for an order for a 2 h PP BS?

   _____

7. What is the difference between a stat order and a routine laboratory order?

   _____

8. List five procedures that require consent forms and are performed by the doctor to obtain specimens for study.

   a. _____

   b. _____

c. _____

d. _____

e. _____

9. What procedure must be performed before some blood components, such as packed red cells, can be ordered for a patient for a transfusion?

_____

10. What is the health unit coordinator's responsibility concerning specimens collected on the unit to be sent to or delivered to the laboratory?

_____

11. What four laboratory studies make up the test called electrolytes?

a. _____

b. _____

c. _____

d. _____

12. Write the abbreviations for the three cardiac enzyme studies.

a. _____

b. _____

c. _____

13. Name six chemistry studies.

a. _____

b. _____

c. _____

d. _____

e. _____

f. _____

14. Name six hematology studies.

a. _____

b. _____

c. _____

d. _____

e. _____

f. _____

15. Name six microbiology studies.

a. _____

b. _____

c. _____

d. _____

e. _____

f. _____

16. Explain the difference between fasting and NPO.

_____

17. Define the following terms:

a. biopsy: _____

b. clean catch: _____

c. fasting: _____

d. lumbar puncture: _____

e. midstream: _____

f. occult blood: _____

g. postprandial: _____

h. sputum: _____

i. sternal puncture: _____

j. urinalysis: _____

k. voided specimen: _____

l. dipstick urine: _____

18. In the space provided, write in the laboratory division that performs each of the following tests:

a. FBS: _____

b. urine for C&S: _____

c. lytes: _____

d. CBC: _____

e. BMP: _____

f. APTT: _____

g. 1 unit of PC: _____

h. Hct & Hgb: _____

i. VDRL: _____

j. triglycerides: _____

k. RA factor: _____

l. sputum for AFB: _____

m. RBC indices: _____

n. T_3: _____

o. GTT: _____

p. Retics: _____

q. WBC & diff: _____

r. 2 h PP BS: _____

s. PT: _____

t. protein electrophoresis: _____

u. T&C: _____

v. Coombs' test: _____

w. Na: _____

x. stool for O&P: _____

y. BNP: _____

z. CMP: _____

19. List three drugs that may have a peak-and-trough ordered to monitor levels:

a. _____

b. _____

c. _____

20. How may errors be avoided in recording of telephoned laboratory results?

_____

21. Rewrite the following doctors' orders using symbols and abbreviations. Or to practice writing doctors' orders, have some-one read the orders to you while you record them. Again, practice using symbols and abbreviations.

a. complete blood count and electrolytes every morning:

_____

b. hemoglobin and hematocrit immediately:

_____

c. type and crossmatch for six units of packed (red blood) cells—hold for surgery in the morning:

_____

d. sputum specimen for culture and sensitivity and acid-fast bacillus:

_____

e. lumbar puncture for cerebrospinal fluid: on tube number one, do protein and glucose levels; on tube number two, do cultures for cytomegalovirus and fungus; on tube number three, do an acid-fast bacillus stain:

_____

f. comprehensive metabolic panel tomorrow morning:

_____

TOPICS FOR DISCUSSION

1. Discuss possible consequences of labeling a laboratory specimen with the wrong patient's label.

2. Discuss the importance of washing your hands after handling laboratory specimens (even bagged specimens).

3. Discuss the importance of reading all of the doctors' orders before ordering laboratory tests.

Diagnostic Imaging Orders

7. List six studies performed by the nuclear medicine department.
8. List seven special instructions about the patient that the health unit coordinator is to include when ordering tests from the diagnostic imaging department.

Vocabulary

Clinical Indications ▲ Notations recorded when ordering diagnostic imaging to indicate the reason for doing the procedure

Computed Tomography ▲ A radiographic process of creating computerized images (scans) of body organs in horizontal slices (referred to as a CT scan)

Contrast Media ▲ Substances (solids, liquids, or gases) used in diagnostic imaging procedures that permit the radiologist to distinguish between the different body densities; they may be injected, swallowed, or introduced by rectum

C-Arm ▲ A mobile fluoroscopy unit used in surgery or at the bedside

Fluoroscopy ▲ The observation of deep body structures made visible by use of a viewing screen instead of film; a contrast medium is required for this procedure

Magnetic Resonance Imaging ▲ A technique used to produce computer images (scans) of the interior of the body using magnetic fields

Nuclear Medicine ▲ A technique that uses radioactive materials to determine function capacity of a organ

"On Call" Medication ▲ Medications prescribed by the doctor to be given prior to the diagnostic imaging procedure; the department notifies the nursing unit of the time the medication is to be administered to the patient

Portable X-ray ▲ An x-ray taken by a mobile x-ray machine, which is moved to the patient's bedside

Position ▲ An alignment of the body on the x-ray table favorable for taking the best view of the part of the body being imaged

Chapter Objectives

Upon completion of this chapter, you will be able to:

1. Define the terms in the vocabulary list.
2. Write the meaning of each abbreviation in the abbreviations list.
3. Name five patient positions that may be included in an x-ray order.
4. Identify x-ray orders that require no preparation and x-ray orders that require preparation.
5. Name five x-ray orders that require a signed patient consent form.
6. List, in order, the four x-rays that should be performed in sequence.

Routine Preparation ▲ The standard preparation suggested by the radiologist to prepare the patient for a diagnostic imaging study

Scan ▲ An image produced by using a moving detector or a sweeping beam (scans are produced by computed tomography, magnetic resonance imaging, and ultrasonography)

Ultrasonography ▲ A technique that uses high-frequency sound waves to create an image (scan) of body organs (may also be referred to as sonography or echography)

Abbreviations

Abbreviation	Meaning	Example of Usage on a Doctor's Order Sheet
AP	anteroposterior	AP view of abd
BE	barium enema	BE tomorrow
CI	clinical indications	BE-CI: R/O tumor
CT	computed tomography	CT scan of abd
CXR	chest x-ray	CXR today
DSA	digital subtraction angiography	Cerebral DSA
F/U	follow-up	F/U KUB in AM
Fx	fracture	x-ray lt femur CI: Fx
GB series	gallbladder series	GB series tomorrow
GI	gastrointestinal	GI study tomorrow
h/o	history of	UGI CI: h/o ulcers
IVP	intravenous pyelogram	IVP c̄ Rt prep
IVU	intravenous urogram; synonymous with IVP	
KUB	kidneys, ureters, and bladder	KUB today
lat	lateral	PA & lat chest
LLQ	left lower quadrant	
LUQ	left upper quadrant	Abd x-ray special attention to LUQ & LLQ
L&S	liver and spleen	L&S scan tomorrow (nuclear medicine)
LS	lumbosacral	X-ray LS spine (x-ray)
MRI	magnetic resonance imaging	MRI of brain
PA	posteroanterior	PA chest x-ray
PCXR	portable chest x-ray	PCXR stat
PET	positron emission tomography	PET tomorrow AM (nuclear medicine)
PTC or PTHC	percutaneous transhepatic cholangiography	PTC or PTHC tomorrow
R/O	rule out	UGI to R/O ulcers

Abbreviation	Meaning	Example of Usage on a Doctor's Order Sheet
RLQ	right lower quadrant	X-ray of abd Compare c̄ x-ray of 12/2/00 Check RUQ and RLQ
RUQ	right upper quadrant	
SBFT	small bowel follow-through	UGI c̄ SBFT
UGI	upper gastrointestinal	UGI p̄ IVU
US	ultrasound	US of GB

EXERCISE 1

Write the abbreviation for each term listed below.

1. intravenous pyelogram _____

2. right lower quadrant _____

3. kidneys, ureters, and bladder _____

4. barium enema _____

5. posteroanterior _____

6. upper gastrointestinal _____

7. lateral _____

8. lumbosacral _____

9. left upper quadrant _____

10. anteroposterior _____

11. gastrointestinal _____

12. right upper quadrant _____

13. computed tomography _____

14. left lower quadrant _____

15. gallbladder _____

16. magnetic resonance imaging _____

17. small bowel follow-through _____

18. chest x-ray _____

19. digital subtraction angiography _____

20. portable chest x-ray _____

21. percutaneous transhepatic cholangiography _____

22. fracture _____

23. history of _____

24. follow-up _____

25. clinical indications _____

26. intravenous urogram _____

27. ultrasound _____

28. rule out _____

29. positron emission tomography _____

30. liver and spleen _____

EXERCISE 2

The following is a list of orders for imaging procedures that may appear on patients' charts. Write the meaning of each underlined abbreviation.

1. <u>BE</u> tomorrow p̄ sigmoidoscopy

_____

2. Stat <u>LS</u> spine x-ray

_____

3. <u>KUB</u> this AM

_____

4. <u>US</u> for fetal age

_____

5. Abdominal x-ray c̄ attention to <u>RLQ</u> & <u>LUQ</u>

_____

6. <u>IVU</u> & <u>UGI</u> tomorrow. Check with radiologist for prep

_____

7. <u>CT</u> scan of brain

_____

8. <u>GI study</u> c̄ barium swallow

_____

9. <u>PA</u> & <u>lat</u> chest now

_____

10. <u>MRI</u> of brain

_____

11. <u>PCXR</u>

_____

12. <u>UGI</u> c̄ <u>SBFT</u>

_____

COMMUNICATION WITH THE DIAGNOSTIC IMAGING DEPARTMENT

Orders for the diagnostic imaging department, which includes radiography, nuclear medicine, ultrasound, computed tomography, and magnetic resonance imaging, are communicated by the ordering step of transcription by using a computer or requisition form (Fig. 15–1). Because the patient usually is transported to the diagnostic imaging department for the procedure, it is important to indicate the mode of transportation—wheelchair or gurney (stretcher). The patient may be transported by the nursing staff, diagnostic imaging department staff, or transport service.

A *portable* or *mobile x-ray* is an exception to the standard transportation procedure. A request for a portable x-ray necessitates the radiographer taking the portable equipment to the patient's room. A portable x-ray is ordered when movement might be detrimental to the patient's condition.

When ordering the diagnostic procedure, indicate the following information about the patient:

■ Clinical indication (reason the doctor is ordering the procedure)
■ Is receiving intravenous fluids
■ Has a seizure disorder
■ Is receiving oxygen
■ Needs isolation precautions
■ Does not speak English
■ Is a diabetic
■ Is sight or hearing impaired

This information will assist personnel in the diagnostic imaging department to provide better care for the patient (see Fig. 15–1). Often doctors will write the name of the radiologist to read the image and/or special instructions in their orders. The health unit coordinator should include this information on the requisition.

Doctor Ordering _____

Date to be done _____ ☐ Stat ☐ Routine ☐ ASAP

Today's Date _____ Requested by _____

┌───┐
│ **Diagnostic Imaging - X-Ray Procedures** │
└───┘

Clinical Indication _____

Transportation ☐ portable ☐ stretcher ☐ wheelchair ☐ ambulatory

O_2 ☐ yes ☐ no   Diabetic ☐ yes ☐ no   Hearing deficit ☐ yes ☐ no

IV ☐ yes ☐ no   Seizure disorder ☐ yes ☐ no   Sight deficit ☐ yes ☐ no

Isolation ☐ yes ☐ no   Non-English speaking ☐ yes ☐ no

Comments: _____

☐ Abdomen _____

☐ Bone x-ray order: _____

☐ Chest order: _____

☐ KUB order: _____

☐ Mammogram _____

☐ Sinus series order: _____

☐ SNAT series _____

☐ Spine order: _____

☐ BE _____

☐ GB _____

☐ IVU _____

☐ SBFT _____

☐ UGI _____

☐ Write-in order _____

FIGURE 15–1 ▲ Diagnostic imaging computer ordering screen for x-ray procedures.

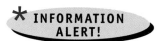

✱ INFORMATION ALERT!

Clinical indications (the reason the doctor is ordering the procedure) must be recorded by the health unit coordinator when ordering a diagnostic imaging procedure. Insurance companies require this information before they will provide reimbursement to the health care facilities. Diagnostic imaging departments will not perform procedures until they have the clinical indications recorded.

■ BACKGROUND INFORMATION FOR RADIOLOGY

In 1895, Wilhelm Roentgen discovered a strange phenomenon that produced a photograph of the bones of his wife's hand. The exact mechanism for the production of the rays was unknown to Roentgen; therefore, he used the algebraic symbol for the unknown, x, to title his discovery.

The x-ray studies performed in the radiology area of the diagnostic imaging department are carried out by a *radiographer,* a person with special education in the area of radiography. The x-ray images are developed in the department and are interpreted by a *radiologist,* a doctor who has specialized in this field. Some studies are done by observing the path of contrast media in the body by means of fluoroscopy.

It should be noted that doctors' orders for radiology do not always have the term *x-ray* in them. An order for "Chest, PA and lat" is an order for a chest x-ray taken from posterior to anterior and laterally. Some studies are also called CT scans and others are identified by the suffix *–gram,* as in *carotid arteriogram.*

The new trend in diagnostic imaging is a computerized radiology or digital system, which will be filmless. In filmless radiology there will be no x-ray films, only images, stored in computer systems and viewed on a monitor.

As you learn more about diagnostic procedures, you will find that some tests scheduled in the radiology area must be carried out in specific sequences so that the contrast medium necessary for one test does not block the image of another.

■ PATIENT POSITIONING

The doctor may wish x-rays to be taken while the patient is placed in a specific position on the x-ray table to allow the best view of the area to be exposed. The health unit coordinator must be careful to include all of the x-ray order without making any changes, and to be absolutely accurate when transcribing such orders. For example, the health unit coordinator should be sure not to write AP (anteroposterior) when the order calls for PA (posteroanterior) positioning. The wrong abbreviation can cause the radiographer to film a different view, which may obscure an abnormality.

Following is a list of the positions used most frequently in writing x-ray orders.

- *AP position:* This view may be taken while the patient is either standing or lying on his or her back (supine); the machine is placed in front of the patient.
- *PA position:* This view may be taken while the patient is either standing or lying on his stomach (prone) with the x-ray machine aimed at the patient's back.
- *Lateral position:* This view is taken from the side.
- *Oblique position:* This picture is taken with the patient lying halfway on his or her side in either the AP or PA position.
- *Decubitus position:* In this view, the patient is lying on his or her side with the x-ray beam positioned horizontally.

■ INFORMED CONSENT FORMS

Diagnostic imaging procedures that are invasive, those requiring the injection of contrast medium, require the patient to sign a consent form after being informed of risks, alternatives, outcomes, etc. It is the responsibility of the health unit coordinator to prepare the consent form for the patient's signature. Diagnostic imaging procedures that require a consent form may vary among health care facilities. Keep a list of procedures requiring a consent form handy to assist you in recalling which tests require informed consents until you have this information committed to memory.

■ RADIOGRAPHIC (X-RAY) PROCEDURES

X-Rays that Do Not Require Preparation

X-rays can penetrate solid material, such as bone, which in turn produces a shadow that is recorded on film. Procedures that require the filming of bone structures or that are ordered to determine the position of other organs in relation to these structures can be performed by qualified radiology personnel without any preparation for the procedure (Fig. 15–2).

Listed below are x-ray studies as they are commonly written on a doctors' order sheet.

✔ *DOCTORS' ORDERS FOR X-RAYS THAT DO NOT REQUIRE PREPARATION*

Sinus series CI: sinusitis
X-ray of the paranasal sinus structures.
   Purpose: Used to determine infection, trauma, or disease in the paranasal sinuses.

PA and lat chest CI: pneumonia
Chest x-ray (frequently *x-ray* is not written on the order because some terms in the order are recognized as directions used only

Communication and Implementation of Diagnostic Imaging

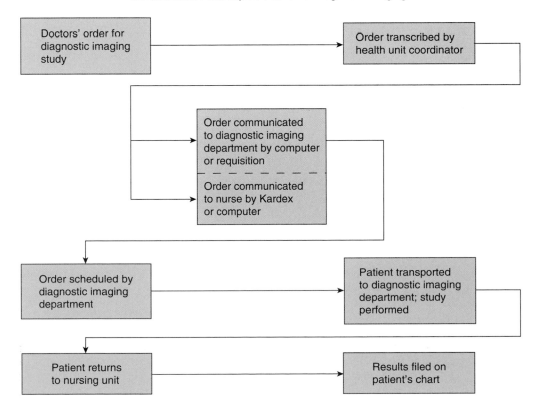

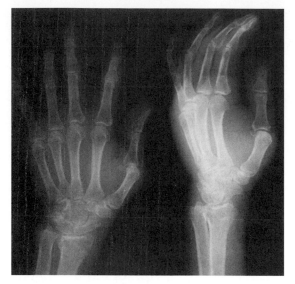

A

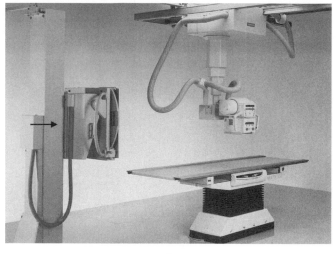

A

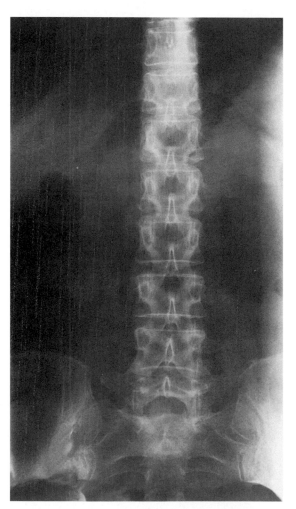

B

FIGURE 15–2 ▲ Images of x-rays that do not require preparation. *A*, PA and oblique of the left hand. *B*, AP of the lumbosacral area. (From Dowd SB, Wilson BG: Encyclopedia of Radiographic Positioning, Vols. I and II, Philadelphia: WB Saunders, 1995, with permission.)

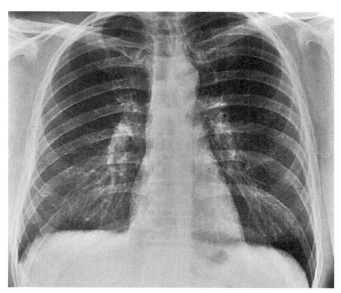

B

FIGURE 15–3 ▲ *A*, Radiographic table with chest unit. *B*, PA x-ray image of normal chest. (From Merrill's *Atlas*, 9th ed., St. Louis, Mosby, 1999.)

in radiography. The terms PA and lat indicate the angles at which the doctor wishes the film to be taken) (Fig. 15–3).

Purpose: Used to diagnose or assess patients with pneumonia, pneumothorax, atelectasis, or check for infiltrates. Also used to determine the size and position of the heart or for the placement of invasive lines or tubes.

LS spine CI: R/O fracture
X-ray of the lumbosacral area of the spine.

Purpose: Used to determine abnormalities of the lumbosacral region.

Mammogram CI: lump 10° lt br
X-ray of the breast.

Purpose: Used to detect cancer or cysts located in the soft tissue of the breast.

X-ray of the tibia with close attention to the distal portion CI: R/O fracture

X-ray of the bone in the patient's lower leg. *Distal* indicates that the radiologist is to observe a particular portion of the bone. Remember to include the entire order on the requisition.

Purpose: Used to determine fractures.

KUB CI: general survey of the abd

X-ray of the abdomen.

Purpose: Used to rule out abnormal calcification.

Portable film of rt femur CI: Fx

A radiographer takes a portable x-ray machine to the patient's bedside to film the right upper leg of the patient. It is important for the health unit coordinator to write *portable* on the requisition form.

Purpose: Used to determine fractures.

Tomogram of lt lung, upper lobe CI: Eval chest lesion

X-ray picture that studies selected levels of the body, in this case levels of the left lung.

Purpose: Used only for further evaluation of a chest lesion.

Postreduction study of the lt forearm

X-ray of the left forearm.

Purpose: Used to evaluate the alignment of a fracture after intervention.

AP and lat rt hip

X-ray of the right hip (*AP* and *lat* indicate the angles at which the doctor wishes the film to be taken).

Purpose: Used to evaluate prosthetic replacement of the hip. Done at the bedside.

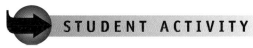

STUDENT ACTIVITY

To practice transcribing radiology (x-ray) orders that require no preparation, complete Activity 15–1 in the *Skills Practice Manual.*

X-Rays that Require Preparation and Contrast Media

When an x-ray is made, images of varying density appear on the exposed image. The differences in density are due to the degree of absorption offered by different tissues and air to the radiation. It is easy to differentiate bony structures, because the bones offer resistance and therefore appear light on the image. The lungs, however, which contain air, do not offer much resistance to radiation and appear black on image.

Certain organs and blood vessels within the body are difficult for the radiologist to see because there is little difference in density between them and their surroundings parts. To increase the contrast, it is necessary for a *contrast medium* to be given to the patient.

The most common types of contrast media are organic iodine compounds and barium preparations. Organic iodine compounds may be injected or taken into the body by mouth, rectum, or other approaches.

Contraindications to the use of iodine compounds include allergy to shellfish or previous reactions to iodinated studies.

For the contrast medium to prove most effective, the patient is prepared for the test before it is scheduled. This process is known as a *routine preparation* and the routine is most often established by the diagnostic imaging department.

The attending doctor may change the routine preparation if the patient's condition does not permit it. Specific preparation orders must be written on the doctors' order sheet by the patient's doctor.

Sometimes a contrast medium used for one test may interfere with results obtained in another scheduled test. Therefore, if multiple x-ray tests are ordered, proper sequencing is necessary to obtain clear results. Sequencing is outlined by the diagnostic imaging department and may vary among hospitals.

Sequencing

The following are typical guidelines for scheduling x-ray studies.

1. X-ray studies of the lower spine and pelvis should be ordered first, before a barium enema or an upper gastrointestinal study is done. The presence of barium in specific parts of the body may obscure the portion of the body that is being studied.
2. Abdominal studies using ultrasound or CT should precede studies using barium.
3. Liver and bone scans and nuclear medicine studies may also conflict with barium studies and should be done first.
4. Four x-ray studies that require contrast media are frequently ordered at the same time for diagnostic reasons. Only one or sometimes two can be done on the same day; thus, the studies may have to be scheduled three or more days in advance. The order of scheduling is listed below.
   a. Intravenous urogram (IVU)
   b. Gallbladder (GB) series
   c. Barium enema (BE)
   d. Upper gastrointestinal (UGI) or UGI and small bowel follow-through (SBFT)

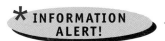

INFORMATION ALERT!

When transcribing diagnostic imaging orders, the health unit coordinator should:

1. Record the clinical indication when entering the order.
2. Record the necessary mode of transportation when entering the order.
3. Record necessary patient information when entering the order.
4. Check if a consent form is necessary; if so, prepare one for signature.
5. Check if patient preparation is required; if so, carry out the communication.
6. Check if scheduling is required; if so, schedule the procedure for the proper day and/or time.

Accuracy in performing these steps is vital to reach the expected outcome.

Preparation Procedure

To visualize internal organs by using contrast media, preparation is usually required. Most of the preparation is done by the nursing staff and may begin the day before the x-ray study is scheduled.

Following are examples of doctors' orders for x-rays that require the patient to have some type of preparation. Each procedure and preparation is explained to help establish its relationship to the others and the role of a health unit coordinator.

Many hospitals have a computer system that will automatically print out the routine preparation when the procedure is entered. Some hospitals have preparation cards—cards listing the tasks to be done to prepare the patient for the x-ray (Fig. 15–4). When a patient is scheduled for one of the x-rays requiring preparation, the computer printout or the preparation card is usually placed in the patient's Kardex form holder to remind the nursing staff of the tasks they need to perform.

Note: It is possible for the preparation procedures to vary among hospitals.

Preparation for IVU

Bowel cathartic

Limit fluids 600 cc PO for 18 hrs

Low residue evening meal

NPO 8–12 hours

No smoking or chewing gum

FIGURE 15–4 ▲ X-ray preparation card.

☑ DOCTORS' ORDERS FOR X-RAYS THAT REQUIRE PREPARATION AND CONTRAST MEDIA

IVU CI: ureterolithiasis (synonymous with IVP; IVU is becoming the more common usage)

A procedure performed to outline the kidney, particularly the renal pelvis, ureters, and urinary bladder (Fig. 15–5). The contrast medium is established by injecting an iodinated contrast medium into the patient's vein. The injection takes place after the patient is transported to the diagnostic imaging department.

Purpose: Used to determine the size and location of the kidneys, ureters, and bladder and to determine the presence of abnormalities such as tumors or strictures.

Patient preparation:
- bowel cathartic
- low-residue evening meal
  - NPO 8 to 12 hours prior to procedure
  - Limit fluids to 600 cc PO for 18 hours

Transcribing the order: In addition to transcribing this order, the health unit coordinator would order the diet changes and alert the nurse to administer bowel cathartics.

GB series (gallbladder series)

X-ray of the gallbladder to determine the ability of the gallbladder to function properly (Fig. 15–6).

Purpose: Used to identify obstruction, such as stones.

Patient preparation:
- Give oral contrast medium PM *before test*
- Light, fat-free PM *meal*
- NPO 8 to 12 hours prior to procedure

Transcribing the order: In addition to transcribing this order, the health unit coordinator initiates diet changes and alerts the

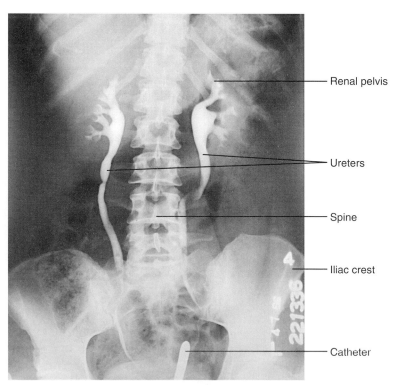

FIGURE 15–5 ▲ Intravenous urogram (IVU) showing renal pelvis and contrast-filled ureters. (From Merrill's Atlas, 9th ed., Vol. II, St. Louis: Mosby, 1999, p. 189.)

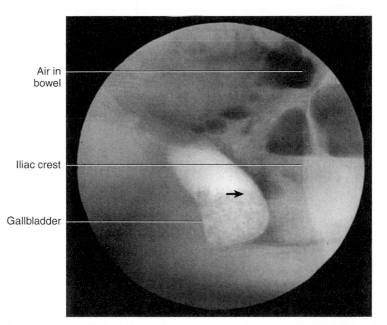

FIGURE 15–6 ▲ X-ray image of AP gallbladder (GB series) showing layering of multiple stones *(arrow)*. (From Merrill's Atlas, 9th ed., Vol. II, St. Louis: Mosby, 1999, p. 70.)

nurse to administer the oral contrast medium, usually after the evening meal.

Note: The gallbladder series is being replaced by ultrasound studies of the gallbladder; however, because the GB series is more cost effective, it continues to be required by some reimbursement programs.

PTC CI: obstruction of the bile ducts

Visualization of the bile ducts by injecting iodine contrast directly into the biliary system.

Purpose: Usually done to determine the cause of jaundice or persistent upper abdominal pain after cholecystectomy.

Patient preparation: Special prep orders may or may not be ordered.

Transcribing the order: Routine transcription

BE CI: lesion of the colon

Visualization of the large intestine (Fig. 15–7). The patient is given an enema using a barium contrast medium in the diagnostic imaging department.

Purpose: Used to identify diseases of the large intestine such as diverticula, cancer, or ulcerative colitis.

Patient preparation:

Day before procedure:

- *2:00 PM—x-prep*
- *7:00 PM—Dulcolax tabs*
- *NPO 2400 hrs*

Day of procedure:

- *NPO*
- *Cleansing enemas*

Transcribing the order: In addition to transcribing the order for a barium enema, the health unit coordinator would initiate diet changes and alert the nurse concerning any medications to be given as preparation. The doctor may wish to order an air contrast barium enema, which requires the same preparation as a barium enema but uses air as well as barium for the contrast medium.

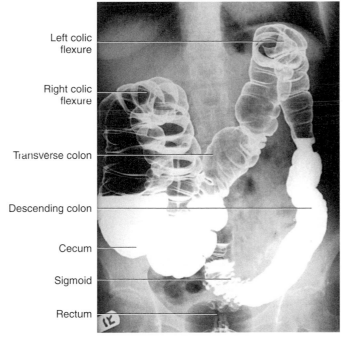

FIGURE 15–7 ▲ X-ray image of barium enema (BE) showing the large intestine. (From Merrill's Atlas, 9th ed., Vol. II, St. Louis: Mosby, 1999, p. 153.)

UGI c SBFT CI: peptic ulcer

Utilizes fluoroscopy, viewing screen, and x-ray machine to examine the upper portion of the esophagus, stomach, and small intestines (Fig. 15–8).

Purpose: Used to detect hiatal hernia, strictures, ulcers, or tumors.

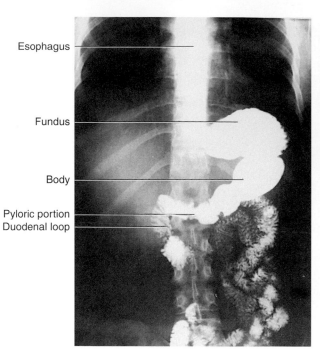
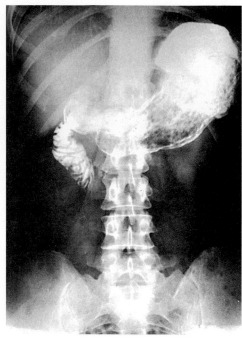

Esophagus

Fundus

Body

Pyloric portion
Duodenal loop

FIGURE 15–8 ▲ Upper gastrointestinal (UGI) showing AP stomach and duodenum. (From Merrill's Atlas, 9th ed., Vol. II, St. Louis: Mosby, 1999, p. 117.)

Patient preparation:
- *NPO 8 to 12 hours prior to procedure*
- *No smoking or gum chewing*

Transcribing the order: The health unit coordinator transcribes the order and initiates the diet change.

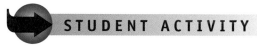

STUDENT ACTIVITY

To practice transcribing radiology (x-ray) orders that require preparation, complete Activity 15–2 in the *Skills Practice Manual.*

■ SPECIAL X-RAY PROCEDURES

Special x-ray procedures are performed under the direction of the radiologist or a surgeon with a radiologist present. A request for the use of a special x-ray room or operating room must be submitted by the doctor in advance, or the procedure may be scheduled by computer as part of the transcription procedure (Fig. 15–9). Before the procedure is done, the patient is requested to sign a patient consent form (see Chapter 8 for use and preparation of a consent form.).

Special x-ray procedures may be performed with or without a general anesthetic. When a general anesthetic is used, the nursing staff follows a preoperative routine (see Chapter 19). Preparations for these studies vary with each hospital.

The radiologist and/or surgeon may prescribe pre-procedure medications to be given at a specific time or "on call." When medications are ordered *on call*, the doctor or department personnel,

at the request of the radiologist and/or surgeon, notify the nursing unit to administer the medication.

☑ DOCTORS' ORDERS FOR SPECIAL X-RAY PROCEDURES

Cerebral angiogram CI: aneurysm
Visualization of vascular structures within the body after injection of a contrast medium (Fig. 15–10). The specific name given to the study is determined by the vascular structure to be studied (e.g., renal angiogram or cerebral angiogram).

Purpose: Used to diagnose vascular aneurysms, malformations, and occluded or leaking blood vessels.

Abdominal arteriogram CI: angiodysplasia
X-ray of an artery after injection of a contrast medium. An arteriogram may be identified according to the anatomic location (e.g., femoral arteriogram).

Purpose: Used to detect obstruction or narrowing of an artery or aneurysm.

Arthrogram of the left knee CI: torn ligament
X-ray of a joint after injection of contrast medium.

Purpose: Used to determine trauma, such as bone chips or torn ligament, from an injury.

Cholangiogram, postoperative (T-tube cholangiogram) CI: retained stones
X-ray taken 6 to 9 days after a cholecystectomy to examine the bile ducts. Examination is done after injection of a contrast medium through T-tube.

Doctor Ordering _____

Date to be done _____ ☐ Stat ☐ Routine ☐ ASAP

Today's Date _____ Requested by _____

| Diagnostic Imaging—Special Procedures |

Clinical Indication _____

Transportation ☐ portable ☐ stretcher ☐ wheelchair ☐ ambulatory

O₂ ☐ yes ☐ no   Diabetic ☐ yes ☐ no   Hearing deficit ☐ yes ☐ no

IV ☐ yes ☐ no   Seizure disorder ☐ yes ☐ no   Sight deficit ☐ yes ☐ no

Isolation ☐ yes ☐ no   Non-English speaking ☐ yes ☐ no

Comments: _____

☐ Abdominal arteriogram_____

☐ Arthrogram_____

☐ Cerebral angiogram_____

☐ Cervical myelogram_____

☐ Hysterosalpingogram_____

☐ Lymphangiogram_____

☐ Spinal myelogram_____

☐ Venogram_____

☐ Voiding cystourethrogram_____

☐ Write-in order_____

FIGURE 15–9 ▲ Computer ordering screen for special x-ray procedures.

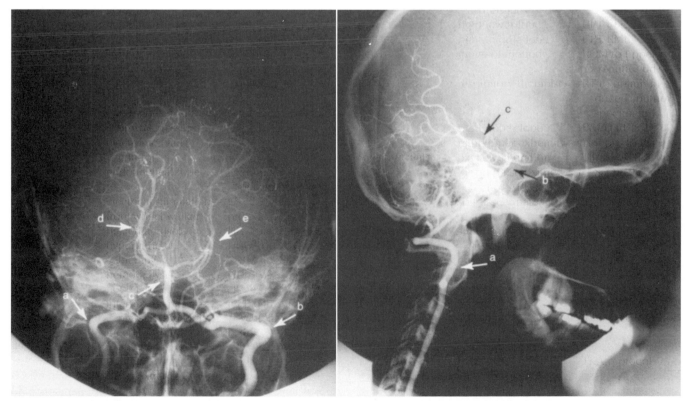

FIGURE 15–10 ▲ Cerebral angiograms. (From Dowd SB, Wilson BG: Encyclopedia of Radiographic Positioning, Vols. I and II, Philadelphia: W. B. Saunders, 1995, with permission.)

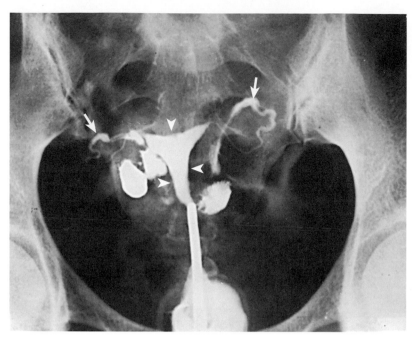

FIGURE 15–11 ▲ Hysterosalpingogram reveals bilateral hysterosalpinx of uterine tubes *(arrows)*. (From Merrill's Atlas, 9th ed., Vol. II, St. Louis: Mosby, p. 117.)

Purpose: Used to rule out residual stones in the biliary tract following a cholecystectomy. It is called *T-tube cholangiogram* because the catheter placed in the biliary ducts during surgery is called a *T-tube.*

Hysterosalpingogram CI: obstruction of fallopian tubes
X-ray of the uterus and fallopian tubes made after injection of a contrast medium (Fig. 15–11).

Purpose: Used in fertility studies and also to confirm abnormalities such as adhesions, fistulas, and so forth.

Lymphangiogram left leg CI: lymphatic obstruction
X-ray of the lymph channels and lymph nodes made after injection of a contrast medium.

Purpose: Used to identify metastatic cancer in the lymph nodes and to evaluate the effectiveness of chemotherapy.

Spinal myelogram CI: cord compression due to HNP
X-ray of the spinal cord after a contrast medium has been injected between lumbar vertebrae into the spinal canal.

Purpose: Used to detect herniated disks, tumors, and spinal nerve root injuries.

Venogram of left leg CI: DVT
X-ray of a vein, usually lower extremities, made after injection of a contrast medium.

Purpose: Used to evaluate veins before and after bypass surgery and to investigate venous function when obstruction is suspected.

Voiding cystourethrogram CI: bladder dysfunction
X-ray films are taken to demonstrate the bladder filling then emptying as the patient voids.

Purpose: Used to demonstrate bladder dysfunction and urethral strictures.

Note: Endoscopies including ERCP are covered in Chapter 16.

 STUDENT ACTIVITY

To practice transcribing orders for special radiology (x-ray) procedures, complete Activity 15–3 in the *Skills Practice Manual.*

■ COMPUTED TOMOGRAPHY

Computed tomography (CT) provides a computerized image that reproduces a section of a body part as if sliced from front to back horizontally (Figs. 15–12, *A* and *B*). Contrast medium is used for most of the studies. When a CT is ordered, the order must indicate whether or not a contrast medium will be used (Fig. 15–13).

DOCTORS' ORDERS FOR CT SCANS

CT scan of the head c̄ DSA CI: aneurysm
Combines angiography, fluoroscopy, and computer technology to visualize the cardiovascular system without the interference of the bone and soft tissue structure to obscure the image.

Purpose: Used to evaluate postoperatively (e.g., endarterectomies) and to detect any cerebrovascular abnormalities.

CT scan of the brain CI: tumor
Computerized analysis of multiple images of brain tissue.

Purpose: Used to diagnose brain tumors, infarction, bleeding, and hematomas.

Patient preparation: The patient is usually NPO for several hours before the test.

FIGURE 15-12 ▲ *A,* Computed tomography scanner. *B,* CT scan of the chest with IV contrast medium. (From Merrill's Atlas, 9th ed., St. Louis: Mosby.)

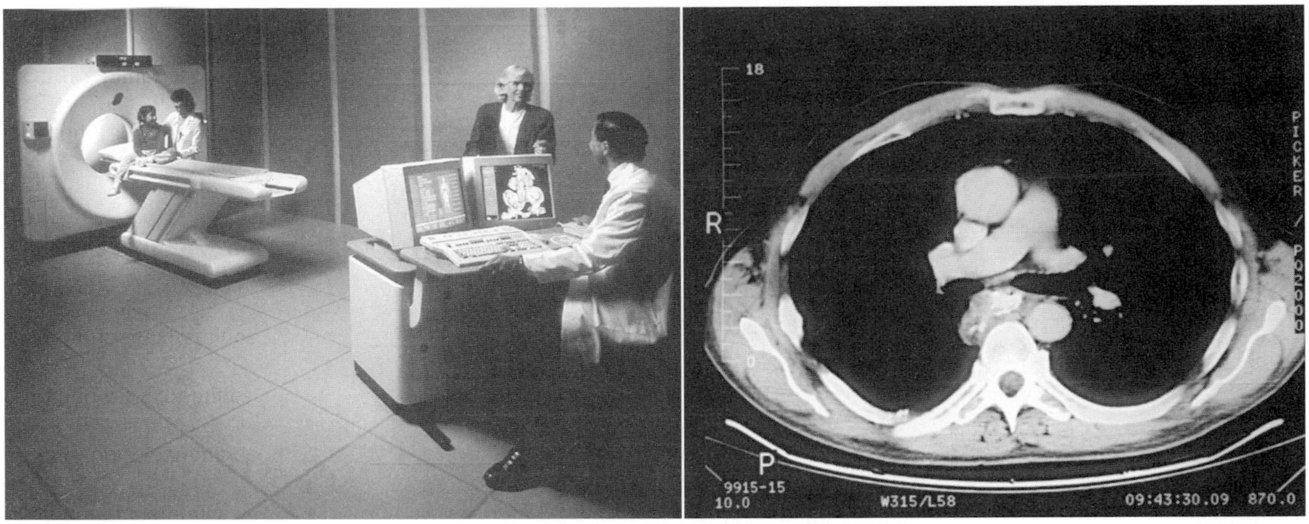

Doctor Ordering _____
Date to be done _____ ☐ Stat ☐ Routine ☐ ASAP
Today's Date _____ Requested by _____

| Diagnostic Imaging—Computed Tomography |

Clinical Indication _____
☐ with contrast   ☐ without contrast

Transportation ☐ portable ☐ stretcher ☐ wheelchair ☐ ambulatory

O_2 ☐ yes ☐ no   Diabetic ☐ yes ☐ no   Hearing deficit   ☐ yes ☐ no
IV ☐ yes ☐ no   Seizure disorder ☐ yes ☐ no   Sight deficit   ☐ yes ☐ no
Isolation ☐ yes ☐ no   Non-English speaking ☐ yes ☐ no

Comments: _____

☐ CT scan of head _____
☐ CT scan of brain _____
☐ CT scan of abdomen _____
☐ CT scan of pelvis _____
☐ CT scan of spine _____
☐ CT of neck _____
☐ CT-guided liver biopsy _____
☐ Write-in order _____

FIGURE 15-13 ▲ Computer ordering screen for computed tomography.

CT scan of abdomen and pelvis CI: retroperitoneal lesion

CT images are obtained from passing x-rays through the abdominal organs from many angles.

Purpose: Used to diagnose tumors, abscesses, and bowel obstruction and to guide needles for biopsy.

Patient preparation: Patient is usually NPO for 4 hours. These studies should be performed before barium studies.

CT of LS spine CI: spinal stenosis

Scan of the lumbosacral area of the spine.

Purpose: Often ordered after myelogram. Used to confirm spinal stenosis, changes in the disk and vertebrae, and to confirm spinal infection.

CT of the neck CI: tumor

Scan of the neck.

Purpose: Used to identify soft tissue masses and/or to evaluate the larynx.

CT of the sinus CI: sinus infection

Scan of the nasal sinus.

Purpose: Used to diagnose infectious processes.

CT-guided liver biopsies

Used to identify the location of tissue to be biopsied so needle placement is precise.

Purpose: Used to obtain tissue of the liver for diagnostic purposes. CT-guided lung and breast biopsies are also performed.

■ ULTRASONOGRAPHY

Ultrasonography uses high-frequency sound waves to create an image of body organs (Figs. 15–14 and 15–15).

☑ DOCTORS' ORDERS FOR ULTRASONOGRAPHY STUDIES

US of abd

Ultrasound of abdomen.

Purpose: Used to detect liver cysts, abscesses, hematomas, and tumors.

Patient preparation:
- *NPO 8 to 12 hours prior to procedure*
- *Full bladder, drink fluids—do not void*
- *No smoking AM of exam*

FIGURE 15–14 ▲ *A,* Ultrasound scanner. *B,* Anatomical drawing of the brain. *C,* Fontal image of ultrasound brain scan with a bleed *(arrow).* (From Merrill's Atlas, 9th edition, Vol. II, St. Louis: Mosby.)

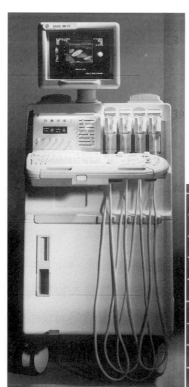

A

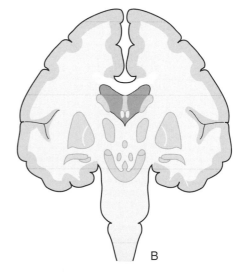

B

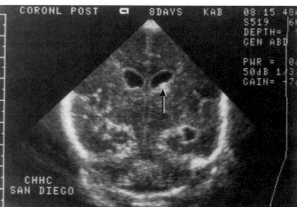

C

Doctor Ordering _____
Date to be done _____ ☐ Stat ☐ Routine ☐ ASAP
Today's Date _____ Requested by _____

| **Diagnostic Imaging—Ultrasonography** |

Clinical Indication _____
Transportation ☐ portable ☐ stretcher ☐ wheelchair ☐ ambulatory

O₂ ☐ yes ☐ no   Diabetic ☐ yes ☐ no   Hearing deficit ☐ yes ☐ no
IV ☐ yes ☐ no   Seizure disorder ☐ yes ☐ no   Sight deficit ☐ yes ☐ no
Isolation ☐ yes ☐ no   Non-English speaking ☐ yes ☐ no

Comments: _____

☐ US of abd _____
☐ US of pelvis _____
☐ US of GB _____
☐ Write-in order _____

FIGURE 15–15 ▲ Computer ordering screen for ultrasonography.

US of pelvis

Ultrasound of pelvis.

Purpose: Used during pregnancy to identify ectopic pregnancy, multiple births, and fetal abnormality. Used otherwise to identify ovarian cancer and other disorders.

Patient preparation:
- *Full bladder—drink fluids, do not void*
- *May require water enema*
- *US of GB*

Purpose: Used to diagnose cholelithiasis, cholecystitis, and to identify obstructive jaundice.

Patient preparation:
- *Fat-free evening meal*
- *Fast 8 to 10 hours*
- *No smoking AM of exam*

Note: Doppler studies are covered in Chapter 16.

■ MAGNETIC RESONANCE IMAGING

Magnetic resonance imaging (MRI) is a technique for viewing the interior of the body using a powerful magnetic field that lines up the protons in the nuclei of the body's cells. The protons spin when a radio frequency is turned on. The protons return to their normal position when the radio signal is discontinued. During proton movement, a computer records cross-sectional images of the part being studied. Bones do not obscure the image as they do in x-rays. Studies are done on selected areas of the body, such as the brain, spinal cord, and bone (Figs. 15–16, 15–17). MRI can distinguish between benign and malignant tumors.

Because of the strength of the magnet and the radiofrequency waves, MRI contraindications exist for patients with the following:

- Pacemakers
- Cerebral aneurysm clips
- Any electrically, magnetically, or mechanically activated implants
- Ferrous-based prosthetic devices
- Pregnancy

The health unit coordinator when transcribing magnetic resonance imaging orders would prepare an interview form for the nurse to complete prior to sending the patient for an MRI. The form lists any contraindications that may prevent the patient from having the procedure.

Dental bridgework may need to be removed prior to the scan but permanent fillings and inlays are acceptable because they are not made of ferrous metals. Prior to the exam, the patient is asked to remove metallic jewelry, wristwatches, eyeglasses, hairpins, or wigs if metal clips are present. Credit cards, bankcards, and similar devices with magnetically coded strips should be removed as well. This is especially important to remember in an outpatient diagnostic setting.

☑ Doctors' Orders for Magnetic Resonance Imaging

- *MRI of brain and spinal cord CI: malignancy*
- *MRI cervical spine CI: HNP*
- *MRI rt shoulder CI: rotator cuff injury*
- *MRI lt knee CI: posterior cruciate ligament tear*

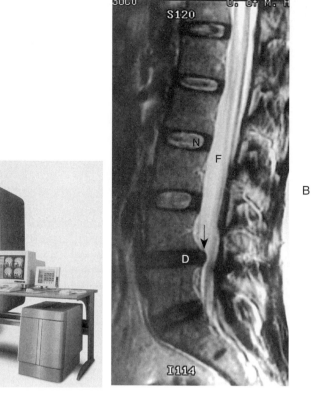

FIGURE 15–16 ▲ *A,* Magnetic resonance scanner. *B,* Sagittal MRI scan of the lumbar spine with herniated disk *(arrow).* (From Merrill's Atlas, 9th ed., Vol. II, St. Louis: Mosby.)

Doctor Ordering _____

Date to be done _____ ☐ Stat ☐ Routine ☐ ASAP

Today's Date _____ Requested by _____

Diagnostic Imaging—Magnetic Resonance Imaging

Clinical Indication _____

Transportation ☐ portable ☐ stretcher ☐ wheelchair ☐ ambulatory

O₂ ☐ yes ☐ no   Diabetic ☐ yes ☐ no   Hearing deficit ☐ yes ☐ no

IV ☐ yes ☐ no   Seizure disorder ☐ yes ☐ no   Sight deficit ☐ yes ☐ no

Isolation ☐ yes ☐ no   Non-English speaking ☐ yes ☐ no

Comments: _____

☐ MRI of brain _____

☐ MRI of spine _____

☐ MRI shoulder_____

☐ MRI knee _____

☐ Write-in order_____

FIGURE 15–17 ▲ Computer ordering screen for magnetic resonance imaging.

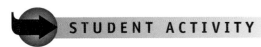

STUDENT ACTIVITY

To practice transcribing orders for computerized tomography scans, ultrasound, and magnetic resonance imaging, complete Activity 15-4 in the *Skills Practice Manual*.

■ NUCLEAR MEDICINE

Background Information

Nuclear medicine utilizes radioactive materials called *radiopharmaceuticals* to determine the functioning capacity of organs. Radioactive scanning materials are used to assist in diagnosing disease because of their ability to give off radiation in the form of gamma rays, which can be traced.

Depending upon the study to be made, the patient may take the radiopharmaceutical by mouth or it may be injected within a vein. A gamma scintillation camera is the instrument used to form an image of the concentration of the radioactive material in a specific organ of the body, thus producing a picture called a *scan*. It is possible to perform organ scans on the following body parts: bone, brain, thyroid, spleen, liver, heart, lungs, kidneys, gallbladder, and pancreas (Fig. 15–18).

Some diseases may be treated with therapeutic doses of radiopharmaceuticals. Cancer of the thyroid and a blood condition called *polycythemia vera* respond to this treatment.

Radioactivity used in nuclear medicine differs from x-rays in that gamma radiation is from an outside source that passes the radiation through the body. In nuclear medicine, the radioactive material is taken internally by mouth or intravenously and emits gamma radiation from the specific organ being studied.

To communicate the doctors' order to the nuclear medicine department, the health unit coordinator must order on the computer or complete a nuclear medicine requisition (Fig. 15–19).

Preparation may be required prior to the test. Check with your health care facility about preparation before scheduling the test.

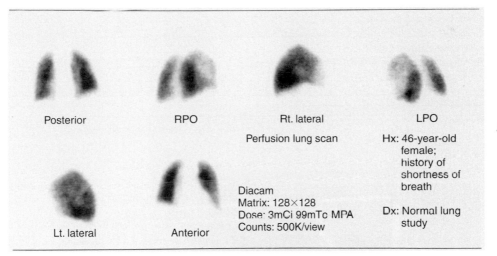

Posterior | RPO | Rt. lateral | LPO

Perfusion lung scan

Lt. lateral | Anterior

Diacam
Matrix: 128×128
Dose: 3mCi 99mTc MPA
Counts: 500K/view

A

Hx: 46-year-old female; history of shortness of breath

Dx: Normal lung study

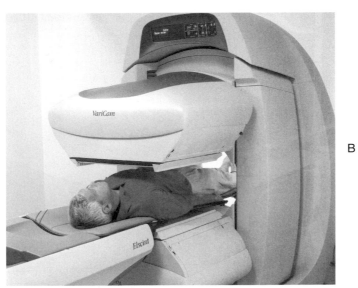

B

FIGURE 15–18 ▲ *A,* Normal perfusion lung scan. *B,* Nuclear medicine scanner. (From Merrill's Atlas, 9th ed., Vol. II, St. Louis: Mosby.)

```
┌─────────────────────────────────────────────────────────┐
│  Doctor Ordering _____              │
│  Date to be done _____ □ Stat □ Routine □ ASAP       │
│  Today's Date _____ Requested by_____          │
│                                                            │
│  ┌──────────────────────────────────────────┐            │
│  │ Diagnostic Imaging—Nuclear Medicine       │            │
│  └──────────────────────────────────────────┘            │
│                                                            │
│  Clinical Indication _____          │
│  Transportation □ portable □ stretcher □ wheelchair □ ambulatory │
│                                                            │
│  O₂ □ yes □ no      Diabetic □ yes □ no       Hearing deficit □ yes □ no │
│  IV □ yes □ no      Seizure disorder □ yes □ no  Sight deficit □ yes □ no │
│  Isolation □ yes □ no  Non-English speaking □ yes □ no     │
│                                                            │
│  Comments: _____                 │
│  □ Bone scan (total)_____                │
│  □ Bone scan (regional)_____                │
│  □ Liver and spleen_____                │
│  □ Gallium scan_____                │
│  □ Thyroid uptake and scan_____                │
│  □ DISIDA_____                │
│  □ PET_____                 │
│  □ MUGA_____                 │
│  □ Thallium stress scan_____                │
│  □ Adenosine/thallium scan_____                │
│  □ Sestamibi stress_____                │
│  □ Write-in order_____                │
└─────────────────────────────────────────────────────────┘
```

FIGURE 15-19 ▲ Computer ordering screen for nuclear medicine.

☑ DOCTORS' ORDERS FOR NUCLEAR MEDICINE STUDIES

Bone scan—total body CI: cancer, prostate-mets
Purpose: Performed to determine the presence of tumors, arthritis, or osteoporosis.

Bone scan—regional CI: cervical Fx
Purpose: Performed to study a particular area of the body, such as vertebral compression fractures or unexplained bone pain.

L&S (liver and spleen) scan CI: cirrhosis
Purpose: Performed to evaluate injury to the spleen, chronic hepatitis, and metastatic processes. It should be done before barium studies. Other body scans may be performed on the brain, heart, lungs, kidneys, gallbladder, and pancreas.

Gallium scan—total body CI: abscess (also may be ordered regionally)
Purpose: Performed to locate the primary site of cancer, as well as to detect an abscess. May be used to examine the brain, liver, and breast tissue if disease is suspected.

Thyroid uptake and scan CI: check for cold nodules
Purpose: Performed to study thyroid gland performance. It demonstrates the ability of the thyroid gland to "take up" radioactive iodine.

Lung perfusion/ventilation study CI: embolism
Purpose: A diagnostic study for pulmonary embolism.

DISIDA scan (formerly PIPIDA scan, also called hepatobiliary scan)
A scan of the biliary tract (gallbladder).
Purpose: Used to identify blockage or abnormal function.

PET (positron emission tomography) scan
Purpose: Used to obtain information about blood flow to the myocardium, metabolism, glucose utilization, and schizophrenia. Isotopes are used.
    Patient preparation: Diet and medication adjustments are required before this procedure.

☑ DOCTORS' ORDERS FOR NUCLEAR CARDIOLOGY TESTS

MUGA scan (also called gated pool imaging) CI: CHF
Scanning of the heart using computers and synchronized electrocardiogram. MUGA (multigated acquisition is the name of computer machinery).
    Purpose: Used to study the function of the heart muscle, especially the left ventricle.

Thallium stress scan CI: evaluate for CAD
Stress is induced by using the treadmill or, if the patient cannot use the treadmill, medications are given to the patient to simulate the effects of exercise in the body. Drugs that simulate the effects of exercise are Persantine, adenosine, and dipyridamole.

Purpose: Used to determine the blood flow to the myocardium while at rest or after normal stress to diagnose coronary artery disease or to evaluate blood flow after a coronary bypass operation.

Adenosine/thallium scan or Persantine/thallium scan

An example of an order for a thallium scan using medication to simulate the effects of exercise.

Sestamibi stress test or Persantine/sestamibi

This is the same test as in thallium stress scan previously mentioned, using sestamibi as a radionuclide instead of thallium.

 STUDENT ACTIVITIES

For practice transcribing the following types of orders, complete the following activities in the *Skills Practice Manual:*
- For practice transcribing nuclear medicine orders, complete activity 15–5.
- For practice transcribing a review set of doctors' orders, complete activity 15–6.
- For practice recording doctors' orders, complete activity 15–7.
- For practice recording telephone messages, complete activity 15–8.

■ SUMMARY

The primary responsibility of the health unit coordinator in the transcription of diagnostic imaging orders, beyond ordering the requested study, is the communication to the nursing staff concerning patient preparation and communication to the dietary department regarding diet changes. Accurate communication of the preparation procedure is vital to the expected outcome. An error may cause a procedure to be postponed or result in an unclear or nonvisible diagnostic image, each costly to the patient and hospital in both time and money. It is important to indicate, as part of the requisitioning process, the date the procedure is to be done (TBD).

★ **INFORMATION ALERT!**

Overview of diagnostic imaging procedures

X-rays Not Requiring Prep	X-rays Requiring Prep
chest	GB series
bones	IVU
mammogram	PTC
sinus	BE
tomogram of lung	UGI

Special X-ray Procedures Requiring a Consent Form	CT Scan
angiogram	brain
arteriogram	abdomen
arthrogram	LS spine
cholangiogram	neck
hysterosalpingogram	sinus
lymphangiogram	CT-guided liver, lung, or
pyelogram	breast biopsy
venogram	CT of head c̄ DSA
voiding cystourethrogram	

Ultrasound	MRI	Nuclear Medicine Scans
abdomen	shoulder	liver and spleen
pelvis	cervical spine	gallium
gallbladder	knee	thyroid uptake
brain	bone	lung perfusion/ ventilation study
		PET
		DISIDA
		MUGA
		thallium
		sestamibi

▼ REVIEW QUESTIONS

1. Write the meaning of each abbreviation listed below:

   a. PA _____

   b. Lat _____

   c. BE _____

   d. IVP _____

   e. IVU _____

   f. AP _____

   g. KUB _____

   h. CT _____

   i. LS (x-ray) _____

   j. UGI _____

   k. GB _____

   l. RUQ _____

   m. R/O _____

   n. MRI _____

   o. L&S (nuclear medicine) _____

   p. SBFT _____

   q. US _____

   r. LLQ _____

   s. CXR _____

   t. DSA _____

   u. PCXR _____

   v. CI _____

   w. PTC _____

   x. PET _____

   y. Fx _____

2. A substance used in x-ray procedures that helps the radiologist to distinguish between various body densities is called a

   _____

3. An x-ray taken at the patient's bedside is called a

   _____

4. A study of deep body structures recorded on a fluorescent screen instead of on film is called a

   _____

5. A technique used for computer imaging of the interior of the body using magnetic fields is called

   _____

6. A procedure that produces a record of echoes made by sound waves that strike different body densities is called

   _____

7. Preparation of patients for x-rays that are performed according to procedures set forth by the radiology department is called

     _____

8. Medications given to a patient by the nursing personnel when notified by the diagnostic department are called

     _____

9. List five positions that may be included in a doctors' order for x-rays:

     a. _____

     b. _____

     c. _____

     d. _____

     e. _____

10. In the event the doctor ordered the following x-rays for the same patient, in what sequence would they be scheduled? GB, BE, IVU, UGI

     a. _____

     b. _____

     c. _____

     d. _____

11. Five x-ray procedures that may require a signed consent form before they may be done are:

     a. _____

     b. _____

     c. _____

     d. _____

     e. _____

12. Seven diagnostic procedures performed by nuclear medicine are:

     a. _____

     b. _____

     c. _____

     d. _____

e. _____

f. _____

g. _____

13. Place a check mark in the proper space to indicate if patient preparation or consent forms are required for the following diagnostic procedures.

	Preparation		Patient Consent Form	
Procedure	Yes	No	Yes	No
a. KUB				
b. IVU				
c. CT-guided liver biopsy				
d. femoral arteriogram				
e. gallium scan				
f. air contrast BE				
g. tomogram rt lung				
h. mammogram				
i. UGI				
j. bronchogram				
k. BE				
l. bone scan				
m. GB				
n. lymphangiogram				
o. thallium stress scan				

14. Rewrite the following doctors' orders using abbreviations.

a. lumbosacral spine, CI: fracture

_____

b. posteroanterior and lateral chest x-ray, CI: pneumonia

_____

c. upper gastrointestinal, intravenous urogram, gallbladder series, and barium enema, CI: abd. mass

_____

d. myelogram tomorrow, CI: spinal tumor

_____

e. magnetic resonance imaging of the right shoulder CI: rotator cuff injury

_____

15. When ordering diagnostic procedures, the clinical indication, or the reason for the test must be recorded. Other information about the patient to be noted is:

a. _____

b. _____

c. _____

d. _____

e. _____

f. _____

g. _____

TOPICS FOR DISCUSSION

1. Discuss why it is important to provide the correct transportation information when ordering a diagnostic procedure for a patient.

2. Discuss other information that may be written in the doctor's orders that you would need to include when entering the order into the computer.

Other Diagnostic Studies

5. State the difference between an invasive procedure and a noninvasive procedure.

6. Name two noninvasive diagnostic studies related to the heart.

7. Name two invasive diagnostic studies related to the heart.

8. Name three drugs that should be noted on an electrocardiogram requisition.

9. Name two devices that may be used to regulate heart rhythm.

10. State two purposes of an electroencephalogram.

11. State what category of medication should be noted on the requisition when ordering an electroencephalogram.

12. Name six endoscopies and the parts of the body visualized by each.

13. Discuss the importance of patient preparation before a sigmoidoscopy or any visual examination of the colon.

14. List four studies related to the gastrointestinal (GI) system performed in the endoscopy department.

15. List four diagnostic pulmonary function tests that are performed by the respiratory care department.

16. Name three medications that should be noted on the requisition when ordering arterial blood gases.

17. Name two studies performed to diagnose vascular diseases by the cardiovascular department.

Chapter Objectives

Upon completion of this chapter, you will be able to:

1. Define the terms in the vocabulary list.

2. State the meaning of each abbreviation in the abbreviations list.

3. Discuss the purpose of the following diagnostic departments: cardiovascular diagnostics, endoscopy, neurodiagnostics, respiratory care, and sleep study.

4. Identify two tests performed by personnel from cardiovascular diagnostics, neurodiagnostics, and the sleep study departments.

Vocabulary

Apnea ▲ The cessation of breathing

Blood Gases ▲ A diagnostic study to determine the exchange of gases in the blood

Cardiac Monitor ▲ Monitor of heart function, providing visual and audible record of heartbeat

Cardiac Monitor Technician (CMT) ▲ A person who observes the cardiac monitors—often a health unit coordinator is cross-trained to this position.

Echoencephalogram (EchoEG) ▲ A graphic recording that indicates (by sound waves) the position of the brain within the skull

Electrocardiogram (EKG or ECG) ▲ A graphic recording produced by the electric impulses of the heart

Electroencephalogram (EEG) ▲ A graphic recording of the electric impulses of the brain

Electromyogram (EMG) ▲ A record of muscle contraction produced by electrical stimulation

Electrophysiological Study (EPS) ▲ An invasive measure of electrical activity

Endoscopy ▲ The visualization of a body cavity or hollow organ by means of an endoscope.

Gastrointestinal (GI) Study ▲ A diagnostic study related to the gastrointestinal system. GI studies are also performed in the endoscopy department

Holter Monitor ▲ A portable device that records the heart's electrical activity and produces a continuous EKG tracing over a specified period

Invasive Cardiac Study ▲ A method of studying the heart by making an entry into the body, such as by placing a cardiac catheter into a blood vessel

Invasive Procedure ▲ A procedure in which the body cavity is entered by use of a tube, needle, device, or even ionizing radiation

Narcolepsy ▲ A chronic ailment consisting of recurrent attacks of drowsiness and sleep during daytime

Nerve Conduction Studies (NCS) ▲ This study measures how well individual nerves can transmit electrical signals (often performed with an electromyogram)

Noninvasive Procedure ▲ A procedure that does not require entering the body, including puncturing the skin

Noninvasive Cardiac Study ▲ A method of studying the heart without entering the body to perform the procedure

Obstructive Sleep Apnea (OSA) ▲ The cessation of breathing during sleep

Pacemaker ▲ An electronic device, either temporary or permanent, that regulates the pace of the heart when the heart is incapable of doing it

Plethysmography ▲ The recording of changes in the size of a part as altered by the circulation of blood in it

Radiopaque Catheter ▲ A catheter coated with a substance that does not allow the passage of x-rays, thus allowing the movement of the catheter to be followed on the viewing screen

Rhythm Strip ▲ A cardiac study that demonstrates the waveform produced by electric impulses from the electrocardiogram

Spirometry ▲ A study to measure the body's lung capacity and function

Telemetry ▲ The transmission of data electronically to a distant location

Abbreviations

Abbreviation	Meaning	Example of Usage on a Doctor's Order Sheet
ABG	arterial blood gases	ABG on RA
BAER	brain stem auditory evoked response	BAER to evaluate hearing loss
CBG	capillary blood gases	CBG @ 10 AM
ECG, EKG	electrocardiogram	ECG before surgery; EKG today
EchoEG	echoencephalogram	Schedule EchoEG
EEG	electroencephalogram	Schedule EEG
EGD	esophagogastroduodenoscopy	EGD
EMG	electromyogram	EMG tomorrow
ENG	electronystagmography	Schedule for an ENG
EPS	electrophysiological study	EPS today
ERCP	endoscopic retrograde cholangiopancreatography	schedule for ERCP in AM
ICD	implantable cardioverter defibrillator	Obtain consent for ICD
IPG	impedance plethysmography	IPG today
LOC	leave on chart (when it follows ECG or EKG)	ECG, LOC
NCS	nerve conduction studies	EMG c̄ NCS
OSA	obstructive sleep apnea	Sleep study to assess pt for OSA
RA	room air	ABG on RA
SEP	somatosensory evoked potential	Schedule for SEP
VEP	visual evoked potential	Schedule VEP in AM

EXERCISE 1

Write the abbreviation for each term listed below.

1. electroencephalogram _____

2. electrocardiogram (2) _____

3. electromyogram _____

4. room air _____

5. leave on chart _____

6. impedance plethysmography _____

7. arterial blood gases _____

8. capillary blood gases _____

9. echoencephalogram _____

10. endoscopic retrograde cholangiopancreatography _____

11. esophagogastroduodenoscopy _____

12. electrophysiological study _____

13. implantable cardioverter defibrillator _____

14. nerve conduction studies _____

15. obstructive sleep apnea _____

16. brainstem auditory response _____

17. electronystagmography _____

18. somatosensory evoked potential _____

19. visual evoked potential _____

EXERCISE 2

Write the meaning of each abbreviation listed below.

1. ABG

_____

2. ECG

_____

3. EEG

_____

4. EKG

_____

5. LOC

_____

6. EMG

_____

7. RA

_____

8. IPG

_____

9. EchoEG

_____

10. EGD

_____

11. ERCP

_____

12. EPS

_____

13. ICD

_____

14. CBG

_____

15. NCS

_____

16. OSA

_____

17. BAER

_____

18. ENG

_____

19. SEP

_____

20. VEP

_____

■ CARDIOVASCULAR DIAGNOSTICS

Background Information

The procedures carried out by this department are related to the performance of the heart and the vascular system. The results of these studies aid the doctor in making a diagnosis and prescribing treatment.

In the following paragraphs the types of tests performed by the cardiovascular studies department are described. They are categorized as either invasive or noninvasive studies. Invasive procedures are those that require entry into the body by some means (such as a catheter into a blood vessel in cardiac catheterization); noninvasive procedures are those that are performed without entering into any body part (such as an electrocardiogram).

The role of the health unit coordinator is to communicate the order to the cardiovascular diagnostics department by computer or by completing a cardiovascular diagnostics requisition (Fig. 16–1).

☑ DOCTORS' ORDERS FOR CARDIAC STUDIES (NONINVASIVE)

EKG, LOC

An electrocardiogram (EKG or ECG) measures the electrical activity of the heart to detect specific cardiac abnormalities. The electric impulses are picked up and conveyed to the electrocardiograph by electrodes or leads that are placed on various points of the body. A regular EKG has 12 leads. The doctor may also use the abbreviation ECG to order this study, which is performed at the bedside. LOC is a request to the EKG technician to leave a copy of the cardiac tracing on the patient's chart (Fig. 16–2). When ordering an EKG, the health unit coordinator should indicate whether the patient has a pacemaker or an automatic implanted cardiac defibrillator (AICD or ICD). Also note whether the patient is on any specific cardiac medications, such as nitroglycerin, quinidine, lidocaine, Lanoxin, etc.

A rhythm strip shows the waveforms produced by electric impulses from the heart. One lead of the electrocardiogram is used (usually lead II) (Fig. 16–3).

Doctor Ordering _____
Date to be done _____ ☐ Stat ☐ Routine ☐ ASAP
Today's Date _____ Requested by_____

Cardiovascular Department

Clinical Indication _____
Cardiac Medications _____
Pacemaker? ☐ yes ☐ no   Type _____   Ht _____Wt_____
Comments: _____
LOC? ☐ yes ☐ no

Noninvasive Studies

☐ Cardiac monitor
☐ Carotid Doppler flow analysis
☐ Carotid phonoangiography
☐ Doppler flow studies_____
☐ Echocardiogram 2D M-Mode
☐ EKG

☐ EKG c̄ Rhythm Strip
☐ Holter monitor_____hours
☐ Impedance plethysmography
   studies_____
☐ Transesophageal electrocardiogram
☐ Treadmill stress test

Invasive Studies

☐ Cardiac catheterization
☐ Write-in order_____

☐ Electrophysiological Studies

Transportation ☐ portable ☐ stretcher ☐ wheelchair ☐ ambulatory
O₂ ☐ yes ☐ no   Diabetic ☐ yes ☐ no   Hearing deficit ☐ yes ☐ no
IV ☐ yes ☐ no   Seizure disorder ☐ yes ☐ no   Sight deficit ☐ yes ☐ no
Isolation ☐ yes ☐ no   Non-English speaking ☐ yes ☐ no

FIGURE 16–1 ▲ Computer ordering screen for cardiovascular diagnostics.

Communication and Implementation of Cardiovascular Diagnostics

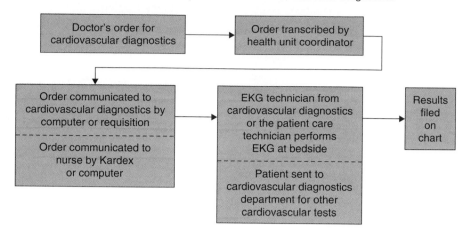

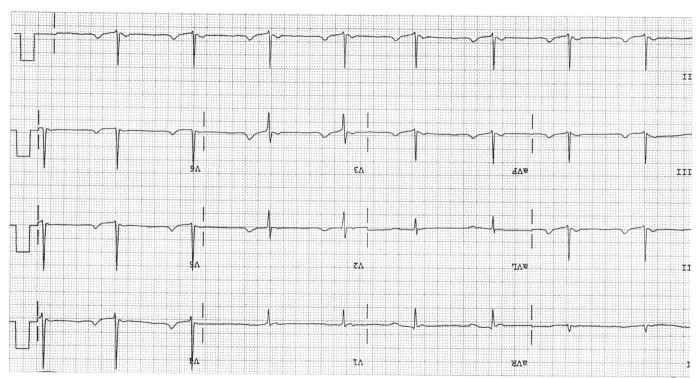

FIGURE 16-2 ▲ An electrocardiogram (EKG) tracing.

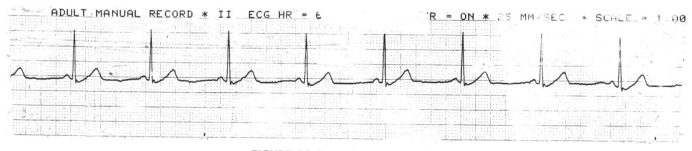

FIGURE 16-3 ▲ Normal rhythm strip.

Echocardiogram or Ultrasonic Cardiogram

The echocardiogram is a graphic recording of the internal structure of the heart and the position and motion of the cardiac walls and valves. This study is made by sending ultra–high-frequency sound waves through the chest wall. This test can also be ordered as M-mode or two- dimensional (2D) mode. The echo M-mode, or motion, uses a narrow beam of sound producing an "ice-pick" view of the cardiac structures. The 2D mode uses a wider sound beam, and images showing both motion and shape are produced.

Transesophageal Electrocardiogram

A transesophageal electrocardiogram examines cardiac function and structure with an ultrasound transducer placed in the esophagus. The transducer provides views of the heart structure and its major blood vessels.

Exercise electrocardiogram (also called **treadmill stress test)**

An exercise electrocardiogram or treadmill stress test is performed by use of a treadmill or stationary bicycle to evaluate the cardiac response to physical stress. These provide information on myocardial response to increased oxygen requirements and determine the adequacy of coronary blood flow.

Holter monitor for 24 hours

A Holter monitor is a portable device that records the heart's electrical activity and produces a continuous ECG tracing over a specified period. It may be used to evaluate chest pain, abnormal heart rhythm, and drug effectiveness. Electrodes are attached to the chest, and the heart sounds are recorded on a cassette tape recorder. The ECG tape recorder is worn in a sling or holder around the chest or waist. The patient usually keeps a 24-hour diary of activities performed while wearing the recorder. A microcomputer analyzes the tape correlating the record of heart activity with the patient's daily activity.

☑ DOCTORS' ORDERS FOR CARDIAC STUDIES (INVASIVE)

The doctor may order a pacemaker for the patient, which is an electronic device, either temporary or permanent (Fig. 16–4), that regulates the pace of the heart when the heart is incapable of doing it. An order for a pacemaker would require that the patient sign a consent form.

Doctors' orders for devices to regulate heart rhythm include:

Insertion of a Pacemaker

A pacemaker is used to jolt the heart into a normal rate and rhythm. Permanent pacemakers are implanted under a chest muscle in surgery. Temporary pacemakers have wires from outside the body leading into the heart.

Insertion of an ICD

An implantable cardioverter defibrillator (ICD) may also be referred to as an automatic implantable cardioverter defibrillator (AICD) and is implanted in the chest. An ICD is a battery-powered device that monitors and if necessary corrects an irregular heart rhythm by sending electrical changes to the heart.

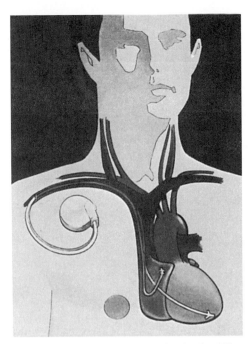

FIGURE 16–4 ▲ Dual-chamber pacemaker implant (Courtesy of Medtronic Inc., Minneapolis, MN).

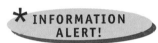

✱ INFORMATION ALERT!

Pacemakers are usually chosen to correct a heart rhythm that is bradycardia (slow heart rhythm), whereas ICDs are used to correct a heart rhythm that is tachycardia (fast heart rhythm).

A telemetry unit is a patient care area where the activity of cardiac monitors worn by patients is registered at the nurses' station. If a nurse or monitor technician detects an abnormality or if the patient complains of chest pain or discomfort, a rhythm strip can be printed of the continuous electrocardiogram for study and interpretation of the occurrence. These rhythm strips are then placed in the patient's chart after interpretation.

☑ DOCTORS' ORDERS FOR VASCULAR STUDIES (NONINVASIVE)

Carotid Doppler flow analysis

A directional Doppler probe is used to detect the flow of blood in the major neck artery.

Carotid phonoangiography

Abnormal sounds from the lumen (opening) of the carotid artery in the neck can be recorded by placing an electronic microphone over this artery for the doctor's interpretation.

Doppler flow studies on lower extremities

In this procedure, an ultrasound probe is placed over the major leg veins or arteries. A graphic tracing is produced, showing flow changes caused by changes within the blood vessels.

Impedance plethysmography studies (IPG)

Changes in the blood volume are shown when electrodes are applied to the leg and electric resistance changes are recorded.

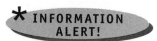

Noninvasive Cardiovascular Diagnostics Tests

- Carotid phonoangiography
- Doppler flow studies
- Echocardiogram
- Electrocardiogram (EKG)
- Exercise electrocardiogram
- Holter or cardiac monitor
- Impedance plethysmography (IPG)
- Transesophageal electrocardiogram

☑ DOCTORS' ORDERS FOR CARDIAC STUDIES (INVASIVE)

Cardiac catheterization at 8 AM tomorrow. Have consent signed.
In this study, a long, flexible radiopaque catheter is passed through a vein in the arm or leg into the heart chambers. The use of a radiopaque catheter (a catheter coated with a substance that does not permit the passage of x-rays) allows the catheter to be followed on a television screen. This procedure is performed to detect cardiac disease or defects, and to study the results of heart surgery.

Cardiac catheterization is performed under surgical conditions. It may be performed in cardiac diagnostics, in a catheterization lab, or in the diagnostic imaging department. A surgical consent form must be signed.

Electrophysiological Studies
An electrophysiological study (EPS) is an invasive measure of electrical activity. An electrode catheter is inserted into the right atrium, usually via the femoral vein. Electrical stimulation is then delivered through the catheter while the ECG monitors and computers record the heart's electrical response to the stimulus.

Swan-Ganz catheter insertion
This is a special procedure performed by a doctor in a critical care unit. A balloon-tipped catheter is inserted through the subclavian vein into the right side of the heart. The catheter goes through the right ventricle past the pulmonic valve and into a branch of the pulmonary artery. The measurements revealed by this procedure are used to guide and evaluate therapy.

Thallium, Sestamibi, and Persantine/sestamibi stress tests
These tests are discussed in Chapter 15, as they are two-step procedures involving both the nuclear medicine and the cardiovascular departments. The health unit coordinator will often call both departments on a conference call to coordinate these tests. If the cardiologist requests a particular time for the scheduling of the test so he or she may be present, the health unit coordinator coordinates that time with the two departments.

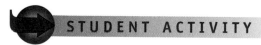

STUDENT ACTIVITY

To practice transcribing cardiovascular diagnostics orders, complete Activity 16–1 in the *Skills Practice Manual*.

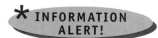

Invasive Cardiovascular Diagnostics Tests

- Cardiac catheterization
- Electrophysiological studies (EPS)
- Nuclear Medicine stress tests (discussed in Chapter 15)
- Swan-Ganz catheter insertion

■ NEURODIAGNOSTICS

Neurodiagnostics may include several tests related to the function of the nervous system (brain and spinal cord). In smaller facilities, the electroencephalography may be the only neurodiagnostic test performed.

Electroencephalography

An electroencephalogram (EEG) is a recording of a patient's brain waves. The procedure is performed to study brain function. The results of the study may be used to diagnose brain tumors, epilepsy, other brain diseases, or injuries, and to confirm brain death or cerebral silence (Fig. 16–5).

The role of the health unit coordinator is to communicate the order to the EEG department by computer or by completing the neurodiagnostics requisition. Anticonvulsant medications such as phenobarbitol, Dilantin, and Tegretol, should be noted when ordering a neurodiagnostics procedure (Fig. 16–6).

Preparation of the patient by the nursing staff is usually required. The patient's hair is washed the night before the test is to be done. The use of cola drinks, coffee, or tea may be restricted because they may act as stimulants; however, food and other fluids are permitted. Some hospitals have special preparation cards that contain information for the preparation of the patient for an EEG. The health unit coordinator places the preparation card in the patient's Kardex holder during the transcription procedure.

An EEG may be ordered to be done portable (an EEG machine would be brought to the patient's bedside) or the patient is transported to the neurodiagnostic department for the test, which is performed by the EEG technician.

To order an electroencephalogram, the doctor usually writes *EEG* on the doctors' order sheet.

Echoencephalography

Echoencephalography (EchoEG) uses ultrasound to produce an image of the brain. It is being replaced in some instances by computed tomography.

Evoked Potentials

Evoked potentials (EPs) are a group of diagnostic tests that measure changes in various parts of the brain produced by visual, auditory, or somatosensory stimuli. Examples of EPs follow.

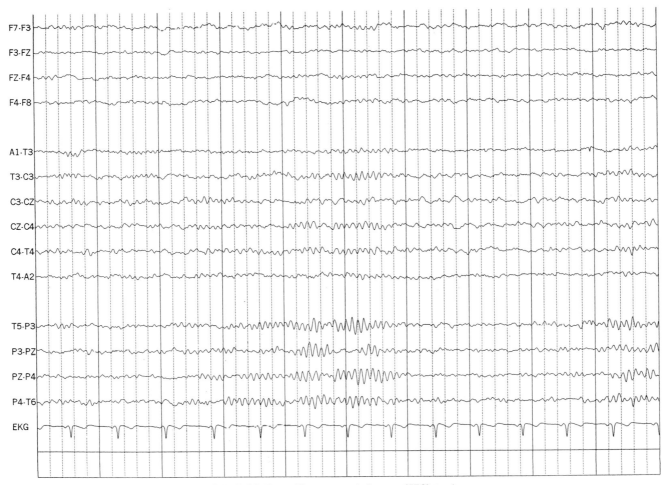

FIGURE 16–5 ▲ Electroencephalogram (EEG) tracing.

Doctor Ordering _____

Date to be done _____ ☐ Stat ☐ Routine ☐ ASAP

Today's Date _____ Requested by _____

| **Neurodiagnostics Department** |

Clinical Indication _____

Transportation ☐ portable ☐ stretcher ☐ wheelchair ☐ ambulatory

O₂ ☐ yes ☐ no   Diabetic ☐ yes ☐ no   Hearing deficit ☐ yes ☐ no

IV ☐ yes ☐ no   Seizure disorder ☐ yes ☐ no   Sight deficit ☐ yes ☐ no

Isolation ☐ yes ☐ no   Non-English speaking ☐ yes ☐ no

Comments: _____

☐ Auditory evoked response
☐ Echoencephalography
☐ Electroencephalography
☐ Electromyography
☐ Electronystagmography
☐ Nerve conduction studies
☐ Somatosensory evoked potential
☐ Visual evoked potential
Write-in order_____

FIGURE 16-6 ▲ Computer ordering screen for neurodiagnostics.

Visual Evoked Potential

The visual evoked potential (VEP) is a response to visual stimuli. It can also be called visual evoked response (VER). It is sometimes used to confirm cerebral silence (brain death).

Auditory Evoked Response

The auditory evoked response (AER) is related to hearing (an auditory stimulus); it is also called the brainstem auditory evoked response (BAER).

Somatosensory Evoked Potential

The somatosensory evoked potentials (SEP) are done to record a response to a painless stimulation of a peripheral nerve.

Electronystagmography

Electronystagmography (ENG) is done by placing electrodes near the patient's eyes and recording involuntary eye movements.

Electromyography and Nerve Conduction Studies

An electromyogram (EMG) is a diagnostic study that measures the electrical discharges made by the muscles. Nerve conduction studies (NCS) measure how well individual nerves can transmit electrical signals. These tests assist in the detection of and severity of diseases that can damage muscle tissue or nerves.

✱ INFORMATION ALERT!

Neurodiagnostics Tests

- Auditory evoked response
- Echoencephalogram (EchoEG)
- Electroencephalogram (EEG)
- Electromyography (EMG)
- Electronystagmography (ENG)
- Evoked potentials (EPs)
- Nerve conduction studies (NCS)
- Somatosensory evoked potential (SEP)
- Visual evoked potential (VEP)

Doctors' Orders for Neurodiagnostics
- *EEG tomorrow*
- *Schedule for ENG*
- *Echoencephalogram today*
- *EMG tomorrow* AM

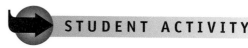

STUDENT ACTIVITY

To practice transcribing a neurodiagnostics order, complete Activity 16–2 in the *Skills Practice Manual*.

■ ENDOSCOPY

Endoscopy is a general term used to indicate the visual examination of a body cavity or hollow organ. It is a diagnostic procedure performed by a doctor. Hospitals have a designated area for these studies. During some endoscopic procedures, biopsies are performed.

To transcribe an endoscopy order, the health unit coordinator schedules the procedure with the responsible department by computer or requisition (Fig. 16–7) may be used to order the study. Endoscopies require a patient to sign a consent form. Some endoscopies require preparation. The doctor writes any pre-procedure preparation orders on the doctors' order sheet.

Types of Endoscopies

There are many types of endoscopic examinations. The name of the procedure and the instruments used depend on the organ being examined. The following is a list of endoscopic examinations commonly performed in a hospital either on an inpatient or outpatient basis.

Bronchoscopy: The visual inspection of the bronchi by means of a bronchoscope

Colonoscopy: The visual examination of the large intestine from the anus to the cecum by means of a fiberoptic colonoscope

Esophagoscopy: The visual examination of the esophagus by means of an esophagoscope

Communication and Implementation of Neurodiagnostic Orders

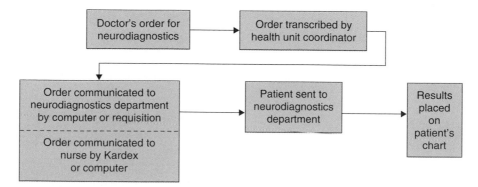

Doctor Ordering _____

Date to be done _____ Time to be done _____

Today's Date _____ Requested by _____

Endoscopy Department

Clinical Indication _____

Transportation ☐ portable ☐ stretcher ☐ wheelchair ☐ ambulatory

O₂ ☐ yes ☐ no   Diabetic ☐ yes ☐ no   Hearing deficit ☐ yes ☐ no

IV ☐ yes ☐ no   Seizure disorder ☐ yes ☐ no   Sight deficit ☐ yes ☐ no

Isolation ☐ yes ☐ no   Non-English speaking ☐ yes ☐ no

Pre-op Medication ☐ yes ☐ no

Time given _____

Comments: _____

☐ Arthroscopy   ☐ Esophagoscopy

☐ Bronchoscopy   ☐ Hysteroscopy

☐ Colonoscopy   ☐ Laparoscopy

☐ Colposcopy   ☐ Pelvioscopy

☐ Cystoscopy   ☐ Peritoneoscopy

☐ Endoscopic retrograde   ☐ Proctoscopy

   cholangiopancreatography (ERCP)   ☐ Sigmoidoscopy

☐ Esophagogastroduodenoscopy (EGD)

☐ Write-in order _____

FIGURE 16–7 ▲ Computer ordering screen for endoscopy.

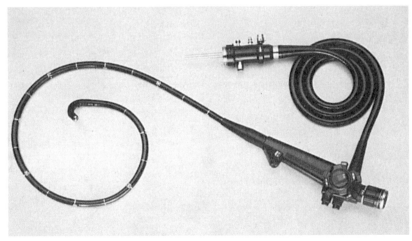

FIGURE 16–8 ▲ Fiberoptic gastroscope (Courtesy of Olympus Corp., Lake Success, NY).

Gastroscopy: The visual examination of the interior of the stomach by means of a gastroscope (Fig. 16–8).

Proctoscopy: The visual inspection of the rectum by means of a proctoscope

Sigmoidoscopy: The visual examination of the sigmoid portion of the large intestine by means of a sigmoidoscope

Other diagnostic procedures related to endoscopy are the following:

Anoscopy: Visual inspection of the anal canal.

Endoscopic retrograde cholangiopancreatography (ERCP): This diagnostic procedure is an inspection of the com-

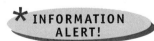
✱ INFORMATION ALERT!

When a patient is scheduled for barium studies, the gastrointestinal endoscopies must be performed prior to the barium studies. The presence of barium would obscure the visualization of the intestinal walls.

mon bile duct, biliary tract, and pancreatic duct; it is done by insertion of a catheter through an endoscope.

Esophagogastroduodenoscopy (EGD): Visual inspection of the esophagus, stomach, and duodenum (Fig. 16–9).

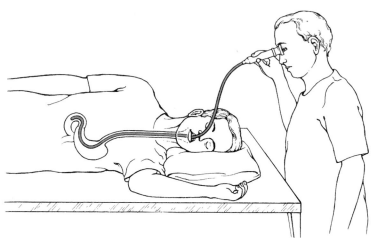

FIGURE 16–9 ▲ Esophagogastroduodenoscopy (EGD) is the visualization of the esophagus, stomach, and duodenum. (From Ignatavicius DD, Workman ML, Mishler MA: Medical-Surgical Nursing: A Nursing Process Approach, 2nd ed. Philadelphia: WB Saunders, 1995.)

☑ DOCTORS' ORDERS FOR ENDOSCOPIES

Sigmoidoscopy tomorrow AM.
· Fleet enema hs and repeat @ 0600

Schedule for gastroscopy tomorrow AM
· NPO p̄ MN

Schedule ERCP for tomorrow
· NPO p̄ MN

Bronchoscopy tomorrow @ 9:30 AM
· Have consent form signed
· Demerol 50 mg
· Atropine 0.8 mg IM @ 8:30 AM

Schedule colonoscopy for 8 AM on Wednesday
· Have consent form signed
· Clear liquids, NPO p̄ MN
· Fleet enema hs and repeat @ 0600

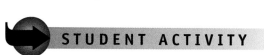

STUDENT ACTIVITY

To practice transcribing endoscopy orders, complete Activity 16–3 in the *Skills Practice Manual*.

✳ INFORMATION ALERT!

Types of Endoscopies	Organ Examination
Anoscopy	Anal canal
Bronchoscopy	Bronchi
Colonoscopy	Large intestine
Endoscopic retrograde cholangiopancreatography (ERCP)	Biliary and pancreatic ducts
Esophagogastroduodenoscopy (EGD)	Gastrointestinal tract
Esophagoscopy	Esophagus
Gastroscopy	Stomach
Proctoscopy	Rectum
Sigmoidoscopy	Sigmoid colon

Gastrointestinal (GI) Studies

Some gastrointestinal (GI) studies are performed in the endoscopy department usually on outpatient basis, whereas others may be performed at the bedside by the nurse. The health unit

Communication and Implementation of Endoscopy Orders

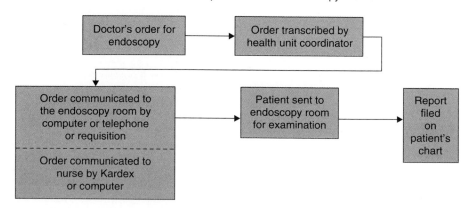

coordinator may be asked to requisition the necessary equipment from the central service department for a bedside collection. Specimens collected by the nurse are sent to the hospital clinical laboratory for study, or they may be sent to a private laboratory.

Gastrointestinal (GI) studies that may be performed in the endoscopy department are listed below.

Gastric analysis

A study performed to measure the stomach's secretion of hydrochloric acid and pepsin as well as for the evaluation of stomach and duodenal ulcers. This test takes approximately 2 ½ hours.

Hollander test for vagotomy

A test performed to determine the amount of hydrochloric acid in the patient's gastric juices after a vagotomy. A vagotomy is the cutting of certain branches of the vagus nerve to reduce the secretion of gastric acid and lessen the chance of a recurrence of a gastric ulcer. The Hollander test takes approximately 3 ½ hours.

Esophageal manometry/motility and reflux

The motility portion of this test studies esophageal function. The reflux study is performed to determine the reason for food and gastric juices flowing back into the esophagus. This test takes approximately 1 hour.

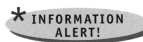

* INFORMATION ALERT!

Gastrointestinal (GI) Studies (Usually performed on outpatient basis)

- Biliary drainage
- Esophageal manometry/motility and reflux
- Gastric analysis
- Hollander test for vagotomy
- Lactose tolerance test
- Secretin test
- Quantitative fecal fat

Biliary drainage

A procedure to obtain duodenal fluids to study for cholesterol crystals, which indicate gallstone formation. This test, which takes approximately 2 hours, also is performed to determine the presence of parasites.

Secretin test

A test of pancreatic function that takes approximately 3 hours.

Lactose tolerance test

A test to determine intolerance to lactose, the sugar in milk. This test takes approximately 2 hours.

Qualitative fecal fat

A study to determine the malabsorption of fat by a patient. The patient's stools are collected for 48 to 72 hours after the patient has eaten a 100 g fat diet for 2 to 3 days.

■ RESPIRATORY CARE DEPARTMENT

Background Information

The respiratory care department (may be called the cardiopulmonary department) performs diagnostic tests to determine lung function and also performs treatments for respiratory disease and conditions. Diagnostic tests that are performed by the respiratory care department will be discussed in this chapter. Blood is analyzed in the pulmonary function laboratory, which is part of the respiratory department. The terms *pulmonary function* and *respiratory function* are used interchangeably. Treatment orders performed by the respiratory care department will be discussed in Chapter 17.

The health unit coordinator communicates the doctors' order to the respiratory care department by computer or by completing a requisition (Fig. 16–10).

No preparation is required for respiratory care tests unless the doctor has included special instructions with the order. For example, the doctor may want the amount of oxygen adjusted or turned off before a study on the patient's blood gases is done, as

---

Doctor Ordering _____

Date to be done _____ ☐ Stat ☐ Routine ☐ ASAP

Today's Date _____ Requested by _____

| Respiratory Care Department—Diagnostics |

Clinical Indication _____

Anticoagulant Medication? ☐ yes   Name of medication _____
                          ☐ no

Room air ☐ yes ☐ no   Oxygen ☐ yes ☐ no

Comments: _____

☐ Arterial blood gases
☐ Capillary blood gases
☐ Pulse oximetry
☐ Spirometry
☐ Write-in order _____

FIGURE 16–10 ▲ Computer ordering screen for respiratory care diagnostics.

Communication and Implementation of Respiratory Care Diagnostic Orders

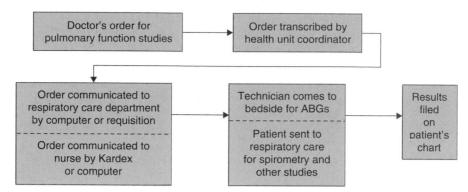

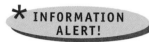

ABGs are used to monitor patients on ventilators, monitor critically ill nonventilator patients, establish preoperative baseline parameters, and to enlighten electrolyte therapy.

If the patient has an arterial line, the specimen may be obtained by the nursing personnel.

in the following orders: DC O_2 at 10 AM, ABG at 11 AM. It is important to note when ordering an arterial blood gas whether the patient is taking an anticoagulant drug, such as Lovenox, Coumadin, or heparin. These medications, which lengthen the time it takes for blood to clot, cause the patient to bleed excessively when the artery is punctured for this test. The doctor may also request that capillary blood (CBG) be used for blood gas determination. The health unit coordinator must be sure to indicate whether the specimen is a capillary specimen when completing the order.

☑ DOCTORS' ORDERS FOR RESPIRATORY CARE

Listed below are examples of doctors' orders for respiratory care studies.

Room air ABGs
The blood sample for this diagnostic study is obtained from the patient's artery by the respiratory care technician while the patient is breathing room air (which is 21% oxygen). The blood is then analyzed in the pulmonary function laboratory. Measurement of ABG provides valuable information in assessing and managing a patient's respiratory (ventilation) and metabolic (renal) acid/base and electrolyte homeostasis. It is also used to assess adequacy of oxygenation.

ABG on O_2 @ 2 L/min
The blood sample for this test is to be drawn while the patient is breathing oxygen (O_2), which is being delivered at a rate of 2 liters per minute.

A point-of-care (POC) ABG portable device may be used in emergency rooms, intensive care units, and doctors' offices or in transport vehicles to perform ABG and pH measurements (Fig. 16-11).

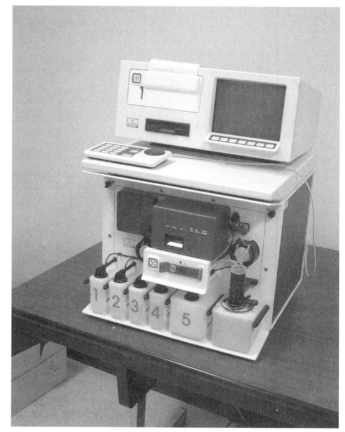

FIGURE 16–11 ▲ Point-of-care blood gas analyzer.

CBG
Capillary blood gases are performed primarily on infants. Blood is obtained from the infant's capillary arterial vessel usually from the heel by the respiratory care technician. The blood is then analyzed in the pulmonary function laboratory. Measurement of CBG also provides valuable information in assessing and managing an infant's respiratory (ventilation) and metabolic (renal) acid/base and electrolyte homeostasis. It is also used to assess adequacy of oxygenation.

Bedside spirometry study
This study measures and records the patient's lung capacity for air to determine certain aspects of lung function.

Pulse oximetry

This study measures the oxygen saturation of the arterial blood. A probe is attached to either the ear or the finger. This noninvasive procedure (Fig. 16–12) is often ordered as a continuous study in the recovery room, intensive care unit, or pediatric unit. The nursing staff may also perform this test.

Pre- and post-spirometry

This test is performed at the bedside before bronchodilator treatment and is repeated after the treatment.

STUDENT ACTIVITIES

For practice transcribing the following types of orders, complete the following activities in the *Skills Practice Manual:*
- To practice transcribing respiratory care orders that relate to lung function, complete Activity 16–4.
- To practice transcribing a review set of doctors' orders, complete Activity 16–5.
- To practice recording doctors' orders, complete Activity 16–6.
- To practice recording telephone messages, complete Activity 16–7.

■ SLEEP STUDY DEPARTMENT

The sleep study department performs studies to assess a patient's sleep patterns to determine nature and severity of insomnia, to reveal presence of obstructive sleep apnea (OSA) and severity of condition, and to assist in the diagnosis of narcolepsy. Many hospitals have a sleep study department and sleep studies are usually performed on an outpatient basis.

Sleep study to assess patient for OSA

During this procedure, electrodes for ECG, EEG, and electromyography are applied to the patient. Excess hair may need to be shaved on male patients. Airflow, oximetry, and impedance mon-

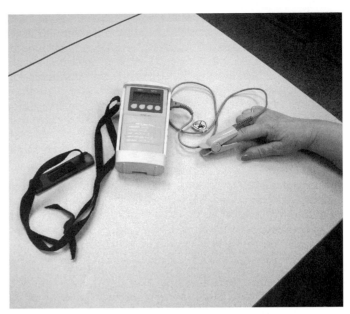

FIGURE 16–12 ▲ Hand-held pulse oximeter.

itors are also applied. The patient is allowed to sleep per normal routine and is monitored for respiratory disturbances such as apnea.

■ SUMMARY

The recognition and proper scheduling of all diagnostic studies are of utmost importance to the patient, the doctor(s), and the hospital. Both the patient who is as yet undiagnosed and the patient awaiting test results that hopefully will show improvement are dependent upon the knowledge and communication skills of the individual coordinating activities on the nursing unit. The health unit coordinator who can identify and order correctly all diagnostic studies is an asset to the unit.

REVIEW QUESTIONS

1. Write out the meaning of each underlined abbreviation appearing in the following sets of doctors' orders.

   a. <u>EMG</u> tomorrow AM

   _____

   b. <u>EKG</u> stat

   _____

   c. <u>ABG</u> on <u>RA</u> @ 4 PM today

   _____

   d. <u>EKG</u> today, <u>LOC</u>

   _____

e. Schedule <u>EEG</u> tomorrow

_____

f. <u>CBG</u> @ 6 AM

_____

2. List two noninvasive cardiac studies the doctor may request to diagnose cardiac abnormalities.

a. _____

b. _____

3. List two invasive cardiac studies the doctor may request to diagnose cardiac abnormalities.

a. _____

b. _____

4. List four cardiovascular medications.

a. _____

b. _____

c. _____

d. _____

5. Name two devices used to regulate heart rhythm.

a. _____

b. _____

6. Name six endoscopic procedures and name the portion of the body that is studied by each procedure.

Procedure	Organ(s) Studied
a.	
b.	
c.	
d.	
e.	
f.	

7. Describe the purpose of each of the following departments:

   a. sleep study lab

   _____

   b. respiratory care department

   _____

   c. neurodiagnostics department

   _____

   d. cardiovascular diagnostic department

   _____

8. Three medications that lengthen clotting time and that should be noted on an arterial blood gas requisition are:

   a. _____

   b. _____

   c. _____

9. Define the following:

   a. GI study

   _____

   b. rhythm strip

   _____

   c. radiopaque catheter

   _____

   d. Holter monitor

   _____

10. List four studies related to the gastrointestinal (GI) system performed (usually on outpatient basis) in the endoscopy department.

   a. _____

   b. _____

   c. _____

   d. _____

11. Using the list in the left-hand column below for reference, identify the department that performs the studies indicated in the following sets of doctors' orders.

Reference List   Doctors' Orders

a. cardiovascular diagnostics
b. endoscopy department
c. neurodiagnostics department
d. respiratory care department

_____ 1. EMG and NCS

_____ 2. spirometry

_____ 3. ABG on RA

_____ 4. sigmoidoscopy at 8 am in clinic

_____ 5. EEG tomorrow

_____ 6. colonoscopy

_____ 7. EKG, LOC

_____ 8. echocardiogram

_____ 9. Doppler flow studies

_____ 10. treadmill stress test

_____ 11. schedule for spirometry study tomorrow

_____ 12. rhythm strip

_____ 13. schedule esophagoscopy for Monday

_____ 14. Holter monitor for 24 hours

_____ 15. IPG—left leg

_____ 16. ERCP tomorrow

_____ 17. schedule BAER

_____ 18. Consent for ICD

12. Rewrite the following doctors' orders using abbreviations. Or to practice writing doctors' orders, have someone read the orders to you while you record them. Again, practice using abbreviations while you do this.

a. impedance plethysmography this morning

_____

b. electrocardiogram now

_____

c. endoscopic retrograde cholangiopancreatography tomorrow morning

_____

d. arterial blood gases on oxygen at two liters per minute

_____

TOPICS FOR DISCUSSION

1. Discuss possible consequences that could result from the health unit coordinator not noting anticoagulant medications on a requisition for an ABG.
2. Discuss the importance of transcribing doctors' orders for diagnostic tests in a timely manner.
3. Discuss the consequences of ordering a diagnostic test on the wrong patient and ways that this could be avoided.
4. Discuss the consequences of missing an order, part of an order, or ordering the wrong test.

Treatment Orders

▶ Chapter Objectives

Upon completion of this chapter, you will be able to:

1. Define the terms in the vocabulary list.

2. Write the meaning of each abbreviation in the abbreviations list.

3. State the purpose of the respiratory care, physical therapy, and occupational therapy departments.

4. List four purposes of traction.

5. Name the traction set-up used by patients to assist them to move in bed.

6. Given a list of treatments, identify which department would perform them.

7. List three treatments performed by physical therapy.

8. List three treatments performed by occupational therapy.

9. List the two main types of dialysis.

▶ Vocabulary

Active Exercise ▲ Exercise performed by the patient without assistance as instructed by physical therapist

Activities of Daily Living ▲ Tasks that enable individuals to meet basic needs (eating, bathing, and so on)

Aerosol ▲ Liquid suspension of particles in a gas stream for inhalation purposes

Dialysis ▲ The removal of wastes in the blood usually excreted by the kidneys

Extubation ▲ Removal of a previously inserted tube (as in an endotracheal tube)

Hydrotherapy ▲ Treatment with water

Hyperbaric Oxygen Therapy (HBOT) ▲ A treatment that involves breathing 100% oxygen while in an enclosed system pressurized to greater than one atmosphere (sea level)

Hypertonic ▲ Concentrated salt solution (>0.9%)

Hypotonic ▲ Dilute salt solution (<0.9%)

Induced Sputum Specimen ▲ A sputum specimen obtained by performing a respiratory treatment to loosen lung secretions

Intervention ▲ Synonymous with treatment

Intubation ▲ Insertion and placement of a tube (within the trachea may be endotracheal or tracheostomy)

Isometric ▲ Of equal dimensions. Holding ends of contracting muscle fixed so that contraction produces increased tension at a constant overall length

Nebulizer ▲ A gas-driven device that produces an aerosol

Passive Exercise ▲ Exercise in which the patient is submissive and the physical therapist moves the patient's limbs

Positive Pressure ▲ Pressure greater than atmospheric pressure

Range of Motion ▲ The range in which a joint can move

Reduction ▲ The correction of a deformity in a bone fracture or dislocation

Resistive Exercise ▲ Exercise using opposition. A T-band or water provides resistance for patient exercises

Titrate ▲ To adjust the amount of treatment to maintain a specific physiologic response

Traction ▲ A mechanical pull to part of the body to maintain alignment and facilitate healing; traction may be static (continuous) or intermittent

Unit Dose ▲ Any premixed or prespecified dose; often administered with SVN or IPPB treatments

Abbreviations

Abbreviation	Meaning	Example of Usage on a Doctor's Order Sheet
AA	active assisted	AA exercises B/L LE
ADL	activities of daily living	OT for ADL
AKA	above-the-knee amputation	AKA protocol
BiPAP	bilevel positive airway pressure	BiPAP 5/15 @hs c̄ 3L/min bleed in O_2
BiW	twice a week	PT BiW
BKA	below-the-knee amputation	consent for BKA
BLE	both lower extremities	HBOT BLE
BUE	both upper extremities	strengthening exercises BUE
CP	cold packs	CP L arm
CPM	continuous passive motion	CPM
CPR	cardiopulmonary resuscitation	CPR training for parents before child's discharge
CPT	chest physiotherapy	DC CPT
CPAP	continuous positive airway pressure	CPAP 5 cm H_2O
EPC	electronic pain control	EPC
ET	endotracheal tube	CXR for ET tube placement
ES	electrical stimulation	ES
FWW	front-wheel walker	provide c̄ FWW
HA	heated aerosol	HA T-piece @ 60%
HBOT	hyperbaric O_2 therapy	HBOT qd 3 × wk for 8 wks
HD	hemodialysis	HD BiW × 3 h
HP	hot packs	HP to neck
IPPB	intermittent positive-pressure breathing	IPPB q4h c̄ 0.5 cc Ventolin in 2 cc NS
IS	incentive spirometry	IS tid
ISOM	isometric	ISOM UE bid
lbs, #	pounds	bucks traction c̄ 5#
LE	lower extremities	ROM LE qd
LLE	left lower extremity	passive exercises LLE
LLL	left lower lobe	CPT—LLL only

Abbreviation	Meaning	Example of Usage on a Doctor's Order Sheet
L/min	liters per minute	↑ O_2 to 4 L/min
LUE	left upper extremities	ROM LUE
LUL	left upper lobe	CPT to LUL
MDI	metered dose inhaler	MDI c̄ Ventolin ii puffs qid
NWB	non–weight-bearing	Crutch-walking NWB
O_2	oxygen	O_2 6 L/min by mask
ORIF	open reduction, internal fixation	ORIF lt femur
OT	occupational therapy or occupational therapist	OT for ADL
PD	peritoneal dialysis	Tenckhoff cath for PD
PEP	positive expiratory pressure	IS c̄ PEP
PROM	passive range of motion	PROM LUE bid
PT	physical therapy or physical therapist	To PT for crutch walking
PTA	physical therapy assistant	PTA to assist patient in amb
P&PD	percussion and postural drainage	P&PD to LUL
RLE	right lower extremities	ISOM to RLE
RLL	right lower lobe	CPT RLL
RML	right middle lobe	CPT RML
ROM	range of motion	ROM to upper extremities tid
RT	respiratory therapist	RT to obtain induced sputum specimen
RUL	right upper lobe	P&PD RUL p̄
RUE	right upper extremity	Hot pks to RUE
SaO or O_2 Sats	oxygen saturation (on pulse oximetry, not ABGs)	Titrate O_2 flow to SaO >95%
STM	soft tissue massage	STM lt shoulder 20 min bid
SVN	small volume nebulizer	Δ SVN to bid
TENS	transcutaneous electrical nerve stimulation	Post-op TENS
TT	tilt table	TT for PT
THR, THA	total hip replacement/ arthroplasty	follow THR protocol
TKR, TKA	total knee replacement/ arthroplasty	TKA protocol
Tx	traction	Buck's Tx
UD	unit dose	UD Ventolin now

Abbreviation	Meaning	Example of Usage on a Doctor's Order Sheet
USN	ultrasonic nebulizer	USN 15 min tid
WBAT	weight bearing as tolerated	amb, WBAT rt leg
WP	whirlpool	WP to L leg bid
>	greater than	Call hospitalist if pH >7.4
<	less than	Call hospitalist if O_2 Sats <70%

EXERCISE 1

Write the abbreviation for each term listed below.

1. left upper lobe _____

2. occupational therapy or occupational therapist _____

3. physical therapy or physical therapist _____

4. liters per minute _____

5. oxygen _____

6. intermittent positive-pressure breathing _____

7. right upper lobe _____

8. range of motion _____

9. right lower lobe _____

10. activities of daily living _____

11. electromyogram _____

12. right middle lobe _____

13. ultrasonic nebulizer _____

14. small volume nebulizer _____

15. left lower lobe _____

16. pounds _____

17. non–weight-bearing _____

18. whirlpool _____

19. hot packs _____

20. transcutaneous electrical nerve stimulation _____

21. electronic pain control _____

22. electrical stimulation _____

23. continuous passive motion _____

24. incentive spirometry _____

25. metered dose inhaler _____

26. chest physiotherapy _____

27. active assisted _____

28. twice weekly _____

29. above-the-knee amputation _____

30. soft tissue massage _____

31. lower extremities _____

32. hemodialysis _____

33. total hip replacement/ arthroplasty _____

34. open reduction, internal fixation _____

35. traction _____

36. tilt table _____

37. isometric _____

38. below-the-knee amputation _____

39. endotracheal tube _____

40. heated aerosol _____

41. positive expiratory pressure _____

42. percussion and postural drainage _____

43. oxygen saturation _____

44. unit dose _____

45. greater than _____

46. total knee replacement/ arthroplasty _____

47. less than _____

48. cold packs _____

49. cardiopulmonary resuscitation _____

50. hyperbaric oxygen therapy _____

51. bilevel positive airway pressure _____

52. continuous positive airway pressure _____

53. both upper extremities _____

54. both lower extremities _____

55. right upper extremity _____

56. left upper extremity _____

57. right lower extremity _____

58. left lower extremity _____

59. physical therapist assistant _____

60. respiratory therapist _____

61. passive range of motion _____

62. weight bearing as tolerated _____

63. front-wheel walker _____

EXERCISE 2

Write the meaning of each abbreviation listed below.

1. O_2

   _____

2. LUL

   _____

3. RLL

   _____

4. OT

   _____

5. PT

   _____

6. EMG

   _____

7. ADL

   _____

8. lbs or #

   _____

9. RUL

   _____

10. RML

    _____

11. NWB

    _____

12. ROM

    _____

13. L/min

    _____

14. SVN

    _____

15. LLL

    _____

16. IPPB

    _____

17. USN

    _____

18. *HP*

_____

19. *WP*

_____

20. *CPM*

_____

21. *ES*

_____

22. *EPC*

_____

23. *TENS*

_____

24. *IS*

_____

25. *CPT*

_____

26. *MDI*

_____

27. *ORIF*

_____

28. *TT*

_____

29. *SaO or O$_2$ Sats*

_____

30. *AKA*

_____

31. *UD*

_____

32. *HA*

_____

33. *ISOM*

_____

34. *LE*

_____

35. *STM*

_____

36. *HD*

_____

37. *Tx*

_____

38. *P&PD*

_____

39. *>*

_____

40. *TKR, TKA*

_____

41. *THR, THA*

_____

42. *ET*

_____

43. *PD*

_____

44. <

_____

45. BiW

_____

46. PEP

_____

47. CP

_____

48. AA

_____

49. CPR

_____

50. HBOT

_____

51. BiPAP

_____

52. CPAP

_____

53. BUE

_____

54. BLE

_____

55. RUE

_____

56. LUE

_____

57. RLE

_____

58. LLE

_____

59. PTA

_____

60. RT

_____

61. PROM

_____

62. WBAT

_____

63. FWW

_____

■ TRACTION

Traction is the mechanical pull applied to a part of the body. The pull is achieved by connecting an apparatus attached to a bed to an apparatus attached to the patient (Fig. 17–1).

Traction may be applied to the arms, legs, neck, backbone, or pelvis. It is used to treat fractures, dislocations, and long-duration muscle spasms, and to prevent or correct deformities. Traction can either be short-term or long-term. Traction serves several purposes: It aligns the ends of a fracture by pulling the limb into a straight position, controls muscle spasm, and relieves pain. It also takes pressure off the bone ends by relaxing the muscle.

Apparatus Set-Up

Bed

The apparatus attached to the patient's bed may include pulleys, rope, weights, and metal bars. The weights (metal disks or sandbags) provide the "pull" to a part of the body. The pulleys, rope, and metal bars are assembled to suspend the weights. Each type of traction requires a different assemblage of these parts; thus a skilled person must perform this task. It is usually the responsibility of the nurse or the orthopedic technician to attach the traction apparatus to the bed. The physical therapy department personnel may assist with setting up traction equipment in smaller hospitals. The health unit coordinator communicates a

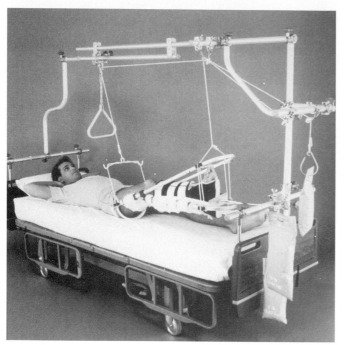

FIGURE 17–1 ▲ Traction and Thomas leg splint with a Pearson attachment. (Courtesy of Zimmer USA.)

traction order to the person responsible for assembling the bed apparatus verbally by telephone or by computer or a requisition (Fig. 17–2).

Patient

The apparatus that is attached to the patient may be an internal attachment, such as a pin, tongs, or wires placed directly into the bone by the surgeon, or an external attachment, such as a halter, belt, or boot. The external apparatus is applied to the patient by the nursing staff, and it sometimes requires the health unit coordinator to order the necessary supplies from the central service department.

Although the kinds of supplies the health unit coordinator orders vary among hospitals, moleskin tape, slings, and sandbags are commonly requisitioned from the central service department. Some hospitals have designated floors for the treatment of patients with orthopedic conditions and who have traction orders.

☑ DOCTORS' ORDERS FOR TRACTION

Traction Orders for Treatment of Bone Fractures

There are two main types of traction: *skin traction* and *skeletal traction*. Skin traction uses 5- to 7-lb weights attached to the skin to indirectly apply the necessary pulling force on the bone. When traction is temporary, or if only a light or discontinuous force is needed, then skin traction is the preferred treatment. Weights are attached either through adhesive or nonadhesive tape, or with straps, boots, or cuffs. Below are examples of doctors' orders for traction that include both types of traction used in the hospital. Illustrations and explanations are provided to assist you in interpreting the orders.

Skeletal traction orders

Cervical traction c̄ Crutchfield tongs
Cervical traction used in the treatment of fractures of the cervical vertebrae. Crutchfield tongs are inserted into the skull bone, and the traction apparatus is applied to the tongs. Other devices used for cervical traction are Gardner-Wells tongs and Vinke tongs. A special bed or Stryker frame may need to be obtained for the patient.

Thomas' leg splint c̄ Steinmann pin 20 lb of traction
This set up is used in the treatment of a fractured hip, femur, or lower leg (see Fig 17–1). A Steinmann pin is driven through the femur or tibia during surgery, and the traction apparatus is applied to the pin. A Thomas splint is frequently used with a Pearson attachment. The doctors' order for these types of external fixator pins may also include nursing treatment orders for care of the pin sites.

Doctor Ordering_____

☐ Stat ☐ Routine ☐ ASAP

Today's Date_____ Requested by_____

| **Orthopedic Equipment** |

Diagnosis_____

Comments:_____

☐ Bucks traction_____
☐ Cervical traction_____
☐ Traction by gravity_____
☐ Skin traction_____
☐ Overhead frame and trapeze
☐ Braun frame
☐ Write-in order_____

FIGURE 17–2 ▲ Computer ordering screen for orthopedic equipment.

Communication and Implementation of Traction Orders

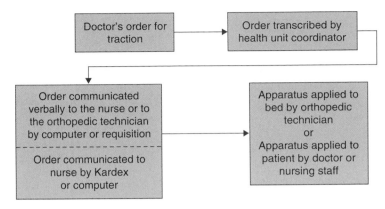

Traction by gravity lt arm
Applies to fractures of the upper limb (hanging cast).

Skin traction orders

Skin traction 5 lb to left arm
Skin traction uses 5- to 7-lb weights attached to the skin to indirectly apply the necessary pulling force on the bone. The doctor may give additional directions regarding positioning.

Skin traction 7 lbs to pelvis
Pelvic traction is applied to the lower spine, with a belt around the waist. This procedure is noninvasive and is the preferred treatment if traction is temporary, or if only a light or discontinuous force is needed. Weights are usually attached through moleskin tape, or with straps, boots, or cuffs.

Left unilateral Buck's traction 5 lb
A traction set up used as temporary treatment of a fractured hip, for sciatica, or for other knee and hip disorders (may also be called Buck's extension). Unilateral indicates that the traction is to be applied to one leg only; bilateral leg traction indicates that the traction is to be applied to both legs. Traction is produced by applying regular or flannel-backed adhesive tape to the skin and keeping it in smooth close contact by circular bandaging of the part to which it is applied. The adhesive strips are aligned with the long axis of the arm or leg, the superior ends being about one inch from the fracture site. Weights sufficient to produce the required extension are fastened to the inferior end of the adhesive strips by a rope that is run over a pulley to permit free motion. (Fig. 17–3).

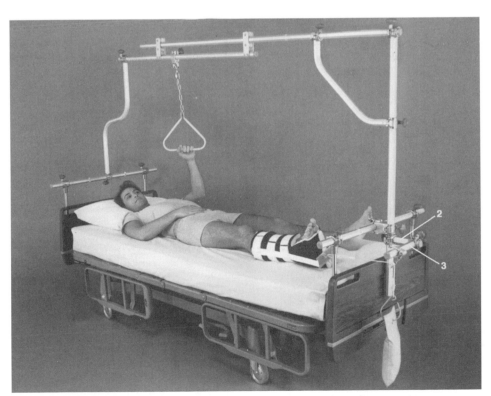

FIGURE 17-3 ▲ Unilateral Buck's traction with overhead frame and trapeze.

Doctor Ordering _____
Date to be done _____ ☐ Stat ☐ Routine ☐ ASAP
Today's Date _____ Requested by_____

| **Respiratory Care Department Treatments** |

Clinical Indication _____

Comments: _____

☐ O₂ _____ L/M   ☐ NP   ☐ Mask   ☐ Tent   ☐ Other_____
☐ SVN _____
☐ CPT _____
☐ IPPB _____
☐ Incentive spirometry _____
☐ USN _____
☐ HA _____
☐ Bi PAP _____
☐ CPAP _____
Write-in order_____

Ventilator orders
IMV mode _____ TV_____ FIO₂_____ PO₂_____ PS_____ Peep_____

Write-in order _____

FIGURE 17–4 ▲ Computer ordering screen for respiratory care treatment.

Other Traction-Related Orders

Overhead frame and trapeze

The overhead frame and trapeze is used by the patient for assistance in moving while in bed (see Fig. 17–3).

Braun frame

This is merely a cradle for the limb but a disadvantage is that the position of the pulleys cannot be altered. The pull is exerted against an opposing force provided by the weight of the body when the foot of the bed is raised.

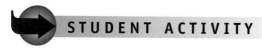

STUDENT ACTIVITY

To practice transcribing traction orders, complete Activity 17–1 in the *Skills Practice Manual*.

■ RESPIRATORY CARE DEPARTMENT

Background Information

The diagnostic tests performed in the Respiratory Care Department were discussed in Chapter 16. In this chapter, treatments ordered by the doctor that are related to the function of the respiratory system will be discussed. The treatments are performed at the patient's bedside by a respiratory therapist. It is important that the health unit coordinator enter all of the information regarding the order into the computer or onto the requisition form. The respiratory therapist will then bring the needed equipment and medication to the unit and will not have to delay the patient's treatment by having to return to obtain necessary items. The therapist will usually read the doctor's order before administering the treatment. Upon completion of the treatment, the therapist records the type of medication and treatment and other pertinent data on a respiratory therapy record sheet on the patient's chart.

To communicate the doctor's order to the respiratory care department, use the computer or complete a respiratory care requisition (Fig. 17–4).

☑ Doctors' Orders for Respiratory Care

Listed below are examples of doctors' orders for the types of treatments performed by the respiratory care department. Explanations and illustrations are provided to promote familiarity with an interpretation of the orders. The orders are written as you may find them on the doctors' order sheet.

O₂ 4 L/min NC cont

Oxygen is piped into the patient's room via a wall outlet. Oxygen is administered under pressure and may have a drying effect upon the respiratory tract; therefore, oxygen is commonly humidified during administration. Oxygen supports combustion; therefore, no smoking is allowed in the room while oxygen is being administered. Most hospitals and other health care facilities have a no smoking policy.

An oxygen order contains the amount of oxygen (flow rate or concentration) the patient is to receive and the type of delivery device (mode of delivery). The flow rate is ordered in liters per minute. In the above order, the flow rate is 4 L/min.

Nasal cannula, frequently referred to as nasal prongs, is a popular method used for oxygen administration. Nasal catheter

Communication and Implementation of
Respiratory Care Treatment/Therapy Orders

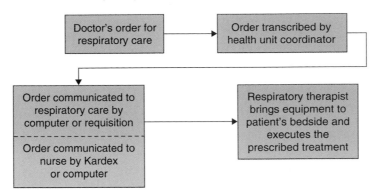

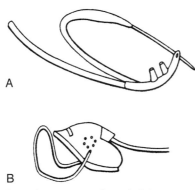

FIGURE 17-5 ▲ Apparatus used to administer oxygen. *A,* Cannula.
B, Mask.

and mask are two other methods also used for the administration
of oxygen (Fig. 17-5).

Plastic tubing is used to carry the oxygen from the wall
outlet to the patient. Although the respiratory care department
personnel usually set up, take down, and handle the equipment for oxygen administration, the nursing staff also monitors
this treatment.

Oxygen tent 40% O₂

The oxygen tent is another method used for administration of
oxygen to the patient. It is used mostly for pediatric patients.

IPPB c̄ 3 cc saline qid

An intermittent positive-pressure breathing (IPPB) machine is
used to administer this treatment order. This treatment is used to
improve ventilation, to help remove secretions from the lungs, to
administer aerosol medications, and for various other reasons
(Fig. 17-6).

The preceding order includes many instructions for the respiratory therapist. It is very important to be accurate in copying
the order onto the respiratory therapy requisition or entering it
into the computer.

IPPB 0.5 mL Ventolin & 3 mL NS tid

This IPPB order includes medication Ventolin and dosage
(0.5 mL). IPPB orders must include frequency and medication;
duration and pressure used may be optional.

The respiratory care department provides any medication
used during treatment. The names of other medications commonly used for IPPB treatments are Vaponefrin, Mucomyst,

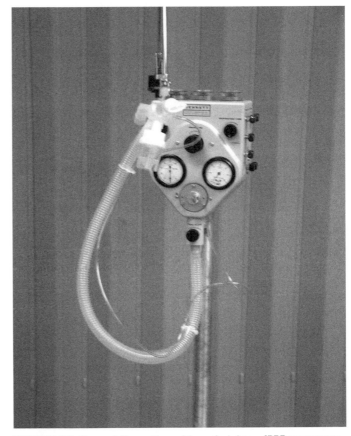

FIGURE 17-6 ▲ A Bennett machine administers IPPB treatments.

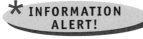
★ INFORMATION ALERT!

Orders for oxygen therapy include the amount of oxygen (flow rate
or concentration) and the type of delivery device.

It is important to recognize a new order for oxygen or a
change in a previous order. An ABG on O₂ @ 4 L/min is *NOT* a new
order for oxygen, but is an arterial blood gas drawn while the patient's oxygen flow rate is at 4 liters per minute. It may be necessary to notify nursing staff or respiratory care of the oxygen
flow rate.

Bronkosol, terbutaline (Monovent), Alupent, albuterol (Ventolin), and Atrovent.

SVN with UD Ventolin tid

This small-volume nebulizer (SVN) order includes a unit dose of Ventolin.

SVN 0.5 cc Bronkosol with 2.5 cc NS qid

This treatment uses a simple device that produces an aerosol from liquid medication to be inhaled into the lungs.

Hypertonic USN for sputum inducement

An ultrasonic nebulizer is used for this treatment. It produces an aerosol that carries further into the airways of the lung to loosen secretions so that the patient may produce a sputum specimen. The solution used is a hypertonic (concentrated) salt solution of 5% sodium chloride (NaCl). This is called an "induced sputum specimen."

A Lukens sputum trap is often used by a respiratory therapist to collect a sterile induced sputum specimen (Fig 17–7).

CPT

Chest physiotherapy includes vibration and percussion, which are hand or mechanical techniques used to loosen secretions within the lung. This treatment is performed in conjunction with postural drainage, a treatment of patient positioning designed to remove secretions from the lung.

Mechanical ventilator

Settings:

Intermittent mechanical ventilation (IMV) mode: resp. rate 8–14
Tidal volume (TV): 10–15 cc/kg ideal body weight
Fracture of inspired oxygen (FIO_2): 0.40–0.60 (initial FIO_2 0.60 to achieve PO_2 32–45, and pH 7.35–7.45)
Pressure support (PS): 10

and/or

Positive end-expiratory pressure (PEEP): 5 (may be added to achieve desired parameters of ABGs/O_2 saturation)

This is an example of a doctors' order to place the patient on a mechanical ventilator, or to provide parameters for a patient already placed on a ventilator. The ventilator assists or replaces respiration of the patient. Servo 900C, PB-840, Drager Evita 4, and Galileo are types of ventilators that may be used for this purpose. You may see these terms included in a doctors' order for mechanical ventilation (Fig. 17–8). Weaning is a term to describe the gradual removal of mechanical ventilation from a patient. ABG will be ordered at intervals on the patient to monitor ventilator settings. Extubation orders will be written when the patient is to be removed from the ventilator. Postextubation orders will be written after the patient has been removed from the ventilator to monitor their respiratory status.

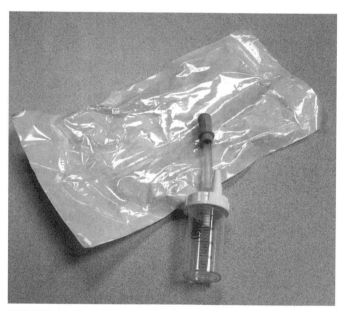

FIGURE 17–7 ▲ A Lukens sputum trap used to collect uncontaminated sputum specimens.

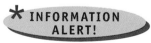
★ INFORMATION ALERT!

The health unit coordinator needs to notify the respiratory care department when the doctor writes an order for an induced sputum specimen. An SVN or hypertonic USN treatment is given by a respiratory therapist to loosen lung secretions. A Lukens trap is often used by a respiratory therapist to collect a sterile sputum specimen.

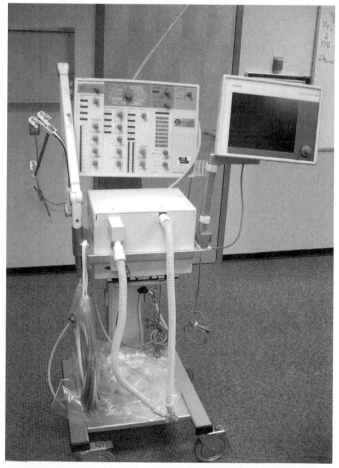

FIGURE 17–8 ▲ A ventilator. (From Ignatavicius DD, Workman ML, Mishler MA: Medical-Surgical Nursing: A Nursing Process Approach, 2nd ed. Philadelphia: WB Saunders, 1995.)

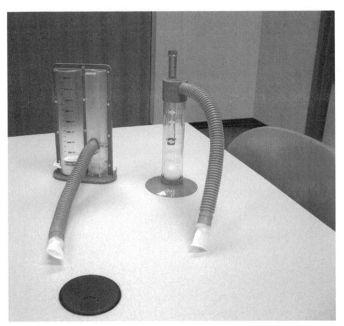

FIGURE 17–9 ▲ Examples of incentive spirometry. (From Ignatavicius DD, Workman ML, Mishler MA: Medical-Surgical Nursing: A Nursing Process Approach, 2nd ed. Philadelphia: WB Saunders, 2002.)

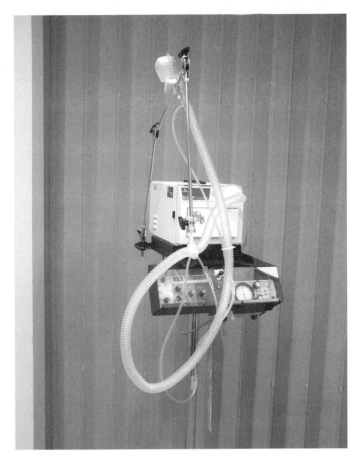

FIGURE 17–10 ▲ BiPa. (From Ignatavicius DD, Workman ML, Mishler MA: Medical-Surgical Nursing: A Nursing Process Approach, 2nd ed. Philadelphia: WB Saunders, 1995.)

HA @ 60% via T-piece

A heated mist (heated aerosol) is produced for the patient to breathe in. It may be ordered for patients who are breathing through a tracheostomy or endotracheal tube.

Incentive spirometry tid (IS)

This technique is often used postoperatively to encourage patients to breathe deeply. Various devices are used (Fig. 17–9).

IS c̄ PEP @ 5 cm H₂0

This incentive spirometry treatment includes positive expiratory pressure (PEP), which supplies resistance against exhalation (keeps air from coming out) in order to reinflate the alveoli in patients with atelectasis. PEP may also be ordered with SVN treatments.

BiPAP I:10 E:5

Biphasic positive airway pressure is a treatment that uses a machine to push air into the lungs during inspiration (such as an IPPB) and expiration (such as CPAP) in order to treat severe atelectasis or sleep apnea (Fig. 17–10).

CPAP 5 cm H₂0

This continuous positive airway pressure treatment provides continuous positive pressure in the airway throughout the entire respiratory cycle. This prevents the lungs from completely returning to resting level, and may be used to treat sleep apnea and other respiratory syndromes. It also can be used in weaning patients from a mechanical ventilator.

MDI c̄ Ventolin qid 111 puffs

MDI is a metered dose inhaler in which the medication is premeasured in the pharmacy.

Respiratory therapy to do pre-op teaching

The respiratory therapist will instruct the patient before surgery about incentive spirometry and other respiratory treatments that the doctor will order to be done after surgery. The patient will then know what to expect and will know what is expected of him or her in the performance of the respiratory treatments.

Respiratory therapy to do CPR training with parents before child's discharge

The respiratory therapist is sometimes asked to teach parents cardiopulmonary resuscitation CPR before a pediatric patient's discharge.

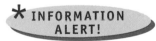

✱ INFORMATION ALERT!

Common medications administered via the respiratory tract are Vaponefrin, Mucomyst, Bronkosol, terbutaline (Monovent), Alupent, albuterol (Ventolin), and Atrovent.

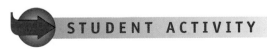

STUDENT ACTIVITY

To practice transcribing respiratory care orders, complete Activity 17–2 in the *Skills Practice Manual*.

■ PHYSICAL MEDICINE AND REHABILITATION

Most hospitals have a physical medicine department consisting of physical therapy, occupational therapy, and speech therapy.

Physical Therapy

Background Information

Physical therapy is the division of the physical medicine department in the hospital that treats patients to improve and restore their functional mobility by methods such as gait training, exercise, water therapy, and heat and ice treatments. Patients include those injured in accidents, sports, or work-related activities. Children affected by cerebral palsy and muscular dystrophy are assisted toward normal physical development through physical therapy. Individuals who suffer strokes, spinal cord injuries, and amputations are assisted back to their highest level of physical function through therapy.

The physical therapist (PT), a person licensed to practice in this field, evaluates the patient and initiates a plan of care. Physical therapy treatments may be carried out in the patient's room or in the physical therapy department by the physical therapist or by the physical therapy assistant (PTA). The physical therapist will read the order before administering the treatment. The phys-

ical therapy assistant may perform certain treatment tasks as directed by the physical therapist. Following treatment, the physical therapist records the treatment and other pertinent data to be included in the patient's chart.

To communicate the order to the physical therapy division, use the computer, or complete a physical therapy requisition form (Fig. 17–11).

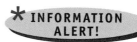

☑ DOCTORS' ORDERS FOR PHYSICAL THERAPY

Below are examples of doctors' orders for physical therapy. Brief descriptions and illustrations are included to assist you with interpreting the orders.

∗ INFORMATION ALERT!

Two common errors that occur when reading doctors' orders is in interpreting the abbreviation "PT." It may be an order for physical therapy, or an order for a prothrombin time, which is a coagulation study (see Chapter 14). PT can also be confused with patient as in the order PT to ambulate daily, which could be interpreted as patient (pt.) to ambulate daily rather than physical therapy (PT) to ambulate the patient daily. It is important to fully understand doctors' orders during transcription.

Doctor Ordering _____

Date to be done _____ Time to be done _____

Today's Date _____ Requested by _____

| Physical Therapy |

Clinical Indication _____

Transportation ☐ portable ☐ stretcher ☐ wheelchair ☐ ambulatory

O₂ ☐ yes ☐ no   Diabetic ☐ yes ☐ no

IV ☐ yes ☐ no   Seizure disorder ☐ yes ☐ no   Hearing deficit ☐ yes ☐ no

Isolation ☐ yes ☐ no   Non-English speaking ☐ yes ☐ no   Sight deficit ☐ yes ☐ no

Comments: _____

☐ CMP _____
☐ Crutch training _____
☐ ES _____
☐ Exercises _____
☐ Evaluation _____
☐ Hot packs _____
☐ Hubbard tank _____
☐ ROM _____
☐ Shortwave diathermy _____
☐ TENs _____
☐ Ultrasound c̄ massage _____
☐ Whirlpool _____
☐ Write-in order _____

FIGURE 17–11 ▲ Computer ordering screen for physical therapy.

Communication and Implementation of Physical Medicine Orders

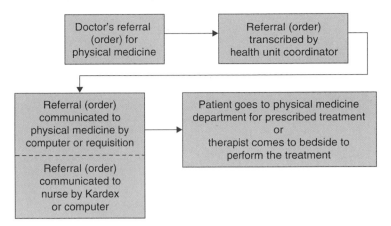

Hydrotherapy Orders

Hubbard tank 30 min qd T 100° F, active underwater exercises to elbows and knees c̄ débridement

This treatment is used for underwater exercises and for cleansing wounds and burns (Fig. 17–12). Hydrotherapy treatments may be ordered to be done with a sterile solution. The physical therapy department will select an appropriate substance to use.

Whirlpool bath LLE bid

The whirlpool is smaller than the Hubbard tank. It is used for the same purposes (Fig. 17–13).

Exercise Orders

Passive, active, resistive, reeducation, coordination, and relaxation are other types of exercises that may be ordered by the doctor.

AA exercise lt shoulder and elbow daily

Active assisted exercises would involve the patient moving an extremity with assistance from the physical therapist as required.

ROM bid to UE

Range-of-motion exercises are frequently ordered for bedridden patients and therefore are usually performed in the patient's room. These exercises involve moving each joint of the upper extremities to the maximum in each direction.

PROM BLE bid

This passive range-of-motion exercise of both lower extremities would require the physical therapist to move each joint of both lower extremities the maximum distance in each direction.

Joint mobilization to lt shoulder bid

The physical therapist will mobilize (stabilize) the patient's left shoulder.

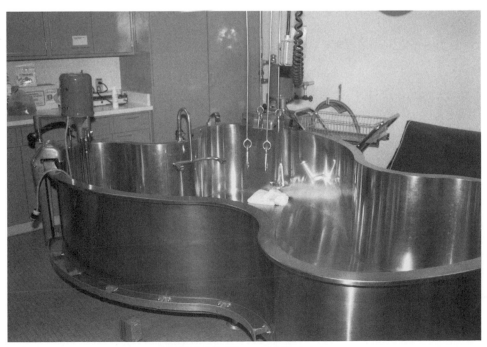

FIGURE 17–12 ▲ Hubbard tank.

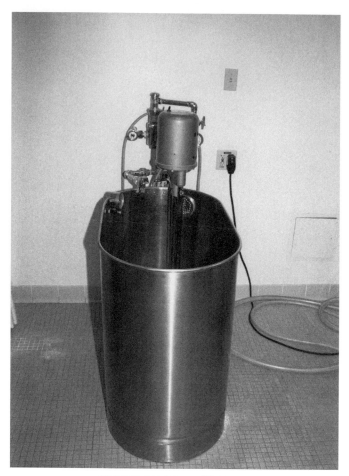

FIGURE 17-13 ▲ Whirlpool.

Strengthening of all four extremities

The physical therapist will evaluate the patient and recommend a series of exercises to strengthen the patient's extremities. The physical therapy assistant (PTA) may help the patient with the exercises.

PT to amb pt with walker as tol

The physical therapy department often decides which equipment is best suited for the patient. For this order the physical therapist would assist the patient in using a walker for walking as tolerated.

PT to eval and treat

PT to evaluate and treat is the most common order written by the doctor. The physical therapist will evaluate the patient and initiates a plan of care.

ACL protocol per Dr. Melzer

Many physicians have preprinted courses of treatment (protocols) on file with the physical therapy department, which are implemented throughout the patient's stay (precluding any complications). These programs of treatment include clinical pathways and goals, and are often named after the orthopedic surgery performed on the patient. Familiarity with orthopedic surgical procedures and abbreviations is helpful. An anterior cruciate ligament (ACL) protocol would follow an ACL repair.

Dr. Jen's BKA protocol

This preprinted protocol is for rehabilitation after a below-the-knee amputation. Another physician's protocol may be different.

THA and TKA protocols

Many physician's have preprinted orders to be used when their patients have a total hip arthroplasty or total knee arthroplasty. The protocol is followed by the physical therapy personnel.

Transfer training, wheelchair mobility

The physical therapist teaches the patient how to transfer from the bed to the wheelchair and how to use the wheelchair; usually ordered for patients who have had an amputation, stroke, or other physical disability.

Gait training with a walker, WBAT LLE

To carry out this order, the physical therapist would train the patient to walk using a walker with weight bearing for the left lower extremity as tolerated. Additional devices such as crutches and different types of canes may be used in patient ambulation.

Crutch walking NWB daily

The physical therapist instructs the patient to walk with crutches. Variations to this order may be noted regarding the amount of weight bearing (such as full weight), any precautions to take, or the type of crutch walking to teach the patient (such as 4-point gait). Additional variations in the amount of weight bearing may be included in the doctor's order.

CPM 0%–45%, progress to 0%–90% by day 5

A continuous passive motion machine is used after joint replacement or total knee arthroplasty. It may be monitored by the physical therapist or by the nursing staff (Fig. 17–14). Additional motion orders may include active assistive range of motion

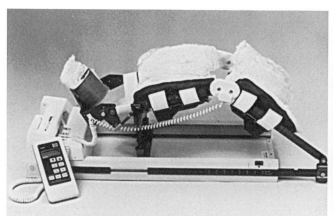

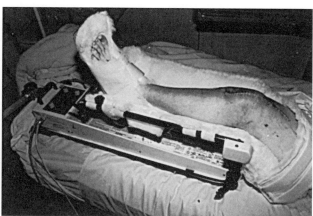

FIGURE 17–14 ▲ Continuous passive motion (CPM) machines. (From Ignatavicius DD, Workman ML, Mishler MA: Medical-Surgical Nursing: A Nursing Process Approach, 2nd ed. Philadelphia: WB Saunders, 1995.)

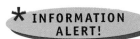

INFORMATION ALERT!

Ultrasound diagnostic procedures are performed in the ultrasound division of diagnostic imaging (see Chapter 15).

An ultrasonic nebulizer is used as a treatment by the respiratory department. An ultrasound treatment is performed by physical therapy. It is important to carefully read the doctor's orders so that the order is sent to the appropriate department.

(AAROM), active range of motion (AROM), and passive range of motion (PROM) (Fig. 17–14).

T-band exercises
These are exercises using a band of rubber, or a theraband for resistance.

Codman's exercises rt shoulder
These exercises for the shoulder are also called pendulum exercises.

Isometrics BUE (bilateral upper extremities)
Isometric exercises flex muscles without allowing actual movement of the limb. This order is performed on both upper extremities.

Heat and Cold Orders

- *Ultrasound and massage to lower back*
- *Hydrocollator packs or hot packs to back bid*
- *Ice or cold packs to left leg bid*

Pain Relief Orders

Post-op TENS
Transcutaneous electrical nerve stimulation (TENS) is used to control pain by blocking transmission of pain impulses to the brain. Electrodes are applied to the skin surrounding the incision during surgery. Thin wires lead from the electrodes to a powered stimulator with a control. Usually the patient is taught before surgery how to use the device. For nonsurgical use, the physical therapist attaches the external electrodes to the skin (Fig. 17–15).

FES or ES
Functional electrical stimulation or electrical stimulation may be used to reduce pain or swelling, promote healing, or assist in exercising muscles. Different types of machines are used to deliver this treatment.

Hyperbaric Oxygen Therapy

Hyperbaric oxygen therapy is defined as breathing 100% oxygen while in an enclosed system pressurized to greater than one atmosphere (sea level). Hyperbaric oxygen therapy delivers oxygen quickly and in high concentrations to injured areas systemically. The increased pressure changes the normal cellular respiration process and causes oxygen to dissolve in the plasma. This stimulates the growth of new blood vessels and a substantial increase in tissue oxygenation that can arrest certain types of infections and enhance wound healing. Hyperbaric oxygen therapy is generally administered on an outpatient basis.

- *Hyperbaric oxygen therapy bid 3 × wk for 8 weeks*

Other Physical Therapy Orders

Apply foam cervical collar
A foam cervical collar is applied to the patient's neck.

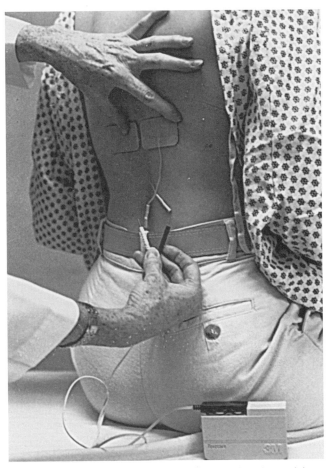

FIGURE 17–15 ▲ TENS unit for pain control. (From Ignatavicius DD, Workman ML, Mishler MA: Medical-Surgical Nursing: A Nursing Process Approach, 2nd ed. Philadelphia: WB Saunders, 1995.)

Use abduction pillow between legs during treatment
An abduction pillow is placed between patient's legs. The pillow is designed to help patients recuperate from hip surgery with minimal discomfort while providing protection from hip dislocation.

Apply knee immobilizer to lt knee
A knee immobilizer is used to stabilize the knee after injury or surgery.

Note: These orders are often included in physical therapy orders or may be performed by nursing personnel.

Occupational Therapy

Background Information

Occupational therapy is the division of the physical medicine department in the hospital that works toward rehabilitation of patients, in conjunction with other health team members, to return the patient to the greatest possible functional independence. Creative, manual, recreational, and prevocational assessment are examples of activities used in rehabilitation of the patient. Occupational therapy activities are ordered by the doctor and administered by a qualified occupational therapist or an occupational therapy technician. To communicate the order to the occupa-

Doctor Ordering _____
Date to be done _____ Time to be done _____
Today's Date _____ Requested by _____

| **Occupational Therapy** |

Clinical Indication _____
Transportation ☐ portable ☐ stretcher ☐ wheelchair ☐ ambulatory

O₂ ☐ yes ☐ no   Diabetic ☐ yes ☐ no
IV ☐ yes ☐ no   Seizure disorder ☐ yes ☐ no   Hearing deficit ☐ yes ☐ no
Isolation ☐ yes ☐ no   Non-English speaking ☐ yes ☐ no   Sight deficit ☐ yes ☐ no

Comments: _____

☐ ADL
☐ Evaluation and treatment as needed
☐ Increase mobility
☐ Supply and train in adaptive equipment (e.g., Use ADL button hooks and feeding utensils)
☐ Write-in order_____

FIGURE 17-16 ▲ Computer ordering screen for occupational therapy.

✱ INFORMATION ALERT!

Examples of basic skills to be achieved as a result of occupational therapy include toileting, bathing, dressing, cooking, and feeding oneself.

tional therapy division, use the computer or complete an occupational therapy requisition form (Fig. 17–16).

☑ DOCTORS' ORDERS FOR OCCUPATIONAL THERAPY

- *OT for evaluation and treatment if needed daily*
- *ADL training*
- *Supply and train in adaptive equipment such as button hooks and feeding utensils for ADL*
- *OT to increase mobility*
- *Fabricate cock-up splint for left upper extremity*

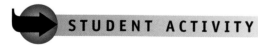

STUDENT ACTIVITY

To practice transcribing physical medicine and rehabilitation orders, complete Activity 17–3 in the *Skills Practice Manual.*

✱ INFORMATION ALERT!

Physical therapy, occupational therapy, and speech therapy are utilized to improve and restore function, and/or increase independence to the patient. Restorative programs may be run out of nursing homes and physical medicine and rehabilitation centers.

■ DIALYSIS

The kidneys are essential organs in the removal of toxic wastes from the blood. When the kidneys fail to remove those wastes, medical intervention is necessary to sustain life. The kidneys may fail temporarily (acute renal failure), or they may be permanently damaged and become nonfunctional (chronic renal failure and end-stage renal disease [ESRD]). There are two main types of dialysis: hemodialysis and peritoneal dialysis.

Hemodialysis (also called extracorporeal dialysis) is the removal of waste products from the blood by the utilization of a machine through which the blood flows. This is regularly performed in a special outpatient dialysis facility, and is commonly done for 3- to 4-hour periods 3 days a week. For the hospitalized patient, hemodialysis is usually performed in a special unit in the hospital. If the patient is too ill to be moved, a portable hemodialysis machine may be used.

Peritoneal dialysis is the introduction of a fluid (dialyzing fluid) into the abdominal cavity that then absorbs the wastes from the blood through the lining of the abdominal cavity, or peritoneum. The dialysate is then emptied from the abdominal cavity. This type of dialysis allows for a greater level of freedom for the patient, as he or she may perform this fluid transfer outside of any health care facility. Some variations of peritoneal dialysis include continuous ambulatory peritoneal dialysis (CAPD), continuous cycling peritoneal dialysis (CCPD), and intermittent peritoneal dialysis (IPD).

☑ DOCTORS' ORDERS FOR DIALYSIS

Hemodialysis 3 × wk for 2 hours
The patient will have hemodialysis for 2 hours per session three times a week.

Consent for Tenckhoff catheter placement for peritoneal dialysis
This procedure is surgical placement of a long-term catheter or tube into the patient's abdomen so that they are able to perform peritoneal dialysis.

Consent for A-V shunt

Hemodialysis requires vascular access. This surgical procedure inserts a cannula into an artery, as well as one into a vein. These are both then connected to tubing that allows for easier needle insertion necessary for hemodialysis.

■ RADIATION TREATMENTS

The area in the hospital where radiation therapy is performed may be a division of the diagnostic imaging department, or it may be a totally separate department.

Many of those undergoing radiation therapies are outpatients. However, the health unit coordinator may be called upon to schedule an appointment for an inpatient that requires treatment for a malignant neoplasm (cancer). Many hospitals require the units to use a requisition form, and others may schedule an appointment by telephone. After the initial visit, radiation therapy usually notifies the nursing unit of the patient's treatment schedule.

STUDENT ACTIVITIES

For practice transcribing the following types of orders, complete the following activities in the *Skills Practice Manual:*

- To practice recording a review set of doctors' orders, complete Activity 17–4.
- To practice recording telephoned doctors' orders, complete Activity 17–5.
- To practice recording telephone messages, complete Activity 17–6.

■ SUMMARY

The transcription of treatment orders involves the communication of the order to the necessary department by computer, or by requisition form and the communication of the order to the nursing staff by the kardexing step of the transcription procedure. Professionals in their respective departments then execute the orders.

▼ REVIEW QUESTIONS

1. State the purpose of each of the following hospital departments:

   a. respiratory care department

   _____

   b. physical therapy department

   _____

   c. occupational therapy department

   _____

2. List the two main types of traction.

   a. _____

   b. _____

3. List four purposes of traction.

   a. _____

   b. _____

   c. _____

   d. _____

4. State the purpose of an overhead frame and trapeze.

   _____

5. Various types of treatments are listed in column 1, including treatments performed by the nursing staff. Write the health care personnel from column 2 that would usually perform each of the treatments.

Column 1

a. IPPB _____

b. SSE _____

c. USN _____

d. ACL protocol _____

e. O₂ _____

f. SVN _____

g. P&PD _____

h. ADL _____

i. IV therapy _____

j. urinary catheterization _____

k. ROM _____

l. K-pad _____

m. whirlpool _____

n. TENS _____

o. MDI _____

p. gait training _____

q. CPT _____

Column 2

Physical Therapy

Respiratory Care

Occupational Therapy

Nursing

6. Define *dialysis*.

_____

7. Two types of dialysis are:

a. _____

b. _____

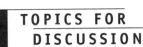
TOPICS FOR DISCUSSION

1. Discuss why it is important to list all of the information regarding a respiratory order when communicating the order to the respiratory department.
2. Discuss why the respiratory therapist should read the doctor's order before administering a treatment.
3. Discuss the reasoning for the patient's chart accompanying the patient when going to the physical therapy department for treatment.

4. Discuss solutions for keeping charts from being scattered and/or taken without your knowledge by personnel from ancillary departments (e.g., physical therapy, occupational therapy, respiratory therapy).

Miscellaneous Orders

Chapter Objectives

Upon completion of this chapter, you will be able to:

1. Define the terms in the vocabulary list.

2. Write the meaning of each abbreviation in the abbreviations list.

3. List seven points of information that should be communicated to the consulting physician's office when transcribing a consultation order.

4. List three reasons why a doctor may wish to transfer a patient to another hospital room.

5. List six tasks the health unit coordinator may have to perform when arranging for a patient to leave the hospital on a pass.

6. Name eight services rendered by the social service department.

7. Identify discharge, transfer, and miscellaneous orders.

Vocabulary

Consultation Order ▲ A request by the patient's attending physician for the opinion of a second physician with respect to diagnosis and treatment of the patient

Discharge Order ▲ A doctor's order that states the patient may leave the hospital. A doctors' order is necessary for a patient to be discharged from the hospital

Microfilm ▲ A film containing a greatly reduced photo image of printed or graphic matter

Transfer Order ▲ A doctor's order that requests a patient to be transferred to another hospital room

Abbreviations

Abbreviation	Meaning	Example of Usage on a Doctor's Order Sheet
appt	appointment	Make appt with dental clinic
disch	discharge	Disch today
DME	durable medical equipment	Contact DME supplier for hospital bed for home
DNR	do not resuscitate	DNR
NINP	no information, no publication	Pt. requests NINP
Rx	take (treatment, medication, etc.)	Disch c̄ Rx
wk	week	Disch see me next wk

EXERCISE 1

Write the abbreviation for each term listed below.

1. appointment _____

2. discharge _____

3. durable medical equipment _____

4. do not resuscitate _____

5. week _____

6. take (treatment, medication, etc.) _____

7. no information, no publication _____

EXERCISE 2

Write the meaning of each abbreviation listed below.

1. *appt*

_____

2. *disch*

_____

3. *DME*

_____

4. *DNR*

_____

5. *wk*

_____

6. *Rx*

_____

7. *NINP*

_____

■ CONSULTATION ORDERS

Background Information

The attending physician may want to have the opinion of another doctor regarding the diagnosis and treatment of a patient. The request for another doctor's opinion is written on the doctors' order sheet by the patient's doctor and is called a consultation order.

The transcription process for consultation orders usually requires the health unit coordinator to notify the consulting doctor's office of the order. Prepare for the call to the doctor's office or answering service by writing the doctor's telephone number on a note pad and having the patient's chart in front of you so you have access to any additional requested information. When calling the doctor's office, insurance information will be requested. If the doctor's office is closed and the consult is called to his or her answering service, the doctor's secretary will call back for insurance information. It is important to document the time of notification and the name of the person or operator number (answering service) you spoke to. Write this information next to the doctors' order on the doctors' order sheet with your initials. Some hospitals may have a policy requiring the requesting doctor to notify the specialist so he or she may provide patient history and additional information.

The following information should be communicated to the consulting doctor's office:

■ Hospital name
■ Patient's name and age
■ Patient's location (unit and room number)
■ Name of the doctor requesting the consultation
■ Patient's diagnosis
■ Urgency of consultation and any additional information provided in order
■ Patient's insurance information located on the patient's fact sheet

After interviewing and evaluating the patient, the consulting doctor will usually dictate his or her findings and recommendations, a hospital medical transcriptionist will type the consultation report, send it to the nursing unit, and the health unit coordinator will file the report in the patient's chart (Fig. 18–1).

☑ DOCTORS' ORDERS FOR CONSULTATION

Doctors' orders for consultation may be expressed in writing on the doctors' order sheet as follows:

▪ *Have Dr. Avery see in consult*
▪ *Call Dr. Reidy for consultation*
▪ *Call Dr. Casey to see patient re radiation therapy*
▪ *Have Dr. Williams see patient today please*

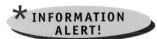
✱ INFORMATION ALERT!

Document the time called and the name or operator number of the person you spoke to when calling a specialist for consultation. Write this information next to the doctors' order on the doctors' order sheet with your initials.

Date of consultation: 01/17/04

Name of cosultant: John P. Rhine, MD

History: This 17-year-old woman was seen in consultation with her mother regarding problems referable to her nose. The patient has had progressive problems of congestion and sniffing, with difficulty moving air through her nose and sensation of pressure. She is a "mouth breather," and has history of allergy to pollens and dust. Patient feels these problems are becoming more severe. Her complaints are fairly consistent.

Examination: She presents with edema of her nasal mucosa, increase in the size of the turbinates, deviation of the nasal septum, and a rather narrow nasal airway.

Diagnosis:
1. Probable allergic rhinitis with hypertrophy of the turbinates.
2. Deviated nasal septum.
3. Narrow, inadequate nasal airway.

Comments:
1. I have discussed with this patient and with her mother the surgical approach to improving her nasal airway with septoplasty, and possible submucous resection of deviated portions of the septum, and possible reduction of the inferior turbinates. At the same time I would be performing a rhinoplasty procedure to smooth out the dorsal nose as well.
2. Because of the history of allergies to pollens, dust, and environmental pollutants, it is quite possible the patient will continue to have some sniffing, and consequently, the degree of improvement of her nasal airway with surgery cannot be precisely determined.

_____

J. P. Rhine, MD

DD:
DT:
jpr/ct

FIGURE 18-1 ▲ Dictated and typed consultation report.

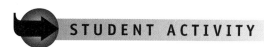

STUDENT ACTIVITY

To practice transcribing a consultation order, complete Activity 18-1 in the *Skills Practice Manual.*

■ HEALTH RECORD ORDERS

Background Information

The health records department, also called medical records or health information management department, stores the charts of patients who have been treated at the health care facility in the past. Usually records from recent hospital admissions will be sent to the unit upon readmission of a patient. The doctor may request records that have been microfilmed and are stored in the health records department. The request is put in writing on the doctors' order sheet by the patient's doctor and is called a health records order.

The order for the microfilmed record is communicated to the health records department either by telephone or by computer by the health unit coordinator. Health records personnel will print a hard copy of the microfilmed record and send it to the nursing unit. While old records are on the nursing unit, they are stored in an envelope labeled with the patient's identification label in a designated area rather than in the current patient's chart holder.

The doctor may also request medical records from the patient's previous stay in another hospital. Because this information is confidential, the patient must give written permission for release of the information from one hospital to another. To transcribe a doctor's order to obtain health records from another hospital, the health unit coordinator places a call to the health records department of the other hospital to request records and initiates a consent form (Fig. 18–2) for the nurse to have the patient sign. When signed, this form may be faxed to the health records department in the other hospital and the requested records may then be faxed to the nursing unit. The faxed records are kept on the nursing unit until the patient is discharged and then are sent to health records with the current chart.

☑ *DOCTORS' ORDERS FOR HEALTH RECORDS*

Doctors' orders for health records may be expressed in writing on the doctors' order sheet as follows:
- *Old charts from admission 5 years ago to floor*
- *Obtain old charts from all previous admissions*
- *Obtain report on total body CT scan from St. Joseph's Hospital (done 2/28/00)*

AUTHORIZATION TO OBTAIN MEDICAL INFORMATION

DATE _1/11/XX_

TO: _Memorial Hospital_   RE. _Marilee Owens_
(NAME OF PATIENT)

1100 Ash St.
(ADDRESS)

Phoenix

_7/7/XX_
(BIRTHDATE)

THE ABOVE NAMED PERSON IS NOW A PATIENT IN THIS HOSPITAL UNDER THE CARE OF
DR. _Roosevelt Conklin_

WE WERE INFORMED THAT THIS PATIENT WAS IN YOUR INSTITUTION ON OR ABOUT
March 10-15 19XX

WOULD YOU PLEASE SEND US A TRANSCRIPT OF ~~HIS~~ HER MEDICAL RECORD AS SOON AS POSSIBLE? WE ARE PARTICULARLY INTERESTED IN THE FOLLOWING REPORTS.

_____HISTORY AND PHYSICAL EXAMINATION

_____OPERATION REPORTS

_____CONSULTATIONS

_____X-RAY REPORTS

_____LABORATORY REPORTS

_____PATHOLOGY REPORTS

__X__ DISCHARGE SUMMARY

__X__ OTHER REPORTS
CT Brain

THANK YOU FOR YOUR COOPERATION

SINCERELY YOURS,

KINDLY ADDRESS YOUR REPLY
ATTENTION OF
MEDICOLEGAL SECRETARY
MEDICAL RECORD DEPARTMENT

DIRECTOR
HEALTH RECORDS SERVICES

I HEREBY AUTHORIZE _Memorial Hospital_ TO GIVE TO THIS HOSPITAL A COPY OF MY HOSPITAL RECORDS OR ANY INFORMATION WHICH MAY HAVE BEEN ACQUIRED IN THE COURSE OF MY EXAMINATION OR TREATMENT.

Marilee Owens
(SIGNATURE OF PATIENT)

_1/11/XX_
(DATE)

FIGURE 18–2 ▲ Consent form to obtain records from another hospital.

Communication and Implementation of Health Record Orders

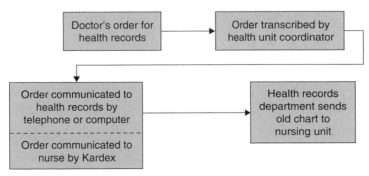

STUDENT ACTIVITY

To practice transcribing a health records order, complete Activity 18-2 in the *Skills Practice Manual*.

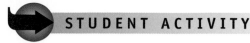

STUDENT ACTIVITY

To practice transcribing an order for case management, complete Activity 18-3 in the *Skills Practice Manual*.

■ CASE MANAGEMENT ORDERS

Background Information

Case management is a nursing care delivery model in which RN case managers coordinate the patient's care to improve quality of care while reducing costs. The case manager interacts on a daily basis with the patient, patient's family, health care team members, and the payer representatives. Case management is not needed for every patient and is usually requested for the chronically ill, seriously ill or injured, and long-term high-cost cases. Case managers act as a patient's advocate in getting the home health services that best suit the patient's needs and coordinate financial coverage through private insurers such as Medicare.

A patient with a life-limiting illness can frequently benefit from the services of Hospice. Hospice is a multidiscipline organization that stresses a holistic approach to care of patients during their final stage of life. The Hospice team comprises a physician, nurses, certified nursing assistants, social workers, a chaplain, and volunteers. Most hospice care can be rendered in the patient's home, although there are hospice units in some hospital and freestanding hospice facilities. The doctor may write orders requesting a case manager to access and prioritize the patient's needs, identify and coordinate available resources, arrange for home care, arrange admission to a long-term care facility, or arrange for hospice.

☑ *Doctors' Orders for Case Managers*

- *Case management for health assessment*
- *Case management to arrange home care with patient's family for discharge in 2 days*
- *Case management to arrange hospice care*

■ SOCIAL SERVICE DEPARTMENT ORDERS

Background Information

Social service provides much-needed information concerning resources available to patients and their families as they transition from the health care facility back to their home. Social workers provide many of the same services as case managers and may also work as case managers. Social workers assist in solving patients' care-related financial matters, transportation home, meals for families staying at the hospital and for in-home meals for patients after discharge, teachers for long-term pediatric patients, living arrangements for families staying with patients, finding custodial care for patients, and support for abuse victims.

☑ *Doctors' Orders for the Social Services Department*

- *Contact family re: plans to place in custodial care facility*
- *Arrange for home-bound teacher for 1 month*
- *Social worker to call child protective services to evaluate home situation*
- *Have social worker evaluate patient's home caregivers*
- *Have social worker arrange for family to stay at Ronald McDonald House*

■ SCHEDULING ORDERS

Background Information

Frequently, while the patient is in a health care facility, the doctor may write an order to schedule the patient for various types of tests or examinations performed in specialized departments or outside of the health care facility.

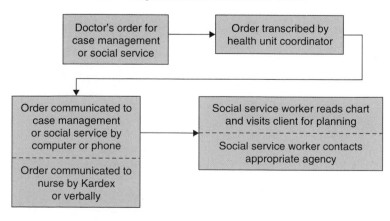

Communication and Implementation of Case Management and Social Service Orders

Communication and Implementation of
a Doctor's Order that Requires Scheduling

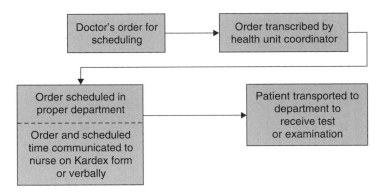

It is the health unit coordinator's task to notify the department or facility that performs the test or examination and schedule a time convenient to both the involved department and the patient. It is important to record the scheduled time on the patient's Kardex form.

☑ DOCTORS' ORDERS THAT REQUIRE SCHEDULING

Below are examples of doctors' orders that require scheduling. These vary greatly among health care facilities, according to the services available.

- *Schedule pt in outpatient department for vaginal examination*
- *Schedule pt for psychological testing*
- *Schedule pt for diabetic classes*
- *Schedule pt for hearing evaluation test*
- *Schedule appt. for dental clinic for evaluation and care*

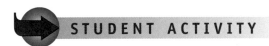
STUDENT ACTIVITY

To practice transcribing an order to schedule an examination, complete Activity 18–4 in the *Skills Practice Manual*.

■ TEMPORARY ABSENCES (PASSES TO LEAVE THE HEALTH CARE FACILITY)

Some long-term patients on rehabilitation units may be allowed to leave for 4 to 10 hours. Patients receive many benefits from visiting their homes or experiencing a recreational outing. A gradual return to society has therapeutic value for rehabilitating patients. A temporary pass requires the health unit coordinator to do the following:

- arrange with the pharmacy for medications the patient is taking
- note on the census when the patient leaves and returns
- cancel meals for the length of the absence
- cancel any hospital treatments for the length of the absence
- arrange for any special equipment that the patient may need
- provide the nurse with a temporary absence release to have the patient sign (Fig. 18–3)

☑ DOCTORS' ORDERS FOR TEMPORARY ABSENCE

- *May have pass for tomorrow from 9 AM to 7 PM*
- *Temporary hospital absence from 8 AM to 6 PM Friday; arrange for rental of wheelchair*
- *May leave hospital from 10 AM to 1 PM today; have patient sign release*

Communication and Implementation of Temporary Absence Orders

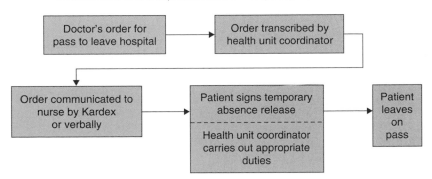

TEMPORARY ABSENCE RELEASE

The undersigned, being a patient of The Above Named Hospital, hereby confirms his (or her) agreement and understanding that neither the hospital, its employees, nor the attending physicians shall be responsible for his (or her) care or condition during any absences of the undersigned from the building or resulting from such absences.

Signed _____
PATIENT / PARENT / GUARDIAN

Date _____

Hour _____

Witness _____

09-0366   **TEMPORARY ABSENCE RELEASE**

FIGURE 18–3 ▲ Temporary absence release form.

■ TRANSFER AND DISCHARGE ORDERS

If the doctor plans to transfer the patient to another room or another unit, or to discharge the patient to his or her home or to another facility, the doctor writes an order for such on the doctors' order sheet.

To transcribe a transfer or discharge order, the health unit coordinator must notify the hospital admitting department (or discharge department) by telephone or computer, or by completing a discharge or transfer slip.

Discharge orders may include information such as instructions for the patient to follow after he or she leaves the hospital, requests for appointments for the patient, and so forth.

The doctor may request a transfer of a patient for various reasons, such as for a different type of room accommodation (to private room), or for more intense nursing care (regular unit to ICU) or less intense nursing care (ICU to regular unit). Another reason for a transfer is if the patient's condition requires that he or she be placed in an isolation room.

The procedures for transferring and discharging a patient are covered in Chapter 20. This section deals only with the transcription procedures for a transfer or discharge order.

☑ DOCTORS' ORDERS FOR TRANSFER OR DISCHARGE OF A PATIENT

Below are examples of how discharge or transfer orders may be expressed by the doctor on the doctors' order sheet.

Transfer
- *Transfer patient to 3E please*
- *Transfer patient to a private room*
- *Transfer patient to ICU after surgery*
- *Transfer patient out of ICU to a medical unit*

Discharge
- *Home today*
- *Discharge p̄ chest x-ray*
- *Home c̄ Rx*
- *Home make appt to see me in 2 wk*
- *Home c̄ crutches*

■ MISCELLANEOUS ORDERS

There are orders that do not relate to any department that are nevertheless deserving of mention. All should be kardexed in their appropriate places. A few of the orders appear below.

- *No visitors, limited number of visitors, or have visitors c̄ nurse before seeing pt*

A sign should be posted on the patient's door to see the nurse for further explanation. The switchboard and information desk should also be notified.

- *DNR (do not resuscitate) or no code*

This order means that no resuscitative measures are to be performed. A do not resuscitate may be requested by a patient upon admission. The order must be written on the patient's chart. A verbal request by a patient or a patient's family is not legal. This order is not a complete refusal of care, simply that a resuscitation code should not be performed in the event of cardiac or respiratory arrest. If the physician writes an order for "do not resuscitate," the order should be visible on the Kardex and on the patient's chart. Some hospitals have DNR forms that specify extent of resuscitative measures to be taken. This information is placed in the front of the patient's chart. The DNR order must also be written on the patient's order sheet by his or her doctor.

- *NINP (no information, no publication)*

Your hospital may use a different abbreviation, but whatever words or abbreviations are used, this order means that the unit personnel denies having the patient when asked by visitors in person or by telephone. This order may also be extended to include family members. Often a code phrase or word is used for persons excluded from this restriction.

- *Notify Dr. Avery of pt's adm. to ICU*

This order is to inform the patient's primary physician of the admission of the patient to the intensive care unit when another physician has admitted the patient.

- *Notify hospitalist (covered in Chapter 2) if systolic BP >190*

This order is to notify the hospitalist if the patient's systolic blood pressure is above 190.

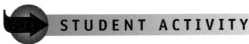

STUDENT ACTIVITY

To practice transcribing a review set of doctors' orders, complete Activity 18–5 in the *Skills Practice Manual*.

■ SUMMARY

This chapter has discussed a variety of doctors' orders. It concludes the transcription practice for all classifications of doctors' orders. Transcribing doctors' orders is a major health unit coordinator task. Repeated performance is necessary to gain expertise in this area.

As you begin transcribing doctors' orders on the nursing unit of the hospital, you will find it helpful to use the transcription procedures presented in this textbook as a reference.

Communication and Implementation of Transfer and Discharge Orders

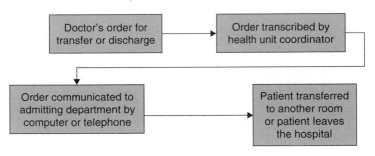

REVIEW QUESTIONS

1. Define the following terms:

   a. transfer order

   _____

   b. discharge order

   _____

   c. consultation order

   _____

2. You are planning to call a doctor's office to notify him or her of a consultation request. You must first gather seven points of information to communicate to the consulting physician's office. These seven points of information are:

   a. _____

   b. _____

   c. _____

   d. _____

   e. _____

   f. _____

   g. _____

3. The doctor may request to transfer a patient to another hospital room because:

   a. _____

   b. _____

   c. _____

4. List six tasks the health unit coordinator may need to perform for a patient having a 10-hour pass:

   a. _____

   b. _____

   c. _____

   d. _____

   e. _____

   f. _____

5. Two services that the case manager may perform for the hospitalized patient are:

   a. _____

   b. _____

6. Which department would assist when a patient is a victim of abuse?

   _____

7. List eight services rendered by the social service department:

   a. _____

   b. _____

   c. _____

   d. _____

   e. _____

   f. _____

   g. _____

   h. _____

8. Can a patient or a patient's family member verbally request that a DNR status be put into practice?

   _____

TOPICS FOR DISCUSSION

1. Discuss why it is so important to document the time of call and the person's name or operator number you spoke to when calling a consultation to a doctor's office or to an answering service.

2. Discuss why documenting the name of the person you receive any report or message from or give a report or message to is so important.

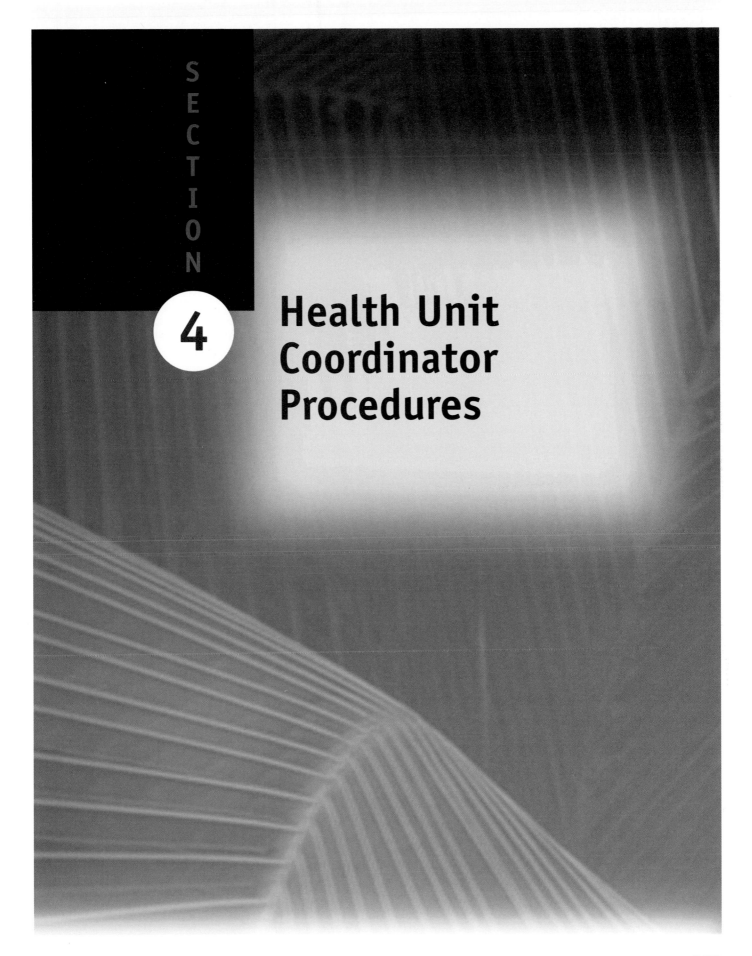

4

Health Unit Coordinator Procedures

Admission, Preoperative, and Postoperative Procedures

> ## Chapter Objectives

Upon completion of this chapter, you will be able to:

1. Define the terms in the vocabulary list.
2. Write the meaning of each abbreviation in the abbreviations list.
3. List eight common components of a set of admission orders.
4. List at least five health unit coordinator tasks regarding the patient's admission.
5. Name three items prepared by the registration department that are sent to the unit as part of the admission procedure.
6. List three types of admission.
7. List at least eight registration tasks.
8. Describe the process for securing patient valuables.
9. Explain the health unit coordinator's responsibilities regarding the preoperative patient's orders and the patient's chart.
10. List seven components that may be a part of a set of preoperative orders.
11. List five records or reports that may be on the patient's chart prior to the patient's surgery.
12. List nine components that may be a part of a set of postoperative orders.
13. List at least three tasks the health unit coordinator may perform concerning the postoperative patient's chart and Kardex.
14. Explain the advance directives options.

> ## Vocabulary

Admission Day Surgery ▲ Surgery in which the patient enters the hospital the day of surgery; it may be called same-day surgery or AM admission

Admission Orders ▲ Written instructions by the doctor for the care and treatment of the patient upon entry into the hospital

Admission Service Agreement or Conditions of Admission Agreement ▲ A form signed upon the patient's admission that sets forth the general services that the hospital will provide; it may also be called the conditions of admission, contract for services, or treatment consent

Advance Directives ▲ Documents that indicate a patient's wishes in the event that the patient becomes incapacitated

Allergy Identification Bracelet ▲ A plastic band with a cardboard insert on which allergy information is printed or a red plastic band that has allergy information written directly on it that the patient wears throughout the hospitalization

Allergy Information ▲ Information obtained from the patient concerning his or her sensitivity to medications and/or food

Blood Transfusion Consent ▲ A patient's written permission to receive or refuse blood or blood products

Census ▲ A list of all occupied and unoccupied hospital beds

Direct Admission ▲ A patient who was not scheduled to be admitted and is admitted from the doctor's office, clinic, or emergency room

Elective Surgery ▲ Surgery that is not emergency or mandatory and can be planned at a time of convenience

Emergency Admission ▲ An admission necessitated by accident or a medical emergency; such an admission is processed through the emergency department

Facesheet ▲ A form initiated by the admitting department included in the inpatient medical record, which contains personal and demographic information, usually computer generated at the time of admission (may also be called the information sheet or front sheet)

Health Records Number ▲ The number assigned to the patient on or before admission; it is used for records identification and is used for all subsequent admissions to that hospital (may also be called medical records number)

Informed Consent ▲ The duty to inform a patient before obtaining a signature of permission (discussed in Chapter 6, pp. 80, 89)

Living Will ▲ A declaration made by the patient to family, medical staff, and all concerned with the patient's care stating what is to be done in the event of a terminal illness; it directs the withholding or withdrawing of life-sustaining procedures

Observation Patient ▲ A patient who is assigned to a bed on the nursing unit to receive care for a period of less than 24 hours; may also be referred to as a medical short-stay or ambulatory patient

Patient Account Number ▲ A number assigned to the patient to access insurance information, usually a unique number is assigned each time the patient is admitted to the hospital

Patient Identification Bracelet ▲ A plastic band with a patient identification label affixed to it, which is worn by the patient throughout hospitalization. In the obstetrics department, the mother and baby would have the same identification label affixed to their ID bracelets

Postoperative Orders ▲ Orders written immediately after surgery. Postoperative orders cancel preoperative orders

Power of Attorney for Health Care ▲ The patient appoints a person (called a proxy or agent) to make health care decisions should the patient be unable to do so

Preadmit ▲ The process of obtaining information and partially preparing admitting forms prior to the patient's arrival at the health care facility

Preoperative Health Unit Coordinator Checklist ▲ A checklist used by the health unit coordinator to ensure that the patient's chart is ready for surgery

Preoperative Nursing Checklist ▲ A checklist used to ensure the chart and the patient are properly prepared for surgery

Preoperative Orders ▲ Orders written by the doctor before surgery to prepare the patient for the surgical procedure

Registrar ▲ The admitting personnel who registers a patient to the hospital

Registration ▲ The process of entering personal information into the hospital information system to enroll a person as a hospital patient and create a patient record; patients may be registered as inpatients, outpatients, or observation patients

Scheduled Admission ▲ A patient admission planned in advance; it may be urgent or elective

Surgery Consent ▲ A patient's written permission for an operation or invasive procedure

Surgery Schedule ▲ A list of all the surgeries to be performed on a particular day; the schedule may be printed from the computer or sent to the nursing unit by the admitting department

Valuables Envelope ▲ A container for storing the patient's jewelry, money, and other valuables, which are placed in the hospital safe for safekeeping

Abbreviations

Abbreviation	Meaning	Example of Usage on a Doctor's Order Sheet
Dx	diagnosis	Dx: anemia
H & P	history and physical	H & P by surgical resident
Hx	history	Resident will do Hx
MSSU	medical short-stay unit	Admit to: MSSU
NKA	no known allergies	Allergies: NKA
OBS	observation	Pt to stay for 2 hrs for OBS
OPS	outpatient surgery (ambulatory surgery)	Send pt to OPS
post-op	after surgery	TCDB q2h post-op
pre-op	before surgery	Call Valley Anesthesia for pre-op orders
SSU	short-stay unit	Pt to remain in SSU for 2°

EXERCISE 1

Write the abbreviation for each term listed below.

1. history and physical _____

2. medical short-stay unit _____

3. after surgery _____

4. observation _____

5. diagnosis _____

6. history _____

7. no known allergies _____

8. before surgery _____

9. outpatient surgery _____

10. short-stay unit _____

EXERCISE 2

Write the meaning of each abbreviation listed below.

1. OPS

_____

2. pre-op

_____

3. NKA

_____

4. Hx

_____

5. Dx

_____

6. OBS

_____

7. post-op

_____

8. MSSU

_____

9. H & P

_____

10. SSU

_____

■ ADMISSION OF THE PATIENT

As a health unit coordinator, your role in the admission procedure is a very important one. You are the first person the new patient encounters on the nursing unit, which will be his or her "home" for several days or longer. You have an opportunity at this time to demonstrate the caring nature of the hospital by greeting the patient warmly and making him or her feel welcome. There may be instances when the health unit coordinator has the responsibility of admitting the patient.

Your ability to perform tasks in an efficient manner enables the health care team to provide, as soon as possible, the care and treatment ordered for the patient.

Types of Admissions

A person may become a hospital patient in a variety of ways. Types of admissions are discussed in the following sections.

Scheduled or planned admissions are admissions that are called into the admitting department before the patient arrives. Patients enter the hospital through the admitting department and are admitted to the service of their primary doctor. Scheduled admissions may be further classified as urgent, direct, or elective. Urgent or direct admissions occur when a doctor sees a patient in his or her office, decides that person should be admitted to the hospital, and calls the hospital to arrange the admission. Another example of a direct admission is a pregnant woman going to the hospital and after evaluation by a doctor, is immediately admitted to labor and delivery. Admission of a patient transported by ambulance or helicopter from another health care facility such as an extended care facility would also be called a direct admission.

Elective scheduled admissions occur when the patient and the doctor elect when to schedule a nonemergency surgery or procedure. Patients may be admitted to the nursing unit on the day before their surgery/procedure or on the day their surgery/procedure is scheduled and will be admitted to a nursing unit after surgery/procedure. A list of scheduled admissions may be available to print from the computer or may be sent to each nursing unit from the admitting department early in the day allowing the nursing unit to plan for the admissions.

Emergency admissions are unplanned and are the result of an accident, sudden illness, or other medical crisis. Patients enter the hospital through the emergency department. These patients are processed through the emergency department and are referred to as emergency admissions. The emergency department personnel prepare an emergency department record (Fig. 19–1). Often old records from the patient's prior admissions are requested from health records if the patient has had previous admissions. Should the patient's condition warrant that he or she remain in the hospital, the patient will be admitted to a nursing unit. The emergency department record is sent to the nursing unit with the patient and placed in the patient's medical record. The patient's old records should also be sent to the nursing unit with the patient and stored on the unit until the patient is discharged or transferred. The health unit coordinator reviews the emergency department record to see if all requested tests have been completed. For example, the emergency room doctor may have ordered a urinalysis, but the patient may not have voided yet. If the tests have not been completed, the health unit coordinator processes those that remain to be done.

EMERGENCY ROOM

MEDICAL RECORD NO. 1	567-435		MED SERVICE Orth	FINANCIAL CL 7	DATE 8 5/23/XX		SOC SEC NO /MEDICARE NO 527-48-XXXX		
PATIENT NAME 2 Lowrey	LAST	Holly FIRST		MIDDLE Elinor		HOSPITALIZATION INSURANCE - 1 Sunstate		POLICY/GROUP NO 100-0000

| PATIENT'S PERMANENT ADDRESS 10001 North Mountain, | CITY Sky, | STATE AZ | ZIP 85000 | TEL 942-XXXX | ADDRESS 2222 N.Tower Pl. Sky, AZ | | POLICY/GROUP NO |
| PATIENT'S TEMPORARY ADDRESS | CITY | STATE | ZIP | TEL | HOSPITALIZATION INSURANCE 2 | | POLICY/GROUP NO |

BIRTHDATE 5/3/XX	AGE 22	HAS PATIENT EVER BEEN TREATED IN THIS HOSPITAL	☐ INPATIENT ☐ OUTPATIENT	WHEN _____ UNDER WHAT NAME _____	ADDRESS	
SEX ☐ MALE ☒ FEMALE	MARITAL STATUS ☐ SINGLE ☒ MARRIED ☐ WIDOWED	☐ SEPARATED ☐ DIVORCED	RACE ☐ WHITE ☒ BLACK ☐ OTHER	☐ INDIAN ☐ ORIENTAL	RELIGION ☐ CATHOLIC ☐ JEWISH	☐ PROTESTANT ☒ OTHER	EFFECTIVE DATE : 1 1/06/XX	EFFECTIVE DATE : 2
							INDUSTRIAL PATIENT'S EMPLOYER ☐ YES ☒ NO	

RESPONSIBLE PARTY NAME 3 SELF		RELATIONSHIP	TEL	ADDRESS		TEL
ADDRESS STREET PO BOX APT NO CITY 4	5	STATE	ZIP 6	RELATIVE NOTIFIED		
SPOUSE OR NEAREST RELATIVE (NEXT OF KIN) Iris Lowrey		RELATIONSHIP Mother	TEL 943-XXXX	TIME 1800	BY WHOM M. Loor	
ADDRESS STREET PO BOX APT NO CITY 211 E. Sun Dr. Sky, AZ		STATE	ZIP 85000	POLICE NOTIFIED		
E R PHYSICIAN Thomas V. Riggs		ATTENDING PHYSICIAN B. Urself		TIME 1730	BY WHOM M. Loor	

EVENTS AND CARE GIVEN PRIOR TO ARRIVAL

Pt. states she was involved in an auto accident 10am to-day - no loss of consciousness - Complaint of pain Right shoulder - right knee - 3 inch lac. to left cheek area - abrasion R hand

CHIEF COMPLAINT

VITAL SIGNS									
TEMP 98⁴	(ORAL) (RECTAL) P 88	R 24	BP 130/80						

ALLERGIES *Codeine*

	ADMIT	EXAM	CALLED	CALLED	CALLED	CONTACTED	ARRIVED		LAB	X RAY 5³⁰p	DISCHG	HOME	ADMIT TO ROOM
INITIAL								CALLED				DR OFF	
TIME	5pm							SPEC TAKEN				OTHER	
LAST TETANUS July 1971	PHYSICIANS NAME B. Urself		5⁴⁵p 5⁵⁵p				6¹⁰p 7pm	RESULTS OBY				WORK	

| BROUGHT IN BY (NAME OF PERSON OR AMBULANCE) Associated ambulance | MEDICAL EXAMINER | DISPOSITION OF VALUABLES to husband | NURSES SIGNATURE Mable Jones RN |

ORDERS	HISTORY: PHYSICAL FINDINGS & TREATMENT
	S. ↓ Rom ✓ R SHOULDER
1. CERVICAL - X TABLE 1ST	2° TO PAIN
2. SKULL	Obj 1. US - STABLE
3 R SHOULDER (done m/)	2. HEAD ① PERLA, EOM's, disc normal
R KNEE	② EAR'S - NO BLOOD
R HAND	③ Ū CRANIAL NERVE SENSATION L=R
4. 1% LIDOCAINE	4. 3" lac FACE
4-0 - NYLON WHITE	3. NECK - SUPPLE
6-0 NYLON - BLACK	4 CHEST - GOOD EXPANSION
done m/ abrasions, laceration cleansed c̄ betadine sol'n dressed c̄ neosporin, dry, dressing.	LUNGS CLEAR P
	5. ABD - GOOD BS, NO HS MESLY, NO TENDERNESS, REBOUND OR REFERRED PAIN.
	6 EXT - R SHOULDER - ECHYMOSIS, ↓ ROM
	R KNEE - CONTUSION + ABRASION
	R-HAND - ABRASION
	7 XRAYS - SKULL, CERVICAL, R SHOULDER - NEG
FINAL DIAGNOSIS A/A, laceration ABRASION + CONTUSION	CODE
FINAL DISPOSITION · DESCRIBE PLAN /HEAD SHEET - STIRRUPS OUT - 4 DAYS ICE T	
SIGNATURE OF E R PHYSICIAN Thomas V. Riggs MD	SIGNATURE OF ATTENDING PHYSICIAN

00-2912 1/77

MEDICAL RECORDS

FIGURE 19-1 ▲ Emergency department record.

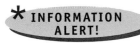

Some emergencies require that a patient receive treatment before being registered by the admitting department. The patient may be unconscious without identification and taken to an intensive care unit. An example is a child that is a near-drowning victim transported by ambulance from a public swimming pool or lake. The health unit coordinator must request that the child be given an alias name, assigned a health record number by the admitting department so tests may be ordered and lab specimens sent. When the patient's family arrives, they are sent to admitting so the patient can be admitted and the correct name will then be entered in the computer. If an invasive procedure or surgery were immediately required to save the life of a patient who is unable to sign an informed consent and has no family present, two medical doctors would sign the consent.

Types of Patients

Patients receiving medical care may also be categorized as to type. Patient type may be categorized according to purpose and length of hospitalization. The three patient types are inpatient, observation patient, and outpatient.

An inpatient is a patient who is admitted to the hospital for longer than 24 hours and assigned to a bed on the nursing unit. A health unit coordinator will prepare a chart and process orders for the patient.

An observation patient is a patient who is assigned to a bed on a nursing unit to receive care for a period of less than 24 hours. An observation patient may also be referred to as a medical short-stay or ambulatory patient. Some hospitals may have a specific unit such as a medical short-stay unit (MSSU) or ambulatory care unit to provide short-term care. If the patient requires further hospital care beyond 24 hours, the doctor must write an order for hospital admission. The criteria for observation patients vary from facility to facility. A health unit coordinator may prepare a chart and process orders for the observation patient. It may be the health unit coordinator's task to monitor the time and notify the nurse that the patient needs to be discharged or an order obtained for admission.

An outpatient is a patient receiving care in a hospital, clinic, or surgicenter but not admitted or staying overnight. An outpatient is usually scheduled to receive treatments, therapies, or tests. The department providing care for the outpatient will process the outpatient's orders. Usually the assembly of a chart is not required, although there may be patients that receive outpatient services on a routine basis that do require a chart.

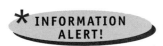

Types of Service

Service type refers to the type of nursing unit (see Chapter 3, "Hospital Nursing Units," pp. 33–34). The patient may also be classified as a teaching or nonteaching patient, indicating whether residents or other health care students will be involved in the patient's care. Patients may be classified according to the type of insurance as well (i.e., Medicare, PPO, HMO, etc.).

Admission Arrangement

In all types of admissions, a doctor with admitting privileges to the hospital must authorize the patient's admission. The attending doctor, the doctor's staff, or the staff of a health maintenance organization acting on instructions of the doctor arranges for the admission of patients. The doctor provides the admitting diagnosis or medical reason for admission. After admission, a hospitalist may be overseeing the patient's care during the hospital stay.

Bed Assignment

Most hospitals are open for admissions 24 hours a day. The admitting department or registration staff performs many tasks in relation to the admission of the patient to the hospital. Most hospitals will have a computerized census in the hospital information system that provides an accurate, up-to-date list of occupied and unoccupied hospital beds. Nursing unit assignments for scheduled admissions are usually determined in advance. A list of scheduled patient admissions may be made available on the computer or may be printed and sent to each nursing unit receiving patients. Nursing assignments are usually determined for scheduled admissions in the morning. Direct admissions or emergency admissions will be assigned beds when the patient arrives at the hospital and is ready for a room. The admitting diagnosis usually determines the type of nursing unit that is suitable and the nursing staff usually determines the specific bed. In many hospitals, the staff on the nursing unit decides bed assignment. The nursing personnel are familiar with staffing and roommate issues and can best decide which bed is appropriate for the new patient. After receiving patient information such as name, diagnosis, age, and sex, the health unit coordinator or nurse may assign the bed number.

Patient Admission/Registration

Registration is the process of entering personal information into the hospital information system to register a person as a hospital patient and create a patient record. A registrar in the admitting department or health unit coordinator may perform the patient admission/registration responsibilities.

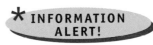

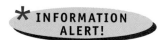

Performing the patient admission/registration tasks may be the responsibility of the health unit coordinator in some health care facilities.

Patient Admission/Registration Tasks

Patient admission/registration tasks include:

- Copy insurance cards
- Verify insurance (may be done in advance when admission is scheduled)
- Ask patient or patient guardian to sign appropriate insurance forms
- Interview patient or family to obtain personal information
- Prepare admission forms (admission service agreement and facesheet) and obtain signatures
- Ask patient if he or she has advanced directives or if he or she would like to create one (required in most states)
- Prepare patient's identification bracelet
- Prepare patient's identification labels
- Secure patient valuables if necessary
- Supply and explain required information including a copy of the hospital privacy laws as required by HIPAA and the *Patient's Bill of Rights*
- Include any test results, prewritten orders, or consents that have been previously sent to the admitting department in the packet that accompanies the patient to the nursing unit

Interview

When admissions are arranged in advance, such as for planned or elective surgery, preadmission information may be obtained by mail, phone, or by computer by the registration staff. This information, such as the patient's name, address, and telephone number; employer's name and address; insurance carrier; doctor's name and diagnosis; is placed on a record called the information sheet or facesheet (Fig. 19–2). If the patient information was not obtained previously, it is done at the time of admission.

Interview Techniques

When interviewing a patient to obtain personal information, it is imperative to utilize the interpersonal skills discussed in Chapter 5. Being admitted to the health care facility is a stressful situation and many patients may also be experiencing physical discomfort. The following guidelines should be observed when interviewing patients.

- Protect confidentiality.
- Ensure privacy when asking for personal information.
- Be proficient and professional.
- Asking if the patient was previously hospitalized can hasten the registration process and reduce the risk of error in as-

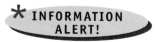

The patient registration tasks should be completed before orders can be processed for the patient unless there is a life-threatening emergency.

signment of health records and patient account numbers (demographics would need to be verified in case of possible changes).

- Treat each patient as an individual.
- Listen carefully.
- Project a friendly, courteous attitude.
- Include family or significant other in the process.

Admission Forms

The admission service agreement or conditions of admission agreement (COA or C of A) lists the general services that the hospital will provide. It is an agreement between the patient and the hospital and provides a legal consent for treatment (Fig. 19–3). This consent may specify financial responsibility also. The patient is to sign the form upon admission. Patients who are unable to sign a condition of admission may have a legal guardian sign for them. A copy of the admission service agreement is given to the patient after it is signed, and the original will become part of the patient's medical record.

The facesheet, front sheet, or information sheet is the form that is generated after the patient information, such as address, telephone number, nearest of kin, insurance carrier, and so on, is entered into the hospital information system. It is usually filed as the first page of the patient's medical record.

Routine admissions may have had tests performed before their admission. Test results are forwarded to the hospital admitting department and sent to the nursing unit with the other chart forms. Doctors may write orders or obtain consents in advance, which are also forwarded to the hospital admitting department and sent to the nursing unit upon admission.

At the time of admission or before admission each patient is assigned a health records number that is unique for that patient. The health records number identifies the patient and all chart forms and will be used for all future admissions to that hospital. The patient account number is assigned at the time of admission and is used to reference insurance information and is usually unique to each admission. The patient account number also serves to identify all charges for equipment, supplies, and procedures. The business office uses the patient account number for billing purposes.

Patient Identification Labels

Patient identification labels are self-adhesive labels used on the patient's identification bracelet, to identify forms, requisitions, specimens, and so on (see Chapter 8, p. 121). The patient identification labels are prepared by the registration staff entering the information into the computer and may then also be printed by staff on nursing unit through the computer.

Patient Identification Bracelet

An identification bracelet or band (Fig. 19–4) is prepared by the registration staff upon admission of the patient to the hospital. The bracelet is a plastic band with the patient's identification label affixed to it. The identifying information may consist of: (1) the patient's name, sex, age, and date of birth, (2) the patient's attending doctor's name, (3) the health records number, (4) the patient account number, (5) type of insurance (i.e., Medicare, PPO, HMO, and so on), (6) date of admission, and (7) assigned room number. Most hospitals have discontinued using the patient's Social Security number for confidentiality purposes. The health records number serves as the main identifier because it is a unique number assigned to

PATIENT HOSP.NO.(M.R.#)	INFO STATUS												ACCOUNT NO. (BUS. OFF.)
1 987-654													123-456

2	PATIENT NAME LAST	FIRST	MIDDLE	ADM. DATE MO. / DAY / YR.	ADM. TIME	HOW BROUGHT TO HOSPITAL
	Andrews	Iver	S.	8 / 7 / XX	1345	Amb.

3	PATIENT'S CURRENT ADDRESS STREET, P.O. BOX, APT. NO.	CITY	STATE	ZIP CODE	TELEPHONE NO.
	701 East Danish Lane	Carpenterville, AZ		85013	246-XXXX

4	PATIENT'S PERMANENT ADDRESS STREET, P.O. BOX, APT. NO.	CITY	STATE	ZIP CODE	TELEPHONE NO.
	Same				

5	SEX 1. MALE 2. FEMALE	MARITAL STATUS 1. SINGLE 4. DIVORCED 2. MARRIED 5. WIDOWED 3. SEPARATED	RACE 1. WHITE 4. ORIENTAL 2. BLACK 5. OTHER 3. INDIAN	RELIGION 3. PROTESTANT 1. CATHOLIC 4. OTHER 2. JEWISH 5. LDS	AREA OF RESIDENCE
	1	5	1	3	

6	BIRTHDATE	AGE	PLACE OF BIRTH	MAIDEN NAME	SOC. SEC. NO./MEDICARE NO.
	10/6/XX	69	N.J.		151-18-XXXX

7	PATIENT'S OCCUPATION	UNION & LOCAL NO.	PATIENT'S EMPLOYER	ADDRESS	TELEPHONE NO.
	Retired				

8	PREVIOUSLY TREATED HERE? ☒ YES ☐ NO	NAME USED Same		PREV. ADM. DATE 2/3/XX MO. DA. YR.	PREV. ADMISSION 1. INPATIENT 2. OUTPATIENT	1	IF NEWBORN, MOTHER'S HOSP. NO.

9	UNIT A5	ROOM NO.	ACCOM. CODES 1. PRI 3. NURSERY 5. ICU 7. CCU 2. SEMI 4. PREMIE 6. RCU 8. VIP	2	ROOM RATE	PAY STATUS	CLASS OF ADMISSION 1. EMERGENCY 3. URGENT 2. ELECTIVE 4. OTHER	3

10	ADMITTING DIAGNOSIS
	Cerebrovascular accident

11	PHYSICIAN NAME	PHYSICIAN NO.	ADM. SERVICE	INFORMATION OBTAINED FROM:
	I.M. Human	432	Med.	daughter

12	SPOUSE OR NEAREST RELATIVE (NEXT OF KIN)	RELATIONSHIP	ADDRESS	TELEPHONE NO.
	Kay Ellis	daugh	301 West Restful Dr. Phoenix	258-XXXX

13	SECOND RELATIVE OR FRIEND	RELATIONSHIP	ADDRESS	TELEPHONE NO.
	Marie Darrow	sister	12 Center St. Danstown, CA	837-XXXX

14	RESPONSIBLE PARTY NAME	RELATIONSHIP	SOC. SEC. NO.
	Self		

15	RESP. PARTY ADDRESS STREET P.O. BOX APT. NO.	CITY	STATE	ZIP CODE	TELEPHONE NO.

16	RESP. PARTY OCCUPATION	NO. YRS. IN THIS EMPLOY	RESP. PARTY EMPLOYER	ADDRESS	TELEPHONE NO.

17	LENGTH OF TIME IN ARIZ. 10 yrs.	1. OWN HOME 2. RENT HOME	1	TYPE OF HOME Single	BANK NAME & BRANCH Desert National - Camelhead	1. SAVINGS 2. CHECKING	1

18	CREDIT	1. NAME Deep River S&L	ADDRESS 9832 N. LasVegas Pl. Phoenix	TELEPHONE NO. 943-XXXX
19	REFERENCES	2. NAME Yucca Federal	ADDRESS 1903 W. Bottletree Ave. Phoenix	TELEPHONE NO. 246-XXXX

20	INDUSTRIAL INJURY	DATE: MO. DA. YR.	CLAIM NO.	EMPLOYER'S NAME AND ADDRESS AT TIME OF INJURY

21	BLUE CROSS	NAME OF PLAN	GROUP NO.	IDENTIFICATION	EFFECTIVE DATE MO. DA. YR.	CITY	STATE

22	CHAMPUS DATA	PATIENT'S ID NO.	CARD EFFECTIVE MO. DA. YR.	CARD EXPIRES ON MO. DA. YR.	PATIENT OR SPONSORS BRANCH OF SERVICE	SERVICE CARD NO.
23		SPONSORS NAME		RANK-SERVICE NO.	DUTY STATION	

24	OTHER INSURANCE (INC. BLOOD BANK & BLUE SHIELD)	INS. CO. NO. 1000	COMPANY NAME Desert State	POLICY HOLDER NAME Iver Andrews	POLICY NO. A657483	DATE ISSUED MO. DA. YR. 2/17/XX	CITY	STATE AZ
25		INS. CO. NO.	COMPANY NAME	POLICY HOLDER NAME	POLICY NO.	DATE ISSUED MO. DA. YR.	CITY	STATE

26	NAME OF HEALTH FACILITY DISCHARGED FROM WITHIN LAST 60 DAYS	ADDRESS
	None	

27	OTHER INFO.	V. A. ☐	COORDINATION OF BENEFITS ☐	INTERVIEWED BY G. Talker	TYPED BY W.K.S.

28 REMARKS:

FIGURE 19–2 ▲ Facesheet or front sheet.

that patient. The bracelet is worn throughout the patient's hospitalization. All personnel performing services for the patient must read the identification bracelet to ensure correct patient identification.

Patients' Valuables

Patients who have a large amount of money, expensive jewelry, or other items of value with them at the time of admission are requested to send them home with family or place them in the hos-

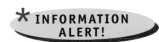
★ INFORMATION ALERT!

Most hospitals have discontinued using the patient's Social Security number on patient identification labels and identification bracelets for confidentiality purposes. The health records number serves as the main identifier because it is assigned to the patient and is unique to that patient. Information contained on patient ID labels may differ slightly among hospitals.

ADMISSION/SERVICE AGREEMENT

PRICE QUOTES: The undersigned understands that any price quotations given are estimates of expected services. The price quotes given do not include the patient's private physician's fees for services and are based on coverages which may vary significantly from actual charges based on physician treatment patterns, secondary or tertiary medical conditions and physicians' interpretations of Patient's private physician's order(s).

_____ **(Patient's initials)**

MONEY, VALUABLES, AND PERSONAL ITEMS: The Hospital has a safe in which money and valuables may be kept, if requested by Patient. **The Hospital will not be responsible for loss or damage to items not deposited in the safe, including personal items retained by the patient such as glasses, dentures, jewelry, hearing aids and contact lenses.**

At time of registration, the patient had these items:

[ ] glasses, [ ] dentures, uppers, [ ] dentures, lowers, [ ] hearing aid, right, [ ] hearing aid, left, [ ] cash $ _____

[ ] jewelry: _____

[ ] other: _____

MEDICARE PATIENTS: The undersigned certifies that the information given in applying for payment under title XVIII of the Social Security Act is correct. **Patient requests that payment of authorized benefits, when received, be made on Patient's behalf to the provider of healthcare services.** Patient authorizes release of any information needed to act on this request.

MEDICARE SECONDARY PAYOR:

[ ] I have provided the information needed for the "Medicare Secondary Payer" screening which is applicable to my hospitalization or hospital services covered by my Medicare health insurance.

MEDICARE - IMPORTANT MESSAGE FROM MEDICARE:

[ ] I acknowledge that I have been provided a copy of the notice entitled "An Important Message From Medicare" detailing my rights as a Medicare hospital patient and procedures for requesting a review by the Peer Review Organization in this area.

HMO MEDICARE - ADDENDUM TO IMPORTANT MESSAGE FROM MEDICARE:

[ ] I acknowledge that I have been provided a copy of the notices entitled "An Important Message From Medicare" and "Addendum to An Important Message From Medicare" detailing my rights as a Medicare hospital patient and procedures for requesting a review by the Peer Review Organization in this area.

PATIENT RIGHTS:

[ ] Copy of Patient Rights provided   [ ] Copy of Patient Rights received previously.

NON-MEDICARE NON-COVERED SERVICES

I have been informed that my insurance will likely deny payment for _____ because:

[ ] This visit/service has not been authorized by my insurance carrier.

[ ] This visit/service is not covered by my insurance. **Further, if payment is not made by my insurance carrier, I agree to be personally and fully responsible for payment.**

_____ **(Patient's initials)**

THE UNDERSIGNED CERTIFIES THAT (1) I HAVE READ AND UNDERSTAND THESE CONDITIONS OF ADMISSION, (2) I HAVE RECEIVED A COPY, AND (3) I AM THE PATIENT OR I AM DULY AUTHORIZED BY THE PATIENT AS PATIENT'S AGENT TO SIGN THIS AGREEMENT AND ACCEPT ITS TERMS.

Patient/Patient's Agent or Representative		Relationship to Patient
Date of Signing	Time of Signing	Witness

FIGURE 19–3 ▲ Admission service agreement; also called a _condition of agreement (C of A or COA)._

ADMISSION/SERVICE AGREEMENT

The patient, or the person acting for the patient, (hereinafter "I" or "Patient") agrees to the following terms of admission:

CONSENT TO TREATMENT: The undersigned understands that Patient is under the control of his/her attending physician, and Patient hereby consents to receive and pay for all medical treatment as ordered by the responsible physician(s), including x-ray, radiological examination, interpretive physician services, nursing services, technical services, laboratory procedures, emergency treatment and room and board services rendered under the general or special instructions of Patient's physician. I understand that Patient's attending physician, and all physicians who provide services to the Patient, are neither employees nor agents of the Hospital and are therefore solely responsible for their own treatment activities. Such physicians include consultants, radiologists, pathologists, cardiologists and anesthesiologists. I agree that the consent to treatment given herein shall be valid and continuing until Patient is finally discharged.

GENERAL DUTY NURSING: The Hospital provides only general duty nursing care. Nurses are called to the bedside by a signal system. The Hospital is not responsible for providing continuous or special duty nursing care. If Patient needs special or private nursing, then Patient or Patient's physician must arrange special nursing care for Patient. Patient hereby releases the Hospital from any and all liability which may arise from the fact that such care is not provided. Patient agrees that Hospital has no responsibility to continuously monitor the Patient's condition, except for physician-ordered special care situations arranged by Patient or Patient's physician.

TEACHING PROGRAMS: The Hospital participates in programs for training health care personnel. Students may participate in, or be present at various times during the Patient's treatment. Patient understands and accepts that such student participation is an integral and appropriate part of the care to be given to Patient, and Patient consents to same.

RELEASE OF INFORMATION: The Provider may release all or any part of the patient's record pertaining to this or any other hospitalization or treatment (INCLUDING ALCOHOL OR DRUG ABUSE, HIV-RELATED, OR COMMUNICABLE DISEASE INFORMATION) to persons or entities engaged in the activities stated below:

A. Insurance and Quality Review: persons or corporations (including insurance companies, worker's compensation payers, hospital or medical service corporations, welfare funds, governmental agencies, or the patient's employer), or their designees, which may be liable under contract to the Provider, any other party, the patient, a family member, or employer of the patient, for purposes of securing payment for all or part of a provider's charges, and quality assurance, utilization review, and peer review committees, accrediting agencies, and Provider and physician liability insurance carriers to enable them to carry out their functions.

B. Billing and Collection: agents or employees of the Provider that process or duplicate medical records for billing and reimbursement purposes.

C. Medical Audit: persons or entities authorized by the Provider for purposes of conducting medical audit activities.

D. Medical Research: authorized persons for the purpose of medical studies or medical research.

E. Other Providers: physicians and personnel involved in the patient's care to provide and manage the patient's health care. Also, information may be given to other health care providers to assure continuity of care.

F. Organ Donation: health facilities, providers, or their designees for the purpose of procuring, processing, or distributing human body or body parts for use in medical education, research, therapy, or transplantation.

The undersigned further consents to the release of the patient's name and address to entities acting on behalf of the Provider, including, but not limited to, affiliated fund-raising agencies.

I understand that I may revoke this authorization at any time, except to the extent the Provider has acted in reliance upon it or the disclosure is authorized by law. This consent to the release of patient information remains valid until expressly revoked by the patient in writing.

PHYSICIAN BILLS: The undersigned understands that Patient's attending, consulting and interpretive physicians will bill separately from the Hospital. These physicians may or may not participate with the same insurance plans as the Hospital, which could result in reduced reimbursement from Patient's insurance carrier for nonparticipating physician bills.

FINANCIAL AGREEMENT: The undersigned, jointly and severally, agree in return for services provided to Patient, to pay the Patient's account in full prior to discharge from the Hospital, or to make arrangements for payment which are satisfactory to the Hospital. To the extent not expressly prohibited by applicable law, the undersigned, jointly and severally, agree to pay all Hospital charges not paid in full by patient's insurance carrier or a third party payor. At the Hospitals option, a delinquent account may be charged interest at the rate of 18% per annum from date of Patient's discharge until paid in full. The undersigned also agrees to pay reasonable attorney's fees and collection expenses if the account is sent to an attorney for collection.

ASSIGNMENT OF INSURANCE BENEFITS: If Patient is entitled to any policy of insurance which insures the Patient, or any party liable to the Patient, then Patient hereby assigns to the Hospital all such benefits to be applied to the Patient's bill. It is understood, however, that the undersigned patient remains responsible for payment of the patient's bill regardless of patient's assignment of insurance coverage. Also, Patient assigns to Hospital any rights to payment for the charges of the physician(s) for whom the Hospital is authorized to bill in connection with its services. I understand that notwithstanding an assignment of insurance benefits, I am responsible for any health insurance deductions and copayments.

FIGURE 19–3, cont'd ▲ Admission service agreement.

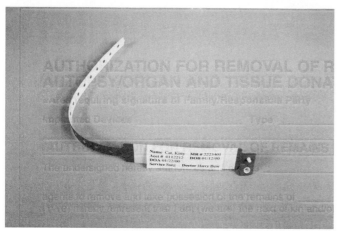

FIGURE 19–4 ▲ Patient identification bracelet.

pital safe. The items are placed in a numbered valuables envelope (Fig. 19–5) and the patient is given a duplicate numbered claim check. This number may also be written on the patient's chart. This serves as a reminder that there are valuables in the hospital safe. A clothing and valuables form is also prepared listing clothing, eyeglasses, false teeth, prosthesis, and any other items of value. The form is signed, witnessed, and placed in the patient's chart (Fig. 19–6).

Patient Information

The registration staff or health unit coordinator will explain the registration process and hospital rules to the patient and/or patient's family. Due to various state laws, the hospital may be required to inform the patient of specific information. Upon admission the patient is usually supplied with a copy of patient rights and may also be given other handouts regarding the hospital stay.

PATIENT'S VALUABLE ENVELOPE

IMPRINT AREA OR PATIENT S NAME AND HOSPITAL NO

01903
ENVELOPE NUMBER

HOSPITAL TAKES ALL POSSIBLE PRECAUTIONS TO SAFEGUARD YOUR PROPERTY BUT DISCLAIMS RESPONSIBILITY FOR VALUABLES SURRENDERED TO WRONGFUL HOLDER OF IDENTIFICATION SLIP AND WILL NOT BE RESPONSIBLE FOR ANY CLAIM FOR LOSS

CONTENTS OF ENVELOPE DEPOSITED WITH HOSPITAL	ARTICLES RETAINED BY PATIENT OR RESPONSIBLE PARTY
[X] CASH $100 ___ $20 *5* $5 *1* LOOSE CHANGE $50 ___ $10 ___ $1 *2* .	[X] CASH $3.00
[ ] CHECKS (LIST SEPARATELY) ___	[ ] WATCH ___
[X] CREDIT CARDS (LIST SEPARATELY) VISA ___	[ ] RINGS ___
[ ] WATCH ___	[ ] WALLET ___
[ ] RINGS ___	[ ] RAZOR ___
[X] WALLET ___	[X] DENTURES PARTIAL LOWER
[ ] OTHER EXPLAIN ___	[X] GLASSES ___
[ ] OTHER EXPLAIN ___	[ ] OTHER EXPLAIN ___

00 1346 REV 5 77

I HAVE CHECKED THE ABOVE AND ACKNOWLEDGE THE LISTS TO BE CORRECT I, THE PATIENT, OR RESPONSIBLE PARTY ASSUME FULL RESPONSIBILITY FOR THOSE ITEMS RETAINED IN MY POSSESSION DURING MY HOSPITALIZATION OR BROUGHT TO PATIENT AFTER SIGNATURES HAVE BEEN OBTAINED

TIME 1400	DATE 11/2/xx	PATIENT S SIGNATURE OR RESPONSIBLE PARTY X Wendy Leign	WITNESSED BY Kay Iver, R.n.
VALUABLE ENVELOPE CHART COPY RECEIVED BY		Kay Iver, R.n.	HOSPITAL EMPLOYEE
CASHIER'S USE ▶	DATE 11/2/xx	RECEIVED AND CERTIFIED Mark Palmer	
EMERGENCY ROOM USE ▶	DATE	PROPERTY COLLECTED BY	WITNESSED BY

WITHDRAWALS

DATE	DESCRIPTION	CASHIER INITIALS	PATIENT SIGNATURE

NOT RESPONSIBLE FOR ARTICLES AFTER 30 DAYS FROM DISCHARGE

LOST RECEIPT DOCUMENTATION

CLAIMANT MUST PROVIDE SOME INDEPENDENT EVIDENCE OF HIS IDENTITY FOR RELEASE OF THE ENVELOPE CONTENTS PLEASE DESCRIBE THIS IDENTIFICATION

FIGURE 19–5 ▲ Valuables envelope.

PATIENT VALUABLES

VALUABLES

QUANTITY   DESCRIPTION

☐ I have been informed that a safe is available in the Patient Accounts Department for the safekeeping of my valuables.

☐ I understand that the Hospital will assume responsibility for eyeglasses, bridgework, dentures and clothing (up to $50) lost or damaged due to negligence of Hospital personnel.

☐ I agree to assume full responsibility for any valuables not turned over to the Hospital for safekeeping in the Hospital safe by myself or my personal representative. I will hold the Hospital responsible for only those valuables listed above.

Signed: _____   Date _____ 19 _____
        (Patient or Representative)

Witnessed by: _____
             (Admission Representative)

Received by: _____   Deposit Envelope No. _____
            (Cashier or Nursing Office Representative)

Verified by: _____
            (Admissions Representative or Other Employee)

    Safe Deposit Envelope No. _____ Date of Deposit _____ 19 _____

    Comments: _____

Patient Valuables

FIGURE 19–6 ▲ Clothing and valuables list. (Courtesy Rockford Memorial Hospital, Rockford, IL.)

Advance Directives

Society now recognizes the individual's right to make decisions regarding care if he or she becomes incapacitated and to die with dignity rather than be kept live indefinitely by artificial life support. As a result, most states have enacted "right to die" laws and laws dealing with advanced directives. The term advance directive refers to an individual's desires regarding care if he or she should become incapacitated and end-of-life care. An adult witness or witnesses or a notary must sign an advance directive. The notary or witness cannot be the person named to make the decisions or the provider of health care. If there is only one witness, it cannot be a relative or someone who will be the beneficiary of property from the patient's estate if the patient dies.

Most states require that the patient be asked if he or she has or would like to have an advanced directive document. Figure 19–7 is an example of an advance directive checklist, which provides documentation that the patient was asked, and what decision was made regarding his or her care. Advanced directives include the documents described here.

A living will is a declaration made by the patient to family, medical staff, and all concerned with the patient's care stating what is to

---

ADVANCE DIRECTIVE CHECKLIST

Patient Name: _____

❏ Advance Directives Brochure Provided   ❏ Advance Directives Brochure Refused

The Following Information Was Obtained From: ❏ Patient   ❏ Other: _____

❏ Patient **HAS** executed the following Advance Directive(s):	COPY RECEIVED		COPY REQUESTED
	THIS ADMIT	PRIOR ADMIT	
❏ Declaration for Health Care Decisions (Living Will)	❏	❏	❏
❏ Medical Power of Attorney (MPOA)	❏	❏	❏
Name: _____			
Relationship: _____			
❏ Mental Healthcare Power of Attorney (MHPOA)	❏	❏	❏
Name: _____			
Relationship: _____			
❏ Combination Power of Attorney (that includes MPOA language)	❏	❏	❏
❏ Other: (specify)	❏	❏	❏

❏ Patient **HAS NOT** executed Advance Directive(s). (Check items below **ONLY** when talking with patient.)	**PATIENT Was Advised On** _____ . (date)
❏ **PATIENT** requests more information.	❏ of the *right to accept or refuse medical treatment.*
❏ Social Services notified.	❏ of the *right to formulate Advance Directives.*
❏ **PATIENT** chooses not to execute Advance Directives at this time.	❏ of the *right to receive medical treatment whether or not there is an Advance Directive.*

For Home Health/Hospice Use Only:

❏ Patient **HAS** EXECUTED Prehospital Medical Care (Arizona's Orange Card).

❏ Patient was advised of the *right to have Advance Directives followed by the health care facility and caregivers to the extent permitted by law.*

Signature of Facility Representative:	Department:	Date:

IF ADVANCED DIRECTIVE IS UNAVAILABLE, the patient indicates that the substance of the directive is as follows: *(see reverse for script)*

Living Will: _____

Medical Power of Attorney: _____

❏ Patient signature (legal representative if applicable): _____

❏ Witness signature (if patient physically unable to sign): _____ Reason: _____

Verification Upon Admit/Re-Admit or Transfer:

Verified with patient/legal representative that Advance Directives in medical record are current.	Verified with patient/legal representative that Advance Directives in medical record are current.	Verified with patient/legal representative that Advance Directives in medical record are current.
Signature:	Signature:	Signature:
Date:	Date:	Date:

PATIENT IDENTIFICATION

FIGURE 19–7 ▲ Advanced directive checklist.

be done in the event of a terminal illness. It directs the withholding or withdrawing of life-sustaining procedures. The patient may also define what she or he means by *meaningful quality of life.*

Power of attorney for health care allows the patient to appoint another person or persons (called a proxy or agent) to make health care decisions for the patient should the patient become incapable of making decisions. The proxy (agent) has a duty to act consistently with the patient's wishes. If the proxy does not know the patient's wishes, the proxy has the duty to act in the patient's best interests. Figure 19–8 is an example of a health care power of attorney and living will combined form.

HEALTH CARE POWER OF ATTORNEY & LIVING WILL
Combined Form

I, _____, as principal, designate _____ as my agent for all matters relating to my health care, including, without limitation, full power to give or to refuse consent to all medical, surgical, hospital, psychiatric and related health care. This power of attorney is effective whenever I am unable to make or to communicate health care decisions. All of my agent's actions under this power have the same effects on my heirs, devisees, and personal representatives as if I were alive, competent and acting for myself.

If my agent is unwilling or unable to serve or to continue to serve, I hereby appoint _____ as my agent.

In acting under this power, I want my agent to give great weight to the following statements: I am in favor of trial treatment. That means I want all necessary medical care to treat my condition until, and only until, my doctors and my agent reasonably decide that I am in an irreversible coma, or a persistent vegetative state, or a locked-in state, or that I cannot be expected to return to a fully conscious state. If, following the guidelines stated above, my doctors and my agent decide that further medical care is inappropriate:

1. I **want** only comfort care and I **do not want** to undergo artificial administration of food or fluids.
2. I **do not want** to be resuscitated in case I stop breathing or my heart stops beating.

If my doctors and my agent reasonably decide that I have a terminal illness, I want all decisions concerning my medical and surgical care to be made in light of the expected length and quality of life which would result from such care and the predictable effects on me of undergoing treatment. **If I cannot be expected to have a significant period of conscious life even after medical or surgical care, then I want comfort care only.** (Examples: I do not want any surgery or other care designed to prolong my life. I do not want artificially administered food or fluids and I do not want to be resuscitated.)

This combined health care directive is made under § 36-3221 and § 36-3261, Arizona Revised Statutes. It continues in effect for all who may rely on it, except those to whom I have given notice of its revocation.

_____   _____
Dated   Signature of Mark of Person Making Living Will or Granting Health Care Power of Attorney

Verification

I affirm that: (1) I was present when this living will was dated and signed or marked or (2) the person making this living will directly indicated to me that the living will expressed that person's wishes and that the person intended to adopt it at that time. The maker of this document appeared to be of sound mind and free from duress.

(If there is only one witness signing this document) I certify that: I have not been designated to make medical decisions for the person who signed this living will, I am not directly involved with providing health care to that person, I am not related to that person by blood, marriage, or adoption and I am not entitled to any part of that person's estate.

_____   _____   _____
Witness   Witness   Date

STATE OF ARIZONA   )
) ss.
County of   )

The maker of this document appears to be of sound mind and free from duress. It was subscribed and sworn to before me this _____ day of _____, 19_____.

_____   My Commission Expires _____
Notary Public

(A health care power of attorney and living will must be signed by a notary or by an adult witness or witnesses, who saw you sign or mark the document and who say that you appear to be of sound mind and free from duress. A notary or witness cannot be the person you name to make your decisions or your provider of health care. If you have only one witness, that witness cannot be related to you or someone who will get any of your property from your estate if you die.)

July 1995 · Arizona Hospital and Healthcare Association

FIGURE 19–8 ▲ Health care power of attorney and living will admission.

An advance directive becomes effective *only* when the patient can no longer make decisions for himself or herself. The patient may change or destroy any directive or living will at any time.

Escort to the Nursing Unit

Once the nursing unit and bed assignment has been made, a volunteer, a member of the hospital transportation department, or admitting personnel will escort the patient to the assigned unit. If the patient has already been registered, the admitting papers are delivered to the receiving unit.

The health unit coordinator will greet the patient and tell the nurse that will be caring for the patient of his or her arrival. The nurse will complete the admitting nurse's notes (Fig. 19–9), which the health unit coordinator will use to complete the patient profile with information such as allergies, height, and weight.

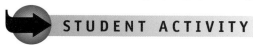

STUDENT ACTIVITY

To practice preparing the newly admitted patient's chart and Kardex forms, complete Activity 19–1 in the *Skills Practice Manual*.

Admission Notes

```
967 896
MART TED
DR Y STOCKS
M 40 MED INS
```

Date: 10/22/XX   Time of arrival: 1300   Admitted to: 711/1

From: home   How arrived: car

Accompanied by: Mother   Relationship:

Orientation to physical environment: Yes

Height: 5'7"   Weight: 140#   T. 37   P. 86   R. 20   B/P 140/80

Valuables brought to floor: None   Disposition:

Allergies and Reaction: All mycins

Admitted by:

ADMISSION ASSESSMENT: S. Mirth, N.A.

Reason for admission: Broken Left radius   Previous adm's: None

MEDS — Medications used at home and why: none

Anticoagulant Therapy No When & Why   Cortisone Therapy ____ When & Why

Disposition: Sent home ____ Retained ____ If retained - identify Rx No. and am't in Nurses Notes

EENT/SENSORY — Patient's vision, hearing, prosthesis (glasses, contacts, hearing aids).
Pt. denies wearing glasses or hearing aid

NEUROLOGICAL — Level of consciousness, alertness and orientation, if indicated.
Alert and oriented to person, place and time. Speech clear. Answers questions appropriately.

CARDIOVASCULAR — B/P, pulse (rate, quality) color, A/R and peripheral pulses as indicated.
No Hx of cardiovascular problems. Skin warm and dry. Pt. able to wiggle L fingers c/o numbness in L thumb

RESPIRATORY — Rate, quality, breath sounds as indicated. Sputum production, cough, dyspnea — influence of activity, smoking Smokes pack of cigarettes a week. Denies constant cough or SOB Breath sounds clear bilaterally. No Hx of asthma or bronchitis.

00-6002 Rev. 3-80   **ADMISSION NOTES**

FIGURE 19–9 ▲ Admission nurse's notes.

▪ ADMISSION ORDERS

Admission orders are written directions by the doctor for the care and treatment of the patient upon entry into the hospital. Most orders are written on the unit by the hospitalist, attending doctor, resident, or nurse practitioner, or received by telephone immediately after the patient's arrival. However, there are times when the admission orders arrive before the patient. Doctors may have preprinted order sets for certain types of admissions, such as cardiac, or total hip or knee replacement surgeries. Some doctors may also write admission orders before the arrival of the patient and leave them on the nursing unit. The health unit coordinator must be sure these orders are identified with the patient's name, which should be written on the order sheet in ink. The orders are labeled with the patient's identification label later when the patient arrives on the nursing unit.

Admission Order Components

The common components of admission orders are:

▪ The admitting diagnosis
▪ Diet
▪ Activity
▪ Diagnostic tests/procedures
▪ Medications. Usually medications are needed for the patient's disease condition, for sleeping, and/or for pain
▪ Treatment orders
▪ Request for old records
▪ Patient care category or code status. The patient care category or code status may be indicated on the patient's admission orders. The patient care category or code status refers to the patient's wishes regarding resuscitation. Code status may be written as full code, modified support, or do not resuscitate. The doctor must follow any state-specific statute and the hospital's policies and procedures when writing a DNR status.

Figure 19–10 is an example of a set of admission orders. See Procedure 19–1 for the health unit coordinator's tasks related to admitting a patient.

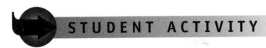

STUDENT ACTIVITY

To practice transcribing a set of admission orders for a medical patient, complete Activity 19–2 in the *Skills Practice Manual.*

PHYSICIANS' ORDER SHEET

DATE	TIME	SYMBOL	ORDERS
5/4/00	1300		Admit to med-surg unit
			DX: acute pulmonary edema
			BRP c̄ help
			VS q 2° for 8° then q4°
			1800 cal ADA NAS diet
			Daily wts
			1 & O
			CBC, lytes & cardiac isoenzymes stat
			CMP in am
			ABG on RA now, then place on O_2 @ 2 L/M
			Repeat ABG in 2 hr—call me c̄ results
			Chest PA & lat today & in am Cl infiltrates
			EKG today & in am
			Lung perfusion/ventilation scan in am Cl embolism
			bepridil hydrochloride 300 mg qd
			bumetanide 2 mg PO now & qd
			Ambien 10 mg qhs prn for sleep
			Old records to floor
			Pt is a full code status
			Dr. John Stewart MD

FIGURE 19–10 ▲ Set of admission orders.

TASK	NOTES
1. Greet the patient upon his or her arrival at the unit	**1.** Introduce yourself and give your status. Example: "I'm Ted Mart, the health unit coordinator for this unit."
2. Inform the patient that you will notify the nurse of his or her arrival.	**2.** Notify the nurse caring for the patient of his or her arrival.
3. Notify the attending doctor and/or hospital resident or the hospitalist of the patient's admission.	
4. Move the patient's name from the admission screen on the computer to the correct bed on the nursing unit.	
5. Record the patient's admission in the admission, discharge, and transfer sheet and the census board.	
6. Check the patient's signature on the admission service agreement form.	**6.** Compare the spelling of the patient's name on the facesheet or front sheet and the patient identification labels with the signature on the admission service agreement form. Also check to see that the doctor's name is correct.
7. Complete the procedure for the preparation of the chart. a. Label all the chart forms with the patient's identification labels b. Fill in all the needed headings c. Place all the forms in the chart behind the proper dividers	
8. Label the outside of the chart.	**8.** Identify the chart with the patient's and the doctor's names and the room number.
9. Prepare any other labels or identification cards used by your facility.	
10. Place the patient identification labels in the correct place in the patient's chart.	
11. Fill in all the necessary information on the patient's Kardex form or into the computer if Kardex is computerized.	**11.** The information is obtained from the front sheet or facesheet prepared by the admitting department and the admission nurse's notes.
12. Place the Kardex form in the proper place in the Kardex file.	
13. Enter appropriate required data into the computer.	**13.** A patient profile requires information found on the facesheet screen: the front sheet or facesheet and the nurse's admission notes such as name, address, nearest of kin, height, weight, etc.
14. Record the data from the admission nurse's notes on the graphic sheet (see Fig. 19–9).	**14.** The admission nurse's notes include data such as vital signs, height, and weight.
15. Place the allergy information in all the designated areas or write "NKA."	**15.** Allergy information (the information obtained from the patient about any sensitivity to medication, food, or other substance) is usually placed on the front of the patient's chart, Kardex form, and medication record. The allergy information is obtained from the admission nurse's notes. Writing "NKA" indicates to the staff that the allergy information has been checked.
16. Prepare an allergy bracelet with allergies written on it to be placed on the patient's wrist if necessary.	
17. Note code status on front of chart if necessary.	
18. Place red tape stating "name alert" on the spine of the chart if there is a patient with same or similar name on the unit.	
19. Transcribe the admission orders according to your hospital's policy.	

■ THE SURGERY PATIENT

Information

The procedure for admission of a medical or surgical patient is the same except that diagnostic tests ordered by the doctor are performed on surgery patients as soon as possible following their arrival to the hospital. This allows the time needed to perform the diagnostic studies and to have the test results on the patient's chart before surgery. An abnormal blood test result or a chest x-ray that is abnormal may require that the surgery be postponed pending further evaluation.

Some surgeries, such as open-heart surgery or organ transplant surgery, may require additional diagnostic studies, patient preparation, preoperative teaching, and careful explanation of the procedure to the patient and the family. A tour of the intensive care unit may be arranged so that the patient will be aware of his or her surroundings and the activities that will take place after surgery.

Admission Day Surgery and Preoperative Care Unit

The purpose of the admission day surgery area is to admit patients the *day of* their scheduled surgery. After the patient's surgery and some time in the postanesthesia care unit (PACU), the patient will be admitted to a surgical nursing unit. Health insurance companies promote this type of area to reduce cost of hospital admission. Other terms for this practice include same-day surgery and AM admission.

The doctor's office, hospital admitting department, and the surgery-scheduling secretary usually coordinate the same-day surgery patient's admission. Laboratory tests, x-rays, and other diagnostic testing may be performed at the doctor's office, outside facility, or the hospital on an outpatient basis before admission. The doctor's office provides the patient's personal information to the hospital admitting department by phone or fax and the patient will sign necessary forms before or on the day of surgery.

On the day of the surgery, the patient reports to the admission area several hours before the scheduled surgery. The patient is taken to the admission day surgery unit with:

- Patient identification bracelet or band
- Doctors' orders
- Laboratory reports (if ordered)
- EKG (if ordered)
- X-ray report (if ordered)
- Patient identification labels
- Admission forms including any consent forms or doctors' orders

After surgery and the recovery room (postanesthesia care unit), the patient is assigned a bed and is transported to an inpatient surgical unit.

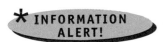

★ INFORMATION ALERT!

Usually admission, pre-op care, post-op care, and surgery are contained in one complete area separate from all inpatient activities.

Preoperative Orders

The doctor who will perform surgery on a patient writes orders relative to the surgery before the surgery is performed. For example, the surgeon who is performing an open-heart surgery may wish the patient to receive preoperative teaching by the respiratory department on the evening before surgery. He or she may also order a heparin lock to be inserted before the patient leaves the nursing unit for surgery.

The surgeon may also designate the anesthesiologist who will write preoperative preparation orders. The surgeon will write the surgical procedure on the physicians' order sheet for the preparation of the surgery consent. If a discrepancy is found between the physicians' written order for the surgery consent, the surgery schedule, or information on the patient's chart, or if there is any confusion for the patient, the patient's nurse should be notified (if unaware) and the correct procedure must be verified by calling the doctor's office immediately. For example, the surgery consent as written on the physicians' order sheet may state that the patient is to have an "open reduction of the *left* femur," whereas the patient's diagnosis and physical examination indicate that the patient has a fracture of the *right* femur; obviously such a discrepancy must be corrected before any orders are carried out. All charting rules must be followed when preparing consent forms. The surgery consent must be written legibly in black ink and written exactly as the doctor wrote it with the exception of abbreviations. Words cannot be added, deleted, or rearranged and all abbreviations must be spelled out on the surgery consent. The first and last names of the patient and the doctor are also required.

The anesthesiologist writes orders on the physician's order sheet before the surgery. His or her orders concern the time food and fluids are to be discontinued and the preoperative medication to be given to help relieve anxiety and aid in the induction of the anesthesia.

Preoperative Order Components

Orders related directly to the surgery have certain common components.

Surgeon's Orders

- *Name of surgery for surgery consent.* The consent must be signed before the patient receives any "mind-clouding" drugs. In the case of surgery that may result in sterility or in loss of a limb (amputation), two permits may be required.
- *Enemas.* The order for an enema depends upon the type of surgery. For surgeries within the abdominal cavity, all wastes must be removed from the intestines. This allows the surgeon more room for exploration, a clear field of vision, and decreases danger of contamination and infection.
- *Shaves, scrubs, or showers.* The site of the surgical incision must be prepared. This order requires the removal of body hair by shaving. The procedure is referred to as a surgical prep. The surgeon may also require a special scrub at the surgical site. In some facilities, the operating room staff may do shaves and scrubs. Often the doctor writes an order for the patient to take a shower before surgery using an antibacterial soap such as Hibiclens.
- *Name of anesthesiologist or anesthesiology group.* It is necessary to know the anesthesiologist's name or specific anesthesiology group in the event that preoperative medication orders are not received. The health unit coordinator may then call the anesthesiologist, group, or person responsible for

writing the preoperative orders. (In hospitals where nurse anesthetists administer the anesthesia, the surgeon may write the preoperative orders.)

■ *Miscellaneous orders.* Other orders may be for Ted hose, additional diagnostic studies, blood components to be given during surgery, or intravenous preparations to be started before surgery. Treatments and additional medications may also be ordered.

Anesthesiologist's Orders

■ *Diet.* When surgery is to be performed during the morning hours, the patient is usually NPO at midnight. A patient having late-afternoon surgery may have an order written for a clear liquid breakfast at 0600 and then NPO. Food and/or fluids by mouth are not allowed for 6 to 8 hours before surgery in which an anesthetic is used that renders the patient unconscious. The NPO rule is maintained to lessen the possibility of the patient aspirating vomitus while under anesthesia.

■ *Preoperative medications.* The anesthesiologist or surgeon usually writes an order for preoperative medication for the patient scheduled for surgery. The preoperative medication order includes a hypnotic to ensure that the patient rests well the night before surgery and an intramuscular injection to be given approximately 1 hour before the surgery to relax the patient. Figure 19–11 is an example of preoperative orders; see Procedure 19–2, Preoperative Procedures.

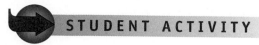

STUDENT ACTIVITY

To practice transcribing a set of preoperative orders, complete Activity 19–3 in the *Skills Practice Manual*.

Preoperative Routine

It is the overall responsibility of the health unit coordinator to see that the surgery chart is properly prepared to send to surgery with the patient. The RN will complete a pre-op checklist; however, the health unit coordinator is involved in preparing the patient's chart. The most important task is to have the following records on the chart, as it is often hospital policy that surgery cannot begin if any of the required reports is missing.

The current history and physical record (H & P): Essential in most health care facilities.
Surgery consent: An informed consent must be obtained prior to surgery that must be accurate, have patient's and surgeon's full names, signed by patient or legal guardian, dated, and witnessed (Fig. 19–12).
Blood consent: A consent form must be signed to accept (Fig. 19–13, *A*) or refuse (Fig. 19–13, *B*) blood products.

PHYSICIANS' ORDER SHEET

DATE	TIME	SYMBOL	ORDERS
5/13/00	1400		Full liq diet tonight
			T & X match 2 u PC & hold for surgery
			CBC, Ua & chest x-ray PA & LAT CI: pre-op
			ECG this pm
			Consent: partial gastrectomy, vagotomy
			& pyloroplasty
			Hibiclens shower this pm
			H & P by surgical resident
			Pre-ops per Dr. A. Sleep
			Start 1000 cc 5% D/W 1 hr prior to surg.
			Dr. G. Astro MD.
5/13/00	1600		NPO 2400
			Restoril 15 mg hs tonight MR x 1
			Demerol 100 mg ⎫
			Vistaril 25 mg ⎬ IM @ 0700
			Dr. A. Sleep MD

FIGURE 19–11 ▲ Set of preoperative orders.

Procedure 19-2: **PREOPERATIVE PROCEDURE**

TASK	NOTES
1. Label the surgery forms with the patient's identification labels and place them within the patient's chart.	1. *The surgery forms include the nurse's preoperative checklist, operating room record, the anesthesiologist's record, the operating room record, recovery room record, etc. (see Fig. 19–17). Forms vary among hospitals.*
2. Check the patient's chart for the history and physical report.	2. *If the history and physical report is not found on the chart, call the health records department to check if it has been dictated. Notify the patient's nurse and doctor if the report is not located.*

3. Check the patient's chart for the following signed consent forms:
  a. Surgical consent
  b. Blood transfusion consent or refusal form
  c. Admission service agreement
	3. *Check the consent forms for the patient and witnesses signature and the correct spelling of the surgical procedure.*

4. Check the patient's chart for any previously ordered diagnostic studies such as laboratory tests, x-rays, and so forth.	4. *If the diagnostic test results are not on the patient's chart, locate the results on the computer, print them, and place in patient's chart. If unable to locate results, notify patient's nurse.*
5. Chart the patient's latest vital signs.	
6. File the current medication administration record in the patient's chart.	
7. Print at least five facesheets to place in chart.	7. *Facesheets are removed and used by doctors and other health care providers to bill patients.*
8. Place at least three sheets of patient identification labels in the patient's chart.	8. *Patient identification labels are used to label specimens.*
9. Notify the appropriate nursing personnel when surgery calls for the patient.	

Admission service agreement (also called *conditions of admission):* Check to see whether signed upon admission.
Nursing preoperative checklist: Should be checked and signed by nursing personnel.
MAR: Current medication administration record should be placed in chart before transport to surgery.
Diagnostic test results: Preoperative tests including laboratory, diagnostic imaging, etc. that were ordered by doctor.

To ensure that each patient's chart is ready to be taken to surgery, a health unit coordinator may choose to create a preoperative checklist (Fig. 19–14). This checklist should not be confused with the nursing preoperative checklist (Fig. 19–15), which is checked and signed by the patient's nurse to ensure proper patient preparation for surgery. The nursing preoperative checklist is a legal chart form in most facilities.

Each nursing unit may print a surgery schedule from the computer or may receive a printed surgery schedule (Fig. 19–16), which lists all the surgeries to be performed on the following day. See Procedure 19–2 for the health unit coordinator tasks to prepare the patient's chart for surgery.

Postoperative Orders and Routine

Immediately after surgery, most patients spend 1 or more hours in the recovery room or postanesthesia care unit (PACU). A record of their progress is kept on the recovery room record. These records along with other surgery records are included in the patient's chart

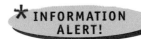

INFORMATION ALERT!

After printing a surgery schedule from the computer or receiving a surgery schedule, the health unit coordinator should highlight the patients going to surgery from that particular nursing unit.

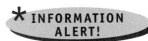

INFORMATION ALERT!

The recovery room personnel (may be a health unit coordinator) will call the surgery waiting room where family is waiting and the nursing unit when the patient arrives in the PACU and again when the patient is ready to return to his or her room.

It is important to notify the patient's nurse of the patient's arrival in the PACU and when the patent is to return to the nursing unit.

(Fig. 19–17, *A* and *B*). The postoperative orders (written by the surgeon to be carried out immediately after surgery) are often initiated here. For example, the recovery room staff may carry out the doctor's order for antiembolism elastic hose (or stockings) to be placed on the patient's legs. The recovery room personnel will indicate on the physicians' order sheet those orders that have already been executed (note order No. 7 on Fig. 19–18).

Health unit coordinator tasks performed during the postoperative procedure are listed at top of p. 391.

┌─────────────────────────┐
│   │
│   │
│   PATIENT LABEL   │
│   │
│   │
└─────────────────────────┘

CONSENT TO OPERATE

1. I authorize the following operation(s) or procedure(s) _____

    _____

    to be performed by Dr. _____ and / or the associates or assistants of
    his / her choice which may include medical or surgical residents.

2. During the course of the operation(s) / procedure(s), unforeseen conditions may arise which may necessitate additional surgery or other therapeutic procedures to promote my well-being. I consent to other surgery / procedures as may be considered necessary or advisable by my physician(s) under the circumstances.

3. I consent to the use of anesthetics, as may be necessary and advisable, except _____.
    I understand that anesthesia may involve serious risk even though administered in a careful manner. I further understand that a patient should not drive, operate equipment or drink alcoholic beverages for at least 24 hours after anesthesia.

4. To further medical and scientific learning, I consent to the photographing and / or video taping of the operation(s) / procedure(s) which may reveal portions of my body, with the understanding that my identity is not to be revealed. To advance medical education, I give my permission for physicians, nurses, medical students, interns, residents and other individuals who are participating in an educational process approved by the hospital to be present during the operation(s) / procedure(s).

5. I consent to the examination for anatomical purposes and disposal by the hospital of any tissue or body parts which may be removed during the operation / procedure.

6. I understand that some physician(s) performing the operation(s) / procedure(s), administering anesthesia and those physicians providing services involving pathology and radiology, may not be the agents, servants or employees of the hospital nor of one another, and may be independent contractors.

7. I have been advised that prosthetic devices including, but not limited to, dentures, bridges, caps, crowns, fillings, dental implants, etc. are more easily damaged than normal teeth. I have been advised to remove all removable prosthetic devices prior to surgery and I agree that responsibility for loss or damage will be mine if I fail to remove such dental or other prosthetic devices.

8. My physician has explained to me the nature, purpose and possible consequences of the operation(s) / procedure(s) as well as significant risks involved, possible complications, expected post operative functional level, expected alterations in lifestyle / health status and alternative methods of treatment. I further understand that the explanation I have received is not exhaustive and that there may be other, more remote, risks and consequences. I have been advised that a more detailed explanation will be given to me if I so desire. I have received no guarantee or warranty concerning the results / outcome and cure and have been given an opportunity to ask and have my questions answered to my satisfaction.

9. In the event a device is implanted during the operation(s) / procedure(s) and federal law requires the tracking of the device, I consent to the release of my social security number to the manufacturer of the device.

    The patient is unable to sign for the following reason:

    ☐ The patient is a minor.

    ☐ The patient lacks the ability to make or communicate medical treatment decisions because of:

    _____

_____   _____   _____
Patient or Legally Authorized Representative   Date   Time

_____
Relationship to Patient

_____   _____   _____
Witness   Date   Time

FIGURE 19–12 ▲ Surgery consent.

PATIENT LABEL

Consent for Transfusion of Blood or Blood Products

1. I HAVE BEEN INFORMED that I need or may need during treatment, a transfusion of blood and/or one of its products in the interest of my health and proper medical care.

2. I HAVE BEEN INFORMED of the risks and benefits of receiving transfusion(s). These risks exist despite the fact that the blood has been carefully tested.

3. The alternatives to transfusion, including the risks and consequences of not receiving this therapy, have been explained to me.

4. I have read, or had read to me, the Blood Transfusion information regarding blood transfusions and have had the opportunity to ask questions.

5. I hereby consent to the transfusion(s).

Patient's Signature	Date	Time

Signature of parent, legally appointed guardian or responsible person
(for patients who cannot sign)

Witness	Date	Time

A

FIGURE 19–13 ▲ *A*, Consent for transfusion of blood or blood products.

PATIENT LABEL

Refusal to Permit Blood Transfusion

1. I request that no blood derivatives be administered to _____
during this hospitalization. (patient name)

2. I hereby release the hospital, its personnel and the attending physician from any responsibility whatever for unfavorable reactions or any untoward results due to my refusal to permit the use of blood or its derivatives.

3. I fully understand the possible consequences of such refusal on my part.

Patient's Signature	Date	Time

Signature of parent, legally appointed guardian or responsible person
(for patients who cannot sign)

Witness	Date	Time

Witness	Date	Time

B

FIGURE 19–13, cont'd ▲ *B*, Refusal to permit blood transfusion.

Surgical Patients   3-C

Rm#	Patient	Surg Time	Service Adm Agreement	H & P	5 Sheets Pt ID Labels	5 Face Sheets	Surgical Consent	Dx Reports
305	Pack, Fanny	0730	X	X	X	X	X	X
311	Juniper, Jack	0800	X	X	X	X	X	X
312	Harris, Susan	1100	X	X	X	X	X	X

FIGURE 19–14 ▲ A preoperative checklist for the health unit coordinator.

PREOPERATIVE CHECK LIST   DATE

NURSING UNIT CHECK LIST	YES	NO
1. Pre-op bath/Oral hygiene given	✓	
2. Make-up/Nail polish removed	✓	
3. Bobby Pins, Combs, Hair Pieces Removed Disposition:	✓	
4. Sanitary Belt removed	—	
5. Jewelry, Rings, Religious Medals, or other items removed (May be worn during cardiac catheterization) when removed disposition is:	✓	
6. Voided/Retention catheter	✓	
7. Preoperative medicine given as ordered	✓	
8. Addressograph with chart	✓	
9. Pre-anesthetic patient questionnaire completed	✓	

10. Where family can be located during and immediately after surgery   *Surgery Waiting room*

NURSING UNIT AND OPERATING ROOM NURSES CHECK LIST

	UNIT NURSE YES	UNIT NURSE NO	O.R. NURSE YES	O.R. NURSE NO
11. Surgical consent for: Rt. (Lt.) *Inguinal herniorrhaphy*	✓			
as obtained from Doctor's Order sheet	✓			
12. Consultation Special Consents				
13. History and Physical — Dictated On Chart	✓			
14. Allergies Noted	✓			
15. Hematology	✓			
16. Urinalysis	✓			
17. Surgical/Cardiac cath prep done	✓			
18. Type and Cross Match — 1 Units P.C.	✓			
19. Culture site: Results:				
20. Admission Chest X-Ray Report	✓			
21. EKG Report if over 40 years	✓			

	REMOVED YES	REMOVED NO	YES	NO
22. Prosthetic Teeth May be worn during cardiac catheterization				
Permanent cap or caps				
Permanent bridge				
Removable bridge				
Removable plate or plates				
Loose teeth				
23. Prosthesis and Disposition:				
Artificial eye in out				
Contact lens in out				
Pacemaker				
Other				

R.N. Signature   O.R. Nurse Signature

00-6015 Rev. 12-79

PATIENT IDENTIFICATION ON UNIT

A. Person from surgery calling for patient

1. Ask for patient by name
2. Check patient's chart
3. Check patient's chart with call slip (not necessary with cardiac catheterization)

B. Person from unit must accompany

1. Ask patient his/her name
   Ask patient his/her doctor's name
2. Check chart face sheet for patient's name and hospital number with patient identiband
3. Check call slip with identiband (not necessary for cardiac catheterization)

Winifred Marshall, R.N.
Signature Nursing Unit Personnel

Bill Standard, Ord.
Signature Surgery Personnel

SPECIAL COMMENTS TO OPERATING ROOM AND RECOVERY ROOM NURSES FROM NURSING UNIT: (PLEASE SIGN YOUR COMMENT)

B.P.:H.S. _130/70_ a Pre-op _140/82_ p Pre-op _136/80_

Pre-op TPR _____ NPO p _Mn_ WT. _136_

Pertinent Drug Therapy:

Demerol 75 mg ⎫ *I.M.*
Atropine 0.4 mg ⎭ *8³⁰ am*

none

none

PREOPERATIVE CHECK LIST

FIGURE 19–15 ▲ Nurse's preoperative checklist.

SURGERY SCHEDULE FRIDAY JUNE 10, 0000

Time	Surgeon	Procedure	Patient's Bed Number
Operating Room 1			
0730	Dr. Singsong	Anterior Colporrhaphy; left Bartholin's cystectomy	412A
0930	Dr. Prossert	Dilatation & curettage; FS, possible vag. hysterectomy, bil. salpingo-oophorectomy	321
1130	Dr. Broad	Laparoscopy	621B
1330	Dr. Street	Rt. breast biopsy, FS, Poss. rt. radical mastectomy	416
Operating Room 2			
0730	Dr. Patellar	Arthrotomy lt. knee, open reduction, internal fixation with plateau medial meniscectomy	502B
0930	Dr. Home	Arthroplasty rt. elbow, insertion of prosthesis; reconstruction rheumatoid rt. hand	511
1330	Dr. Bowl	Bone graft lt. radius	516A
Operating Room 3			
0730	Dr. Branch	Cystoscopy, TURP	212
0930	Dr. Signe	Cystoscopy, manipulation ureteral stone	222A
1130	Dr. Blake	Circumcision	316B
Operating Room 4			
0730	Dr. Throat	Tonsillectomy	304A
0930	Dr. Ober	Hemorrhoidectomy	601
Operating Room 5			
0730	Dr. Love	Cholecystectomy, biopsy rib cage	617B
0930	Dr. Solano	Repair of lt. inguinal hernia	600

FIGURE 19–16 ▲ Surgery schedule.

Postoperative Order Components

The postoperative orders that relate to the patient's treatment after surgery usually contain the following components:

Diet: The patient may remain NPO or be given sips of water or ice chips ("sips and chips"). The diet is then increased as tolerated.

Intake and output: The patient's intake and output is closely watched for 24 to 48 hours (Fig. 19–19).

Intravenous fluids: Most surgery patients have at least one bag of intravenous fluids ordered after surgery. A record of the intake of intravenous fluids is maintained on a parenteral fluid sheet (see Chapter 8, p. 148).

Vital signs: The patient's vital signs are monitored carefully after surgery—usually every 4 hours for 24 to 48 hours.

Catheters, tubes, and drains: Postoperative patients may have a retention or indwelling urinary catheter. Other orders may pertain to intermittent catheterization of the patient, as necessary. Some patients may require suctioning when nasogastric or other tubes are in place.

Activity: Activity after surgery may be only bedrest, and will be increased as the patient continues to recuperate.

Positioning: Some surgeons require the patient's position to be changed frequently. The elevation of the bed may also be very important.

Observation of the operative site: It is imperative that the site of the operation or the bandages be observed closely for bleeding, excessive drainage, redness, and swelling.

Medications: Orders for medications to relieve pain (narcotics) and nausea and vomiting (antiemetics), and to help the patient to sleep or rest (hypnotics) may be prescribed for a period after surgery. Other medications are ordered as needed (see Fig. 19–18, which is an example of postoperative orders).

Postoperative orders cancel all previous orders. See Procedure 19–3, Postoperative Procedure, for health unit coordinator's tasks involved in postoperative procedures.

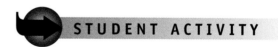

STUDENT ACTIVITY

To practice transcribing a set of postoperative orders, complete Activity 19–4 in the *Skills Practice Manual*.

■ SUMMARY

For most patients, admission to the hospital is a stressful experience. The health unit coordinator can do much in the field of public relations for the hospital at this time. The health unit coordinator is usually the first person with whom the new patient has contact on the nursing unit. A warm welcome and a pleasant smile may help to relieve some anxiety. The expediency with which the patient's chart is prepared and the new orders transcribed allows the health care team to initiate care and treatment sooner.

The health unit coordinator needs to recognize the common components in the admission, preoperative, and postoperative order sets. As in all orders, the quick yet accurate and thorough transcription of orders is a must.

OPERATING ROOM NURSES NOTES

Date: 11 / 06 / XX
     Mo.   Day   Yr.

Operating Room # 4

Anesthesia Method:
☒ General   ☐ Caudal
☐ Local Infiltrate   ☐ Regional Blk.
☐ Spinal   ☐ Epidural

Begin Anesthesia _0740_
Begin Surgery _0810_
End Surgery _0910_
Leave Room _0925_

Administered By: _Gerald Sleep, M.D._

Surgeon: _Robert Cutt, M.D._

Assistant: _Rufus String, M.D._

Perfusionist: _____

Observers: _____

Scrub Nurse: _L. Smythe O.R.T._

Circulating Nurse: _P. Bridge, R.N._

Relief: _____ @ _____

Relief: _____ @ _____

Pre-Operative Diagnosis: _Left Rotator Cuff Tendonitis_

Post-Operative Diagnosis: _Same_

Operation: _Exploratory arthrotomy left shoulder, Bristow procedure_

Radiopaque Sponges 4x4		Laparotomy Sponges	No Sponge Count Taken ☐		
		5 5		Yes	No
			Sponge Count Correct		
			Before Incision Made	☑	☐
			Cavity Closure	☐	☐
			Skin Closure	☑	☐
Rondic	Laminectomy	Cottoniods	Wound Classificaiton	A	☑
				B	☐
				C	☐
Dissect.				D	☐
				E	☐

Tissue: _____
Culture: _____
Implants: Manufacturer: _Zimmer_
       Type: _Bone screw_

To Path Lab By: _____
To Bacteriology By: _____
Serial # _____ Size: _1 inch_

Date	Time	Comments/Complications
		T+C 3 PC.
		Adhesive for Closure caused skin reaction near incision

RN Signature: _Phoebe Bridge, R.N._

A   **OPERATING ROOM NURSE'S NOTES**

FIGURE 19-17 ▲ Surgery forms. A, Operating room nurse's notes.

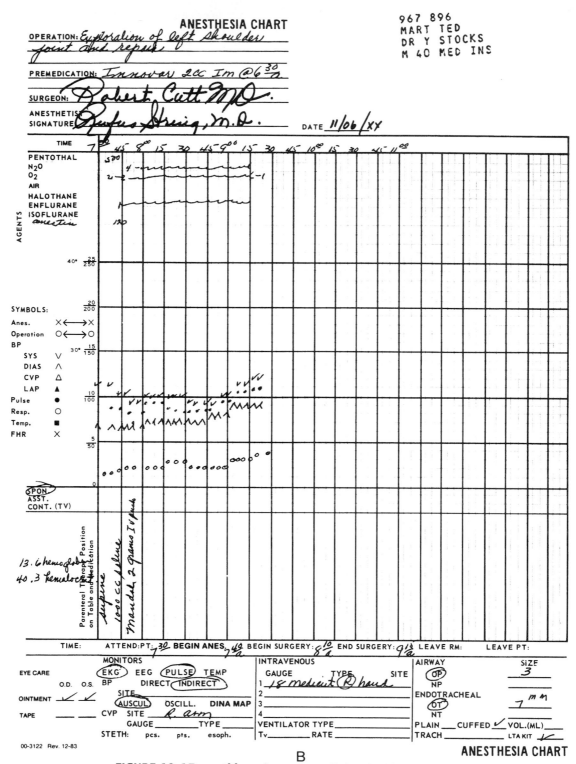

FIGURE 19–17, cont'd ▲ Surgery forms. *B,* Anesthesiologist's record.

PHYSICIANS' ORDER SHEET

DATE	TIME	SYMBOL	ORDERS
6/7/03			*Post op*
			NPO
			NG tube to Low Suction
			Follow present IV c̄ 5% D/LR @ 125cc/h
			Demerol 75 mg IM q 4 h prn pain
			Compazine 10 mg IM q 4 h prn N/V
			Encourage to TCDB
			Knee length elastic hose ✓done / RR @1050
			May dangle this evening
			Dr. G. Astro

FIGURE 19–18 ▲ Set of postoperative orders.

24 - Hour Intake & Output

Name _Rose Philips_
Room _316' West_
Date _5/13/XX_

Shift	Fluid Intake			Fluid Output		Other	Stools
	Oral	I.V.	Piggy Back	Urine	Emesis	Suction ☐	
0700-1500	NPO	Credit _150cc_ Add _1000cc_ Add _____	50cc	100 cc 200 cc 200 cc	50 cc		
8 Hr.		1150	50cc	500cc	50cc		
1500-2300	50cc 50cc 100cc 50cc 100 cc 100 cc 50 cc	Credit _____ Add _____ Add _____	50cc	225cc 200cc			
8 Hr.	500cc		50cc	450cc			
2300-0700		Credit _____ Add _____ Add _____					
8 Hr.							
24 Hr.							

Iced Tea - 6 oz. (180 cc)	Cup of Coffee or Tea - 7 oz. (210 cc)
Water Glass - 6 oz. (180 cc)	Styrofoam Cup - 150 cc
Milk (carton) - 8 oz. (240 cc)	Paper Cup - 150 cc
Fruit Juice - 4 oz. (120 cc)	Coffee Creamer - ½ oz. (15 cc)
Soup - 4 oz. (120 cc)	Cereal Creamer - 2 oz. (60 cc)
Ice Cream - 3 oz. (90 cc)	Coca Cola and Sprite - 12 oz. (360 cc)
Jello - 3½ oz. (105 cc)	H_2O Pitcher - 30 oz. (900 cc)

FIGURE 19–19 ▲ Intake and output record.

Procedure 19-3: POSTOPERATIVE PROCEDURE

TASK	NOTES
1. Inform the patient's nurse of the patient's arrival in the PACU as soon as possible.	1. *PACU personnel will notify the unit when the patient arrives from the operating room. The nurse may then plan his or her work and be prepared for the patient's return to the unit.*
2. Inform the patient's nurse of the expected arrival of the patient from the recovery room.	2. *The recovery room personnel will notify the nursing unit before returning the patient to his or her room.*
3. Place all operating records behind the proper divider in the patient's chart.	
4. Write the date of surgery and the surgical procedure in the designated place on the patient's Kardex form or in the computer.	
5. Write in the date of the surgery on the patient's graphic sheet.	
6. Transcribe the doctors' postoperative orders. Notify the nurse caring for the patient of stat doctors' orders.	6. *All preoperative orders are automatically discontinued postoperatively. The health unit coordinator will usually start a new Kardex form for the patient.*

▼ REVIEW QUESTIONS

1. Place the letter of the correct answer in the second column in the space provided in the first column.

_____ 1. admission orders	a. admission necessitated by an accident or a medical emergency
_____ 2. admission service agreement	b. entry into hospital planned in advance
_____ 3. emergency admission	c. directions for care and treatment written by the doctor on patient's entry into hospital
_____ 4. scheduled admission	d. contains general services the hospital will provide
_____ 5. direct admission	e. a patient who was not scheduled to be admitted and is admitted from the doctor's office, clinic, or emergency room

2. Define the following:

   a. patient health records number

   _____

   b. patient identification bracelet

   _____

   c. preoperative nursing checklist

   _____

   d. surgery schedule

   _____

   e. patient account number

   _____

f. valuables envelope

_____

g. preoperative orders

_____

h. postoperative orders

_____

i. allergy information

_____

j. facesheet or front sheet

_____

k. preoperative health unit coordinator checklist

_____

l. elective surgery

_____

m. allergy identification bracelet

_____

n. preadmit

_____

o. registration

_____

3. List at least six common components of a set of admission orders.

a. _____

b. _____

c. _____

d. _____

e. _____

f. _____

4. Three items prepared by the registration staff that are sent to the unit as part of the admission procedure are:

a. _____

b. _____

c. _____

5. List at least five health unit coordinator tasks regarding the patient's admission.

   a. _____

   b. _____

   c. _____

   d. _____

   e. _____

6. Explain the health unit coordinator's responsibilities regarding the preoperative patient's chart.

   _____

   _____

7. Five records or reports that might be on the patient's chart before surgery are:

   a. _____

   b. _____

   c. _____

   d. _____

   e. _____

8. List seven components that may be part of preoperative orders.

   a. _____

   b. _____

   c. _____

   d. _____

   e. _____

   f. _____

   g. _____

9. List nine components that may be part of a set of postoperative orders.

   a. _____

   b. _____

   c. _____

   d. _____

   e. _____

   f. _____

g. _____

h. _____

i. _____

10. List three tasks the health unit coordinator may perform concerning the postoperative patient's chart and Kardex.

a. _____

b. _____

c. _____

11. Define advance directives.

_____

_____

12. List at least eight patient registration tasks.

a. _____

b. _____

c. _____

d. _____

e. _____

f. _____

g. _____

h. _____

13. What is the difference between a living will and power of attorney for health care?

_____

_____

14. When does an advance directive become effective?

_____

_____

TOPICS FOR DISCUSSION

1. Discuss the consequences of a surgery being canceled due to the discovery of the surgical consent form not being accurate or the condition of admission form not being signed after the patient was sedated.

2. Discuss how the first person you encountered in a health care facility or doctor's office influenced your overall opinion of that facility. Can you think of positive examples as well as negative examples?

3. Discuss what you would do if John Brown's nurse is at lunch and you receive a call that he is ready to return to his room from PACU.

Discharge, Transfer, and Postmortem Procedures

► Chapter Objectives

Upon completion of this chapter, you will be able to:

1. Define the terms in the vocabulary list.
2. Write the meaning of each abbreviation in the abbreviations list.
3. List 14 tasks that may be required to complete a routine discharge.
4. List the additional tasks that may be required when a patient is discharged to a nursing home.
5. Describe the tasks necessary to prepare the discharged patient's chart for the health records department.
6. Explain what the health unit coordinator should do if a patient approaches the nursing station and states that he or she is unhappy with his or her care and is leaving.
7. List nine tasks performed by the health unit coordinator upon the death of a patient.
8. List 13 tasks that are performed in the transfer of a patient from one unit to another.
9. Describe the tasks of the health unit coordinator in the transfer of a patient from one room to another room on the same unit.
10. List nine tasks performed by the health unit coordinator when a transferred patient is received on the unit.

► Vocabulary

Autopsy ▲ An examination of a body after death; it may be performed to determine the cause of death or for medical research

Census Sheet ▲ A daily listing of all patient activity (admissions, discharges, transfers, and deaths) within the hospital; may also be called the admissions, discharges, and transfers sheet (ADT)

Coroner's Case ▲ A death that occurs due to sudden, violent, or unexplained circumstances or a patient that expires during the first 24 hours after admission to the hospital

Custodial Care ▲ Care and services of a nonmedical nature, which consist of feeding, bathing, watching, and protecting the patient

Discharge Planning ▲ Centralized, coordinated, multidisciplinary process that ensures that the patient has a plan for continuing care after leaving the hospital

Expiration ▲ A death

Extended Care Facility ▲ A medical facility caring for patients requiring expert nursing care or custodial care

Organ Donation ▲ Donating or giving one's organs and/or tissues after death; one may designate specific organs (e.g., only cornea) or any needed organs

Organ Procurement ▲ The process of removing donated organs; it may be referred to as harvesting

Patient Care Conference ▲ A meeting that will include the doctor or doctors caring for the patient, the primary nurses, the case manager or social worker, and other caregivers involved with the patient's care

Postmortem ▲ After death (a postmortem examination is the same as an autopsy)

Release of Remains ▲ A signed consent that authorizes a specific funeral home or agency to remove the deceased from a health care facility

Terminal Illness ▲ An illness ending in death

> ## Abbreviations

Abbreviation	Meaning	Example of Usage on a Doctor's Order Sheet
AMA	against medical advice	Patient D/C AMA
ECF	extended care facility	Pls. have case mgt arrange for transfer to ECF

EXERCISE 1

Write the abbreviation for each term listed below.

1. against medical advice _____

2. extended care facility _____

EXERCISE 2

Write the meaning of each abbreviation listed below.
1. AMA

_____

2. ECF

_____

■ DISCHARGE PLANNING

Discharge planning is a centralized, coordinated, multidisciplinary process that ensures that the patient has a plan for continuing care after leaving the hospital. Discharge planning begins the moment a patient is admitted to the hospital. A patient care conference is a meeting that will include the doctor or doctors caring for the patient, the primary nurses, the case manager or social worker, and other caregivers involved with the patient's care. The health unit coordinator should be made aware when the patient's chart is taken into the conference room.

■ DISCHARGE OF A PATIENT

Once it is written by the doctor, the order for the discharge of a patient from the hospital requires the prompt attention of the health unit coordinator. Most patients wish to leave the hospital as soon as possible after the discharge order is written. Environmental Services (or housekeeping) must also prepare the vacated room and bed for the admission of a new patient. There are five types of discharges:

1. Discharge home
2. Discharge to another facility
3. Discharge home with assistance
4. Discharge against medical advice (AMA)
5. Expiration

All discharges require a doctor's order. When a patient insists on leaving AMA, the doctor will usually write a discharge order with documentation that the patient is leaving against medical advice.

Routine Discharge Procedure

Most discharges from the hospital are routine in nature; that is, the patient is discharged alive to go home in the company of a family member, a friend, or alone. See Procedure 20–1 and Figures 20–1 through 20–4.

Procedure 20-1: DISCHARGE PROCEDURE

TASK	NOTES
1. Read the entire order when transcribing the discharge order. Check for any Rx that may have been left in chart by doctor.	**1.** *The order may be written on the doctor's order sheet the day before or the day of the expected discharge. Read the order carefully. Sometimes the doctor will write dc p̄ chest x-ray or other diagnostic test.*
2. Notify the discharged patient's nurse.	**2.** *The patient's nurse will provide the patient with discharge instructions.*
3. Enter a "pending discharge" with the expected departure time into the computer.	**3.** *Notification may be by telephone. Entering a "pending discharge" with expected departure time notifies the admitting department to prepare the patient's bill. Some patients may be required to stop at the business office before leaving the hospital.*

Procedure 20–1: DISCHARGE PROCEDURE—cont'd

TASK	NOTES
4. Explain the procedure for discharge to the patient and/or the patient's relatives.	**4.** *The explanation of the discharge procedure may also be given by the nurse; however, many patients come to the health unit coordinator in the nurse's station for the explanation.*
5. Notify other departments that may be giving the patient daily treatments.	**5.** *Departments such as physical therapy and respiratory care may need to be notified. This may be communicated by telephone or by computer.*
6. Communicate the patient's discharge to the dietary department by computer.	**6.** *If the patient is not planning to leave the hospital during the regular discharge hours (usually before lunch), type in the expected departure time.*
7. Arrange for any appointments requested by doctor.	**7.** *Write out the appointment date and the time on a piece of paper and give it to the patient. A discharge instruction sheet is prepared by the nurse and is given to the patient (see Fig. 20–1).*
8. Arrange transportation if needed.	**8.** *Patients who do not have family or friends available to provide transportation may need to have a call made for a taxi.*
9. Prepare credit slips for medications returned to the pharmacy or equipment and supplies to CSD.	**9.** *Supplies specifically ordered for the patient from CSD and not used by the patient must be returned to CSD with a credit slip (see Fig. 20–2).*
10. Notify nursing personnel or transportation service to transport patient to the discharge area when patient is ready to leave.	**10.** *Patients should never be allowed to go to the discharge area without an escort from the hospital staff. Also, the patient should be transported via a wheelchair.*
11. Write the patient's name on the admission, discharge, and transfer sheet (see Fig. 20–3).	
12. Delete the patient's name from the unit census board and TPR sheet.	**12.** *Draw a line through the patient's name on TPR sheet and erase name on census board.*
13. Notify environmental services to clean the discharged patient's room.	**13.** *Notification may be by telephone, computer, or by telling the environmental services personnel on the unit.*
14. Prepare the chart for the health records department:	**14.** *Many hospitals issue a discharge checklist (see Fig. 20–4) to prepare the chart for the health records department.*

14. Prepare the chart for the health records department:
   a. Check the summary/DRG worksheet for the doctor's summation and the patient's final diagnosis. It is important to have this information upon patient discharge so that coding of the diagnosis-related groups may be placed on the chart by the health records department.
   b. Check for the correct patient identification labels on the chart forms.
   c. Shred all chart forms that have been labeled and do not have any documentation on them.
   d. Check for old records or split records and send with the chart to health records.
   e. Arrange the chart forms in discharge sequence according to your hospital policy.
   f. Send the chart of the discharged patient to the health records department along with any old records of the patient. Charts of discharged patients must be sent to health records on the day of discharge.

DISCHARGE
INSTRUCTIONS

DIAGNOSIS: _____

_____

SURGERY/PROCEDURE: _____

1. **ACTIVITY**	NO LIMIT	LIMIT
Bathing		
Driving		
Sexual		
Work		
Exercise		
Ambulation		

2. **MEDICATION:**

_____ Patient/family knows what medications are for.

_____ Prescriptions sent with patient or family.

NAME OF MEDICATION	**DOSAGE**	**FREQUENCY/TIMES**

3. **DIET:**

Your diet will be _____

Please call dietition at _____ if you have any questions.

4. **SPECIAL INFORMATION:** (include wound care, further treatments, referrals, equipment, etc.)

5. **RETURN VISIT TO PHYSICIAN:** Please call Dr. _____Phone: _____

to make an appointment in _____ days. Please call the doctor if you cannot take your medicine

or to answer any questions.

6. **INSTRUCTION SHEETS GIVEN:** (Please list pamphlets, written instructions or other standardized information.)

The above was discussed with me and
I understand all of the information.

_____
Signature of R.N.

_____
Date

_____
Signature of Patient/Guardian

Patient (original)   Medical Records (yellow)   Other (pink)   DISCHARGE INSTRUCTIONS

FIGURE 20–1 ▲ Discharge instruction sheet. (From Rockford Memorial Hospital, Rockford, IL, with permission.)

MISCELLANEOUS CREDIT

CREDIT

PATIENT NO.	C	DR. NO.	DATE	NUR. STA.	99	9 C	SERV. DEPT.	CODE	PRICE	SERV. DEPT.	CODE	PRICE

TECH.

EXPLANATION OF CREDIT	CODE	PRICE

MISCELLANEOUS CREDIT

ORIGINATING DEPT.

FORM NO. 53-02

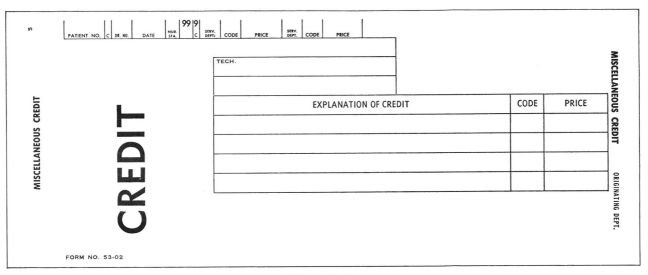

FIGURE 20–2 ▲ Credit requisition.

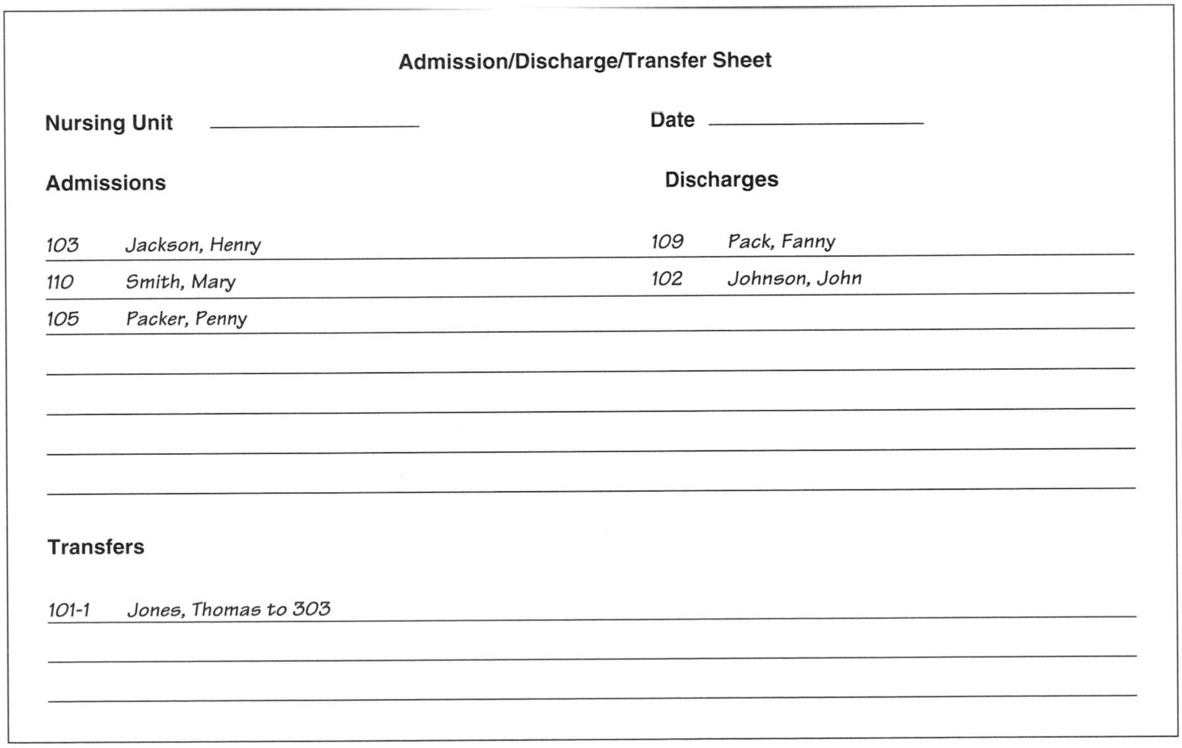

Admission/Discharge/Transfer Sheet

Nursing Unit ____________ **Date** ____________

Admissions		**Discharges**	
103	*Jackson, Henry*	*109*	*Pack, Fanny*
110	*Smith, Mary*	*102*	*Johnson, John*
105	*Packer, Penny*		

Transfers

101-1 *Jones, Thomas to 303*

FIGURE 20–3 ▲ Census sheet or admission, discharge, and transfer sheet.

DISCHARGE CHECKLIST

(To be completed and sent with chart to the Medical Records Department by end of shift on which the patient is discharged. Check Yes or No box.)

Date of Admission ___12/4/XX___

Check List

HISTORY & PHYSICAL

Yes No

☒ ☐ 1. History and Physical on chart within 48 hours. Due ___12/6/XX___
       (IF NO, ANSWER NUMBER TWO.)

☐ ☐ 2. History and Physical Notification Form # 00-0531 sent to Medical Records. Date sent _____

Health Unit Coordinator Signature ___Ina Clerke___

Check List

FINAL DISPOSITION OF CHART

Yes No

☐ ☐ 1. All sheets embossed with correct patient master card and legible, and all reports are for this patient.

☐ ☐ 2. Portions of chart which have been removed are replaced in proper order, with chart dividers removed.

☐ ☐ 3. Reports are correctly inserted or attached.

      4. FRONT SHEET:

☐ ☐   a. Discharge diagnosis written on Front Sheet by Doctor. If No, answer 4b.

☐ ☐   b. Final diagnosis noted on Telephone Tentative or Final Discharge Diagnosis Form #00-0523 attached to chart and send to Medical Records with check list. If unable to complete, state reason on form.

☐ ☐ 5. Previous Medical Records return to Medical Record Department.

☐ ☐ 6. Accordion folders used for sending records to Medical Record Department.

☐ ☐ 7. Discharge entered in Unit Transit Book.

Date of Discharge _____

Health Unit Coordinator Signature _____

☐ ☐ 8. Nurses notes are complete.

R.N. or L.P.N. Signature: _____

FIGURE 20–4 ▲ Discharge checklist.

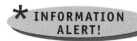
★ INFORMATION ALERT!

It is important to read a discharge order carefully prior to a patient leaving the unit. The doctor may write "discharge after chest x-ray" or other directions and may leave a prescription on the chart to give to the patient.

Discharge to Another Facility

Insurance reviewers are employed by the insurance companies to review hospitalized patients' charts to advise doctors what the insurance will cover and how many hospital days will be covered. When the patient no longer needs expert nursing care but still requires custodial care, the doctor is requested to transfer the patient from the hospital to an assisted living facility or nursing care home. Custodial care is care of a nonmedical nature, such as feeding, bathing, watching, and protecting the patient. The insurance reviewer will place a

Procedure 20-2: ADDITIONAL STEPS TO DISCHARGE PATIENT TO ANOTHER FACILITY

TASK	NOTES
1. Notify case management or social service of the doctor's orders to discharge to another facility.	
2. Transportation will usually be arranged by the case manager or social worker.	2. *The patient who is confined to bed may require an ambulance when requested.*
3. Complete the continuing care form or transfer form.	3. *The continuing care form requires some information that the health unit coordinator may fill in from the facesheet. The nurse and doctor complete their sections of the form (see Fig. 20–5).*
4. Photocopy patient chart forms as indicated in the doctor's orders.	4. *Requirement of forms will vary from facility to facility. It is also necessary to check hospital policy to determine who is responsible for making copies—the health unit coordinator or the health records department. Once the copies are made, it is important to place the originals back in the chart in proper sequence.*
5. Distribute continuing care form and copies as required.	5. *The photocopies and a copy of the continuing care form are placed in a sealed envelope to be given to the ambulance driver or a family member. This person delivers the envelope to the nurse at the nursing care facility.*
6. Now perform all routine steps as shown in Procedure 20-1.	

Procedure 20-3: ADDITIONAL STEPS FOR DISCHARGE HOME WITH ASSISTANCE

TASK	NOTES
1. Notify case management or social service of the doctor's order.	1. *The responsible personnel will vary depending on patient type.*
2. Prepare the continuing care form.	2. *Health unit coordinator to complete personal information section.*
3. Obtain a release of information signature from patient.	
4. Photocopy forms as indicated in the doctor's order.	
5. Distribute continuing care form and copies as required.	
6. Now perform routine discharge steps.	

sticker on the cover of the patient's chart binder indicating how many more days will be covered by the patient's insurance. If the doctor feels that the patient needs additional hospitalization, he or she will document the reasons for the additional days.

Other patients may be discharged to an assisted living facility, nursing care home, or an extended care facility (ECF). Frequently, the hospital case manager or social service worker makes the arrangements for long-term care. The discharge of a patient to another facility is the same as a routine discharge with additional steps (Procedure 20–2).

Many patients need care or assistance at home as part of their recovery process. Additional steps are required when a patient needs home health care. The hospital case manager or social service worker arranges home health care and home health equipment. See Procedure 20–3 and Figure 20–5.

(Use Typewriter or Ballpoint Pen – Press Firmly)   *(See Instructions on back of Page 3)*

CONTINUING CARE TRANSFER INFORMATION

TO BE COMPLETED AND SIGNED BY NURSING SERVICE (Please attach a copy of the Nursing Care Plan)

PATIENT'S NAME	Last	First	MI	DATE OF BIRTH	SEX	RELIGION	HEALTH INSURANCE CLAIM NUMBER

PATIENT'S ADDRESS (Street number, City, State and Zip Code) | ATTENDING PHYSICIAN   Name   Address

RELATIVE OR GUARDIAN   Name   Address   Phone Number

Name and Address of Facility Transferring FROM | Dates of Stay at Facility Transferring FROM — Admission / Discharge | Facility Name and Address Transferring TO

PAYMENT SOURCE FOR CHARGES TO PATIENT:

☐ Self or Family   ☐ Private Insurance ID Number _____   ☐ Blue Cross/Blue Shield ID Number _____   ☐ Employer or Union

☐ Public Agency _____   ☐ Other (specify) _____

PATIENT EVALUATION:

SPEECH: ☐ Normal ☐ Impaired ☐ Unable to speak

HEARING: ☐ Normal ☐ Impaired ☐ Deaf

SIGHT: ☐ Normal ☐ Impaired ☐ Blind

MENTAL STATUS: ☐ Always Alert ☐ Occasionally Confused ☐ Always Confused

FEEDING: ☐ Independent ☐ Help with Feeding ☐ Cannot Feed Self

DRESSING: ☐ Independent ☐ Help with Dressing ☐ Cannot Dress Self

ELIMINATION: ☐ Independent ☐ Help to Bathroom ☐ Bedpan or Urinal ☐ Incontinent

BATHING: ☐ Independent ☐ Bathing with Help ☐ Bed Bath with Help ☐ Bed Bath

AMBULATORY STATUS: ☐ Independent ☐ Walks with Help ☐ Help from Bed to Chair ☐ Bed Bound

NURSING ASSESSMENT AND RECOMMENDATIONS:

TREATMENTS:

Last Medication: _____ / Dose: _____

Date: _____   Time: _____

APPLIANCES OR SUPPORTS: or check none ☐

Signature   Title   Date

TO BE COMPLETED AND SIGNED BY THE ATTENDING PHYSICIAN

ECF Admitting Diagnosis:

Please send a copy of the following records with patient:

☐ Summary Sheet (face sheet)
☐ Discharge Summary
☐ Physical Examination and History
☐ Consultation
☐ Other (specify) _____

Patient knows diagnosis: ☐ Yes ☐ No

Surgical Procedures: (current admission)

Transfer by: ☐ Ambulance ☐ Car ☐ Other (specify) _____

Allergies: ☐ No ☐ Yes (specify) _____

VDRL: ☐ Positive ☐ Negative

Anticoagulant: ☐ Taking now ☐ Previously

Orders: Diet, medication and special therapy *(To be renewed in 48 hours)*

Chest X-Ray Diagnosis: _____

I will care for this patient after admission to new facility: ☐ Yes ☐ No

Medication Regimen is stabilized: ☐ Yes ☐ No

Anticipated length of stay for extended care _____ days

Physician's Signature   Date

If necessary, attach order sheet – The above constitutes valid temporary orders only if signed by a physician.

Address   Telephone Number

FIGURE 20–5 ▲ Continuing care transfer form.

■ DISCHARGE AGAINST MEDICAL ADVICE

A patient may feel that he or she is not receiving the care that is needed. Or perhaps the patient believes that there is no improvement in the condition for which he or she is hospitalized. Whatever the reason, the patient may decide to leave the hospital without the doctor's approval.

The patient may appear at the nurse's station and announce that he or she is leaving the hospital. The health unit coordinator should ask the patient to be seated until his or her nurse is advised. The hospitalist, resident, or admitting doctor may be called to speak with the patient. The patient may be advised that his or her insurance will not cover the hospital bill if he or she leaves against medical advice. Everything possible is done to encourage the patient to

LEAVING HOSPITAL AGAINST ADVICE

Date_____

This is to certify that_____,
a patient in The Above Named Hospital, is leaving the hospital against the advice
of the attending physician and the hospital administration. I acknowledge that I
have been informed of the risk involved and hereby release the attending physician,
and the hospital, from all responsibility and any ill effects which may result from
this action.

_____
PATIENT

_____
OTHER PERSON RESPONSIBLE

_____
RELATIONSHIP

Witness_____

Witness_____

00-0434   LEAVING HOSPITAL AGAINST ADVICE

FIGURE 20–6 ▲ Form for discharge against medical advice.

remain in the hospital until the treatment is completed. However, if the patient does not pose a threat to self or others, the patient cannot be restrained from leaving and usually the admitting doctor, resident, or hospitalist will write a discharge order with the documentation that the patient is leaving against medical advice.

In the event that the patient is not convinced to stay, a release form (see Fig. 20–6) is prepared. The form is signed by the

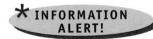

INFORMATION ALERT!

A patient may be restrained from leaving the hospital if two doctors certify that the patient poses a threat to self or others.

AUTHORIZATION FOR REMOVAL OF REMAINS/ AUTOPSY/ORGAN AND TISSUE DONATION

*Area requiring signature of Family/Responsible Party

Implanted Devices _____ Type _____
(i.e., Epidural or Venous access, implanted pump, etc.)

AUTHORIZATION FOR REMOVAL OF REMAINS

The undersigned hereby authorizes and directs _____ and/or its
(Funeral Home)

agents to remove and take possesion of the remains of _____.
I (We) hereby represent that I am (we are) the next of kin and/or are legally authorized with this responsibility.

_____ _____ _____ _____ 19 _____
*(Signature)   (Relationship)   (Witness)   (Date)

Please ask that dentures remain with the deceased.
The Funeral Director would appreciate a phone number where the family can be reached:

Name: _____ **Phone** _____

☐ Infection Control Precautions should be followed if an "Infection Hazard" tag is attached.

AUTHORIZATION FOR AUTOPSY

Autopsy Requested ☐ NO   ☐ YES   **If Yes, by** _____

I (We) request and authorize the physicians and surgeons in attendance at _____ . Hospital to perform a complete

autopsy on the remains of _____,
and I (we) authorize removal and retention or use for diagnostic, scientific or therapeutic purposes, of such organs, tissues and
parts, at this hospital, and at such other institutions as such physicians and surgeons deem appropriate. This authority is granted

subject to the following restrictions: _____

_____
(If no restrictions, write "None")

I (We) hereby represent that I am (we are) the next of kin and/or legally authorized by law to control the disposition of the remains.

_____ _____ _____ _____ 19 _____
*(Signature)   (Relationship)   (Witness)   (Date)

_____ _____ _____ _____ 19 _____
*(Signature)   (Relationship)   (Witness)   (Date)

When consent is given by telephone, two auditing witnesses must sign.

Name of person obtaining authorization:

AM
_____ Date _____ 19 ___ Time _____ PM

Autopsy performed _____ by _____ M.D.

ORGAN/TISSUE DONATION REQUEST

1. Please complete the Organ/Tissue Donation Screening Record   One copy is for the
   patient's medical record and one copy for   Administration.

2. In addition to completing the Authorization for the Removal of the Remains
   please complete the   Consent Record

3.   donor manual available for reference.

Nursing Office notified		**Coroner notified**	_____
			(Name) (Date/Time)
		Coroner to Autopsy ☐ Yes ☐ No _____	
_____	_____		
(Name)	(Date/Time)		
Primary physician notified		**Possessions and belongings released to**	
_____	_____	_____	_____
(Name)	(Date/Time)	*(Signature)	(Date/Time)

Authorization for Removal of Remains/Autopsy/Organ and Tissue Donation
Original – Med. Records   Copy – Patient

FIGURE 20–7 ▲ Expiration form, release of remains, authorization for autopsy, and organ donation request. (From Rockford Memorial Hospital, Rockford, IL, with permission.)

patient or his or her representative, and witnessed by an appropriate member of the hospital staff. The patient is then permitted to leave the hospital, and the discharge procedure is the same as for a routine discharge.

DISCHARGE OF THE DECEASED PATIENT

Patient Deaths

Not all patients who enter the hospital for care and treatment are discharged alive. Some patients who enter the hospital are well advanced in age. Other patients, in any age group, may have a terminal illness that results in expected death. Sometimes, death is unexpected, as in the case of complications from surgery. Frequently, the patient's death is slow, and there is an opportunity to offer support to family members as time permits.

You may be requested to call a religious counselor to speak with the patient or perform final rites. Many hospitals have counselors of various denominations and also nondenominations to assist patients and families. A notation should be made on the patient's Kardex form of any final rites that have been performed.

Certification of Death

In cases in which a death is expected, the nurse or family members may be with the patient at the time of expiration (death). At other times, the patient may die unexpectedly. In either instance, the doctor must be notified to pronounce the patient dead. The patient is examined for any signs of life. If none can be determined, the patient is pronounced dead and the official time is recorded on the doctors' progress notes. The doctor must also complete a death certificate, and a report of the death filed with the bureau of vital statistics.

Release of Remains

The patient's family or guardian must indicate the funeral home to which the body will be released. Usually, the family must sign a form (Fig. 20-7) before the patient can be released to the funeral home. The nursing staff may notify the funeral home of the expiration. The funeral home personnel may pick up the patient from the unit or the hospital morgue. A hospital security officer may need to accompany the funeral home personnel.

Organ Donation

Many patients indicate their wishes for organ donation before their death. A patient may designate specific organs (e.g., only cornea) or any needed organs or tissues. Due to state laws, the nursing staff may be required to ask the family about organ donation. It will be necessary to check the hospital's policies regarding organ donation. Additional consent forms (Fig. 20-8) will be necessary in the harvesting of an organ (organ procurement).

AUTOPSY OR POSTMORTEM EXAMINATION

An autopsy, or postmortem examination, of the body is performed to determine the cause of death or for medical research (see Fig. 20-7). The family may ask that an autopsy be done, or the doctor may request it. Before an autopsy can be performed, however, the family must grant permission. A consent for autopsy form must be signed by the next of kin.

Coroner's Cases

A coroner's case is one in which the patient's death is due to sudden, violent, or unexplained circumstances, such as an accident, a poisoning, or a gunshot wound. Deaths that occur less than 24 hours after hospitalization may also be termed coroner's cases. State, county, and local governments have regulations defining a coroner's case in their particular locality. The law gives the coroner permission to study the body by dissection to determine whether there is evidence of foul play. A signed consent by the nearest of kin is not required when a death is ruled a coroner's case. See Procedure 20-4 for tasks related to the death of a patient, which may be performed by the health unit coordinator.

TRANSFER OF A PATIENT

A variety of circumstances may necessitate a patient transfer. A patient's condition may change; a patient improves and is transferred out of intensive care. A patient may need a private room for infection control or isolation. A patient may be transferred if his or her original room request becomes available; the patient wanted a private room that is now available. A patient may be transferred because of roommate incompatibilities.

The duties performed in a series of tasks allow for an orderly transfer of the patient from one area to another. Transfer may be from one unit of the hospital to another, or it may be from one room to another on the same nursing unit.

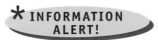

✶ INFORMATION ALERT!

Five Types of Discharges

Home
To another facility
Home with assistance
Against medical advice
Expiration

AUTHORIZATION FOR DISPOSITION
OF BODY OR PARTS THEREOF

NAME OF PATIENT:_____ DATE:_____

STATUS OF SIGNER: Patient ☐   Surviving Spouse ☐   Parent ☐   Child ☐   Brother ☐

Sister ☐   Other person entitled by law to control disposition of remains ☐   Specify:

_____

ORGAN OR TISSUE DONATED (Should be specified unless whole body is donated):_____

_____

DONEE: (a) University of Arizona ☐   (b) Arizona Eye Bank, Inc. ☐   (c) to be determined by hospital or any

available physician ☐   (d) specify if other ☐ _____

    The Undersigned hereby donates the body of the above-named patient, or the parts thereof above specified, to the donee above specified for such humanitarian, research, educational, or transplant purposes or other disposition or use as the donee may in its discretion determine. If the entire body is donated, it is to be delivered unembalmed and without autopsy other than such as may be required by law.

_____   _____
         WITNESS   SIGNATURE

_____
         WITNESS

IF SIGNER IS THE PATIENT THIS FORM MUST BE SIGNED BY A NOTARY PUBLIC.

STATE OF ARIZONA   )
) ss.
County of Maricopa   )

    This instrument was acknowledged before me this_____day of_____, 19_____.

_____
         NOTARY PUBLIC

My Commission Expires:

_____

AUTHORIZATION FOR DISPOSITION
OF BODY OR PARTS THEREOF

FIGURE 20–8 ▲ Consent form for donation of body organs.

Procedure 20-4: **POSTMORTEM PROCEDURE**

STEP TASK	NOTES
1. Contact the attending doctor, hospitalist, or resident when asked by the nurse to do so to verify the patient's death.	
2. Notify the hospital operator of the patient's death.	
3. Prepare any forms that may be needed.	**3.** *These forms may consist of a release of remains/request for autopsy (see Fig. 20–7) and/ or a consent for donation of body organs (see Fig. 20–8). Some hospitals use a postmortem checklist (Fig. 20–9) to ascertain that all postmortem tasks have been completed.*
4. Notify the mortuary that has been requested by the family.	**4.** *If the family is not familiar with mortuaries in the area, a list of mortuaries is usually available from the hospital telephone switchboard operator. The nursing office personnel may notify the funeral home.*
5. Call the hospital to determine if the body is to be taken for autopsy or is to remain there until the mortuary arrives.	
6. The nurse will gather the deceased's clothes, place them in a paper sack to be labeled with the patient's name, the room number, and the date.	**6.** *The clothing is given to the family or to the mortician.*
7. Obtain the mortuary book from the nursing office or have a mortuary form prepared when the mortician arrives.	**7.** *The mortician claiming the body must complete forms to show that he or she has claimed the body, the clothing, or any valuables (Fig. 20–10).*
8. Notify all doctors who were involved with the patient's care.	
9. Now perform routine discharge steps shown in Procedure 20–1.	

The tasks that may be performed for the transfer of a patient from one hospital unit to another are listed in Procedure 20–5. Tasks to be performed when transferring a patient from one room to another on the same unit are listed in Procedure 20–6. Tasks to be performed when receiving a transferred patient on a nursing unit are listed in Procedure 20–7.

■ SUMMARY

The health unit coordinator's tasks for discharge and transfer procedures are many. If you learn these procedures in a particular order and do not deviate from them, you can be sure that you will always perform the tasks thoroughly and completely.

CHECK LIST
Post-Mortem Care

1) Telephone Notification
☐ Family
☐ ALL physicians involved in patient care
☐ Whether or not an autopsy is to be done
☐ Switch Board (name, room number, time, mortuary)
☐ Police in event of Coroner's Case (check to see if physician called)
☐ Mortuary if known - and if mortician is to come to the unit.

2) Forms
Mortuary Form
When mortician comes to unit
☐ white copy to chart
☐ yellow to mortician
☐ pink to Business office with discharge requisition
☐ Patient Information Form remains on the unit
When patient goes to morgue
☐ entire completed form goes with patient
☐ Patient Information Form attached to mortuary form
Autopsy
☐ single copy remains on chart - send to Medical Records as soon as possible

3) Preparation of Body
When patient goes to Morgue
☐ Shroud and tag properly
☐ Mark on the shroud tag if patient is in isolation and causative organism, if known
☐ Complete #1 and 2
If a Coroner's Case
☐ Do not remove drains, IV's, etc., until police come. They may take the body with them.
☐ Notify mortuary of this
When patient goes to mortuary from the unit
☐ Do not shroud unless isolated
☐ Mark on tag causative organism

4) Transport Patient
☐ Patient elevator on E Wing 7:00 a.m. to 3:30 p.m., Mon. thru Fri.
☐ A, B, and C to 5th floor and cross to elevator #8 to 1st floor of S Building, S-4
☐ If body goes to refrigerator, mark 3 x 5 card on door
☐ Two people go with patient and their names are charted

5) Chart
☐ Complete all of Check List for Medical Records
☐ All of items noted in "Telephone Notification"
☐ Who takes body to morgue
☐ Name of mortuary
☐ Follow Discharge Procedure

6) Please refer to Procedure Book for clarification of any and all of the above points, especially in reference to Coroner's Case, fetal death and autopsy.

_____ R.N.
Signature

00-0585

FIGURE 20–9 ▲ Postmortem checklist.

MORTUARY FORM

Name _____

Address _____

Doctor _____ Religion _____

☐ Date Admitted _____

Religious Rites Performed ☐ desired ☐ Date of Death _____ Time _____ Home Phone _____

I. Clothing and Valuables from Room:	II. Jewelry and/or Valuables sent to safe.	III. Items on body:
		IV. Number_____ Valuables envelope on admission (in safe).
	Valuables Envelope Number_____	
Listed by_____ Registered Nurse	Witness_____ Registered Nurse	

Disposition of possessions

To Family:

Items:

Received by _____

Relationship _____

Witness_____
Registered Nurse

To Mortuary:

Items:

Received by _____

Mortuary _____

Witness_____
Hospital Representative Title

I accept the body and valuables (as listed above) of the patient named above. The identity has been verified by:

_____
Mortuary

_____
Mortuary Representative

Telephone number of nearest
relative or responsible party _____

Miscellaneous:

Witness_____

Title _____

Autopsy: Yes _____ No _____   Time _____ Date _____

DISPOSITION: 1. When body goes to the Morgue, send all 3 copies with the body.

2. When the Mortician comes to the unit, distribute copies as follows:

00-0308   WHITE – To Patient's Chart ● YELLOW – To Mortician ● PINK – To Business Office

FIGURE 20–10 ▲ Mortuary form.

Procedure 20–5: PROCEDURE FOR TRANSFER FROM ONE UNIT TO ANOTHER

TASK	NOTES
1. Transcribe order for a transfer.	
2. Notify the nurse caring for the patient of the transfer order.	
3. Notify admitting department of transfer order to obtain a new room assignment.	
4. Communicate new unit and room assignment to the nurse caring for the patient.	
5. Notify the receiving unit of the transfer.	
6. Record the transfer on the unit admission, discharge, and transfer sheet.	
7. Send all thinned records, old records, and x-rays with the patient to the receiving unit.	
8. Send the patient's chart, Kardex form, and current MAR with the patient to the receiving unit.	8. *An empty chart will be given in exchange for the patient's chart by the receiving unit.*
9. Usually the nurse will put medications in a bag and place them with the chart.	
10. Erase patient's name on the census board.	
11. Notify all departments that perform regularly scheduled treatments on the patient.	
12. Indicate the transfer on the diet sheet or in the computer and on the TPR sheet.	
13. Notify environmental services to clean the room.	13. *Environmental services may be notified by telephone, computer, or in person.*
14. Notify the attending doctor, all other doctors involved with the patient's care, and the information desk of the transfer.	

Procedure 20–6: PROCEDURE TO TRANSFER TO ANOTHER ROOM ON THE SAME UNIT

STEP TASK	NOTES
1. Transcribe the order for the transfer.	
2. Notify the nurse caring for the patient when request for transfer is granted.	
3. Place patient's chart in correct slot in the chart holder after replacing patient ID labels with corrected labels.	
4. Place Kardex form in its new place in the Kardex form file.	
5. Move the patient's name to the correct bed on the computer census screen. Send change to the dietary department. Change room number on the TPR sheet.	
6. Record the transfer on the unit admission, discharge, and transfer sheet.	
7. Notify environmental services to clean the room.	7. *Environmental services may be notified by telephone, computer, or in person.*
8. Notify the switchboard and the information center of the change.	

Procedure 20-7: PROCEDURE FOR RECEIVING A TRANSFERRED PATIENT

STEP / TASK	NOTES
1. Notify the nurse caring for the patient of the expected arrival of a transferred patient.	
2. Introduce yourself to the transferred patient upon his or her arrival on the unit.	
3. Notify the nurse caring for the patient of the transferred patient's arrival.	
4. Place the patient's chart in the correct slot in the chart holder, print corrected patient ID labels, and label patient's chart.	4. *Provide empty chart to unit from which the patient was transferred.*
5. Place Kardex form in the proper place.	
6. Record the receiving of a transfer patient on the unit admission, discharge, and transfer sheet, and write the patient's name on the census board.	
7. Place the patient's name on the TPR sheet and notify the dietary department of the patient's transfer.	
8. Move the patient's name from the unit the patient came from and place in correct bed on the computer census screen.	
9. Transcribe any new doctors' orders.	9. *When the patient is transferred from an intensive care unit to a regular unit, or a regular unit to an intensive care unit, the doctor must write new orders. The intensive care unit orders are no longer valid.*

REVIEW QUESTIONS

1. List 14 tasks performed in a routine discharge of a patient from the hospital.

   a. _____

   b. _____

   c. _____

   d. _____

   e. _____

   f. _____

   g. _____

   h. _____

   i. _____

   j. _____

   k. _____

   l. _____

m. _____

n. _____

2. What would you do if a patient advises you that he or she is unhappy with the care received and is leaving the hospital?

_____

_____

3. Describe the tasks of the health unit coordinator in the preparation of the discharged patient's chart for the health records department.

_____

_____

4. List the additional tasks performed when a patient is discharged to another facility.

_____

_____

5. List the additional tasks when a patient is discharged home with assistance.

_____

_____

6. Define the following:

a. terminal illness

_____

b. expiration

_____

c. postmortem

_____

d. custodial care

_____

e. autopsy

_____

f. organ donation

_____

g. release of remains

_____

h. coroner's case

_____

i. extended care facility

_____

j. patient care conference

_____

k. discharge planning

_____

7. List nine tasks performed upon the death of a patient.

a. _____

b. _____

c. _____

d. _____

e. _____

f. _____

g. _____

h. _____

i. _____

8. Describe the duties performed in the transfer of a patient from one room to another room on the same unit.

_____

_____

9. List 13 tasks that are performed in the transfer of a patient from one unit to another unit.

a. _____

b. _____

c. _____

d. _____

e. _____

f. _____

g. _____

h. _____

i. _____

j. _____

k. _____

l. _____

m. _____

n. _____

10. List nine tasks performed when a transferred patient is received on the unit.

a. _____

b. _____

c. _____

d. _____

e. _____

f. _____

g. _____

h. _____

i. _____

TOPICS FOR DISCUSSION

1. Discuss the consequences of not reading the entire doctor's order when discharging a patient.
2. Discuss what actions you would take if a patient approached the nurse's station and angrily states that he is very dissatisfied with the care and is leaving.
3. Discuss what you would do when a patient expires.
4. Discuss the importance of communicating orders for the case manager or social worker regarding a patient's discharge or transfer.

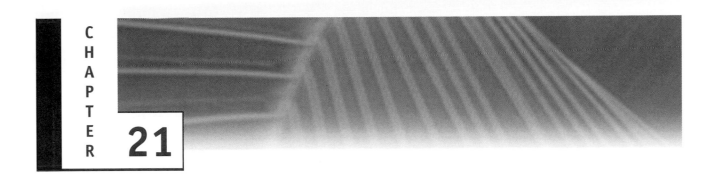

C H A P T E R

21

Recording Vital Signs, Ordering Supplies, Daily Diagnostic Tests, and Filing

Chapter Objectives

Upon completion of this chapter, you will be able to:

1. Define the terms in the vocabulary list.
2. Write the meaning of each abbreviation in the abbreviations list.
3. Describe the health unit coordinator's responsibilities for recording the vital signs and other information on the patient's graphic sheet.
4. Demonstrate the correct procedure for correcting three kinds of errors on the graphic sheet.
5. Convert Fahrenheit scale to Celsius scale, and Celsius scale to Fahrenheit scale.
6. List two reasons for efficient, accurate filing of the records on the patient's chart.
7. List five guidelines for filing the records on the patient's chart.
8. Describe the health unit coordinator's responsibilities for ordering daily diagnostic tests.
9. Explain the process of retrieving diagnostic test results using the computer.
10. Name five hospital departments that may provide supplies to the nursing unit, and write the type of supplies that may be obtained from each department.

Vocabulary

Bowel Movement ▲ The passage of stool

Celsius ▲ A scale used to measure temperature in which the freezing point of water is 0° and the boiling point is 100° (formerly called centigrade)

Daily TPRs ▲ Taking each patient's temperature, pulse, and respiration at a certain time(s) each day

Fahrenheit ▲ A scale used to measure temperature in which 32° is the freezing point of water and 212° is the boiling point

Pulse Deficit ▲ The difference between the radial pulse and the apical heartbeat

Stool ▲ The body wastes from the digestive tract that are discharged from the body through the anus

Abbreviations	
Abbreviation	**Meaning**
BM	bowel movement
C	Celsius
F	Fahrenheit
PO Day	postoperative day
PP	postpartum
TPR(s)	temperature, pulse, and respiration

TABLE 21–1	Celsius–Fahrenheit Conversion	
Conversion from Fahrenheit to Celsius	**Conversion from Celsius to Fahrenheit**	
Subtract 32	Multiply by 9	
Multiply by 5	Divide by 5	
Divide by 9	Add 32	

■ RECORDING VITAL SIGNS AND OTHER DATA ON THE GRAPHIC RECORD

In Chapter 10 we discussed what vital signs are, different methods for obtaining them, and doctors' orders relating to vital signs.

Review the terms and abbreviations relating to vital signs presented in the vocabulary and abbreviations lists, and the doctors' orders relating to vital signs written in the Doctors' Orders for Nursing Observation section (Chapter 10).

It is hospital routine to take each patient's temperature, pulse, respiration (TPR), and blood pressure (BP) usually three times each day or according to specific hospital policy to monitor patient condition. This process is often referred to as routine vital signs. If the doctor wishes the vital signs to be observed more often than the routine set forth by the hospital, he or she writes the order for such and a frequent vital sign record is used to record them.

The normal vital signs vary from one person to another; however, the following values are considered normal: temperature—98.6°F or 37°C; pulse—60 to 80; respiration—16 to 20; and blood pressure below 120/80.

It is hospital routine to record each patient's bowel movements along with the daily vital signs. If the doctor has ordered the patient to be weighed daily, this is also done routinely with the morning vital signs. The patient's intake and output is also recorded on the graphic record.

Vital signs are often included in the nursing record, and the nurse or certified nursing assistant is responsible for recording his or her patient's vital signs (Fig. 21–1). In some hospitals, the nursing personnel record patient vital signs on a TPN sheet. It is then the health unit coordinator's task to record the data from the TPR sheet onto each patient's graphic record form. The process is often referred to as recording vital signs.

The health unit coordinator should record the vital signs and other data as soon as it is recorded on the TPR sheet so that the information is readily available to the doctors when they make their hospital rounds. *Accuracy in the transfer of the vital signs is a must,* as the doctor may use this information to prescribe treatment for the patient.

Most often the temperature is taken and recorded using the Fahrenheit scale, but is sometimes taken and recorded on the Celsius scale, also known as the centigrade scale. There may be times when the health unit coordinator will have to convert the temperature from one scale to another. The conversion formulae above (Table 21–1) are used to convert Fahrenheit to Celsius and Celsius to Fahrenheit. Using this formula, a temperature of 98.6° Fahrenheit converts to 37.0° on the Celsius scale.

Method for Correcting Errors on the Graphic Record

Minor graphic errors may be corrected on the original graphic record. However, correction of major errors may require that the original graphic record be recopied. The following procedure for correcting errors should be followed.

1. To correct a *minor error on the graphic portion* of the graphic record, write "mistaken entry" in ink on the incorrect connecting line, record your first initial, your last name, and status about the error, then graph the correct value (Fig. 21–2).
2. To correct a *numbered entry,* such as the respiration value, draw a line through the entry in ink and write in ink "mistaken entry," your first initial, your last name, and status near it. As close as possible, insert the correct numbers (see Fig. 21–2).
3. To correct a *series of errors* on the graphic record, the entire record needs to be recopied showing the correct data (see Fig. 21–3, A).
   a. Prepare a new graphic record and label with the patient's ID label (Fig. 21–3, B).
   b. Transfer in ink *all* the information onto the new graphic record, including the correction of errors (see Fig. 21–3, B).
   c. Draw a diagonal line through the old graphic record in ink and record in ink "mistaken entry" on the line (see Fig. 21–3, A).
   d. Write that the graphic record was recopied, and write in ink your name, your status, and the date on the old graphic record (see Fig. 21–3, A).
   e. Place the old record behind the recopied record; it remains a permanent part of the chart.
   f. Write "recopied" followed by your name, status, and the date in ink on the new graphic record (see Fig. 21–3, B), and place it behind the correct divider in the patient's chart.

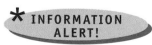

INFORMATION ALERT!

Accuracy in the transfer of the vital signs is a must, because the doctor may use this information to prescribe treatment for the patient.

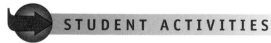

STUDENT ACTIVITIES

To practice recording the vital signs and other data on the graphic record, complete Activities 21–1 and 21–2 in the *Skills Practice Manual.*

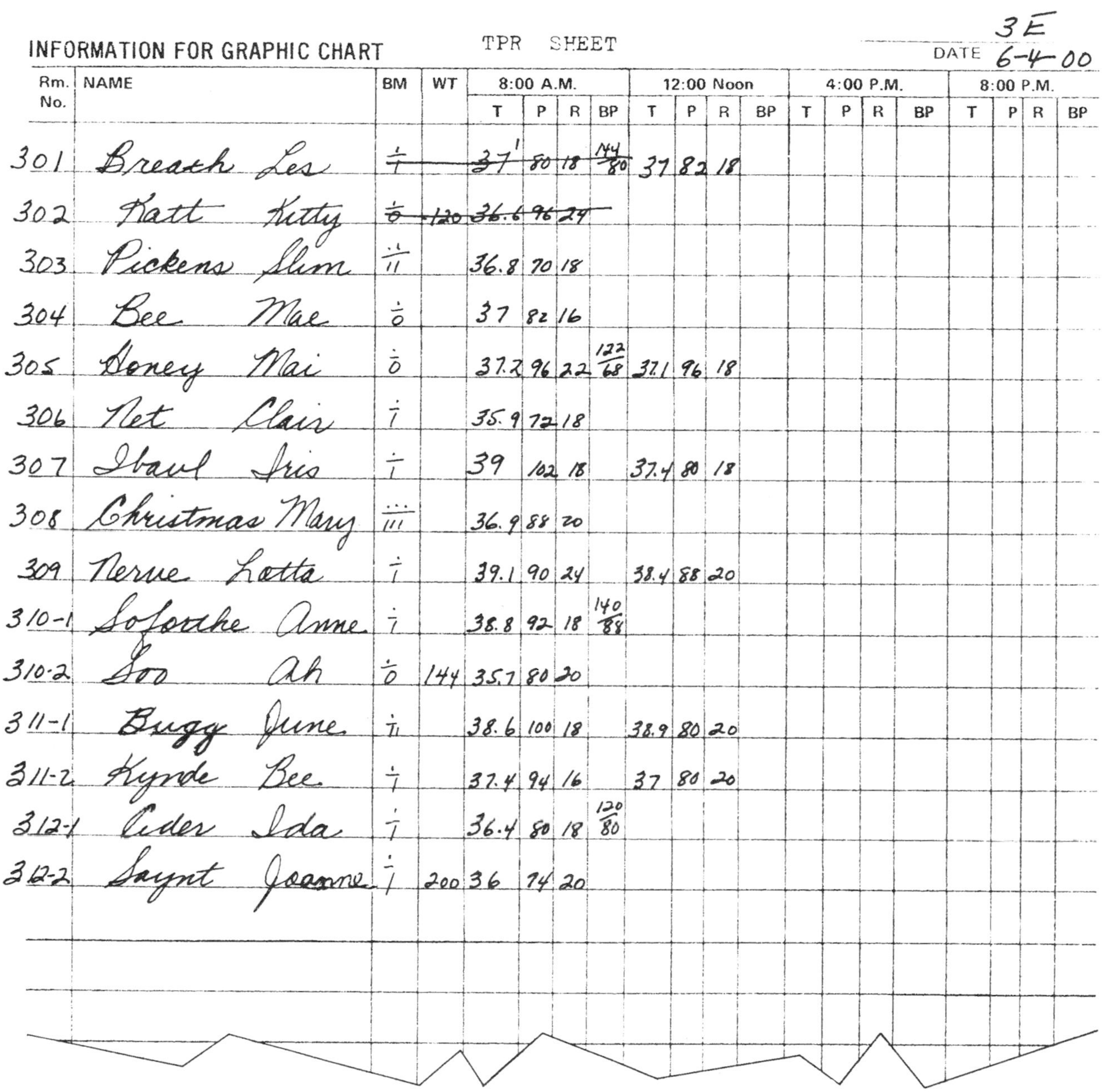

INFORMATION FOR GRAPHIC CHART TPR SHEET

3E

DATE 6-4-00

Rm. No.	NAME	BM	WT	8:00 A.M.				12:00 Noon				4:00 P.M.				8:00 P.M.			
				T	P	R	BP	T	P	R	BP	T	P	R	BP	T	P	R	BP
301	Breach Les	÷		37¹	80	18	144/80	37	82	18									
302	Katt Kitty	ö	120	36.6	96	24													
303	Pickens Slim	÷̈		36.8	70	18													
304	Bee Mae	ö		37	82	16													
305	Honey Mai	ö		37.2	96	22	122/68	37.1	96	18									
306	Net Clair	÷		35.9	72	18													
307	Ibaul Iris	÷		39	102	18		37.4	80	18									
308	Christmas Mary	⃛		36.9	88	20													
309	Nerve Latta	÷		39.1	90	24		38.4	88	20									
310-1	Soforthe Anne	÷		38.8	92	18	140/88												
310-2	Soo Ah	ö	144	35.7	80	20													
311-1	Bugg June	÷̈		38.6	100	18		38.9	80	20									
311-2	Kynde Bee	÷		37.4	94	16		37	80	20									
312-1	Cider Ida	÷		36.4	80	18	120/80												
312-2	Saynt Joanne	÷	200	36	74	20													

FIGURE 21-1 ▲ A TPR sheet with 8:00 AM and 12:00 noon data recorded on it. The straight line drawn through the values indicates that the information has been recorded (Celsius temperature scale).

FILING RECORDS ON THE PATIENT'S CHART

Each day the nursing unit receives many typed and computer-generated records, such as diagnostic results, history and physical reports, pathology reports, and others to be filed on the patient's chart. Efficient, accurate filing on the patient's chart is necessary for two reasons. First, during the patient's hospital stay, the filed written records are readily available for use by the attending doctor and other hospital personnel. Second, upon the patient's discharge, the health records department personnel have the legal responsibility of assembling and storing *all* records produced during the patient's hospital stay. Correct filing

methods used during the patient's hospitalization assist the health records personnel to complete this task.

Below are listed guidelines for filing records on the patient's chart on the nursing unit.

Guidelines for Filing Records on the Patient's Chart

File at the same time each day. Filing near the end of the shift allows you to file all the records received during the shift at one time. It is important for the nurse in charge to see all laboratory results as soon as they arrive on the nursing unit.

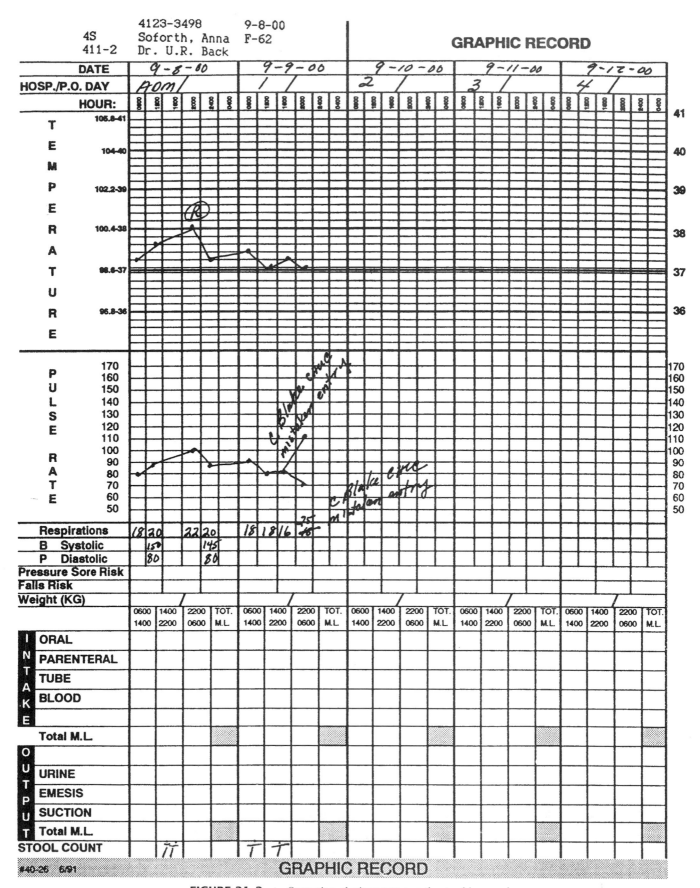

FIGURE 21–2 ▲ Correction of minor errors on the graphic record.

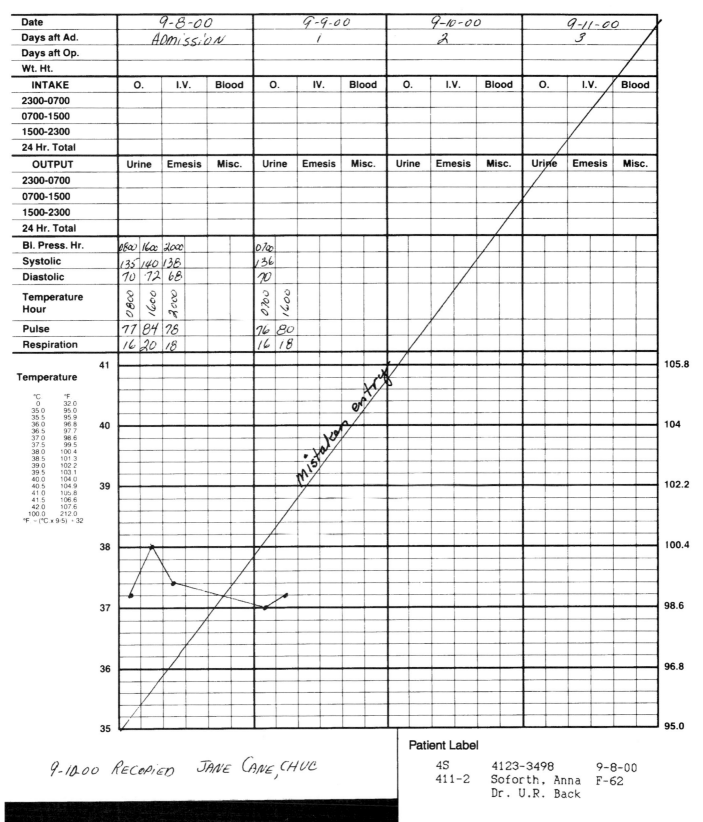

Date	9-8-00			9-9-00			9-10-00			9-11-00		
Days aft Ad.	ADMISSION			1			2			3		
Days aft Op.												
Wt. Ht.												
INTAKE	O.	I.V.	Blood	O.	IV.	Blood	O.	I.V.	Blood	O.	I.V.	Blood
2300-0700												
0700-1500												
1500-2300												
24 Hr. Total												
OUTPUT	Urine	Emesis	Misc.	Urine	Emesis	Misc.	Urine	Emesis	Misc.	Urine	Emesis	Misc.
2300-0700												
0700-1500												
1500-2300												
24 Hr. Total												
Bl. Press. Hr.	0800	1600	2000	0700								
Systolic	135	140	138	136								
Diastolic	70	72	68	70								
Temperature Hour	0800	1600	2000	0700	1600							
Pulse	77	84	78	76	80							
Respiration	16	20	18	16	18							

Temperature

°C	°F
0	32.0
35.0	95.0
35.5	95.9
36.0	96.8
36.5	97.7
37.0	98.6
37.5	99.5
38.0	100.4
38.5	101.3
39.0	102.2
39.5	103.1
40.0	104.0
40.5	104.9
41.0	105.8
41.5	106.6
42.0	107.6
100.0	212.0

°F = (°C x 9/5) + 32

mistaken entry

9-10-00 RECOPIED JANE CANE, CHUC

GRAPHIC RECORD

Patient Label

4S 4123-3498 9-8-00
411-2 Soforth, Anna F-62
Dr. U.R. Back

A

FIGURE 21–3 ▲ Recopied graphic record used to correct a series of errors. *A,* The original graphic record.

Date	9-8-00			9-9-00			9-10-00			9-11-00		
Days aft Ad.	*Admission*			1			2			3		
Days aft Op.												
Wt. Ht.												
INTAKE	O.	I.V.	Blood	O.	IV.	Blood	O.	I.V.	Blood	O.	I.V.	Blood
2300-0700												
0700-1500												
1500-2300												
24 Hr. Total												
OUTPUT	Urine	Emesis	Misc.	Urine	Emesis	Misc.	Urine	Emesis	Misc.	Urine	Emesis	Misc.
2300-0700												
0700-1500												
1500-2300												
24 Hr. Total												
Bl. Press. Hr.	0800 1600 2000			0700								
Systolic	135 140 160			125								
Diastolic	70 72 80			90								
Temperature Hour				0800 0900								
Pulse				80 60								
Respiration				20 22								

Temperature

°C	°F
0	32.0
35.0	95.0
35.5	95.9
36.0	96.8
36.5	97.7
37.0	98.6
37.5	99.5
38.0	100.4
38.5	101.3
39.0	102.2
39.5	103.1
40.0	104.0
40.5	104.9
41.0	105.8
41.5	106.6
42.0	107.6
100.0	212.0

°F = (°C x 9/5) + 32

9-10-00 RECOPIED JANE CRANE, CHUC

Patient Label

4S   4123-3498   9-8-00
411-2   Soforth, Anna F-62
        Dr. U.R. Back

GRAPHIC RECORD

B

FIGURE 21-3 cont'd ▲ Recopied graphic record used to correct a series of errors. *B,* A copied graphic record.

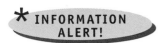

Some nursing units require reports to be filed when received.

Separate the records according to the patient's name.
This prepares you to file all the records for a given patient at
one time, so that you need to obtain and open the chart holder
only once.

**Always check the patient's name on the chart back with
the name on the record before filing it.** Never select the
chart by the room number recorded on the record, because the
room number on the record is incorrect if the patient has been
transferred to another bed on the nursing unit after the records
were initiated. Often a doctor prescribes treatment according to
test results.

**Be especially alert when there are two patients on the
unit with the same name.** When this happens, both patients'
charts are flagged with a "name alert" sticker. File all medical
records by their health records number. Many times you will
have patients with the same or very similar names on your nursing unit. The medical records number will never be duplicated.

Place the record behind the correct chart divider. Use
consistent sequencing in filing the reports on the patient's
charts to make it easier for the doctor and other health care
personnel to locate them. Reports are filed either to read like a
book, or the reverse—that is, the latest report is filed in front,
right behind the divider.

Initial all records you file. Follow the policy in your health
care facility about *where* on the form you should place your
initials.

Never discard any patient's record. If in doubt, check with
the nurse in charge or with the health records department. Unfiled records for patients who have been discharged should be
forwarded to the health records department. Unfiled records for
patients who have been transferred within the hospital should
be forwarded to the receiving unit.

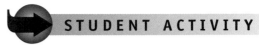

To practice filing records on the patient's charts, complete
Activity 21–3 in the *Skills Practice Manual*.

■ ORDERING DAILY DIAGNOSTIC TESTS

In Chapters 14 through 16 you practiced transcription of many
different types of diagnostic orders, including doctors' orders for
daily laboratory tests. Chest x-rays and electrocardiograms may
also be ordered to be performed daily.

The doctor may specify the number of days, such as chest x-
ray or EKG × 3 days or may write a standing order, such as daily
FBS. Daily diagnostic tests may be ordered for several days in advance on most computer systems or may be ordered each day
until the doctor cancels the order.

To order daily laboratory tests or diagnostic imaging procedures each day, check each patient's Kardex form (Fig. 21–4) and
enter the test or procedure in the computer every day. Note on
the Kardex that the daily laboratory test or diagnostic imaging
procedure has been ordered for the following day. Each unit has
a method of indicating that daily orders have been entered and
sent. "Order inquiry" is a computer screen that may be used to
verify whether a patient's order has been entered and sent. This
computer screen will display all of the patient's orders from the
time of his or her admission. The health unit coordinator chooses
"order inquiry" from the master or home screen and then
chooses a patient from the census screen to locate a list of all the
orders entered on the chosen patient.

Ordering daily tests may be the task of either the day or
the evening shift health unit coordinator. The ordering should

DATE ORD.	TREATMENTS	DATE ORD.	DIAGNOSTIC STUDIES	TO BE DONE
6-1	K-pad to left shoulder	6-1	CBC UA Chest xray	
		6-2	T3 uptake	
		6-1	✻ Daily Hgb & Hct	
		DATE	DIAGNOSTIC RESULTS	

FIGURE 21–4 ▲ Kardex form with a daily laboratory order recorded on it.

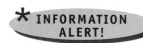

✳ INFORMATION ALERT!

Daily laboratory tests should be ordered for the first laboratory draw in the morning so the patient will not have eaten breakfast and the results will be available when the doctors make their AM rounds.

✳ INFORMATION ALERT!

Daily diagnostic tests may be ordered in advance on most hospital computer systems. When that is not possible or preferable, each nursing unit has a method of indicating that daily diagnostic tests have been ordered. When ordering a test in advance, the date the order was written by the doctor is entered on the Kardex form, a 3 × 5 card with patient label affixed to it, or a separate book for daily diagnostic tests. A series of dates are written next to or below the test and each day when the health unit coordinator orders the test for the following morning she or he will place a diagonal line across that date to indicate that it has been ordered.

Example: 2/14 Daily H & H 2/15, 2/16, 2/17, 2/18.

This would indicate that the H & H was ordered for 2/15 and 2/16.

To verify that a test has been ordered, choose "order inquiry" from the computer master screen (which will show the patient census on your nursing unit), and choose the patient's name. All of that patient's orders will be displayed on the computer screen.

be done at a certain time each day to avoid omission; if done on the day shift, it should be scheduled toward the end of the shift, to allow for possible cancellation of the order by the doctor. Daily diagnostic tests are ordered until the doctor writes an order to discontinue the test.

■ RETRIEVING DIAGNOSTIC TEST RESULTS

Most diagnostic test results may be retrieved from the computer by selecting "laboratory results" or "diagnostic imaging results" and then selecting the patient's name. The results will be displayed on the computer screen and may be printed. The health unit coordinator can print daily lab or diagnostic imaging results to place on the outside of the patient's chart before the doctors make their AM rounds. Printing the diagnostic test results will save the doctors time and eliminate the need for them to use the computer or ask the health unit coordinator to obtain the results while making rounds. Printing diagnostic test results is also helpful for the patient's nurses in assessing the patient's condition. Recorded diagnostic test results may also be obtained by telephone in some hospitals by calling a specified number.

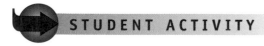

STUDENT ACTIVITY

To practice ordering daily diagnostic tests, complete Activity 21–4 in the *Skills Practice Manual*.

■ ORDERING SUPPLIES FOR THE NURSING UNIT

A busy nursing unit stocks a variety of supplies to keep the unit functioning smoothly. Nursing unit supplies are obtained from the purchasing department, the central service department, the dietary department, the pharmacy, and the laundry department.

Two systems for restocking the supplies are used. One system is for the health unit coordinator or a unit aide to determine the supplies needed and order them from the supplying department; the other is for the supplying department to make daily rounds throughout the hospital and restock the supply as needed (similar to restocking shelves in a grocery store).

An aspect to be considered regarding supplies is who pays for them. The patient usually pays for some items, such as catheter trays and medications, whereas other items, such as requisition forms, hand soap, paper clips, and so forth, are paid for from the nursing unit budget. Requisition forms are often used for items charged to the patient for billing and restocking purposes. Failure to complete the requisition form on items normally charged to the patient usually results in the cost being deducted from the nursing unit's budget. Carelessness in this area may play havoc with the overall management of money for the nursing unit supplies.

Purchasing Department Supplies

Purchasing department supplies consist of nonnursing items, such as chart and requisition forms, pencils, staples, flashlights, and numerous other items. Figure 21–5 illustrates an example of a purchasing department order form. Items received from the purchasing department are usually paid for from the nursing unit budget. A cost control center number for the nursing unit is placed on all requisitions issued from the unit. Restocking of purchasing department supplies is done weekly or bimonthly and is the most demanding of all the supply areas. It is important to order what is needed in a timely manner.

Central Service Department Supplies

Central service department supplies consist of items used for nursing procedures that are either charged to the patient or charged to the nursing unit's budget. Items charged to the patient, such as catheter trays and irrigation trays, usually have a requisition form with them. (See Fig. 11–2 for an example of CSD computer screen.) Smaller items, such as Band-Aids, tongue blades, alcohol, and sponges, are a part of the nursing unit's budget.

A recent trend is for many frequently used disposable-nursing items (such as catheter trays and enema bags), usually supplied by the central service department, to be obtained directly from the purchasing department. As you know, the purchasing department originally buys all hospital supplies; therefore, this method of bypassing the central service department is both efficient and economical.

STANDARD REGISTER
STOCKLESS FORMS REQUISITION

NO. 01132

| NAME OF REQUESTOR | | TELEPHONE NO. | | AUTHORIZED SIGNATURE | | DATE ORDERED | |
| DEPARTMENT NAME | | BUILDING/LOCATION | | FLOOR | | COST CENTER .460 | |

QTY	UNIT OF MEASURE	FORM NUMBER	DESCRIPTION
	500/BX	2044	ENV BLUE #9 SPEC WINDOW
	500/BX	2045	ENV INTER OFFICE BLUE #10
	1/EA	2046	ENV INTER OFFICE MAN/10x13
	500/BX	2051	ENV MANILLA PAYROLL WIND
	500/BX	2061	ENV WHITE ST JOSEPH #10
	1000/ROLL	2093	LABEL WHT 2-7/8 x 1-7/16
	500/BX	2177	ST JOSEPH LETTERHEAD
	500/BX	2881	ENV WHITE #9 OUTGOING
	1000/CTN	3224	PURCH 5 PT PAPER COLOR
	500/BX	3387	ENV WT WINDOW #10 PAT ACT
	2000/PK	3481	LABEL-ADDRESSOGRAPH-PACK
	25/PK	3623	HIV CONSENT FORM
	3000/CTN	61911G	WARD REPORT
	25/PK	ADM-1-4	CLASS ATTENDANCE SHEET
	25/PK	ADM-1-104	ST JOE OCCURRENCE RPT
	10/PK	ADM-1-196	ESP GRAM
	25/PK	ADM-1-426	EMPL EXP REINBURSE
	50/PK	ADM-1-775	PATIENT COMPLAINT SHEET
	100/PD	ADM-3-140	WHILE YOU WERE OUT PAD
	100/PD	ADM-503-127	REQ SPEC FOOD SERV
	100/PK	ADM-505	SPEED MEMO
	1930/CTN	ADMIT 1271	PATIENT INFO
	1000/CTN	ADMIT-1637	4 PT REQ INFO
	100/PD	BUS-1-222	OCCUPATIONAL THPY CHG
	100/PK	BUS-10	222 X-RAY CHGS
	200/PK	BUS-1000	RADIOLOGY CONSULT
	100/PK	BUS-1002	SP PROC X-RAY
	100/PK	BUS-1007	DEPT RAD CARDIO NUC MED
	100/PD	BUS-1008	GEN SERG DRUG CHGS
	50/PK	BUS-1016	CDV DIAG LAB
	50/PK	BUS-15	BLOOD GAS LAB
	100/PK	BUS-15	EEG CHARGE SLIP
	100/PK	BUS-1597	PERINATAL AMNI BLOOD TEST
	100/PD	BUS-16-134	PHYS MED CHGE SLIP
	100/PD	BUS-178	CONDITIONS FOR TREATMENT
	100/PD	BUS-18	PHARMACY CHARGE SLIP
	100/PD	BUS-29-2	MISC CHARGE SLIP

QTY	UNIT OF MEASURE	FORM NUMBER	DESCRIPTION
	100/PD	BUS-30-135	CREDIT SLIP
	100/PK	BUS-33	SPEECH OTOLOGY CHARGE
	100/PK	BUS-35-295	FULL SIZE MEMO PAD
	100/PD	BUS-35-295A	MEMO PADS
	100/PD	BUS-42	BLOOD BANK CONTINUOUS
	4950/CTN	BUS-42B	OUTPT LAB REQUISITION
	100/PK	BUS-447	NEW INV CODING SHEET
	100/PD	BUS-448	PREPAID A/C CODE
	100/PK	BUS-50B	MICRO URNE FLDS LAB REQ
	100/PD	BUS-510-143	REQ FOR CK OR CASH
	100/PK	BUS-53B	CHEM, HEMA, SEROLO LAB REQ
	50/PK	BUS-60A	CYTOLOGY
	100/PK	BUS-61	TISSUES FORM
	100/PK	BUS-63	GENERAL SURGERY CHARGES
	250/PK	BUS-641	SPD CHARGE CARD
	100/PK	BUS-674	ER MEDICATION CHARGES
	100/PK	BUS-677	DELIVERY ROOM CHARGES
	100/PD	BUS-817	OCCUP THERAPY CHG SLIP
	100/PK	CRS-1421	GENERAL DIAGNOSTIC-CRS
	950/CTN	CRS-1483	CRS MTST PAPER
	100/PD	CS-3-291	NURSING CARE PLAN
	100/PK	DORM-508	DORM VISITATION SLIP
	100/PK	DP-2-163	BATCH HEADER/TRAILER
	250/PK	DP-2-163C	BATCH HEADER/TRAILER BLUE
	100/PD	DP-960	CREDIT/DEBIT RECORD
	100/PD	DP-962	BALANCE TRANSFER
	100/PD	DP-963	CREDIT/DEBIT SHEET
	250/PK	DP2-163B	BATCH HEADER/TRAILER PBS
	100/PD	EEG-609	PHYSICIAN TRANSCRIPTION
	100/PD	ENG-445	PLANT SERV SERVICE CALL
	100/PK	ERA-508-172	PHONE REPORT OF LAB
	500/PK	ER-514	ER C/SERV ITEMS CHG SLIP
	5000/CTN	FS-1427	MENU LABEL
	100/PD	HB-17-96	WORK ORDERS
	1450/CTN	HB-1720	A/P BLUE
	200/PK	HB-54	RECEIPTS-PEGBOARD
	250/PK	HB-55	JOURNAL-PEGBOARD
	100/PK	HRS-2027	OPERATING ROOM PATH CONST
	2500/CTN	LAB-1684	1 PART LAB REPORT
	5000/CTN	LAB-1352	LAB LABEL-GREEN, MULTI-CUT
	5000/CTN	LAB-1353	LAB LABEL-WHT, SINGLE CUT
	2500/CTN	LAB-1354	LAB LABEL-RED
	1600/CTN	LAB-1428	12 PART CANARY-CONTINUOUS

QTY	UNIT OF MEASURE	FORM NUMBER	DESCRIPTION
	5700/CTN	LAB-1557	HEMO-CONTINUOUS
	1300/CTN	LAB-1621	3 PART LAB REPORT
	3000/CTN	LAB-1979	PATHOLOGY REPORT-LASER
	100/PD	LAB-501-79	PATHOLOGY CONSULTATION
	2500/CTN	LABEL 2-7/16 x 4	WHITE LABEL 2-7/16 x 4
	100/PK	ME-17	ADULT MCC ENCOUNTER
	100/PK	MD-300-01	MD PED HEME CHARGE
	200/PK	MR-5	LAB REPORT
	100/PD	MR-i-303	SUMMARY SHEETS
	100/PK	MF-1012	ICU MEDICATION RECORD
	200/PK	MF-1016	MEDICATION REC UNIT DOSE
	100/PK	MF-1017	RESP THERAPY MOUNT SHEET
	100/PK	MR-1-219-232	24-HR NWBRN NURSERY OBS
	100/PK	MR-1-225-248	N3 DEFICIENCY SLIP
	100/PD	MR-1C30-270	OB DEFICIENCY SLIP
	100/PK	MF-11-41	GEN/BNI ANESTHESIA RECORD
	100/PK	MR-1117	MEDICATION ADMIN RECORD
	1350/PD	MR-1134	MED ADMINISTRATION REC
	100/PK	MR-1142	MATERNITY PT CARE PLAN
	100/PD	MR-1156	PHYSICIAN IN CHARGE
	100/PK	MR-116	PED ADMISSION ASSESSMENT
	100/PD	MR-1262	MATERNITY PT CARE SUP
	100/PK	MR-1490	NURSES CARE PLAN
	100/PD	MR-1542	DISCHG PLAN WORKSHEET
	100/PK	MR-18-304	NURSES RECORD
	100/PD	MR-19-305	PROGRESS REPORT
	50/PK	MR-1904	BLANK FORM CARRIER
	25/PK	MR-1904A	ATRIAL LABEL
	25/PK	MR-1904ART	ARTERIAL LABEL
	25/PK	MR-1904CVP	CVP LABEL
	25/PK	MR-1904GP	GENERAL PURPOSE LABEL
	25/PK	MR-1904ICP	ICP LABEL
	50/PK	MR-1904IV	IV LABEL
	10/PK	MF-1904PA	PA LABEL
	250/PK	MR-20B-306	BLUE MD ORDERS
	200/PK	MR-20W-507	WHITE MD ORDERS
	100/PK	MR-210	ADMISS STATUS REC DORM
	100/PK	MR-245	PRE ADMIT PHYS ORDERS
	200/PK	MR-27	FOLLOW UP INSTRUCTIONS
	100/PK	MR-275	LABOR-DELIVERY FORM
	100/PD	MR-283	HEMODYNAMIC FLOWSHEET
	100/PK	MR-32	ER CLINICAL RECORD
	200/PK	MR-34-309	RECOVERY RM RECORD
	100/PK	MR-34A-318	RECOVERY RM REC CONT

QTY	UNIT OF MEASURE	FORM NUMBER	DESCRIPTION
	50/PD	MR-41-282	CONSENT PHOTOG-PUBLS
	100/PK	MR-417	REQ FOR PRIOR ORDERS
	100/PK	MR-43-216	MEDICATION RECORD
	100/PD	MR-46-158	DIABETIC CHART
	2850/CTN	MR-47	DISCHARGE FINAL REPORT
	2850/CTN	MR-48	WEEKLY LAB SUMMARY
	100/PK	MR-480	PHYS PARENTERAL NUT ORDER
	100/PK	MR-509-98	ADMISSION ASSESSMENT
	500/CTN	MR-522	6-PLY MTST PAPER/CBNLESS
	650/CTN	MR-522	MTST 5-PT PAPER CBN
	50/PK	MR-533	MEDICAL RECORD OUT CARD
	100/PK	MR-581	VENTILATOR RESP THERAPY
	100/PK	MR-581	PATIENT RECORD
	100/PK	MR-563	CDV ICU FLOW SHEET
	100/PD	MR-593	DEFICIENCY RECORD
	100/PK	MR-595-179	PROBLEM SHEET
	100/PD	MR-600-643	PREOP CHECK LIST
	100/CTN	MR-616	PULMONARY LAB REPORT
	2500/CTN	MR-616A	PULMONARY LAB REPORT 1-PT
	100/PK	MR-650	VITAL SIGNS
	100/PK	MR-671-730	PRE-ANESTHESIA QUES
	100/PK	MR-675	NEONATAL RECORD I
	100/PK	MR-676	NEONATAL II
	100/PK	MR-677	OB SUMMARY
	100/PK	MR-684	CONDITIONS OF ADMISSION
	100/PK	MR-685-755	NURSING DISCHARGE ASSESS
	100/PC	MR-692-783	X-RAY CASSETTES
	100/PK	MR-717	PERIOPERATIVE RECORD
	100/PC	MR-803	DIET SERVICE PROG NOTE
	100/PK	MR-895	CRITICAL CARE FLOWSHEET
	100/PK	MRS-1157	BACKING SHEET
	100/PD	NS-12-240	NOURISHMENT ORDER FORM
	100/PD	NS-507-114W	WEEKLY SCHEDULES
	100/PD	NS-510-215	REV TEAM ASSIGNMENT
	200/PK	NS-518-14	RN CLINICAL REPORT
	50/PK	NS-529-478	TREAT AND TEST PLAN
	100/PD	NS-530-115	FLUID FORMS
	100/PD	NS-7-100	TPR RECORD
	100/PD	NS-9-21	INTAKE/OUTPUT SHEETS
	1/EA	NSY-325	INFO ABOUT YOUR BABY
	50/PK	NSY-761	NURSERY ICU KARDEX
	200/PK	OPD-19	CLINICAL PRESCRIPTIONS
	100/PK	OPD-60-253	PED-PROGRESS NOTES

QTY	UNIT OF MEASURE	FORM NUMBER	DESCRIPTION
	100/PK	PER-1-196	EMPLOYMENT APPLICATION
	25/PD	PER-13-37	ACCIDENT EXPOSURE RC
	50/PK	PER-663-793	EMP/POS CHG REQUEST
	100/PD	PH-1-299	PRESCRIPTION BLANKS
	100/PD	PH-2-637	PHONE ORDER FOR MEDS
	4900/CTN	PRD-1923	NOTICE OF DEPOSIT
	100/PD	PULF-526	PULF TELEPHONE REPORTS
	100/PD	PUR-1	PURCHASE ORDERS
	25/PK	PUR-1622	OFFICE SUPPLY REQ
	25/PK	PUR-203	REQUISITION TO PURCHASE
	100/PD	PUR-4-53	GEN REQUISITION SM
	100/PK	PUR-IV	PURCHASE ORDER TOP COPY
	25/PK	PUR-9	FORMS REQUISITION
	2500/CTN	QA-1247	RSQUM WORKSHEET
	10/PK	QA-842	MONITORING SYSTEMS
	1/EA	RO-11-214	RADIATION ONCOLOGY BROCH
	25/PD	RAD-18	CAT HISTORY FORM
	100/PK	RAD-511-667	RADIOLOGY PRELIM REPT
	250/PK	RAD-516	DAYLIGHT FLASHER CARD
	250/PK	RAD-516A	BLANK DAYLIGHT FLASHER
	200/PK	RTD-504	RESP THERAPY CHG
	400/CTN	RTD-507	RESP THERAPY SCHEDULE
	100/PD	SSD-104-283	MED RECORD
	100/PD	TRAN-363	TUBE ROOM ROUTE SLIP
	100/PD	TRAN-564	TRAN CALL SLIP

PROCEDURE FOR COMPLETING FORM

1. FILL IN QUANTITY OF FORMS DESIRED. COMPLETE ALL BLANKS AT TOP OF FORM.
2. FOR ITEMS NOT APPEARING ON THIS REQUISITION, CONSULT FORMS CATALOG AND WRITE IN BELOW. (FOR NON-CATALOG FORMS, SPECIAL ORDERS OR NEW FORMS, CONTACT PURCHASING).
3. KEEP "REQUESTOR'S COPY" FOR YOUR RECORDS.
4. SEND ALL REMAINING COPIES TO PURCHASING.
5. FOR ASSISTANCE, CALL EXT. 3443.

QTY	UNIT OF MEASURE	FORM NUMBER	DESCRIPTION

FIGURE 21-5 ▲ Purchasing department order form.

```
         NOURISHMENT ORDER FROM FOOD SERVICE

UNIT_____ORDERED BY_____

DATE_____
```

DESCRIPTION	ORDER
Homogenized Milk	
Skim Milk	
Chocolate Milk	
Orange Juice (unsw) (qts)	
Apple Juice	
Cranberry Juice	
Prune Juice	
Tomato Juice	
Nectar	
Decaffeinated Coffee (pkg of 20)	
Tea Bags (pkg of 30)	
Graham Crackers (pkg of 12)	
Saltines (pkg of 20)	
Powdered non-dairy Creamers (50 per box)	
Sugar (per 100 ind.)	
Ice Cream	
Sherbet	
Jello	
Custard	
Oleo (ind.)	
Bread (pkg of 10 ind.)	
Bouillon -Beef or Chicken (pkg/12)	
7-Up (6 pk)	
Cola (6 pk)	

```
NOTE: BETWEEN MEAL FEEDINGS, TUBE FEEDINGS OR
LIQUID SUPPLEMENTS ARE TO BE ORDERED ON THE
"DIET CHANGE SHEET" AND ON THE "SPECIAL DIET"
CARD.
NS-12-240    Received by_____
```

FIGURE 21–6 ▲ Dietary department stock supply order form.

Pharmacy Supplies

The pharmacy supplies include all medications administered to the patients. Medications are kept on the nursing unit in three classifications: (1) the controlled substances, which are locked in the narcotics cupboard or in a computerized dispensing cart; (2) the other daily and prn medications currently being administered to the patients according to doctors' orders; and (3) a unit stock supply of frequently used medications, such as aspirin. Restocking of daily medications is usually performed on a daily basis and the stock supply is replenished as needed. The patient is charged for medications that he or she has received, and therefore pharmacy supplies are not a part of the nursing unit's budget. The charges, which cover the cost of administration supplies, such as needles and syringes, are usually determined from the patient's medication record sheet.

Dietary Department Supplies

Dietary department supplies include food items such as milk, orange juice, and ginger ale that are stored in the nursing unit kitchen and issued to the patients as needed. These supplies are restocked daily and are usually charged to the nursing unit's budget. Figure 21–6 illustrates an example of a dietary department stock supply order form.

Laundry Department Supplies

Laundry department supplies include linens and bedding such as pillows, sheets, blankets, towels, washcloths, and patient gowns. The cost of linen supplies is usually absorbed in the charge for the patient's room. Most hospitals employ a laundry service to supply linen that is then delivered to each nursing unit by hospital personnel. If supplies run low during the day, the health unit coordinator may need to call the linen department or page personnel from the laundry department for more items.

■ PREPARING DAILY FORMS

As a health unit coordinator, it may be your task to prepare forms for use by the nurse manager and nursing team members, such as the patient assignment sheet (see Fig. 3–8, p. 40) and work schedules. Because preparing these forms usually involves recording data pertinent to your nursing unit, we will not discuss it further. Daily tasks may also include: preparing nurse's progress records by labeling with patient ID labels and filling in the headings, labeling CSD cards and recopying MARs as needed. Find out what your responsibilities are regarding filling out forms. If filling out forms is a daily health unit coordinator task on your unit, plan to fill them out at the same time each day.

■ SUMMARY

All the tasks included in this chapter, except for ordering the nursing unit supplies, are performed daily; therefore, you will soon become skilled at performing them.

Accuracy and efficiency are extremely important in charting the vital signs, filing reports on the patients' charts, ordering daily tests and procedures. Performing these tasks at the same time each day is necessary for efficient management of your time.

▼ REVIEW QUESTIONS

1. If it is the health unit coordinator's task to transfer information from the TPR sheet onto each patient's graphic sheet, at what time should you perform this task? Why?

   _____

2. Why is accuracy important in the recording of vital signs?

   _____

3. You have recorded an incorrect temperature on the graphic sheet. How would you correct this error?

   _____

4. You are recording a set of vital signs and you notice that an error was made in the recording of a set of vital signs 2 days previously, which resulted in the following day's entries being incorrect. To correct this series of errors, you need to:

   _____

5. If it is necessary to recopy a patient's graphic record, what is done with the original?

   _____

6. Convert the following Fahrenheit temperatures to Celsius.

   a. 98.6° _____   b. 101.4° _____   c. 99.8° _____   d. 96.7° _____

7. Convert the following Celsius temperatures to Fahrenheit.

   a. 38.2° _____   b. 39.5° _____   c. 36.4° _____   d. 37.8° _____

8. List two reasons for the need for efficient, accurate filing of records on the patient's chart.

   a. _____

   b. _____

9. List five guidelines for filing records on the patient's chart.

   a. _____

   b. _____

   c. _____

   d. _____

   e. _____

10. Name five hospital departments that may provide the nursing unit supplies, and list the type of supplies that may be obtained from each department.

a. _____

b. _____

c. _____

d. _____

e. _____

11. Define the following terms:

a. pulse deficit:

_____

b. Celsius:

_____

c. stool:

_____

d. Fahrenheit:

_____

12. Write the meaning of each of the following abbreviations:

a. BM _____

b. TPR _____

c. C _____

d. F _____

e. PP _____

f. PO day _____

TOPICS FOR DISCUSSION

1. Discuss the problems that carelessness in charting vital signs could cause.

2. Discuss the possible consequences of reports being filed in the wrong patient's chart or behind the incorrect divider.

3. Discuss the importance of restocking supplies on the nursing unit.

Reports, Infection Control, Emergencies, and Special Services

Chapter Objectives

Upon completion of this chapter, you will be able to:

1. Define the terms in the vocabulary list.
2. Write the meaning of each abbreviation in the abbreviations list.
3. List three conditions that may cause a patient to become immunocompromised.
4. List four categories of incidents that require a written report.
5. Explain the importance of incident reports.
6. Name three methods by which bacteria may be spread.
7. Name three pathogenic microorganisms that are frequently responsible for hospital-acquired infections.
8. List four types of personal protective equipment used with standard precautions.
9. Explain how HIV is transmitted.
10. Name two opportunistic diseases related to AIDS.
11. List nine tasks that the health unit coordinator may perform in a medical emergency.
12. Explain the duties carried out during a fire or fire drill.
13. List six guidelines to follow for electrical safety.
14. Describe how to handle mail and flowers delivered to the unit.

Vocabulary

Airborne Precautions/Isolation ▲ The required use of mask and ventilated room, in conjunction with standard precautions

Cardiac Arrest ▲ The patient's heart contractions are absent or insufficient to produce a pulse or blood pressure (may also be referred to as *code arrest*)

Centers for Disease Control and Prevention (CDC) ▲ Division of the U.S. Public Health Service that investigates and controls diseases that have epidemic potential

Communicable Disease ▲ A disease that may be transmitted from one person to another

Disaster Procedure ▲ A planned procedure that is carried out by hospital personnel when a large number of people have been injured

Epidemiology ▲ The study of the occurrence, distribution, and causes of health and disease in humans; the specialist is called an *epidemiologist*

Hepatitis B Virus (HBV) ▲ An infectious bloodborne disease that is a major occupational hazard for health care workers

Human Immunodeficiency Virus (HIV) ▲ The virus that causes acquired immunodeficiency syndrome (AIDS)

Incident ▲ An episode that does not normally occur within the regular hospital routine

Isolation ▲ The placement of a patient apart from other patients insofar as movement and social contact are concerned, for the purpose of preventing the spread of infection

Material Safety Data Sheet (MSDS) ▲ A basic hazard communication tool which gives details on chemical dangers and safety procedures

Medical Emergency ▲ An emergency that is life threatening

Nosocomial Infections ▲ Infections that are acquired from within the health care facility

Occupational Safety and Health Administration (OSHA) ▲ A U.S. governmental regulatory agency concerned with the health and safety of workers

Pathogenic Microorganisms ▲ Disease-carrying organisms too small to be seen with the naked eye

Protective Care ▲ Another term for isolation

Respiratory Arrest ▲ When the patient ceases to breathe or when respirations are so depressed that the blood cannot receive sufficient oxygen and therefore the body cells die (may also be referred to as *code arrest*)

Reverse Isolation ▲ A precautionary measure taken to prevent a patient with low resistance to disease from becoming infected

Risk Management ▲ A department in the hospital that addresses the prevention and containment of liability regarding patient care incidents

Standard Precautions ▲ The creation of a barrier between the health care worker and the patient's blood and body fluids (may also be called universal precautions)

Tuberculosis (TB) ▲ A disease caused by *Mycobacterium tuberculosis*, an airborne pathogen

Abbreviations

Abbreviation	Meaning
AIDS	acquired immunodeficiency syndrome
ARC	AIDS-related complex
CDC	Centers for Disease Control and Prevention

Abbreviation	Meaning
HBV	hepatitis B virus
HIV	human immunodeficiency virus
OSHA	Occupational Safety and Health Administration
PPE	personal protective equipment
R *A *C *E	*R*escue individuals in danger
	*A*larm: sound the alarm
	*C*onfine the fire by closing all doors and windows
	*E*xtinguish the fire with the nearest suitable fire extinguisher
TB	tuberculosis

■ INCIDENT REPORTS

An incident is an episode that does not normally occur within the regular health care facility routine. The incident may be an accident, such as a patient falling while on the way to the bathroom. It also may be a situation, such as spilled liquids in a hospital corridor that causes someone to slip and sustain an injury.

Incidents may occur to patients, visitors, or health care facility personnel and students. Events other than accidents that occur within the hospital or on hospital property are also reportable.

Examples of incidents that require written reports are:

- Accidents
- Thefts from persons on hospital property
- Errors of omission of patient treatment or errors of administration of patient treatment
- Exposure to blood and body fluids such as caused by a needlestick

Many incidents occur in the patient's room and are not viewed by the health unit coordinator. In such cases, the health unit coordinator prepares the incident report form for the nurse by completing the initial information such as date, name of patient, etc. The nurse and/or any witnesses complete the report. However, anything that is seen or that you have knowledge of regarding an incident should be written up immediately so that all details can be communicated as they occurred.

An incident report form (Fig. 22–1) should be written for all incidents occurring to anyone, no matter how insignificant they may seem. Documentation of all incidents is important to identify hazards and to prevent continuing problems and in the case of a lawsuit arising from them. Names and home addresses of witnesses are required in case the incident would become a lawsuit and the witnesses are no longer employed at the hospital when the case is brought to court.

The hospitalist, attending doctor, or resident may be called to examine the patient involved in an incident. All incidents involving patients are reported to their attending doctor. A copy of the incident report is sent to the nurse manager, a copy is sent to risk management, and a copy is sent to quality assurance. If the incident involves another department, such as transport, a copy will be sent to that department's manager. The incident report never becomes part of the patient's permanent record.

Employee hospital incidents must be documented and the employee seen by the employee health nurse or doctor for him or her to be eligible for coverage by the state workman's com-

Confidential Information
INCIDENT REPORT
(Patient or Visitor)
Not a Part of Patient's Permanent Chart

1. Date of Admission _____

2. Diagnosis _____

3. Date of Incident _____ Time _____ M | Room No., Name, Age, Sex, Hospital Number, Attending Physician

4. Were Bed Rails up? _____   5. Hi Lo Bed Position _____
                 (YES OR NO)   (UP OR DOWN)

6. Was Safety Belt or Restraints in use? _____
                                       DESIGNATE SPECIFICALLY

7. Activity (Complete Bed Rest, Bathroom Privileges, Etc.) _____

8. Sedatives _____ Dose _____ Time _____ M ⎫
                                                    Given
9. Narcotics _____ Dose _____ Time _____ M within
                                                    12 hours
10. Tranquilizers _____ Dose _____ Time _____ M previous
                                                    to incident ⎭

11. Nurse's Account of Incident (State incident, where discovered, condition of patient, etc.)

_____

_____

_____

_____

_____

_____

_____

_____

12. History of Incident as related by Patient

_____

_____

_____

13. List Witnesses or Persons Familiar with Details of Incident (Include roommate's name and hospital number.)

Name _____ Address _____

Name _____ Address _____

Name _____ Address _____

14. Time Doctor was called _____ AM _____ PM   15. Time Doctor Responded _____ AM _____ PM

16. Time Supervisor called _____ AM _____ PM

17. Date of Report _____

18. _____
             SIGNATURE OF PERSON REPORTING

19. _____
             SIGNATURE OF DEPARTMENT SUPERVISOR

20. _____
             SIGNATURE OF DEPARTMENT HEAD

A   Complete **IMMEDIATELY** for **EVERY** incident and send to Administrator via Department Head.

FIGURE 22–1 ▲ An incident report. *A*, General information.

Continued

PHYSICIAN'S STATEMENT

21. State injuries or other result, if any, from this incident _____

_____

_____

22. How, if at all, did the results of this incident affect the patient's original condition? _____

_____

_____

23. What treatment was given? _____

_____

24. Were X-rays or other tests ordered (specify) _____

_____

_____

25. Results of X-ray or other tests _____

_____

_____

26. Patient Examined: Date _____ Hour _____ AM _____ PM

27. Signed _____ M.D. (House Physician)

B

28. Signed _____ M.D. (Attending Physician)

FIGURE 22–1, cont'd ▲ An incident report. *B,* Doctor's statement.

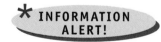

★ INFORMATION ALERT!

Patient incident reports are not a part of the patient's chart.

pensation commission. Hospital employees who fail to put into writing something which may appear trivial, such as a finger puncture with a needle, have no evidence to present should an infection follow the injury.

Risk management personnel may interview witnesses to a patient incident to be prepared for a lawsuit. Risk management will also study patient incidents looking for any trends and to prevent future similar incidents.

The health unit coordinator is also responsible for maintaining a supply of incident report forms for the nursing unit.

■ INFECTION CONTROL

For statistical purposes, records must be kept of infectious diseases. A report should be submitted to the infectious disease department or personnel in the hospital (Fig. 22–2). Most hos-

pitals employ an epidemiologist or infection-control officer who maintains all infection records and investigates all hospital-acquired infections. Infection control is essential to provide a safe environment for both patients and health care workers. Patients are at risk for acquiring infections because of lower resistance to infectious microorganisms, increased exposure to numbers and types of disease-causing microorganisms, and invasive procedures. The presence of a pathogen does not mean that an infection will begin. Development of an infection depends on six components called the *chain of infection,* as listed below (Fig. 22–3).

1. Infectious agent or pathogen (bacteria)
2. Reservoir or source for pathogen to live and grow (human body, contaminated water or food, animals, insects, etc.)
3. Means of escape (blood, urine, feces, wound drainage, etc.)
4. Route of transmission (air, contact, and body excretions)
5. Entryway (mouth, nostrils, and breaks in the skin)
6. Susceptible host (individual who does not have adequate resistance to the invading pathogen)

To prevent infection from developing, the chain must be broken. By following infection prevention and control techniques, health care workers can prevent the spread of microorganisms to

Report # _____

REPORT OF INFECTION

COMPLETE ALL BLANKS IN TOP SECTION   UNIT

1. Diagnosis is: _____

_____

_____

2. Date of admission: _____

3. Evidence of Infection on admission?
   Yes ☐   No ☐

4. Date of last previous admission here:

_____

5. Hospitalized at another hospital?
   Yes ☐   No ☐
   If yes, name hospital?

_____

   Date:_____

6. Date of surgery/delivery _____

7. Procedure done: _____

_____

8. Culture sent? Yes ☐   No ☐
   (If yes, what was cultured?)
   _____ Blood
   _____ Urine
   _____ Sputum
   _____ Drainage from _____
   _____ Other(specify)_____

9. *Fever?   Yes ☐   No ☐
   NOTE: *Fever = temp. greater than
   100.4°F (38°C) Oral
   101°F (38.4°C) Rectal

10. Pt. Isolated? Yes ☐   No ☐
    If yes, enter date next to type initiated
    _____ a. Limited
    _____ b. Respiratory
    _____ c. Wound & Skin
    _____ d. Enteric
    _____ e. Strict
    _____ f. Protective

11. Date of Discharge: _____

CHECK ALL THAT APPLY:

DIARRHEA:
_____ Over 3 stools/24 hrs. for more than 2 days s̄ laxatives, enemas, x-rays preps, cardiac drugs or antibiotics

PHLEBITIS: Location _____

Non-Suppurative:
_____ Mechanical Intracath
_____ Drug
_____ Possible focal site of infection
_____ Observed by Nurse
_____ Diagnosis by Physician

Suppurative:
_____ Purulent drainage

POST PARTUM:
_____ *Fever(exclude 1st PP day)
_____ Purulent vaginal discharge
_____ Diagnosis by Physician

POST-OP:
_____ Continuous *Fever for 2 consecutive days
_____ Abscess(usually documented at time of surgery)

RESPIRATORY TRACT:
Upper
_____ Coryza(profuse nasal drainage)
_____ Pharyngitis
_____ Diagnosis by Physician

Lower:
_____ Sudden on set of cough
_____ Purulent sputum
_____ Suppuration of trachea
_____ X-ray Dx - Pneumonia
_____ Diagnosis by Physician

SKIN:
_____ Abscess
_____ Boil
_____ Cellulitis
_____ Purulent decubiti
_____ Suppuration

BLOOD:
_____ HAA Pos.
_____ HAA Neg.
_____ Positive Culture

URINARY TRACT:
Asymptomatic:
_____ No clinical symptoms
_____ Positive bacteriology X 100,000/ml
_____ Positive bacteriology X 10,000/ml c̄ previous urine culture negative
_____ Pyuria X 10 WBC

Symptomatic:
_____ Frequency
_____ Burning
_____ Urgency
_____ CVT(costo-vertebral tenderness)

WOUND:
_____ Abscess(usually documented at surgery time)
_____ Continuous *Fever for 2 consecutive days
_____ Stitch abscess
_____ Suppuration of wound
_____ Diagnosis by Physican
_____ Other _____

Report completed by: _____   Date:_____

COMMENTS: _____

_____

_____

(DO NOT WRITE IN THIS SECTION. FOR USE BY INFECTION CONTROL OFFICER ONLY)

FIGURE 22–2 ▲ Infection report.

patients and also protect themselves. Prevention and control techniques include standard precautions, airborne precautions, and good handwashing technique.

Standard Precautions

In 1987 the CDC developed and presented a concept to protect health care providers from bloodborne pathogens such as human immunodeficiency virus (HIV), hepatitis B virus, and hepatitis C virus. During that time there was a quiet panic among

health care providers. They were not sure of how HIV was spread or how they could protect themselves. The CDC called this new concept "universal precautions" (for blood and body fluids). Nationwide, hospitals and other health care facilities accepted and taught this new concept to their employees and have changed the name to "standard precautions."

Standard precautions are the creation of a barrier between the practitioner (health care worker) and the patient's body fluids. Body fluids considered potentially infectious include blood, semen, vaginal secretions, peritoneal fluid, pleural fluid, pericardial fluid, synovial fluid, cerebrospinal

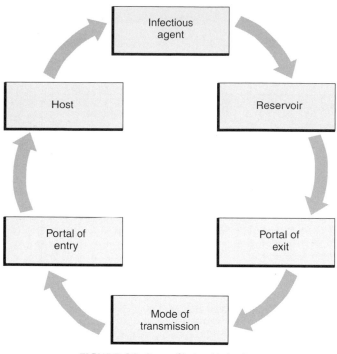

FIGURE 22-3 ▲ Chain of infection.

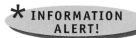

Hands should be washed when arriving at work, before and after personal breaks, and after handling any patient specimen (even if bagged). Microorganisms can also be transmitted through handling objects in the nursing station. Handwashing is the number one method to reduce the spread of infection.

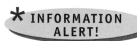

Avoid putting your hands on your face, in your eyes, or in your mouth while on the nursing station.

Handwashing

Handwashing should be practiced when arriving at work, before and after taking a personal break and prior to eating, and after handling any patient specimens (even if bagged). Use soap and scrub between fingers. Rinse each hand thoroughly with running water from the wrists down to fingertips. Dry with clean paper towel and use towel to turn off faucet.

■ DISEASES THAT COULD BE TRANSMITTED THROUGH CONTACT WITH BLOOD AND BODY FLUIDS

AIDS

AIDS stands for *acquired immunodeficiency syndrome.* AIDS is caused by a virus called human immunodeficiency virus, also called HIV or the AIDS virus. The AIDS virus attacks the immune system and thereby reduces the body's ability to defend itself against infection and disease. Persons who have AIDS become open to many opportunistic infections that are not usually a threat to persons with a normal functioning immune system. These infections are called *opportunistic* because the organisms take advantage of the patient's weakened immune system. As the immune system becomes weaker, these opportunistic illnesses may overwhelm the AIDS patient and cause death.

AIDS is transmitted by blood, vaginal fluids, and semen and is not spread though casual contact. There are four main ways AIDS is spread. The first is by sexual contact. The second is by using needles previously injected into someone carrying the AIDS virus. The third is from an infected mother to her infant during pregnancy or birth. The fourth is transmission of the virus through blood transfusions; this mode is especially common if the patient received the transfusion before blood was routinely tested for the virus (prior to the late-1980s). Surgical patients, hemophiliac patients, and mothers who received transfusions during or after birth have contracted the HIV virus this way. AIDS may also be transmitted through the blood of an infected person entering another person's bloodstream either through a cut, open sore, or blood being splashed into the mouth or eye. Appropriate PPE must be worn when coming in contact with body fluids from all patients.

An *AIDS virus carrier* is a person who carries the AIDS virus in his or her blood, but who may stay healthy for a long time.

fluid, amniotic fluid, urine, feces, sputum, saliva, wound drainage, and vomitus.

The *barrier* in standard precautions is created by wearing personal protective equipment (PPE) consisting of such items as gloves, gown, mask, goggles or glasses, pocket masks with one-way valves, and moisture-resistant gowns. *Every health care employee should practice standard precautions with every single patient.*

Airborne Precautions/Isolation

Airborne precautions/isolation is used to reduce risk of droplet nuclei or contaminated dust particles from traveling over short distances (less than three feet) and landing in the nose or mouth of a susceptible person. The patient is placed in a private room with monitored negative air pressure and high-efficiency filtration. The room usually has a door, an entryway, and another door with both doors remaining closed. Individuals entering the room are required to wear masks, gloves, and gowns. Handwashing is also required. Linen and trash are bagged to prevent contamination.

Examples of patients who would be placed in airborne isolation are those with active tuberculosis (TB), measles, chicken pox, or meningitis.

Reverse Isolation

Reverse isolation is used to protect patients with a decreased immune system function by reducing their risks of exposure to potentially infectious organisms. Reverse isolation is also known as immunocompromised isolation. Examples of patients who are immunocompromised are organ transplant recipients, burn victims, or patients receiving chemotherapy.

Some may never get sick. The only indication of AIDS infection in the carrier is usually a positive blood test for antibodies to the AIDS virus. Once a person has been infected with the AIDS virus, he or she remains infected for life.

Months or years after the initial infection, some people carrying the virus develop symptoms that may include tiredness, fevers, night sweats, swollen lymph glands, or mental deterioration resembling Alzheimer's disease. Often the symptoms are recurrent and disable the person. This person is said to have ARC or AIDS-related complex.

AIDS is the most severe form of the infection. A full-blown case may not appear until months or years after the initial infection. ARC symptoms may or may not have appeared. The two most frequent opportunistic illnesses that may overtake the AIDS patient are (1) *Pneumocystis carinii* pneumonia (PCP), a pneumonia caused by *Pneumocystis carinii*; and (2) Kaposi's sarcoma (KS), an otherwise rare skin cancer.

Hepatitis B Virus

Hepatitis B is an inflammation of the liver caused by the hepatitis B virus (HBV). It was formerly called serum hepatitis. Like AIDS, hepatitis B is spread by body fluids but it is even more contagious than AIDS. Health care providers are at risk for exposure. Standard blood and body fluid precautions must be practiced.

OSHA mandates that employers provide hepatitis B vaccine for all employees who have an occupational exposure risk. The vaccines are given in three doses over a 6-month period. An employee has the right to refuse the hepatitis B vaccine, but must sign a form stating his or her refusal.

Tuberculosis

Tuberculosis (TB) is caused by *Mycobacterium tuberculosis*, an airborne pathogen. Working with patients who have tuberculosis requires the use of special PPE, such as special masks fitted to the individual health care worker, to avoid inhaling the tiny droplets that carry the virus through the air. TB has increased in the United States and some viruses have become resistant to drug therapy.

Nosocomial Infections

Nosocomial infections are infections acquired from within the health care facility and are often transmitted to the patient by health care workers. Three pathogenic microorganisms that are frequently responsible for hospital-acquired infections are *Streptococcus*, *Staphylococcus*, and *Pseudomonas*. Excellent handwashing technique is the best way for health care workers to stop the spread of nosocomial infections.

■ HEALTH UNIT COORDINATOR TASKS TO CONTROL INFECTION

The health unit coordinator tasks for infection control and isolation vary from institution to institution. It is necessary in any health care facility for the health unit coordinator to have a ba-

sic understanding of infection-control policies and standard precautions. *Accurate* information must be given to inquiring visitors. If you are unable to answer a question or are unsure of what to say, ask a nurse to speak with the visitor. All infectious or communicable diseases on the unit must be reported to infection control. The nurses will ask the health unit coordinator to order PPE and isolation packs as needed. The health unit coordinator should wear gloves when handling or transporting specimens and should practice good handwashing techniques throughout the working day. Eating, drinking (open cups), or handling contact lenses should not be done in the nursing station. Food should not be stored in refrigerators with specimens. The health unit coordinator transcribes laboratory orders pertaining to infection control. Below is a list of doctors' orders and the division of the laboratory to which they are sent:

- CSF for:
  cell count—hematology
  protein—chemistry
  glucose—chemistry
- LDH—chemistry
- KOH and fungus culture—microbiology
- AFB and TB—microbiology
- Lyme titer—chemistry

Another area in which the health unit coordinator must be fully aware of institution policy is in disclosure of information such as in cases of AIDS. Laws regarding AIDS and confidentiality vary from state to state, as do laws regarding disclosure of HIV-positive persons. When in doubt, *do not disclose information*. In many health care facilities, guidelines have been established to assist the health care worker. Examples of some of these guidelines include:

- *Not* putting "diagnosis of AIDS" or "rule out AIDS" on the computer; the primary diagnosis is the infection, symptoms, or cancer. AIDS becomes the secondary diagnosis and appears on the medical record but not in the computer.
- Family, friends, and other persons may not know about the AIDS diagnosis and must not be told by any health care employee unless so advised by the doctor. Confidentiality and knowledge of the health care facility's policies and guidelines is essential information for the health unit coordinator to complete tasks and offer quality patient care in the area of infection control.

■ EMERGENCIES

Chemical Safety

All employees will receive chemical safety training during orientation regarding OSHA requirements for hazardous chemicals. Chemicals must be labeled with a statement of warning, and a statement of what the hazard is to eliminate risk and help in first aid measures in the event of a spill or exposure. A material safety data sheet (MSDS) is a communication tool that gives details on chemical dangers and safety procedures. Chemicals should not be stored above eye level or in unlabeled containers. Never add water to acid or mix chemicals indiscriminately. Never use chemicals in ways other than intended. Appropriate PPE should be worn when using chemicals. Spill kits must be available and comply with OSHA guidelines. As a health unit coordinator it is unlikely that you will be handling chemicals but may need to know what to do in case of a spill or an employee incident involving chemicals.

Fire and Electrical Safety

Fire and electrical safety is also part of the employee orientation. The term *fire* is not used, as it may trigger responses that could be fatal to a patient or create panic among patients. A code number, such as Code 1000, or a name such as "Code Red," is usually announced by the hospital telephone operator to alert all hospital personnel when a fire or fire drill takes place. It is essential that all employees be aware of the location of fire extinguishers. The health unit coordinator may be expected to assist with the evacuation of patients who are endangered by the fire. If the fire is not on the unit, the health unit coordinator may help the nursing personnel to close the doors to the patient rooms. Each hospital unit or section of the hospital is separated by fire doors. These doors are constructed to help contain the fire in one area. They must also be closed during a fire. Most hospitals teach the RACE system because it is easy to remember:

R   Rescue individuals in danger
A   Alarm: sound the alarm
C   Confine the fire by closing all doors and windows
E   Extinguish the fire with the nearest suitable fire extinguisher

Classes of Fire:

Class A: wood, paper, clothing
Class B: flammable liquids and vapors
Class C: electrical equipment
Class D: combustible or reactive metals

The health unit coordinator is often asked to call maintenance when electrical equipment used for patient care needs repair. Electrical equipment used in the nursing station must also be well maintained for safety purposes.

Guidelines for Electrical Safety:

- Avoid the use of extension cords
- Do not overload electrical circuits
- Inspect cords and plugs for breaks and fraying
- Unplug equipment when servicing
- Unplug equipment that has liquid spilled in it
- Unplug and do not use equipment that is malfunctioning

Medical Emergencies

Two medical emergencies—that is, life-threatening situations—that require remaining calm, swift action, and good communication by the health unit coordinator are cardiac arrest and respiratory arrest. (It is common hospital terminology to refer to these as *code arrests*.) The hospital telephone operator is notified immediately to announce the code. In a cardiac arrest the patient's heart contractions are absent or grossly insufficient, and there is no pulse and no blood pressure. In respiratory arrest, the patient may cease to breathe or the respirations become so depressed that the patient does not receive enough oxygen to sustain life. Both conditions require quick action by hospital personnel and the use of emergency equipment. Treatment must be

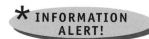

It is helpful when the health unit coordinator working on a nearby nursing unit offers assistance to the health unit coordinator on the unit where the code is announced.

instituted within 3 to 4 minutes, because the brain cells deteriorate rapidly from lack of oxygen.

Each hospital nursing unit and department maintains a code or crash cart. This is taken to the code arrest patient's room immediately. It is important for health unit coordinators to know the location of the code or crash cart and any other emergency equipment so that it can be brought quickly to their nursing unit when needed.

Hospitals have designated hospital personnel who report to each code arrest. They are members of the code arrest team. They may be employed in various hospital departments, such as intensive or coronary care, other nursing units, the respiratory care department, pulmonary function department, surgery, and so forth.

As a member of the health care team, the health unit coordinator may be asked to perform the tasks outlined in Procedure 22–1.

Disaster Procedure

A disaster procedure is a planned procedure that is carried out by hospital personnel when a large number of persons have been injured. The disaster may occur during a flood, a fire, a bombing, or an accident such as a train derailment, or plane crash. Each hospital maintains a disaster plan book. Disaster drills are held once or twice a year to keep the hospital personnel informed and in practice. Announcing a code such as "Code 5000" on the hospital public address system activates the disaster procedure.

The health unit coordinator is usually designated to handle communication and to call off-duty health care personnel to assist in caring for the hospital patients and disaster victims and handle communications. The role of the health unit coordinator may vary among hospitals.

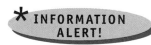

Fire and disaster drills must be taken seriously so that all personnel will be prepared in case a fire or disaster actually happens.

■ SPECIAL SERVICES

Flowers

When a health care facility is large enough to have a specific area where all flowers are delivered, the task of delivering the flowers to patients may be assigned to a hospital volunteer. In that case, the health unit coordinator may need only to direct the volunteer to the correct room.

In hospitals in which the representative from the florist delivers the flowers directly to the unit, the health unit coordinator

Procedure 22-1: PROCEDURE FOR PERFORMING TASKS RELATED TO MEDICAL EMERGENCIES

TASK	NOTES
1. Notify the hospital telephone operator to announce the code.	1. *Notification is made by pressing a special button on the telephone, stating code arrest, and giving the location. Be very specific when stating unit, such as 4A-Apple, 4B-Boy, 4C-Charlie, or 4D-David. Some health care facilities use the expression "Code Blue" to designate a cardiac or respiratory arrest.*
2. Direct the code arrest team to the patient's room.	
3. Remove the patient information sheet from the patient's chart and take or send the chart to the patient's room.	
4. Notify all doctors connected with the patient's case (attending doctor, consultants, and residents).	
5. Notify the patient's family of the situation if requested to do so.	5. *If the health unit coordinator does communicate with the family, the conversation should be carried on in as controlled a manner as possible, so as to not cause panic. The dialogue might be, "Mr. Whetstone, your brother's condition has changed, and the doctor thought you would like to know. The doctors are with him now. Will you be coming to the hospital?"*
6. Label any laboratory specimens with the patient's ID label, enter the test ordered in the computer, and send the specimen to the laboratory stat.	
7. Call the appropriate departments for treatments and supplies as needed.	7. *Usually respiratory care, diagnostic imaging, and CSD are the departments involved.*
8. Alert the admissions department and the ICU for possibility of transfer to ICU.	8. *If the code procedure is successful, the patient is transferred to ICU or possibly CCU, where he or she can be closely monitored.*
9. For a successful code, follow Procedure 20-5 for a transfer to another unit.	9. *See Chapter 20, p. 410.*
10. For an unsuccessful code procedure, follow Procedure 20-4 for postmortem care.	10. *See Chapter 20, p. 407.*

should ascertain that the patient is still on the unit or within the hospital before signing for and accepting the flowers. After signing the delivery slip, the health unit coordinator may deliver the flowers to the patient's room.

The health unit coordinator must be aware of any restrictions. For example, flowers are not allowed on some nursing units, such as intensive care or on respiratory units, and rubber balloons are not allowed on pediatric units. If family members are present, flowers and balloons may be sent home with them.

Mail

Mail is delivered to the nursing unit daily. The mail is checked and the patient's room and bed numbers are written on each envelope. In the event that the patient has been discharged, you write "discharged" in pencil on the envelope and return it to the mailroom. The mail may be distributed to the patients as time allows or the task may be designated to a hospital volunteer.

■ SUMMARY

Although there are many things the new health unit coordinator needs to learn upon employment, it is important to know the routines and be able to perform the tasks related to medical emergencies, fires, and disasters. When emergencies occur, there is no time to look in a book for directions about what you must do.

The other tasks discussed in this chapter may not be part of your regular routine, and therefore it is necessary for you to review the procedures in your hospital as time permits.

REVIEW
QUESTIONS

1. Write the meaning of each abbreviation listed below in the space provided.

   a. AIDS

   _____

   b. ARC

   _____

   c. CDC

   _____

   d. HBV

   _____

   e. HIV

   _____

   f. OSHA

   _____

   g. PPE

   _____

   h. TB

   _____

   i. RACE

   _____

   _____

2. List four categories of incidents that require a report to administration.

   a. _____

   b. _____

   c. _____

   d. _____

3. Describe the duties of a health unit coordinator during a fire drill.

   _____

   _____

4. List six guidelines to follow for electrical safety:

    a. _____

    b. _____

    c. _____

    d. _____

    e. _____

    f. _____

5. Name three pathogenic microorganisms that are frequently responsible for hospital-acquired infections.

    a. _____

    b. _____

    c. _____

6. Define the following:

    a. Centers for Disease Control and Prevention

    _____

    b. reverse isolation

    _____

    c. respiratory arrest

    _____

    d. protective care

    _____

    e. pathogenic microorganisms

    _____

    f. medical emergency

    _____

    g. isolation

    _____

    h. incident

    _____

    i. communicable disease

    _____

    j. material safety data sheet

_____

    k. cardiac arrest

_____

    l. disaster procedure

_____

    m. nosocomial infections

_____

    n. standard precautions

_____

    o. risk management

_____

    p. airborne precautions

_____

7. List nine tasks that the health unit coordinator may perform during a medical emergency.

    a. _____

    b. _____

    c. _____

    d. _____

    e. _____

    f. _____

    g. _____

    h. _____

    i. _____

8. What should the health unit coordinator do when handling or transporting specimens?

_____

_____

9. Why is reporting in writing of each hospital incident important?

_____

_____

10. List six components that comprise the chain of infection.

    a. _____

    b. _____

    c. _____

    d. _____

    e. _____

    f. _____

11. Three methods by which bacteria may be transmitted are:

    a. _____

    b. _____

    c. _____

12. Name three conditions that may cause a patient to become immunocompromised.

    a. _____

    b. _____

    c. _____

13. List four types of PPE used with standard precautions.

    a. _____

    b. _____

    c. _____

    d. _____

14. In AIDS, what is meant by an "opportunistic infection"?

    _____

15. Name the two opportunistic diseases related to AIDS.

    a. _____

    b. _____

16. Describe the process for acceptance and delivery of:

    a. patient mail

_____

    b. patient flowers

_____

TOPICS FOR DISCUSSION

1. Discuss the importance of fire and disaster drills.
2. Discuss the consequences of not using good handwashing techniques and not adhering to standard precautions.

WEBSITES OF INTEREST

Centers for Disease Control and Prevention: www.cdc.gov.
OSHA: www.osha-slc.gov
World Health Organization: www.who.int/en

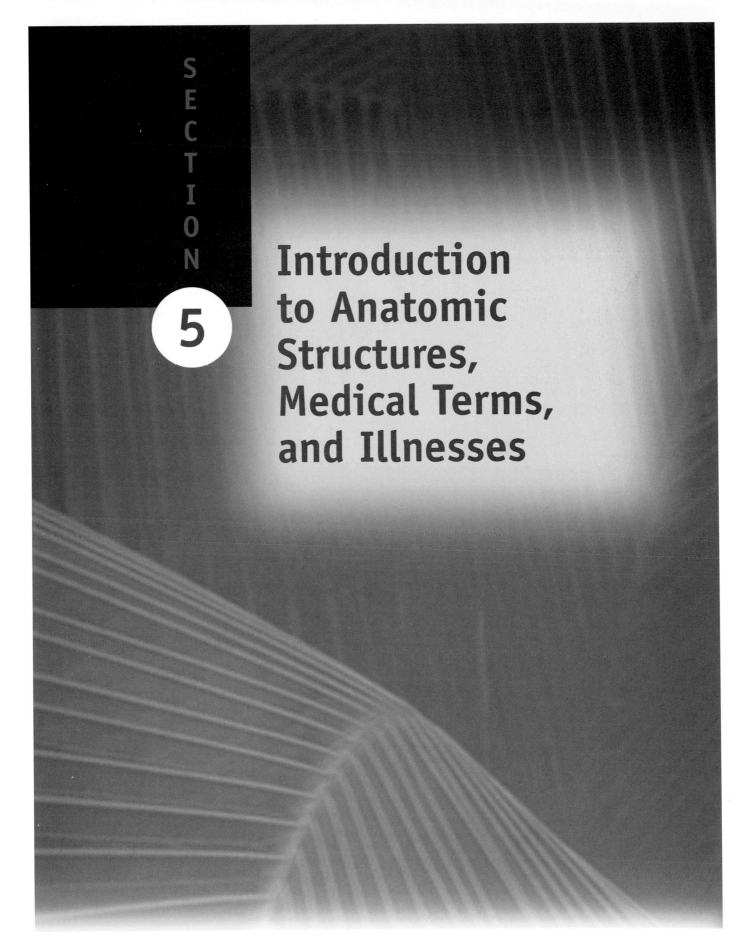

5

Introduction to Anatomic Structures, Medical Terms, and Illnesses

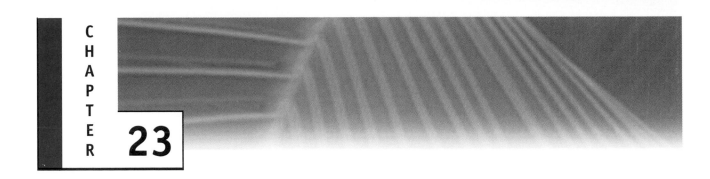

C H A P T E R

23

Medical Terminology, Basic Human Structure, Diseases, and Disorders

UNIT 1

Medical Terminology: Word Parts, Analyzing, and Word Building

Unit Objectives

Upon completion of this unit, you will be able to:

1. Identify the three main origins of medical terms.
2. Name and define the four word parts that are commonly used in building medical terms.

3. List three guidelines to follow when connecting word parts to form a medical term.
4. Define *analysis of medical terms* and *word building.*
5. Given a list of medical terms and a list of word parts, divide the medical terms into their component parts—that is, word roots, prefixes, suffixes, and combining vowels—and identify the kinds of word parts present in each term by name.
6. Given a description of the medical condition and a list of word parts—that is, word roots, prefixes, suffixes, and combining vowels—write out the medical term that represents a stated medical condition.

■ INTRODUCTION TO MEDICAL TERMS

Most medical terms are made up of Greek (e.g., *nephrology*) and Latin (e.g., *maternal*) words; however, some have been adapted from modern languages, such as *triage* and *lavage* from French. Two other sources of medical terms include acronyms and eponyms. An acronym is a word formed from the first letters of major terms in a descriptive phrase, such as *laser* (*l*ight *a*mplification by *s*timulated *e*mission of *r*adiation).

An eponym is a name given to something that was discovered by or is identified with an individual. The Pap smear (Dr. Papanicolaou) and Lou Gehrig's disease (amyotrophic lateral sclerosis) are two examples of eponyms. Although a background of Greek or Latin is not necessary to learn the meaning of medical terms, it is necessary to learn the English translation of the Greek or Latin word parts. In this course of study the parts of the word are memorized rather than the whole word. By learning word parts you will be able to build words according to a given definition and break down words into word parts to determine their meaning.

For example, in the medical term

nephr / ectomy

nephr- is the word part that means "kidney" and *-ectomy* is the word part meaning "surgical removal." Thus *nephrectomy* means "surgical removal of the kidney." Once you have memorized the meanings of the word parts (*nephr-* and *-ectomy*), you will know their meanings when they appear in other medical terms.

In the preceding example, you can define the term by literally translating it. However, a few medical terms have implied meanings. For example, the word

an / emia

literally translated, means "without" (*an-*) "blood condition" (*-emia*). However, the correct interpretation of anemia—an implied meaning—is a deficiency of red blood cells (RBCs). Knowledge of the meanings of the word parts for a medical term with an implied meaning takes you almost, but not quite, to the exact meaning of the term.

Medical terms are used instead of English words because one word says what it would take many English words to say. For example, nephrectomy means "surgical removal of the kidney." Medical terms are efficient and factual, they save space, and they often describe a situation or procedure more exactly.

Pronunciation of medical terms varies. What is acceptable pronunciation in one part of the country may not be used in another part of the country; therefore, flexibility is necessary in the pronunciation of medical terms.

Correct spelling is absolutely necessary to avoid the incorrect use of a term. *Ileum* (portion of small intestine) and *ilium* (part of the hip bone) are two examples of terms close in spelling, yet anatomically diverse in meaning.

As you begin working with medical terminology, you may feel overwhelmed at the task of learning this new language. However, repeated use of the word parts will assist you in building your vocabulary, and you will soon be using medical terms fluently in your everyday speech. Many students employ the use of mnemonics (memory-aiding devices) to remember the word parts. For example, *entero* is the word part for "intestine." One might think of "digested food *entering* the intestine" and more easily recall the meaning of *entero*. Similarly, ileum of the small intestine is spelled with an *e* and one might associate "eating" with the intestine and not mistake this term with ilium, a part of the hipbone.

This unit deals with the word parts and how they are used together to form medical terms. *Remember:* it is important for you to master Unit 1 before proceeding to Unit 2, and so forth, because each unit is a continuation of the previously studied units.

■ WORD PARTS

In this course of study the development of a medical vocabulary is based upon memorizing parts of words rather than the whole word. *Word part* is the term we will use to describe the components of words. To build or analyze (divide into parts) medical terms, you must first learn the following four word parts:

1. Word root
2. Prefix
3. Suffix
4. Combining vowel

Word Root

The word root is the basic part of the word; it expresses the principal meaning of the word. For example, in the medical term

gastr / ic

gastr (stomach) is the word root.

Prefix

The prefix is the part of the word placed before the word root to alter its meaning. For example, in the medical term

intra / gastr / ic

intra (within) is the prefix.

Suffix

The suffix is the part of the word added after the word root to alter its meaning. For example, in the medical term

gastr / ic

ic (pertaining to) is the suffix.

Combining Vowel

The combining vowel, usually an *o*, is used between two word roots or between a word root and a suffix to ease pronunciation. Three guidelines are followed in using a combining vowel.

1. When connecting a word root to a suffix, a combining vowel is usually not used if the suffix begins with a vowel. For example, in the word [gastr / ectomy], *ectomy* (surgical removal) begins with the vowel *e*; thus the combining vowel *o* is not used.
2. When connecting two word roots, the combining vowel is usually used even if the second root begins with a vowel. For example, in the word [gastr / o / enter / itis], the second word root *enter* (intestine) begins with the vowel *e*, but the combining vowel *o* is still used.
3. A combining vowel is not used when connecting a prefix and word root. For example, in the medical term [sub / hepat / ic], a combining vowel is not used between the prefix, *sub,* and the word root, *hepat.*

Note: A combining form, not a true word part, is simply the word root separated from its combining vowel with a slash mark. For example, gastr/o is a combining form. Although *o* is the most commonly used combining vowel, *a*, *e*, and *i* may also be used. Throughout this chapter the word roots are listed in combining forms.

Word Root	Meaning
cardi / o	heart
cyt / o	cell
electr / o	electricity, electrical activity
enter / o	intestine
gastr / o	stomach
hepat / o	liver
nephr / o	kidney

Prefixes	Meaning
intra-	within
sub-	under, below
trans-	through, across, beyond

Suffixes	Meaning
-ectomy	excision, surgical removal
-gram	record, x-ray image
-ic	pertaining to
-itis	inflammation
-logy	study of

■ ANALYZING MEDICAL TERMS

To analyze medical terms means to divide the term into word parts and identify each word part. Divide the word into word parts by use of vertical slashes and identify the word part by labeling it as follows:

P   prefix
WR   word root
S   suffix
CV   combining vowel.

EXERCISE 1

Analyzing Medical Terms: Analyze the following medical terms by dividing each into word parts and writing *P, WR, S,* or *CV* above the appropriate part, as in the following examples. Use the list above to help you identify word parts.

Examples:

WR	CV	WR	S		P	WR	S
gastr	/ o	/ enter	/ itis		intra	/ gastr	/ ic

1. *cytology* _____

2. *gastrectomy* _____

3. *subhepatic* _____

4. *electrocardiogram* _____

5. *cardiology* _____

6. *transhepatic* _____

■ WORD BUILDING

Word building is the process of creating a medical term using word parts. In building medical terms from a given definition, keep in mind that the beginning of the definition usually indicates the suffix that is needed to build the term.

EXERCISE 2

Word Building: Build medical terms from the following definitions. Use the above list to assist you.
Example: study of the kidney   nephrology

1. the study of the heart _____

2. the study of cells _____

3. surgical removal of the stomach _____

4. inflammation of the stomach and intestines _____

5. pertaining to the stomach _____

6. pertaining to within the stomach _____

7. surgical removal of the kidney _____

REVIEW
QUESTIONS

1. Name the three main origins of medical terms and give an example for each.

    a. _____

    b. _____

    c. _____

2. List the four word parts. Define and give an example of each.

    a. _____

    Example: _____

    b. _____

    Example: _____

    c. _____

    Example: _____

    d. _____

    Example: _____

3. List the guidelines followed in connecting:

    a. prefix and word root

    _____

    b. word root and word root

    _____

    c. word root and suffix

    _____

4. Define:

    a. analysis of medical terms

    _____

    b. word building

    _____

UNIT 2

Body Structure, Integumentary System, and Oncology

▶ Outline

▶ Unit Objectives

Upon completion of this unit, you will be able to:

1. Define the terms *cell, tissue, organ,* and *system.*
2. Briefly describe the structure of the living cell.
3. Name four types of tissue.
4. List five body cavities and name a body organ contained in each.
5. List the four quadrants and nine regions of the abdomino-pelvic cavity.
6. Define anatomical position and the directional terms outlined in this unit.
7. Describe the structure and function of skin.
8. Describe cancer, burns, abscess, laceration, abrasion, gangrene, infection, and decubitus ulcer.

■ BODY STRUCTURE (ANATOMY) AND FUNCTION (PHYSIOLOGY)

Body Cells

The cell is the basic unit of all living things (Fig. 23-1). The human body is made up of trillions of cells. Cells perform specific functions, and their size and shape vary according to function. Bones, muscles, skin, and blood are each made up of different kinds of cells. Body cells are microscopic; approximately 2,000 are needed to make an inch. Cells are constantly growing and reproducing. Such growth is responsible for the development of an embryo into a child and a child into an adult. This growth is also responsible for the replacement of cells that have a relative short life span and for cells that are injured, diseased, or worn out.

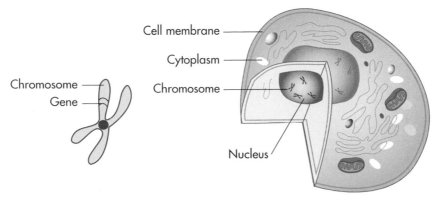

Cell membrane
Cytoplasm
Chromosome
Chromosome
Gene
Nucleus

FIGURE 23–1 ▲ Parts of a body cell.

To visualize the structure of a cell we can compare the three main parts of the cell with the three parts of an egg: the egg shell, the egg white, and the egg yolk.

Cell Membrane

The cell membrane (egg shell), the boundary of the cell, is porous, flexible, and elastic. The protective cell membrane actively or passively regulates the movement of a substance in and out. The cell membrane keeps the cell intact. The cell dies if the cell membrane can no longer carry out this function.

Cytoplasm

Cytoplasm (egg white) is the main body of the cell in which are found various organelles, such as the mitochondria, specialized structures that carry out activities necessary for the cell's survival. For example, in the muscle cell the basic contracting is done by the sarcomere within its cytoplasm, called *sarcoplasm.*

Nucleus

The nucleus (egg yolk), a small structure, is located near the center of the cell. It is the control center of the cell and plays an important role in reproduction. Chromosomes located in the nucleus contain the genes that determine hereditary characteristics. Not all cells contain a nucleus, such as the mature RBC. Some other cells, such as certain bone cells and skeletal muscle cells, contain several nuclei.

Body Tissues (Fig. 23–2)

A tissue is made up of a group of similar cells that work together to perform particular functions. Four types of tissues are:

1. *Epithelial Tissue:* Epithelial tissue forms protective coverings (skin), lines body cavities (e.g., digestive, respiratory and urinary tracts), and forms many glands.
2. *Connective Tissue:* The main functions of the connective tissue are to connect and hold tissues to one another, transport substances, and protect against foreign invaders. Connective tissue forms and protects bones, fat, blood cells, and cartilage and provides immunity.
3. *Muscle Tissue:* Muscle tissue forms the muscles of the body, which contract and relax to produce movement.
4. *Nerve Tissue:* Nerve tissue forms parts of the nervous system, which conducts electrical impulses and helps to coordinate body activities.

Body Organs

An organ is made up of two or more kinds of tissues that perform one or more common functions. The stomach is an organ. It is made up of muscle, nerve, connective, and epithelial tissue.

Body Systems

A *system* is a group of organs that work closely together in a common purpose to perform complex body functions (Fig. 23–3). For example, the urinary system is made up of the following organs: kidneys, ureters, urinary bladder, and urethra. Its main function is to remove wastes from the blood and eliminate them from the body. Other body systems are digestive, musculoskeletal, nervous, reproductive, endocrine, circulatory, respiratory, sensory, and integumentary. Some organs are a part of more than one system. The pharynx, for example, is part of both the digestive and respiratory

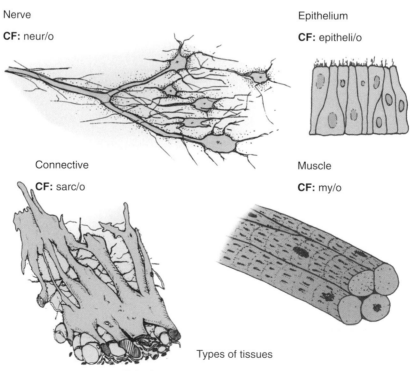

Nerve

CF: neur/o

Epithelium

CF: epitheli/o

Connective

CF: sarc/o

Muscle

CF: my/o

Types of tissues

FIGURE 23–2 ▲ Types of tissues.

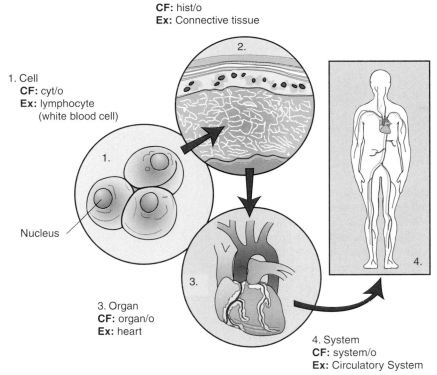

FIGURE 23–3 ▲ Organization of the body.

systems. In the digestive system the pharynx allows for the passage of food; in the respiratory system it allows for the passage of air.

Homeostasis is the maintenance of a stable, relatively constant environment in the body cells and tissues. Stability of the body's normal volume, temperature, and chemicals is effected by the successful harmony of the organ systems and is regulated by the nervous and endocrine systems. Failure to keep the body systems in homeostasis results in disease.

Body Cavities

Large spaces within the body that contain internal organs, or viscera, are called *body cavities* (Fig. 23–4). The two major body cavities are the *dorsal cavity* (near the back) and the *ventral cavity* (near the front).

Dorsal Cavity

The dorsal cavity is composed of the cranial cavity and the spinal cavity, which form a continuous space.

Cranial cavity: Space in the skull; contains the brain.
Spinal cavity: Space in the spinal column; contains the spinal cord.

Ventral Cavity

The ventral cavity is composed of the thoracic (or chest) cavity and the abdominopelvic cavity.

Thoracic cavity: This space is divided into a right and left pleural cavity and the mediastinum. Organs within the thoracic

cavity include the heart, lungs, trachea, esophagus, thymus gland, and major blood vessels.
Right and left pleural cavity: Spaces containing the lungs.
Mediastinum: Space containing the heart, trachea, esophagus, thymus gland, and major blood vessels.
Abdominopelvic cavity: This space is divided into the abdominal cavity and the pelvic cavity.
Abdominal cavity: Upper portion of the abdominopelvic cavity; this space contains the stomach, most of the intestines, kidneys, ureters, liver, pancreas, gallbladder, and spleen. The abdominal cavity is separated from the thoracic cavity by a muscle called the diaphragm.
Pelvic cavity: Lower portion of the abdominopelvic cavity; this space contains the bladder, urethra, reproductive organs, part of the large intestine (sigmoid colon), and the rectum. The abdominopelvic cavity is divided into four quadrants and nine regions (Fig. 23–5). You will frequently encounter these descriptive terms in your health care employment.

Body Directional Terms

Directional terms, used to describe a location on or within the body, refer to the patient in the *anatomical position.* Anatomical position is the point of reference to ensure proper description: body erect, face and feet forward, arms at side, and palms facing forward. In Fig. 23–11 (in Unit 3 of this chapter, page 466), the skeletal orientation is in anatomical position.

Superior (cranial): Pertaining to *above.* (The eye is located superior to the mouth.)

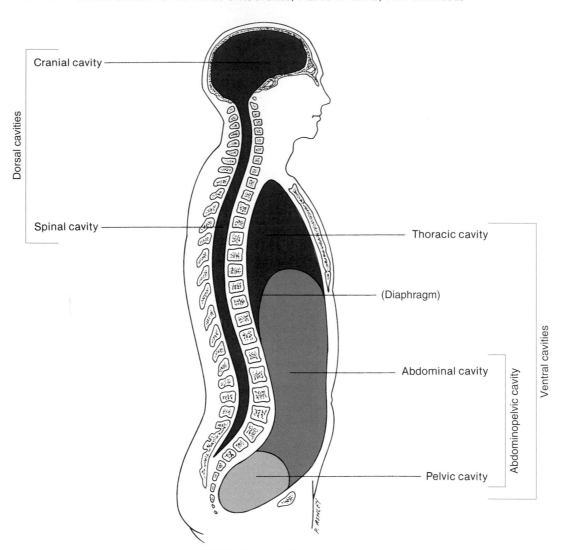

FIGURE 23–4 ▲ The body cavities.

Inferior (caudal): Pertaining to *below*. (The mouth is located inferior to the nose.)

Anterior (ventral): Pertaining to *in front of*. (The eyes are located on the anterior of the head.)

Posterior (dorsal): Pertaining to *in back of*. (The gluteus maximus is posterior to the navel.)

Lateral: Pertaining to the *side*. (The little toe is lateral to the big toe.)

Medial: Pertaining to the *middle*. (The nose is medial to the ears.)

Abduction: Pertaining to *away from*. (Spreading the fingers wide apart is an example of abduction.)

Adduction: Pertaining to *toward*. (Bringing the fingers together from being spread out shows adduction.)

Proximal: Pertaining to *closer than* another structure to the point of attachment (The elbow is proximal to the wrist.)

Distal: Pertaining to *farther than* another structure from the point of attachment (The fingers are distal to the elbow.)

Superficial: Toward the surface (Hair follicles are superficial structures.)

Deep: Farther from the surface (The femur is deep to the skin.)

Prone: Lying with the face downward (The patient is placed in a prone position to suture the back of her head.)

Supine: Lying on the back (Supine positioning was required for his sternal puncture.)

■ INTEGUMENTARY SYSTEM

The integumentary system consists of the skin (the largest organ of the body) and accessory structures (hair, nails, and sweat and oil glands) (Fig. 23–6). The skin of an adult may weigh 20 pounds or more. The skin has many functions. The main one is to protect underlying tissues from pathogenic (disease-causing) microorganisms and other environmental hazards. The skin also assists in the regulation of body temperature and the synthesis of vitamin D. As a sensory organ, the specialized receptors of the skin pass messages of pain, temperature, pressure, and touch to the brain.

The thin outer layer of skin is called the *epidermis* and is composed of epithelial tissue. The cells of the innermost layer produce themselves. As they move toward the surface, the outer-

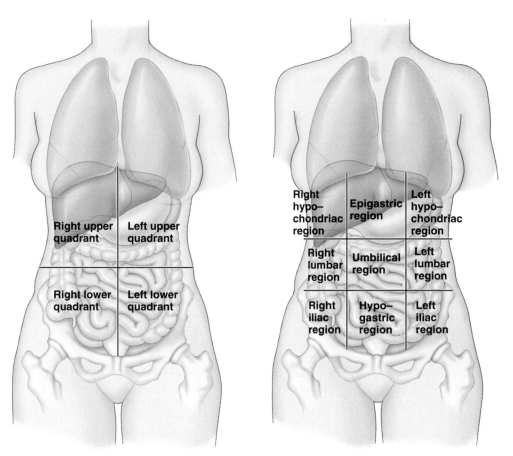

FIGURE 23–5 ▲ Division of the abdominopelvic cavity into four quadrants and nine regions.

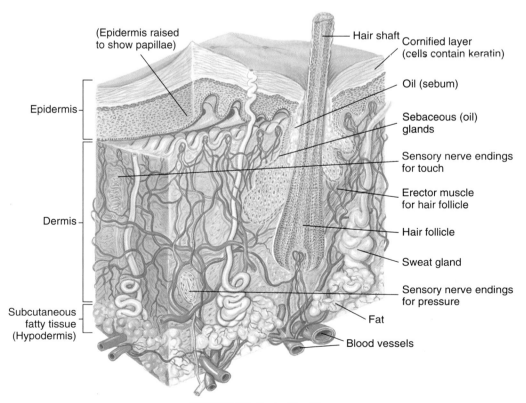

FIGURE 23–6 ▲ The skin.

most cells are shed. Millions of cells are produced and shed each day. The epidermis contains no blood vessels.

The thick layer directly below the epidermis is called the *dermis,* or *true skin.* It is made up of connective tissue and contains blood vessels, nerve endings, hair follicles, and sweat and oil glands.

The subcutaneous tissue (or *hypodermis*), a thick, fat-containing tissue located below the dermis, serves to connect the skin to underlying muscles, bone, and organs.

Hair provides a protective function; for example, nasal hairs trap foreign particles to prevent their being inhaled into the lungs. The hair follicle is a pouchlike depression in the skin from which the hair grows to extend above the skin surface. Oil glands (sebaceous glands) connect to the hair follicle by tiny ducts. Each sebaceous gland produces oil (sebum), which lubricates the hair and skin and inhibits bacterial growth.

The *sweat glands* (sudoriferous glands) are coiled, tubelike structures located mainly in the dermis. Each extends to the surface in the form of a tiny opening called a *pore.* There are approximately 3000 pores in the palm of a hand and 2,000,000 on the body surface. Sweat, a saline fluid, is produced by the sweat glands. As sweat evaporates on the body surface, it cools the body.

Skin color is determined by the amount of melanin in the epidermis of the skin. Skin color varies from pale yellow to black. A condition called *albinism* results when melanin cannot be formed by the melanocytes. An albino can be recognized by the characteristic absence of pigment in the hair, eyes, and skin.

■ DISEASES AND CONDITIONS OF THE SKIN AND BODY CELLS

Cancer

Cancer (often abbreviated as *CA*) is a disease in which unregulated new growth of abnormal cells occur. It is normal for worn-out body cells to be replaced by new cell growth and also for new cells to form to repair tissue damage. Normal cell growth is regulated; in cancer this cell division is unregulated, and it continues to reproduce until a mass known as a *tumor,* or *neoplasm,* forms. Skin cancer arises from cell changes in the epidermis and is the most common form of human cancer. Exposure to broad-spectrum ultraviolet (UV) rays of the sun and artificial sources is thought to be an important factor in development of skin cancer. Basal cell carcinoma and squamous cell carcinoma, two major types of skin cancers, are both very responsive to treatment and seldom metastasize (spread) to other body systems.

Cancerous tumors are malignant, which means they become progressively worse, whereas noncancerous tumors are benign or nonrecurrent. Malignant tumors grow in a disorganized fashion, interrupting body function and interfering with the food and blood supply to normal cells. Malignant cells may metastasize from one organ to another through the bloodstream or lymphatic system.

Cancer is many different diseases, and one cause of this abnormal cell division cannot be pinpointed. Genetic factors, steroidal estrogens, cigarette smoking, exposure to carcinogenic substances, and UV rays are believed to be among the causes of cancer.

Detection of cancer includes self-examination, x-ray imaging, blood tests, and microscopic tissue examination. Treatments of cancer include surgery, chemotherapy, and radiation therapy.

Cancer's Seven Warning Signals

The seven warning signals of cancer may easily be recalled by the mnemonic CAUTION.

Change in bowel or bladder habits
A sore that does not heal
Unusual bleeding or discharge
Thickening or lump in the breast, testes, or elsewhere
Indigestion or difficulty in swallowing
Obvious change in a wart or mole
Nagging cough or hoarseness

Burns

All burns are dangerous if not treated properly because infection can occur and because shock is possible in more serious burns as a result of fluid loss from the skin. Burns are classified according to degrees of severity, which includes depth of burn (full or partial thickness) (Fig. 23–7) and extent of surface area involvement (Fig. 23–8).

1. *First-degree burns* damage the epidermis. Also called *partial thickness* burn, sunburn is an example of a first-degree burn in which redness, minor discomfort; and slight edema may be present.
2. *Second-degree burns* damage the epidermis and the dermis. Also called partial thickness burns, presenting symptoms are redness, pain, edema, and blisters.
3. *Third-degree burns* destroy the epidermis, dermis, and subcutaneous tissue. Also called full thickness burn, there is no pain because of destruction of the skin's sensory receptors. Third-degree burns heal only from the edges and debridement (removal of dead skin) and skin grafts are necessary.

Abscesses

An *abscess* is a cavity containing pus. Abscesses are usually caused by pathogenic microorganisms that invade the tissue through a break in the skin. As the microorganisms destroy the tissue an increased blood supply is rushed to the area, causing inflammation in the surrounding tissue. Abscesses are formed by the body to wall off the pathogenic microorganisms and keep them from spreading throughout the body.

Lacerations and Abrasions

A *laceration* is a wound produced by tearing body tissue. An *abrasion* is a scraping away of the skin. Cleaning lacerations and abrasions is important because of the danger of infection. Suturing may be required to repair lacerations.

Gangrene

Gangrene, a serious medical condition, is the death of body tissue caused by lack of blood supply to an area of the body; often it is the result of infection or injury. Symptoms include fever, pain, darkening of the skin, and an unpleasant

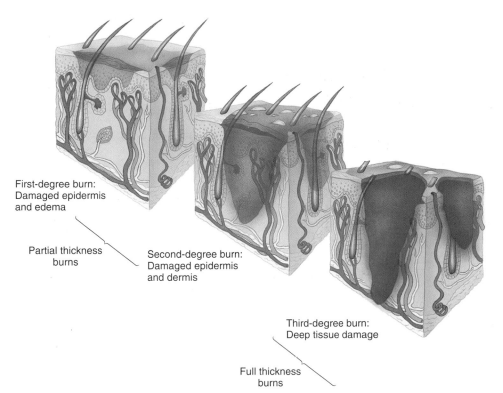

First-degree burn:
Damaged epidermis
and edema

Partial thickness
burns

Second-degree burn:
Damaged epidermis
and dermis

Third-degree burn:
Deep tissue damage

Full thickness
burns

FIGURE 23–7 ▲ First-degree burns damage the epidermis; second-degree burns damage the epidermis and the dermis; third-degree burns damage the epidermis, the dermis, and the subcutaneous tissue.

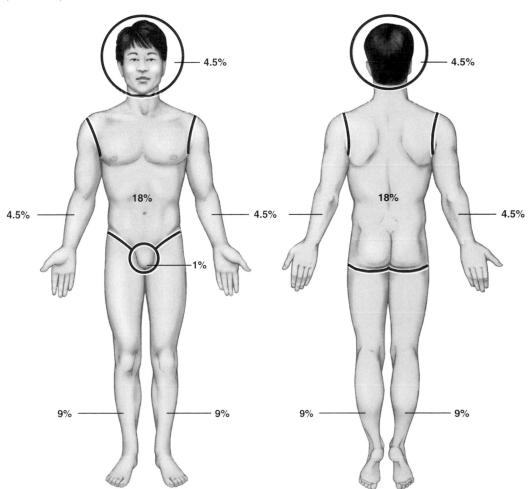

4.5%

4.5%

4.5%

18%

4.5%

4.5%

18%

4.5%

1%

9%

9%

9%

9%

FIGURE 23–8 ▲ Surface area involvement of burns. The *rule of nines* is one method used to estimate the total body surface area (TBSA) burned in an adult. This method divides the TBSA into multiples of 9% (1% for the groin). The Lund-Browder Chart is used for infants and children because the surface area of the head and neck is greater than for adults, and the limbs are smaller.

odor. Treatment, depending on the underlying cause, includes surgical debridement (removal with a sharp instrument) of the necrotic tissue or amputation, intravenous (IV) antibiotics, and hyperbaric oxygen therapy to help kill the bacteria.

Infection

Infection is the invasion of the body by pathogenic microorganisms that reproduce and multiply, causing disease. Infections may be caused by streptococcal, staphylococcal, or *Pseudomonas* bacteria; by viruses; or by other organisms. Bacterial infections are treated with antibiotic therapy. Methicillin-resistant *Staphylococcus aureus* (MRSA) has become a widespread nosocomial (hospital- or health care setting-acquired) pathogen. The main mode of transmission of MRSA in the clinical setting is from the hands of health care workers. MRSA can be found on the skin, in the nose, and in blood and urine. Proper hand cleansing techniques are normally reviewed with new employees by the Infection Control Department of the clinical setting to avoid transmission of MRSA.

Decubitus Ulcer

Decubitus ulcer, also known as *bedsore* or *pressure sore,* is a vascular condition arising in patients who sit or lie in one position for long periods of time. The weight of the body, typically over bony projections such as the hips, heels, and ankles, slows blood flow, causing ulcers to form and possibly infections to develop when microorganisms enter the affected area. The decubitus ulcer, like the burn, is categorized according to severity with the use of stages (stage I to stage IV). Beginning as a reddened, sensitive, unbroken patch of skin termed *stage I,* the pressure sore may progress to an open sore (ulcer) requiring strict attention to wound care. In stage IV, the patient may experience full-thickness skin loss with damage to muscle, bone, or other body structures. Periodic body position changes and soft support cushions may help to prevent the onset of pressure sores.

▼ REVIEW QUESTIONS

1. Define the following terms:

   a. cell: _____

   b. tissue: _____

   c. organ: _____

   d. system: _____

2. Name four kinds of tissues.

   a. _____

   b. _____

   c. _____

   d. _____

3. List five body cavities and name one internal organ contained in each.

   a. _____

   b. _____

   c. _____

   d. _____

   e. _____

4. Match the following directional terms in Column 1 with the correct meaning in Column 2.

Column 1

a. superior

b. inferior

c. lateral

d. medial

e. anterior

f. posterior

g. adduction

h. abduction

i. proximal

j. distal

k. deep

l. superficial

m. supine

n. prone

Column 2

_____ 1. in front of

_____ 2. pertaining to the middle

_____ 3. pertaining to away from

_____ 4. pertaining to the side

_____ 5. above

_____ 6. below

_____ 7. pertaining to towards

_____ 8. in back of

_____ 9. farther from the surface

_____ 10. nearer (point of reference)

_____ 11. closer to the surface

_____ 12. farther from (point of reference)

_____ 13. lying with face downward

_____ 14. lying on the back

5. List four functions of the skin.

a. _____

b. _____

c. _____

d. _____

6. The thin outermost layer of the skin is called the _____. The thick layer of skin directly below this layer is called the _____. The innermost layer of fat-containing tissue is called the _____ tissue.

7. Skin color is determined by the amount of _____ in the skin. Absence of this results in _____.

8. _____ glands produce oil that lubricates the skin and hair.

9. _____ open to the surface of the skin in tiny openings called *pores*.

10. Describe the three main structures of a living cell.

_____

_____

_____

11. Match the terms in Column 1 with the phrases in Column 2.

Column 1	Column 2
a. burns	_____ 1. cavity containing pus
b. abscess	_____ 2. classified according to degree of severity
c. laceration	_____ 3. invasion of the body by pathogenic microorganisms
d. gangrene	_____ 4. new growth of abnormal cells
e. infection	_____ 5. death of body tissue
f. cancer	_____ 6. wound produced by tearing
g. abrasion	_____ 7. pressure sore
h. decubitus ulcer	_____ 8. scraping away of skin

MEDICAL TERMINOLOGY RELATING TO BODY STRUCTURE, INTEGUMENTARY SYSTEM, AND ONCOLOGY

Upon mastery of medical terminology for this unit, you will be able to:

1. Define, spell, and pronounce the medical terms listed in this unit.

2. Analyze the medical terms that are built from word parts.

3. Given a meaning of a medical condition, build the corresponding medical terms, using word parts.

Word Parts

Listed below are the word parts you will be working with in this Unit. You will need to memorize each one because you will continue to use them in this chapter and in your work environment. The exercises following the lists will assist you in this task. Practice pronouncing each word part aloud.

To review, a word root is the basic part of the word; a combining form is the word root plus a combining vowel (generally an _o_); a prefix is the modifying word part added to the beginning of a word, and a suffix is the modifying word part added on to the end of a word root.

Word Roots/ Combining Forms	Meaning
cancer/o, carcin/o (kar´-sĭn-ō), onc/o (ŏn´-kō)	cancer
cutane/o (kyū-tā´-nē-ō), dermat/o (dĕr´-mĕ-tō), derm/o (dĕr´-mō)	skin
cyt/o (sī´-tō)	cell
epitheli/o (ĕp-ĭ-thē´-lē-ō)	epithelium
hist/o (hĭs´-tō)	tissue
lip/o (lĭp´-ō)	fat
path/o (păth´-ō)	disease
sarc/o (sar´-cō)	connective tissue, flesh
trich/o (trĭk´-ō)	hair
ungu/o (ŭng´-ŭō)	nail
viscer/o (vĭs´-ĕr-ō)	internal organs

Many of the suffixes presented in this course of study are made up of word roots and suffixes. For example, the suffix _-logy_ is built from _log_ (word root for "study") plus _y_ (suffix). For learning purposes, these will be studied as suffixes and analyzed as one word part.

Prefixes	Meaning
sub-	under, below
trans- (trăns)	through, across, beyond

Suffixes	Meaning
-al, -ous	pertaining to
-genic (jĕn'-ĭk)	producing, originating, causing
-itis (ī'-tĭs)	inflammation
-oid (oyd)	resembling
-ologist (ŏl'-ō-jĭst)	one who specializes in the diagnosis and treatment of (doctor)
-ology (ŏl'-ō-jē)	study of
-oma (ō'-mah)	tumor

EXERCISE 1

Define each combining form listed below.

1. viscer/o

   _____

2. dermat/o

   _____

3. cyt/o

   _____

4. hist/o

   _____

5. derm/o

   _____

6. trich/o

   _____

7. path/o

   _____

8. carcin/o

   _____

9. sarc/o

   _____

10. epitheli/o

    _____

11. lip/o

    _____

12. onc/o

    _____

13. cutane/o

    _____

14. cancer/o

    _____

15. ungu/o

    _____

EXERCISE 2

Define each suffix and prefix listed below.

1. -al   _____

2. -logy   _____

3. -logist   _____

4. -oid   _____

5. -itis   _____

6. -oma   _____

7. -genic   _____

8. trans-   _____

9. -ous   _____

10. sub-   _____

EXERCISE ③

Write the word parts for each definition below. Indicate which word parts are suffixes by writing *S* in the space provided, indicate which word parts are word roots or combining forms by writing *WR* in the space provided, and indicate which word parts are prefixes by writing *P* in the space provided.

Meaning	Word Part	Type of Word Part
Example: inflammation	-itis	S
1. cell	_____	_____
2. skin		
a.	_____	_____
b.	_____	_____
c.	_____	_____
3. specialist	_____	_____
4. resembling	_____	_____
5. internal organs	_____	_____
6. tissues	_____	_____
7. pertaining to		
a.	_____	_____
b.	_____	_____
8. study of	_____	_____
9. through, across, beyond	_____	_____
10. cancer		
a.	_____	_____
b.	_____	_____
c.	_____	_____
11. under, below	_____	_____

■ MEDICAL TERMS RELATING TO BODY STRUCTURE AND SKIN

Listed below are the medical terms you need to know for this unit. Practice pronouncing these words aloud. Following the list are exercises that will assist you in learning these terms.

General Terms	Meaning
carcinogenic (kar'-sĭn-ō-jĕn'-ik)	producing cancer
cytoid (sī'-toyd)	resembling a cell
cytology (sī-tŏl'-ō-jē)	study of cells
dermal (dĕr'-mal)	pertaining to the skin (may also use the term *cutaneous*)
dermatoid (dĕr'-măh-toyd)	resembling skin
dermatologist (dĕr-măh-tŏl'-ō-jĭst)	one who specializes in the diagnosis and treatment of skin (diseases)
dermatology (dĕr-măh-tŏl'-ō-jē)	study of skin (branch of medicine that deals with diagnosis and treatment of skin disease)
dermoid (dĕrm'-ōid)	resembling skin
epithelial (ĕp-ĭ-thē'-lē-al)	pertaining to epithelium
histology (hĭs-tŏl-ō-jē)	study of tissues
oncology (short o]n-kol'-ō-jē)	study of cancer
pathogenic (păth-ō-jĕn'-ĭk)	producing disease
pathologist (pă-thŏl'-ō-jĭst)	one who specializes in the diagnosis and treatment of disease (body changes caused by disease)
pathology (pă-thŏl'-ō-jē)	the study of disease
subcutaneous (sŭb-cŭ-tān'-ē-ŭs)	pertaining to under the skin
subungual (sŭb-ŭng'-ŭăl)	pertaining to under the nail
transdermal (trăns-dĕr'-mal), or transcutaneous	pertaining to (entering) through the skin
trichoid (trĭk'-oyd)	resembling hair
visceral (vĭs'-er-al)	pertaining to internal organs

Diagnostic Terms	Meaning
carcinoma (kăr-sĭ-nō'-mah)	cancerous tumor (malignant)
dermatitis (dĕr-mah-tī'-tĭs)	inflammation of the skin
epithelioma (ĕp-ĭ-thē-lē-ō'-mah)	tumor (composed of) epithelial cells
lipoma (lī-pō'-mah)	tumor (containing) fat
sarcoma (sar-kō'-mah)	tumor (composed of) connective tissue (highly malignant)

EXERCISE 4

Analyze and define each term listed below.

Example: pathologist

Analyze:
WR / CV / S
Path / o / logist

Define:
Specialist in the diagnosis and treatment of disease

1. cytology

_____

_____

2. trichoid

_____

_____

3. pathology

_____

_____

4. *pathogenic*

_____

_____

5. *dermal*

_____

_____

6. *cytoid*

_____

_____

7. *visceral*

_____

_____

8. *histology*

_____

_____

9. *dermatologist*

_____

_____

10. *dermatitis*

_____

_____

11. *carcinogenic*

_____

_____

12. *epithelial*

_____

_____

13. *carcinoma*

_____

_____

14. *epithelioma*

_____

_____

15. *sarcoma*

_____

_____

16. *lipoma*

_____

_____

17. *pathologist*

_____

_____

18. *dermatoid*

_____

_____

19. *dermatology*

_____

_____

20. *transdermal*

_____

_____

21. *oncology*

_____

_____

22. *subungual*

_____

_____

23. *subcutaneous*

_____

_____

EXERCISE 5

Build the medical terms that correspond with the definitions listed here. Remember that the *beginning* of the definition usually indicates the *suffix* that is needed to build the term.

1. *resembling a cell*

_____

2. *resembling hair*

_____

3. *resembling skin*

   a. _____

   b. _____

4. *one who specializes in the diagnosis and treatment of disease (body changes caused by disease)*

_____

5. *one who specializes in the diagnosis and treatment of skin (diseases)*

_____

6. *pertaining to the skin*

   a. _____

   b. _____

7. *pertaining to the internal organs*

_____

8. *study of tissues*

_____

9. *study of disease*

_____

10. *study of skin*

_____

11. *producing disease*

_____

12. *study of cells*

_____

13. *inflammation of the skin*

_____

14. *tumor containing fat*

_____

15. *tumor composed of epithelial cells*

_____

16. *pertaining to epithelium*

_____

17. *producing cancer*

_____

18. *a tumor composed of connective tissue*

_____

19. *cancerous tumor*

_____

20. *pertaining to through the skin*

_____

_____

21. *study of cancer*

_____

22. *pertaining to under the nail*

_____

23. *pertaining to under the skin*

_____

EXERCISE 6

Write each medical term studied in this unit by having someone dictate the terms to you.

1. _____

2. _____

3. _____

4. _____

5. _____

6. _____

7. _____

8. _____

9. _____

10. _____

11. _____

12. _____

13. _____

14. _____

15. _____

16. _____

17. _____

18. _____

19. _____

20. _____

21. _____

22. _____

23. _____

24. _____

25. _____

UNIT 3

The Musculoskeletal System

▶ **Unit Objectives**

Upon completion of this unit, you will be able to:

1. Describe five functions of the skeletal system.
2. Describe bone structure.
3. Name, number, and spell correctly the bones of the body.
4. Distinguish between the axial and appendicular skeleton.
5. Define joint, ligament, and tendon.
6. Describe the four main functions of the muscular system.
7. Describe three types of muscles.
8. Describe arthritis, herniated disk, osteoporosis, Paget's disease, types of fractures, and joint replacement.

■ THE SKELETAL SYSTEM

Organs of the Skeletal System

An adult skeleton has 206 bones.

Functions of the Skeletal System

Protection: To protect the internal organs from injury
Support: To provide a framework for the body
Movement: To act with the muscles to produce body movement
Blood cell production: To produce blood cells (hematopoiesis) in the red marrow of certain bones
Mineral storage: To store calcium and phosphorus, minerals essential for cellular activities

Bone Structure

■ There are four types of bones: long, short, flat, and irregular.
■ Bones have their own system of blood vessels and nerves.
■ Bones contain *red bone marrow* (produces red and white blood cells) and *yellow bone marrow* (consists mostly of adipose tissue, or fat).
■ Bones are covered with a thin membrane called *periosteum*, which is necessary for growth and repair and is the attachment point for ligaments and tendons.

Axial Skeleton

The axial skeleton (80 bones) consists of skull, hyoid bone, vertebral column, and rib cage, so named because the bones revolve around the vertical *axis* of the skeleton.

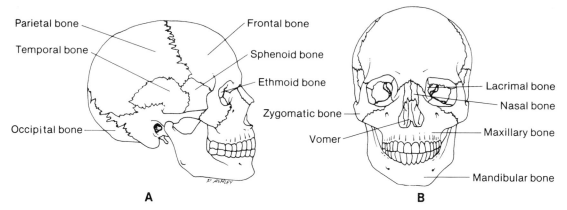

FIGURE 23–9 ▲ The bones of the skull. *A*, Cranial bones. *B*, Facial bones.

Bone Framework of the Head (Fig. 23–9)

Skull/Cranium (8 Bones)

Frontal bone (1): Framework of the forehead and roof of the eye socket

Parietal bones (2): Form the upper sides of the cranium

Temporal bones (2): Form the lower sides of the cranium and contain parts of the ear

Ethmoid bone (1): Forms part of the cranial floor and part of the nasal cavity

Sphenoid bone (1): Bat-shaped bone that extends behind the eyes and forms part of the base of the skull

Occipital bone (1): Composes the back and most of the base of the skull. It connects with the parietal and temporal bones

Facial Bones (14 Bones)

Maxillary bones (2): Upper jaw bones

Mandible (1): Lower jaw bone; the only movable bone in the skull

Nasal bones (2): Support the bridge of the nose

Lacrimal bones (2): Corner of the eye sockets

Zygomatic bones (2): Cheek bones

Vomer (1): Lower portion of the nasal septum

Inferior Nasal Concha (2): Lateral walls of nasal cavity

Palatine (2): Hard palate and part of nasal cavities and orbit walls

Hyoid bone (1): U-shaped bone in throat; anchors tongue

Auditory Ossicles (6): In middle ear; transmit sound
  Malleus (2)—hammer
  Incus (2)—anvil
  Stapes (2)—stirrup

Vertebral Column (26 Vertebrae) *(Fig. 23–10)*

Cervical (7): The first seven vertebrae; form the neck

Thoracic (12): The next 12 vertebrae; form the outward curve of the spine and join with 12 pairs of ribs

Lumbar (5): The next five vertebrae, the largest and strongest; form the inward curvature of the spine

Sacrum (1): The next five vertebrae; these fuse together to form one sacrum in the adult

Coccyx (1): The last three to five vertebrae; in the adult, these fuse together to form one coccyx

The vertebrae form the spinal column. Openings in the vertebrae provide a continuous space through which the spinal cord travels. The vertebrae are separated by disks (plates of cartilage). The central portion of the disk is filled with a pulpy elastic substance called *nucleus pulposus*. The disks allow for flexibility and absorb shock. The lamina is located on the posterior arch of the vertebra.

Rib Cage (24 Bones; Fig. 23–11)

All 24 ribs (12 pairs) are attached posteriorly to the thoracic vertebrae. The first seven pairs of ribs *(true ribs)* attach anteriorly to the sternum; the next three pairs converge and join the seventh rib anteriorly; and the last two pairs remain free at the anterior ends. The last five pairs of ribs are called *false ribs* because they do not attach directly to the sternum. The last two pairs are often referred to as *free* or *floating ribs*.

Sternum (1 Bone)

The sternum is the breastbone.

Appendicular Skeleton (126 Bones)

The appendicular skeleton consists of the limbs that have been appended to the axial skeleton.

Upper Extremities (64 Bones)

Clavicle (2): Collar bone

Scapula (2): Shoulder blade

Arm and Hand Bones (60 Bones)

Humerus (2): Upper arm bone

Ulna (2): Smaller lower arm bone, small finger side

FIGURE 23-10 ▲ The vertebral column.

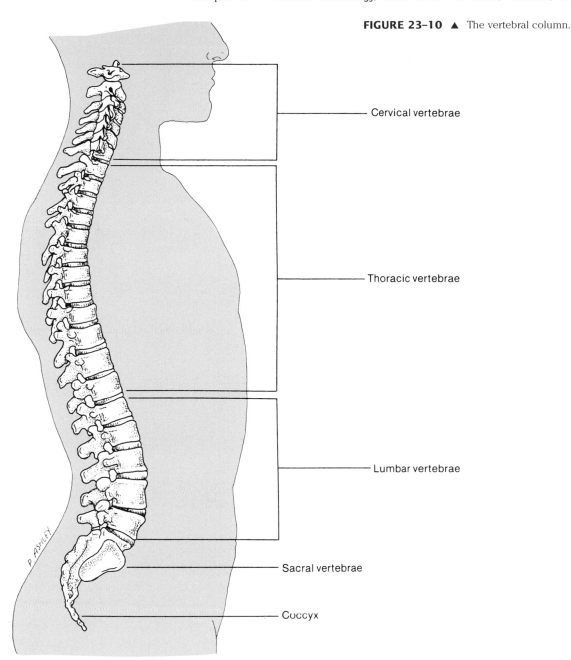

Cervical vertebrae

Thoracic vertebrae

Lumbar vertebrae

Sacral vertebrae

Coccyx

Radius (2): Larger lower arm bone, thumb side
Carpals (16): Wrist bones
Metacarpals (10): Bones of the hand
Phalanges (28): Three bones in each finger and two bones in each thumb

Lower Extremities (62 bones)

In the child, the pelvic girdle consists of three pairs of separate bones: a superior element (the ilium), and two inferior elements (the ischium posteriorly and the pubis anteriorly). These bones

fuse during adolescence and form the single coxal bone on either side characteristic of the adult.

Coxal bone (2): Pelvic or hip bones

Leg and Foot Bones

Femur (2): Thigh bone; largest bone in the body
Patella (2): Kneecap
Tibia (2): Larger, inner lower leg bone (shin bone)
Fibula (2): Smaller, outer lower leg bone
Tarsals (14): Instep bones; form heel and back portion of foot

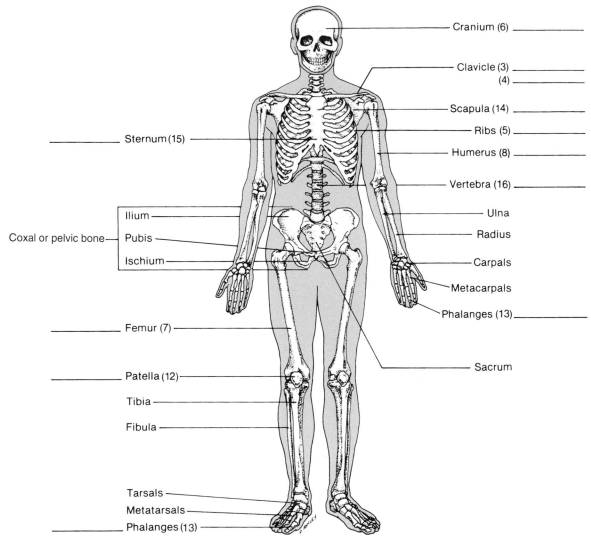

Cranium (6) _____

Clavicle (3) _____

(4) _____

Scapula (14) _____

Ribs (5) _____

Humerus (8) _____

Vertebra (16) _____

Ulna

Radius

Carpals

Metacarpals

Phalanges (13)_____

Sacrum

Sternum (15)

_____ Sternum (15)

Ilium

Coxal or pelvic bone— Pubis

Ischium

_____ Femur (7)

_____ Patella (12)

Tibia

Fibula

Tarsals

Metatarsals

_____ Phalanges (13)

FIGURE 23–11 ▲ The skeleton.

Metatarsals (10): Bones of the foot
Phalanges (28): Three bones in each toe, except for two in each big toe

Joints

A joint is that place on the skeleton where two or more bones meet. Joints allow for movement and hold bones together. Immovable joints, only found in the skull, are called *sutures*. In the newborn, the sutures not yet entirely closed, are called fontanels or soft spots, which allow for "give" in the skull during the birth process. Ligaments are tough bands of tissue that connect one bone with another bone at a joint.

■ THE MUSCULAR SYSTEM

Organs of the Muscular System

Muscles: There are more than 600 muscles in the human body.

Muscular Function

Muscles enable movement of body parts (including blood through blood vessels, food through the digestive system, and glandular secretions through ducts), maintain posture, stabilize joints, and generate heat. Oxygen and nerve supply to the muscle are necessary for muscle function.

Types of Muscles

Skeletal Muscle: Skeletal muscles enable the body to move. The muscles are attached to the bones by tendons. Muscle action is produced by a pulling motion, and muscles work in pairs. Skeletal muscle is a voluntary muscle because it is controlled by the conscious portion of the brain.
Cardiac Muscle: The cardiac muscle, found only in the heart, is an involuntary muscle because it is not under the control of the conscious part of the brain but responds to impulses from the autonomic nerves.

Smooth Muscle: Smooth muscles generally line the walls of hollow organs and serve to propel substances through body passageways and adjust the pupil. Smooth muscles, which are involuntary muscles, may be found in the walls of blood vessels, the eye, and the digestive, urinary, and reproductive tracts.

■ DISEASES AND CONDITIONS OF THE MUSCULOSKELETAL SYSTEM

Arthritis

Over 100 types of joint diseases exist; the two most common types are rheumatoid arthritis and osteoarthritis. Much is still unknown about the cause of arthritis; however, it has been observed that emotional upset can aggravate the disease.

Rheumatoid Arthritis

Rheumatoid arthritis, thought to be an autoimmune disease, usually occurs between the ages of 35 and 50 years, more commonly in women. The onset of symptoms, which include malaise, fever, weight loss, and stiffness of the joints, is gradual. The symptoms come and go. If the disease becomes chronic, degeneration of the joints, with permanent damage, occurs. Treatment consists of heat and drugs, such as aspirin, nonsteroidal antiinflammatory drugs (NSAIDS), and corticosteroids, to reduce inflammation and pain.

Osteoarthritis

Osteoarthritis, the most common form of arthritis, usually occurs in weight-bearing joints, such as the hips or knees. It is the chronic inflammation of the bone and joints caused by degenerative changes in the cartilage covering the surface of the joints. It occurs mostly in older individuals. Treatment consists of drugs to reduce pain and inflammation and physical therapy to loosen the impaired joints.

Ruptured Disk

A *ruptured disk* may also be referred to as a slipped or herniated disk or as a herniated nucleus pulposus (HNP). It is the abnormal protrusion of the soft, gelatinous core of an intervertebral disk (nucleus pulposus) into the neural canal that causes pressure on the spinal cord. Such herniation occurs generally in the lumbar spine (lower back). Treatment consists of bedrest, physical therapy, and analgesics. A laminectomy may be performed to remove a portion of the vertebra, creating more room for the protruding portion of the disk, or a diskectomy may be performed, in which the disk is removed and two or more of the vertebrae are fused together (Fig. 23–12).

Osteoporosis

Osteoporosis, an abnormal decrease in the amount of bone mass, is the leading cause of fractures because the bone tissue becomes porous, thin, and brittle. It is the most prevalent bone disease in the world. Over 20 million people in the United States have osteoporosis. Postmenopausal estrogen-deficient women are the most likely to be affected. Age-related osteoporosis affects both men and women equally. Osteoporosis is known as the "silent crippler," resulting in a virtually symptomless process. Symptoms occur after the disease has progressed. The most common symptoms are pain and loss of height due to the bent-over position that the person assumes. The disease can cause up to an 8-inch loss in height. Fractures can occur in all parts of the skeletal system.

Osteoporosis is diagnosed by radiologic and laboratory studies to measure the bone density and serum calcium levels. Because the onset of the disease is virtually symptom free, the focus is on prevention to minimize bone loss. Preventive and therapeutic measures, aimed at improving bone density, include taking calcium supplements and Vitamin D, weight-bearing exercise, hormone replacement therapy (if appropriate), and correct posture. Bisphosphonates and calcitonin, drugs that slow

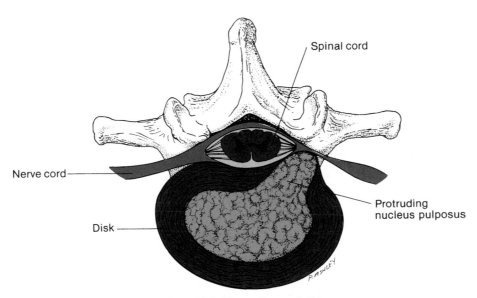

FIGURE 23–12 ▲ Ruptured disk.

down the dissolving process of the osteoclasts, are also useful in treating osteoporosis.

Paget's Disease (Osteitis Deformans)

Paget's disease, the second most common bone disease in the world, causes bones to become extremely weak. Affected individuals are generally older than 40 years of age. The bone may fracture with a very slight blow. If the vertebrae are involved, they may collapse. Bones are living substances that are in a constant process of dissolving and rebuilding. Osteoblasts are the cells that rebuild bone, and osteoclasts are the cells that dissolve bone. An imbalance of this dissolving and rebuilding process results in weak areas or lesions of the bone.

The symptoms of Paget's disease depend on the bones that are affected. Lesions in long bones cause pain, bowing, and arthritic changes of the extremities. When the disease affects the skull, the patient may have headaches, ringing in the ears, hearing loss, and dizziness. If the skull involvement affects the occipital region, pressure is placed on the cerebellum that may compress the spinal cord. Pressure on the spinal cord causes neurologic changes such as muscle weakness, loss of coordination, and ataxia.

Diagnosis is confirmed by abnormal radiologic studies characteristic of Paget's disease and by elevated laboratory values for serum alkaline phosphatase, an enzyme produced by the osteoblasts during bone formation. The treatment for Paget's disease includes using a bisphosphonate or calcitonin to slow down the dissolving process of the osteoclasts.

Fractures

Fracture, the medical term for break (often abbreviated *FX*), is an injury to a bone in which the bone is broken (Fig. 23–13). A fracture is classified by the bone that is injured, such as fractured radius. Some types of fractures are:

Closed (simple): A broken bone but no open wound
Open (compound): A broken bone and an open wound in the skin
Greenstick (incomplete): A bone partially bent and partially broken, more commonly seen in children where the bone is more pliable than in an adult
Comminuted: The bone is splintered or crushed
Spiral: The bone has been twisted apart
Compression: Occurs when the vertebra collapse by trauma or pathology

An *open* or *closed reduction* is used to correct a displaced fracture to restore the fractured ends into normal alignment. In a closed reduction, the bone is realigned with manipulation and/or traction without an incision, whereas an open reduction (and internal fixation—ORIF) is performed after an incision is made into the fracture site. Internal or external devices (plates, nails, screws, or rods) may be applied to maintain proper alignment of the bone during healing.

Joint Replacement

Joint replacement, a surgical procedure known as *arthroplasty,* is performed to replace an arthritic or damaged joint. An artificial joint, or *prosthesis,* is used to replace the patient's hip or knee joint. In a total or partial arthroplasty, hip and knee joints, and less commonly, ankle, elbow, shoulder, wrist, and finger joints are replaced in cases of advanced osteoarthritis and improperly healed fractures, or to relieve a chronically painful or stiff joint.

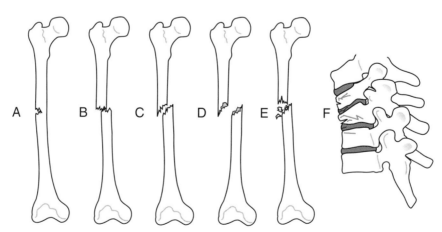

FIGURE 23–13 ▲ Types of fractures. *A,* Greenstick. *B,* Transverse. *C,* Oblique. *D,* Spiral. *E,* Comminuted. *F,* Compression.

REVIEW QUESTIONS

1. List five functions of the skeletal system.

   a. _____

   b. _____

   c. _____

   d. _____

   e. _____

2. _____ is a thin membrane that covers bones.

3. Write the names of the bones that make up the cranium and the face. Indicate the number of each.

   Cranium

   a. _____   d. _____

   b. _____   e. _____

   c. _____   f. _____

   Face

   a. _____   e. _____

   b. _____   f. _____

   c. _____   g. _____

   d. _____   h. _____

4. Name the bone in the throat that anchors the tongue.

   _____

5. Name the middle ear bones and the number of each.

   a. _____   c. _____

   b. _____

6. List the five regions of the vertebral column and number of vertebrae in each region.

   a. _____   d. _____

   b. _____   e. _____

   c. _____

7. Write the name of the bone to match the definitions written below.

   a. shoulder blade _____

   b. collar bone _____

   c. upper arm bone _____

   d. lower arm bone, thumb side _____

   e. lower arm bone, finger side _____

   f. wrist bones _____

   g. bones of the hand _____

   h. finger bones _____

8. Write the names of three pairs of bones that are fused together to form the pelvic bones.

   a. _____   c. _____

   b. _____

9. List the bones of the leg and foot.

   a. _____   e. _____

   b. _____   f. _____

   c. _____   g. _____

   d. _____

10. Name the three types of muscles and give an example of each. Note if the muscle type is voluntary or involuntary.

   a. _____   c. _____

   b. _____

11. Define:

   a. joint _____

   b. tendon _____

   c. ligament _____

12. Two types of arthritis are:

   a. _____

   b. _____

13. Two operations that may be performed for a herniated disk are:

    a. _____

    b. _____

14. Define:

    a. closed fracture _____

    b. open fracture _____

    c. spiral fracture _____

    d. comminuted fracture _____

    e. greenstick fracture _____

    f. compression fracture _____

15. Joint replacement is also called:

    _____

16. Cells that dissolve bone are called _____ and cells that rebuild bone are called

    _____.

17. When Paget's disease affects the skull the symptoms are:

    a. _____

    b. _____

    c. _____

    d. _____

18. An abnormal decrease in the amount of bone mass is called:

    _____

19. In osteoporosis, preventive interventions include:

    a. _____   d. _____

    b. _____   e. _____

    c. _____

■ MEDICAL TERMINOLOGY RELATING TO THE MUSCULOSKELETAL SYSTEM— PREFIXES AND SUFFIXES

Upon mastery of the medical terminology for this unit, you will be able to:

1. Define and spell the word parts and medical terms presented in this unit of study.

2. Analyze the medical terms built from word parts.

3. Given the meaning of a medical condition relating to the musculoskeletal system, build with word parts the corresponding medical term.

4. Given descriptions of hospital situations in which the health unit coordinator may encounter medical terminology, apply the correct medical terms to the situation.

■ WORD PARTS

Listed below are the word parts you need to memorize for the skeletal system. The exercises included in this unit will help you with this task. You will continue to use these word parts throughout the course and during employment. Practice pronouncing each word element aloud.

Skeletal System	Meaning
1. arthr/o (ar′-thrō)	joint
2. chondr/o (kŏn′-drō)	cartilage
3. clavic/o (klăv-ĭ-kō)	clavicle (collar bone)
4. clavicul/o (klah-vĭk′-ū-lō)	clavicle (collar bone)
5. cost/o (kŏs′-tō)	rib
6. crani/o (krā′-nē-ō)	cranium (skull)
7. femor/o (fĕm′-or-ō)	femur (thigh bone)
8. humer/o (hūm′-er-ō)	humerus (upper arm bone)
9. lamin/o (lăm′-ĭ-nō)	lamina (bony arch of the vertebrae)
10. menisc/o (mĕ-nĭs′-kō)	meniscus (cartilage of the knee joint)
11. oste/o (ŏs′-tē-ō)	bone
12. patell/o (pah-tĕl′-ō)	patella (kneecap)
13. phalang/o (fah-lăn′-jō)	phalange (finger or toe bone)
14. scapul/o (skăp′-ū-lō)	scapula (shoulder blade)
15. stern/o (ster′-nō)	sternum (breast bone)
16. vertebr/o (ver′-tĕ-brō)	vertebra (s), vertebrae (pl) (bones of the spine)

Muscular System	Meaning
my/o (mī′-ō)	muscle

Other	Meaning
electr/o (ē-lĕk′-trō)	electricity, electrical activity

EXERCISE 1

Write the combining forms for the skeletal system in the spaces provided on the diagram in Figure 23–11 (p. 466). The number preceding the combining form in the list above matches the number of the body parts in the diagram.

EXERCISE 2

Define each combining form listed below.

1. *arthr/o*

_____

2. *oste/o*

_____

3. *cost/o*

_____

4. *crani/o*

_____

5. *femor/o*

_____

6. *my/o*

_____

7. *humer/o*

_____

8. *patell/o*

_____

9. *stern/o*

_____

10. *clavicul/o*

_____

11. *scapul/o*

_____

12. *phalang/o*

_____

13. *vertebr/o*

_____

14. *clavic/o*

_____

15. *electr/o*

_____

16. *lamin/o*

_____

17. *chondr/o*

_____

18. *menisc/o*

_____

13. muscle _____

14. lamina _____

15. cartilage _____

16. meniscus _____

Recall from Units 1 and 2 that suffixes are letters that may be added to the end of a word root. Listed below are the suffixes you need to know for this unit. Continue to use these throughout the chapter. The exercises will assist you in learning each suffix.

Suffix	Meaning
-algia (ăl′-jē-ah)	pain
-ar, -ic	pertaining to *(Recall you have already learned -al, -ous)*
-centesis (sĕn-tē-sĭs)	surgical puncture to aspirate fluid
-ectomy (ĕk′-tō-mē)	surgical removal or excision
-gram	record, x-ray image
-graph	instrument used to record
-graphy	process of recording, x-ray imaging
-osis (ō′-sĭs)	abnormal condition
-plasty (plăs′-tē)	surgical repair
-scope (skōp)	instrument used for visual examination
-scopy (skōp′-ē)	visual examination
-tomy (ŏt′-ō-mē)	surgical incision or to cut into
-trophy (trōf′-ē) (may also be used as a word root)	development, nourishment

EXERCISE 3

Write the combining forms for each part of the body listed below.

1. finger bone _____
2. joint _____
3. bone _____
4. thigh bone _____
5. kneecap _____
6. shoulder blade _____
7. bones of the spine _____
8. collar bone
   a. _____
   b. _____
9. skull _____
10. breast bone _____
11. upper arm bone _____
12. rib _____

EXERCISE 4

Write the suffix for each term listed below.

1. surgical repair _____
2. pain _____
3. pertaining to
   a. _____
   b. _____
   c. _____
   d. _____
4. surgical incision _____
5. surgical removal _____
6. instrument to record _____
7. process of recording _____
8. record, x-ray image _____
9. development, nourishment _____
10. abnormal condition _____

11. instrument used for visual
    examination   _____

12. visual examination   _____

13. surgical puncture to aspirate fluid _____

EXERCISE 5

Write the definition for each suffix listed below.

1. -algia

   _____

2. -graph

   _____

3. -gram

   _____

4. -graphy

   _____

5. -tomy

   _____

6. -trophy

   _____

7. -ic

   _____

8. -plasty

   _____

9. -ectomy

   _____

10. -ar

    _____

11. -osis

    _____

12. -scopy

    _____

13. -scope

    _____

14. -centesis

    _____

Recall from Unit 1 that prefixes are letters that may be added to the beginning of a word root to modify its meaning. Listed below are six prefixes you need to memorize in this unit.

Prefix	Meaning
a-, an-	without or absence of (if used with a word root that begins with a vowel, use *an;* if used with a word root that begins with a consonant, use *a*)
dys- (dĭs)	difficult, painful, labored, abnormal
inter-	between
intra-	within
supra-	above

EXERCISE 6

Write the prefix for each term listed below.

1. within   _____

2. painful   _____

3. under   _____

4. without

   a.   _____

   b.   _____

5. between   _____

6. above   _____

EXERCISE 7

Write the definition for each prefix listed below. You may be asked to recall a prefix from previous study.

1. *intra-*

   _____

2. *supra-*

   _____

3. sub-

_____

4. dys-

_____

5. a-, an-

_____

6. inter-

_____

■ MEDICAL TERMS RELATING TO THE MUSCULOSKELETAL SYSTEM

Listed below are the medical terms you need to know for the musculoskeletal system. Most are made up of the word roots, prefixes, and suffixes you have been working with; however, there are some words that relate to the musculoskeletal system that are not made up of the word parts you have studied thus far. These are also included in the list. Following the list are exercises that will assist you in learning the meaning and spelling of each word. Practice pronouncing each word aloud.

General Terms	Meaning
atrophy (ăt'-rō-fē)	without development (decrease in the size of a normally developed organ)
chondrogenic (kŏn-drō-jĕn'-ĭk)	producing cartilage
cranial (krā'-nē-al)	pertaining to the cranium
dystrophy (dĭs'-trō-fē)	abnormal development
femoral (fĕm'-ō-ral)	pertaining to the femur (or thigh bone)
humeral (hū'-mĕr-al)	pertaining to the humerus
intervertebral (ĭn-tĕr-vĕr'-tĕ-bral)	pertaining to between the vertebrae
intracranial (ĭn-trah-krā'-nē-al)	pertaining to within the cranium
orthopedics (or-thō-pē'-dĭks)	branch of medicine dealing with the diagnosis and treatment of disease, abnormalities, or fractures of the musculoskeletal system
orthopedist (or-thō-pē'-dist)	a doctor who specializes in orthopedics
osteoma (ŏs-tē-ō'-mah)	a tumor (composed of) bone
sternal (stĕr'-nal)	pertaining to the sternum
sternoclavicular (stĕr'-nō-klah-vĭk'-ū-lar)	pertaining to the sternum and clavicle
sternocostal (stĕr nō kŏs' tal)	pertaining to the sternum and ribs
sternoid (stĕr'-noyd)	resembling the sternum
subcostal (sŭb-kŏs'-tal)	pertaining to below a rib or ribs
subscapular (sŭb-skăp'-ū-lar)	pertaining to below the scapula
suprascapular (soo-prah-skăp'-ū-lar)	pertaining to above the scapula
vertebrocostal (vĕr'-tĕ-brō-kŏs'-tal)	pertaining to the vertebrae and ribs

Surgical Terms	Meaning
arthroplasty (ar'-thrō-plăs-tē)	surgical repair of a joint
arthrotomy (ar-thrŏt'-ō-mē)	surgical incision of a joint
chondrectomy (kŏn-drĕk'-tō-mē)	excision of a cartilage
clavicotomy (klăv-ĭ-kŏt'-ō-mē)	surgical incision into the clavicle
costectomy (kŏs-tĕk'-tō-mē)	excision of a rib
cranioplasty (krā'-nē-ō-plăs-tē)	surgical repair of the cranium
craniotomy (krā-nē-ŏt'-ō-mē)	surgical incision into the cranium
laminectomy (lăm-ĭ-nĕk'-tō-mē)	surgical removal of lamina (often performed to relieve symptoms of a ruptured [slipped] disk)
meniscectomy (mĕn-ĭ-sĕk'-tō-mē)	excision of the meniscus (of the knee joint)
patellectomy (păt-ĕ-lĕk'-tō-mē)	excision of the patella
vertebrectomy (vĕr-tĕ-brĕk'-tō-mē)	excision of a vertebra

Diagnostic Terms	Meaning
arthralgia (ar-thrăl'-jē-ah)	pain in a joint
arthritis (ar-thrī'-tĭs)	inflammation of a joint
arthrosis (ar-thrŏ'-sĭs)	abnormal condition of a joint

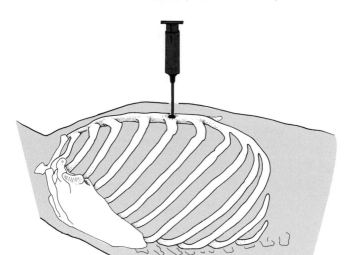

FIGURE 23–14 ▲ Sternal puncture. (From LaFleur M and Starr W: Exploring Medical Language, St. Louis: Mosby, 1985, with permission.)

chondritis (krŏn-drī′-tĭs)	inflammation of the cartilage
meniscitis (mĕn-ĭ-sī′-tĭs)	inflammation of the meniscus (of the knee joint)
muscular dystrophy (mŭs′-kū-lar) (dĭs′-trō-fē)	a number of muscle disorders characterized by a progressive, degenerative disease of the muscles
myoma (mī-ō′-mah)	a tumor (formed) of muscle (tissue)

Terms Relating to Diagnostic Procedures

Terms Relating to Diagnostic Procedures	Meaning
arthrocentesis (ar-thrō-sĕn-tē′-sĭs)	surgical puncture to aspirate a joint
arthrogram (ar′-thrō-grăm)	x-ray image of a joint (contrast medium, dye, or air is used)
arthroscope (ar′-thrō-scōpe)	instrument used to visualize a joint (commonly the knee and shoulder)
arthroscopy (ar-thrŏs′-kō-pē)	visual examination of a joint (for diagnosing, identifying, and correcting problems)
electromyogram (EMG) (ē-lĕk′-trō-mī′-ō-grăm)	record of electrical activity of a muscle
electromyograph (ē-lĕk′-trō-mī′-ō-grăph)	instrument used to record the electrical activity of a muscle
electromyography (ē-lĕk′-trō-mī′-ŏg′-rah-fē)	process of recording the electrical activity of muscle
sternal puncture (stĕr′-nal) (pŭngk′-chŭr)	insertion of a hollow needle into the sternum to obtain a sample of bone marrow to be studied in the laboratory (Fig. 23–14) (used for diagnosing blood disorders such as anemia and leukemia)

EXERCISE 8

Analyze and define each medical term listed below.

1. electromyogram

_____

2. myoma

_____

3. sternoclavicular

_____

4. cranial

_____

5. vertebrocostal

_____

6. arthritis

_____

7. intervertebral

_____

8. humeral

_____

9. dystrophy

_____

10. subscapular

_____

11. arthrosis

_____

12. electromyography

_____

13. arthrogram

_____

14. electromyograph

_____

15. sternocostal

_____

16. arthralgia

_____

17. subcostal

_____

18. femoral

_____

19. clavicotomy

_____

20. arthrotomy

_____

21. intracranial

_____

22. atrophy

_____

23. arthroplasty

_____

24. osteoma

_____

25. costectomy

_____

26. cranioplasty

_____

27. patellectomy

_____

28. vertebrectomy

_____

29. craniotomy

_____

30. suprascapular

_____

31. sternoid

_____

32. chondrogenic

_____

33. arthroscopy

_____

34. chondritis

_____

35. *arthroscope*

_____

36. *chondrectomy*

_____

37. *laminectomy*

_____

38. *sternal*

_____

39. *meniscectomy*

_____

40. *arthrocentesis*

_____

41. *meniscitis*

_____

EXERCISE ⑨

Using the word roots, prefixes, suffixes, and combining vowels as needed, build medical terms from each definition listed below.

1. pertaining to the cranium _____

2. resembling the sternum _____

3. pertaining to below the scapula _____

4. pertaining to the femur _____

5. surgical incision into a joint _____

6. excision of a cartilage _____

7. pain of a joint _____

8. inflammation of a joint _____

9. abnormal condition of a joint _____

10. pertaining to the humerus _____

11. without development _____

12. pertaining to the vertebrae and ribs _____

13. surgical incision into the cranium _____

14. surgical removal of a rib _____

15. pertaining to below the rib _____

16. x-ray image of a joint _____

17. surgical removal of a vertebra _____

18. record of the electrical activity of a muscle _____

19. surgical incision into the clavicle _____

20. process of recording electrical activity of a muscle _____

21. abnormal development _____

22. a tumor (formed) of muscle (tissue) _____

23. machine used to record electrical activity of a muscle _____

24. pertaining to the sternum and clavicle _____

25. pertaining to between the vertebrae _____

26. pertaining to within the cranium _____

27. pertaining to the sternum and rib _____

28. surgical removal of the patella _____

29. surgical repair of the cranium _____

30. a tumor composed of bone _____

31. surgical incision into the clavicle _____

32. producing cartilage _____

33. visual examination of a joint _____

34. instrument used for visual examination of a joint _____

35. inflammation of cartilage _____

36. excision of cartilage _____

37. surgical removal of the lamina _____

38. pertaining to the sternum _____

39. puncture and aspiration of _____
    a joint

40. excision of the meniscus _____

41. inflammation of the meniscus _____

EXERCISE 10

Define each medical term listed below.
1. orthopedics

_____

2. orthopedist

_____

3. muscular dystrophy

_____

4. sternal puncture

_____

EXERCISE 11

Spell each medical term studied in this unit by having someone dictate the terms to you.

1. _____
2. _____
3. _____
4. _____
5. _____
6. _____
7. _____
8. _____

9. _____
10. _____
11. _____
12. _____
13. _____
14. _____
15. _____
16. _____
17. _____
18. _____
19. _____
20. _____
21. _____
22. _____
23. _____
24. _____
25. _____
26. _____
27. _____
28. _____
29. _____
30. _____
31. _____
32. _____
33. _____
34. _____
35. _____
36. _____
37. _____
38. _____
39. _____

40. _____

41. _____

42. _____

43. _____

44. _____

45. _____

a. fractured tibia   a. _____

b. fractured humerus   b. _____

c. fractured cervical 6 (C6)   c. _____

d. fractured ilium   d. _____

e. fractured clavicle   e. _____

f. fractured radius   f. _____

EXERCISE 12

Answer the following questions.

1. _____ is the name of the nursing unit in the hospital that cares for the patients with *fractures, abnormalities,* or *diseases of the bone.* _____ is the name of the doctor who specializes in this area of medicine.

2. A _____ _____ tray is used by the doctor to obtain a *sample of bone marrow from the sternum.* The tray is named after the procedure.

3. The doctor ordered a procedure to determine the *electrical activity of a muscle.* The procedure is called a(an) _____.

4. The following is a list of diagnostic phrases. In the space provided, write the name of the fractured bone.

   Example: fractured femur   thigh bone

5. A surgery schedule is a list of operations to be performed on a given day in the hospital. The following are types of operations recorded on the surgery schedule. Indicate the terms that are incorrectly spelled by rewriting the term correctly in the space provided.

   a. castectomy _____

   b. craniotomy _____

   c. lamonectomy _____

   d. clavictamy _____

   e. cranioplasty _____

   f. patelectomy _____

   g. ostoarthrotomy _____

   h. meniscectomy _____

6. The doctor ordered a procedure to x-ray a joint that requires the use of contrast medium. The procedure is called a(an) _____. Puncture and aspiration of a joint is called _____.

UNIT 4

The Nervous System

Outline

Unit Objectives
The Nervous System
  Organs of the Nervous System
  Functions of the Nervous System
  Nerves
  Brain

  Spinal Cord
  Meninges
Diseases and Conditions of the Nervous System
  Cerebrovascular Accident
  Transient Ischemic Attack
  Parkinson's Disease
  Alzheimer's Disease
  Epilepsy

Review Questions
Medical Terminology Relating to the Nervous System and Psychology

> ## Unit Objectives

Upon completion of this unit, you will be able to:

1. Name the organs of the nervous system.
2. Describe the overall function of the nervous system.
3. List and describe the organs of the nervous system covered in this unit.
4. Describe the function of the meninges and locate and name the three layers of tissue that make up the meninges.
5. Describe cerebrovascular accident, Parkinson's disease, transient ischemic attack, Alzheimer's disease, and epilepsy.

■ THE NERVOUS SYSTEM

Organs of the Nervous System

1. Nerves
2. Brain
3. Spinal cord

The nervous system is commonly divided into two parts:

1. The central nervous system (CNS) consists of the brain and spinal cord.
2. The peripheral nervous system (PNS) consists of the nerves of the body (12 pairs of cranial nerves and 31 pairs of spinal nerves). The autonomic (involuntary) and somatic (voluntary) nervous systems are subdivisions of the PNS. The autonomic nervous system is further divided into the sympathetic (fight or flight) and parasympathetic (tranquil: rest and digestion) nervous systems.

Functions of the Nervous System

All body parts and systems must work together to maintain a healthy body. The nervous system monitors, regulates, and controls the functions of body organs and body systems by using nerve impulses to transmit information from one part of the body to another (Fig. 23–15). The nervous system works in concert with the endocrine system in maintaining homeostasis, a constant internal environment, by inhibiting or stimulating the release of hormones.

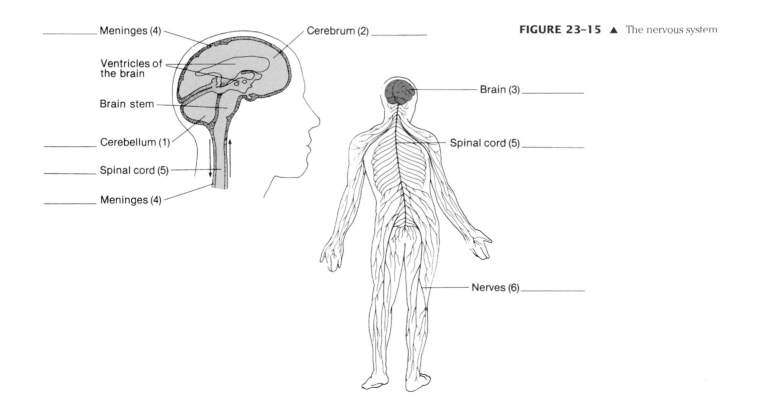

Meninges (4)
Ventricles of the brain
Brain stem
Cerebellum (1)
Spinal cord (5)
Meninges (4)
Cerebrum (2)
Brain (3)
Spinal cord (5)
Nerves (6)

FIGURE 23–15 ▲ The nervous system

Nerves

A *nerve* is a cordlike structure located outside of the CNS. It contains nerve cells called *neurons*. The neuron transmits nerve impulses from one part of the body to another. Two types of neurons are:

1. Sensory neurons, which transmit impulses to the brain and spinal cord.
2. Motor neurons, which transmit impulses from the brain and spinal cord to muscles or glands.

Brain

The brain is located in the cranial cavity and is the main center for coordinating body activities. The brain is divided into three parts: the cerebrum, the cerebellum, and the brain stem. Each part of the brain is responsible for controlling certain body functions.

The *cerebrum* is the largest part of the brain. It is located in the upper portion of the cranium. The cerebrum is divided into the right and left hemispheres, which are connected only at the lower middle portion. The cerebrum contains the sensory, motor, sight, and hearing centers. Memory, intellect, judgment, and emotional reactions also take place in the cerebrum.

Four spaces within the brain, called *ventricles*, produce a watery fluid known as *cerebrospinal fluid (CSF)*. This cushion of fluid surrounds the brain and spinal cord. Its function is to absorb shocks that may occur to the spinal cord or brain and to nourish and remove waste from the nervous tissue. The *cerebellum*, or "little brain," is situated below the posterior portion of the cerebrum. Its functions are to assist in the coordination of voluntary muscles and to maintain balance. The *brain stem* has three main parts: the midbrain, pons, and medulla oblongata. It contains the nerve fibers that form the connecting links between the different parts of the brain and the centers that control three vital functions: blood pressure, respiration, and heartbeat.

Spinal Cord

The spinal cord extends from the brain stem and passes through the spinal cavity to between the first and second lumbar vertebrae (Figure 23–17, *A*, p. 489). The spinal cord is the pathway for conducting *sensory impulses* up to the brain and *motor impulses* down from the brain. Injury to the spinal cord can result in paralysis, the loss of voluntary muscle function.

Meninges

The meninges are made up of three layers of connective tissue that completely surround and protect the spinal cord and brain. The outer tough layer is called the *dura mater*. The middle layer is the *arachnoid (mater)*, a weblike structure. The inner thin, tender layer, the *pia mater*, carries blood vessels that provide nourishment to the nervous tissue. The cerebrospinal fluid flows through a space between the arachnoid and the pia mater called the *subarachnoid space* (see Fig. 23–17, *C*, p. 489).

■ DISEASES AND CONDITIONS OF THE NERVOUS SYSTEM

Cerebrovascular Accident

Cerebrovascular accident (CVA), also called a *stroke*, is the interference of blood flow to the brain, which reduces the supply of oxygen and nutrients, causing damage to the brain tissue. The major causes of CVA are embolism, thrombosis, and hemorrhage (Fig. 23–16). Strokes affect about 700,000 people each year, causing death in one quarter of them.

Damage to the brain tissue varies according to the artery affected. Paralysis is a result of the damage, and it may range from slight to complete hemiplegia (paralysis of one side of the body). CVA of the left hemisphere of the brain produces symptoms on the right side of the body, and CVA of the right side of the brain produces symptoms on the left side of the body. The more quickly the circulation returns, the better the chance for recovery.

Transient Ischemic Attack

Transient ischemic attacks (TIA) are recurrent episodes of decreased neurologic function such as double vision, slurred speech, weakness in the legs, and dizziness lasting from seconds to 24 hours, then clearing. TIAs are considered warning signs for strokes. TIAs are caused by small emboli that temporarily interrupt blood flow to the brain. Treatment includes the administra-

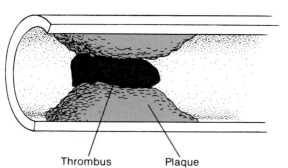
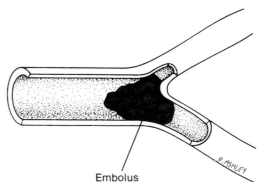

Thrombus   Plaque   Embolus

FIGURE 23–16 ▲ Thrombus (blood clot) or embolus (floating mass that blocks a vessel) in a cerebral artery can cause a cerebrovascular accident (CVA).

tion of aspirin and anticoagulants to minimize thrombosis in the hope of preventing a CVA. Preventive treatment may include a *carotid endarterectomy,* a surgical procedure to remove the thickened inner area of the carotid artery.

Parkinson's Disease

Parkinson's disease, also called *shaking palsy, parkinsonism,* and *paralysis agitans,* is one of the most common crippling diseases in the United States. Parkinson's disease, a gradual progressive disorder of the central nervous system, occurs with degeneration of the dopamine-releasing neurons in the *substantia nigra,* an area of the brain. Dopamine, one of the chemical messengers *(neurotransmitters)* responsible for transmitting signals within the brain, initiates and controls movement and balance. The cause of Parkinson's disease is most often unknown, but is thought to be the result of genetic factors, viral infection, exposure to toxins, or cerebral arteriosclerosis. Symptoms include muscle rigidity, tremors, and a shifting gait. Deterioration is progressive. There is no cure; treatment is aimed at relieving symptoms and promoting function as long as possible. Parkinson's disease does not impair intellect.

Alzheimer's Disease

Alzheimer's disease, also called *presenile dementia,* is characterized by confusion, mental deterioration (dementia), restlessness, hallucinations, and the inability to carry out purposeful speech and movement. The patient may lose bowel and bladder control and refuse to eat. The disease is progressive and usually begins in later midlife. Because the precise cause of Alzheimer's disease has not been identified, definitive treatment has not been established. Care of the patient generally includes maintaining proper hygiene, nutrition, preventing injury, and promoting purposeful activity.

Epilepsy

Epilepsy, a group of chronic disorders of the CNS, is a result of abnormal electrical (neuron) activity in the brain. It is common to hear epilepsy and seizure used synonymously; the difference is that epilepsy is the disease and the seizure is the result of the disease. Epilepsy usually occurs in childhood or after age 50. The disease can be classified as idiopathic (etiology unknown) or acquired. Some of the known causes of acquired epilepsy are brain tumors, brain injury, and endocrine disorders. Seizures resulting

from fever, otitis media, or drug toxicity are usually isolated incidents and do not warrant the diagnosis of epilepsy.

Seizures are classified according to the origin of the abnormal brain signals. Involvement of the entire brain is known as *generalized seizure,* whereas a *partial seizure* is one which abnormal electrical activity occurs in a particular region of the brain.

Seizure activity is divided into three stages: during the *preictal* stage the patient may experience abnormal somatic and psychic sensations and a strange-sounding cry. These sensations and/or cry are called an *aura.* The second stage is called *interictal* and includes violent jerking of some parts or total body. The patient may experience a grand mal seizure characterized by incontinence of urine and stool, foaming or frothing from the mouth, changes in skin color, tongue biting, arching of the back, and turning of the head to one side. The period immediately after the seizure is called the *postictal stage.* During this stage the patient may be confused and lethargic, and reports headache and sore muscles. The petit mal seizure, another form of generalized seizure, is marked by a brief loss of consciousness with unresponsive behaviors.

Diagnosis is confirmed by observation of the seizure activity, blood testing to rule out other ailments, and magnetic resonance imaging (MRI) or computed tomography scan (CT) of the brain to look for a lesion. An electroencephalogram (EEG) and/or an echoencephalogram (EchoEG) may also locate the site and possible cause of the disorder.

Treatment requires stabilization on anticonvulsant drugs (see Chapter 13 for a list of these drugs); 95% of the population responds to drug therapy. The other 5% is treated surgically to remove the affected brain tissue. Patient education is included in the treatment regimen. Information about seizure triggers and how to avoid those triggers are an important part of the patient education. There is a national association that helps the patient deal with self-esteem issues and the stigma that is still attached to epilepsy. Because of the stigmatization many people who have epilepsy will not wear an identification bracelet, and they will not inform others of their illness.

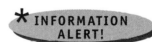

✱ INFORMATION ALERT!

Patients who are experiencing a seizure need to be protected from injury, especially head injuries. Remove any furniture or other objects that the patient may strike. If possible put a pillow under the patient's head. Call for help. *Do not try to restrain the movements of the patient.* Protect the patient's privacy. Ask those that are uninvolved with the care of the patients to please leave the area.

REVIEW QUESTIONS

1. Name the organs of the nervous system. Write the function of each organ.

a. _____

b. _____

c. _____

2. A nerve cell is called a(an) _____. The two types of nerve cells are _____ and

_____.

3. Name three parts of the brain and describe the functions of each.

   a. _____

   b. _____

   c. _____

4. Describe the location and function of the spinal cord.

   _____

5. The meninges are made up of three layers of tissue. The tough outer layer is called the _____ ; the

   middle layer is called the _____ ; and the inner layer is called the _____ .

6. Match the terms in Column 1 with the phrases in Column 2.

   Column 1   **Column 2**

   a. Parkinson's disease   _____ 1. also called shaking palsy

   b. Alzheimer's disease   _____ 2. may be idiopathic or acquired

   c. transient ischemic attack   _____ 3. may result in hemiplegia

   d. cerebrovascular accident   _____ 4. warning sign for strokes

   e. cerebral palsy   _____ 5. symptoms include confusion and hallucinations

   f. epilepsy

7. Name the three stages of a seizure.

   a. _____

   b. _____

   c. _____

■ MEDICAL TERMINOLOGY RELATING TO THE NERVOUS SYSTEM AND PSYCHOLOGY

Upon mastery of the medical terminology for this unit, you will be able to:

1. Spell and define the word parts and medical terms that relate to the nervous system.

2. Analyze the medical terms relating to the nervous system that are built from word parts.

3. Given the meaning of a medical condition relating to the nervous system, build with word parts the corresponding medical term.

4. Spell and use in sentence form the psychology terminology represented in this unit.

5. Given descriptions of hospital situations in which the health unit coordinator may encounter medical terminology, apply the correct medical terms to the situations.

Word Parts

Listed below are the word parts you need to memorize for the nervous system. The exercises included in this unit will help you with this task. You will continue to use these word parts throughout the course and during employment. Practice pronouncing each word element aloud.

Word Roots/Combining Forms

Word Roots/Combining Forms	Meaning
1. cerebell/o (sĕr-ĕ-bĕl'-ō)	cerebellum (little brain)
2. cerebr/o (sĕr'-ē-brō)	cerebrum (main portion of the brain)
3. encephal/o (ĕn-sĕf'-ah-lō)	brain
4. mening/o (mĕ-nĭng'-gō)	meninges (spinal cord covering)
5. myel/o (mī'-ĕl-ō)	spinal cord (also means *bone marrow*)
6. neur/o (nū'-rō)	nerve
7. phas/o (f-āz'-ō)	speech
8. psych/o (sī'-kō)	mind
9. spin/o (spī'-nō)	spine

Other Word Roots/Combining Forms

Other Word Roots/Combining Forms	Meaning
pneum/o (nŭ'-mō)	air
poli/o (pō'-lē-ō)	gray matter

Suffixes

Suffixes	Meaning
-cele (sēl)	herniation or protrusion
-plegia (plē'-jē-ah)	paralysis, stroke
-rrhagia (or-ah'-jē-ah)	rapid flow of blood
-rrhaphy (or'-ah-fē)	to suture (surgical), repair
-rrhea (o-rē'-ah)	excessive discharge, flow

 EXERCISE 1

Write the combining forms for the nervous system in the spaces provided on the diagram in Figure 23–15 (p. 481). The number preceding the combining form in the list above matches the number of the body part on the diagram.

EXERCISE 2

Define each combining form listed below.

1. *cerebr/o*

_____

2. *encephal/o*

_____

3. *neur/o*

_____

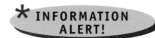 **✻ INFORMATION ALERT!**

Cerebrovascular Accident (Stroke) Warning Signs and Treatment

Warning Signs

- Sudden numbness, weakness, or paralysis of the face, arm, or leg, especially on one side of the body
- Sudden confusion; problems with memory or perception
- Sudden loss of speech, difficulty speaking or understanding
- Sudden trouble seeing out of one or both eyes; blurred or double vision
- Sudden difficulty walking, dizziness, or loss of balance or co-ordination
- Sudden, severe headache with no known cause

Thrombolytic Treatment

Tissue plasminogen activator (tPA) is a thrombolytic agent (clot-busting drug) approved for use in certain patients having a heart attack or stroke caused by blood clots that block blood flow. This class of drugs may dissolve blood clots, which cause most heart attacks and ischemic strokes, if given within three hours of the onset of symptoms. tPA, administered by hospital personnel through an IV line, can significantly reduce the effects of stroke, including permanent disability.

4. *poli/o*

_____

5. *mening/o*

_____

6. *spin/o*

_____

7. *myel/o*

_____

8. *cerebell/o*

_____

9. *pneum/o*

_____

10. *phas/o*

_____

11. *psych/o*

_____

EXERCISE 3

Write the combining forms for each term listed below.

1. nerve _____

2. cerebrum _____

3. meninges _____

4. spinal cord _____

5. cerebellum _____

6. brain _____

7. spine _____

8. air _____

9. gray matter _____

10. speech _____

11. mind _____

EXERCISE 4

Write the suffix(es) that match each definition written below. (*Note*: This exercise includes suffixes from this unit and previous units. Refer back as needed.)

1. tumor _____

2. surgical repair _____

3. pertaining to _____

_____

_____

_____

4. to suture _____

5. excessive discharge _____

6. inflammation _____

7. specialist _____

8. record, x-ray image _____

9. study of _____

10. rapid discharge _____

11. herniation _____

12. surgical removal _____

13. incision _____

14. pain _____

EXERCISE 5

Write the definition for each suffix listed below. (*Note*: This exercise includes suffixes from this unit and previous units. Refer back as needed.)

1. *-gram*

_____

2. *-itis*

_____

3. *-logy*

_____

4. *-rrhea*

_____

5. *-rrhagia*

_____

6. *-rrhaphy*

_____

7. *-cele*

_____

8. -ar

_____

9. -ectomy

_____

10. -plasty

_____

11. -tomy

_____

12. -algia

_____

13. -osis

_____

■ MEDICAL TERMS RELATING TO THE NERVOUS SYSTEM

Listed below are medical terms you will need to know for the nervous system. Exercises following this list will assist you in learning these terms. Practice pronouncing these terms aloud.

General Terms	Meaning
aphasia (ah-fā'-zē-ah)	without speech (loss of expression or understanding of speech or writing)
cerebrospinal (ser'-ē-brō-spī'-nal)	pertaining to the brain and spine
hemiplegia (hĕm ĭ plē-jē-ah)	paralysis of the right or left side of the body (usually caused by a stroke)
myelorrhagia (mī-ĕ-lō-rā'-jē-ah)	rapid flow of blood into spinal cord
neurologist (nū-rŏl'-ō-jĭst)	one who specializes in the diagnosis and treatment of nerves
neurology (nū-rŏl'-ō-jē)	study of nerves (the branch of medicine that deals with the diagnosis and treatment of disorders or diseases of the nervous system)
paraplegia (păr-ăh-plē'-jē-ah)	paralysis of the legs and sometimes the lower part of the body, usually caused by an injury to the spinal cord
quadriplegia (kwăd-rĕ-plē'-jē-ah)	paralysis that affects all four limbs

Surgical Terms	Meaning
neuroplasty (nū'-rō-plăs-tē)	surgical repair of a nerve
neurorrhaphy (nū-rŏr'-ah-fē)	suturing of a nerve

Diagnostic Terms	Meaning
cerebral palsy (ser'-ē-bral) (paul'-zē)	partial paralysis and lack of muscle coordination from a defect, injury, or disease of the brain, which is present at birth or shortly thereafter
cerebrovascular accident (CVA) (ser'-ē-brō-văs'-kū-lăr)	impaired blood supply to parts of the brain; also called a stroke
cerebellitis (ser-ĕ-bĕl-ī'-tĭs)	inflammation of the cerebellum
cerebrosis (ser-ĕ-brō'-sĭs)	abnormal condition of the brain
encephalitis (ĕn-sĕf-ah-lī'-tĭs)	inflammation of the brain
encephalocele (ĕn-sĕf'-ah-lō-sēl)	herniation of brain (tissue through a gap in the skull)
epilepsy (ĕp'-ĭ-lĕp-sē)	convulsive disorder of the nervous system characterized by chronic or recurrent seizures

General Terms	Meaning
meningitis (mĕn-ĭn-jī′-tĭs)	inflammation of the meninges
meningomyelocele (mĕ-nĭng-gō-mī′-ĕ-lō-sĕl)	protrusion of the spinal cord and meninges (through the vertebral column)
multiple sclerosis (MS) (mŭl′-tĭ-pl) (sklĕ-rō′-sĭs)	a degenerative disease of the nerves controlling muscles, characterized by hardening patches along the brain and spinal cord
neuralgia (nū-răl′-jē-ah)	pain in a nerve
neuritis (nū-rī′-tĭs)	inflammation of a nerve
neuroma (nū-rō′-mah)	a tumor made up of nerve (cells)
poliomyelitis (pō′-lē-ō-mī-ĕ-lī′-tĭs)	inflammation of the gray matter of spinal cord (virally caused disease, commonly known as polio)
subdural hematoma (sŭb-dū′-ral) (hēm-ah-tō′-mah)	blood tumor pertaining to below the dura mater (accumulation of blood in the subdural space)

Terms Relating to Diagnostic Procedures	Meaning
CT scan (computed tomography)	use of radiologic imaging that produces images of bloodless "slices" of the body. CT scanning can detect hemorrhages, tumors, and brain abnormalities
echoencephalogram (EchoEG) (ĕk′-ō-ĕn-sĕf′-ă-lō-grăm)	record of brain (structures) by use of sound (recorded on a graph)
electroencephalogram (EEG) (ē-lĕk′-trō-ĕn-sĕf′-ăh-lō-grăm)	record of the electrical activity of the brain
magnetic resonance imaging (MRI)	noninvasive procedure for imaging tissues that cannot be seen by other radiologic techniques. Also called *nuclear magnetic resonance* (NMR) imaging; the advantage of this diagnostic procedure is not only the avoidance of harmful radiation by its use of magnetic fields and radio frequencies, but also the ability to detect small brain abnormalities. Patients with pacemakers or cranial metallic foreign bodies generally cannot undergo this procedure
myelogram (mī′-ĕ-lō-grăm)	x-ray image of the spinal cord (injected dye is used as the contrast medium)
pneumoencephalogram (nū′-mō-ĕn-sĕf′-ăh-lō-grăm)	x-ray image (of the ventricles) in the brain using air (as the contrast medium)
spinal puncture (lumbar puncture) (LP) (spī′-năl) (pŭngk′-chŭr)	removal of cerebrospinal fluid (CSF) for diagnostic and therapeutic purposes. A hollow needle is inserted into the subarachnoid space between the third and fourth lumbar vertebrae (Fig. 23–17)

EXERCISE 6

Analyze and define each medical term listed below.

1. neurology

_____

_____

2. cerebrospinal

_____

_____

3. neuralgia

_____

_____

4. poliomyelitis

_____

_____

5. neuroplasty

_____

_____

6. encephalitis

_____

_____

FIGURE 23–17 ▲ *A*, Location and length of spinal cord. *B, C*, Lumbar or spinal puncture (spinal tap).

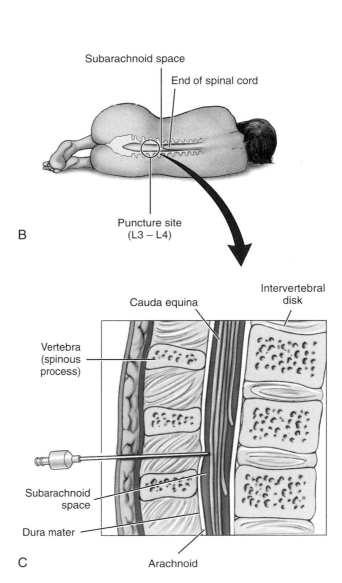

Foramen magnum

L1

End of spinal cord

Cauda equina

A

Subarachnoid space

End of spinal cord

Puncture site (L3 – L4)

B

Cauda equina

Intervertebral disk

Vertebra (spinous process)

Subarachnoid space

Dura mater

Arachnoid

C

7. *meningitis*

_____

_____

8. *pneumoencephalogram*

_____

_____

9. *neurorrhaphy*

_____

_____

10. *neurologist*

_____

_____

11. *encephalocele*

_____

_____

12. *electroencephalogram*

_____

_____

13. *meningomyelocele*

_____

_____

14. *cerebellitis*

_____

_____

15. *cerebrosis*

_____

_____

16. *neuroma*

_____

_____

17. *myelorrhagia*

_____

_____

18. *myelogram*

_____

_____

19. *neuritis*

_____

_____

EXERCISE 7

Define each medical term listed below.

1. *multiple sclerosis*

_____

2. *epilepsy*

_____

3. *cerebral palsy*

_____

4. *cerebrovascular accident*

_____

5. *echoencephalogram*

_____

6. *hemiplegia*

_____

7. *paraplegia*

_____

8. *quadriplegia*

_____

9. *spinal puncture*

_____

10. *subdural hematoma*

_____

11. *CT scan*

_____

12. *MRI*

_____

13. *aphasia*

_____

10. herniation of the meninges   _____
    and spinal cord (through the
    vertebral column)

11. inflammation of the cerebellum   _____

12. herniation of the brain (through   _____
    a gap in the skull)

13. x-ray image of the ventricles of   _____
    the brain with the use of air
    (as contrast medium)

14. rapid flow of blood from the   _____
    spine

15. record of the electrical activity   _____
    of the brain

16. x-ray image of the spinal cord   _____

EXERCISE 9

Spell each medical term studied in this unit by having someone dictate the terms to you.

1. _____
2. _____
3. _____
4. _____
5. _____
6. _____
7. _____
8. _____
9. _____
10. _____
11. _____
12. _____
13. _____
14. _____
15. _____
16. _____
17. _____

EXERCISE 8

Using the word elements studied in this unit and previous units, build medical terms from each of the definitions listed below.

1. inflammation of a nerve   _____

2. inflammation of the brain   _____

3. inflammation of the meninges   _____

4. surgical repair of a nerve   _____

5. one who specializes in the   _____
   diagnosis and treatment
   of nerves

6. suture of a nerve   _____

7. tumor made of nerve cells   _____

8. pain in a nerve   _____

9. pertaining to the cerebrum   _____
   and spine

18. _____

19. _____

20. _____

21. _____

22. _____

23. _____

24. _____

25. _____

26. _____

27. _____

28. _____

29. _____

30. _____

31. _____

32. _____

33. _____

■ TERMS RELATING TO PSYCHOLOGY

An extensive knowledge of psychology vocabulary is not necessary for general hospital employment; therefore, we will discuss only those terms that you as a health unit coordinator may encounter in general medical and surgical areas of employment.

Psych/o is a combining form meaning mind. The following words are developed from the word root *psych* and suffixes, most of which you have already studied.

Psychology Terms	Meaning
psychiatrist (sī-kī′-ah-trĭst)	a doctor who specializes in the mind
psychiatry (sī-kī′-ah-trē)	treatment of the mind (a branch of medicine that deals with the study, treatment, and prevention of mental illness)
psychologist (sī-kŏl′-ō-jĭst)	one who specializes in the diagnosis and treatment of the mind (a person trained to perform psychological analysis, therapy, or research, generally at a master's level of education or Ph.D.)
psychology (sī-kŏl′-ō-jē)	study of the mind (behavior)
psychosis (sī-kō′-sĭs)	abnormal condition of the mind

Psychology Terms	Meaning
psychosomatic (sī′-kō-sō-măt′-ĭk)	pertaining to the mind and body (relationship)
neur/o	*the combining form that means nerve; it may be used to describe certain psychiatric disorders, as in the following terms*
neurosis (nŭ-rō′-sĭs)	an emotional disorder considered less serious than a psychosis
neurotic (nŭ-rŏt′-ĭk)	having a neurosis

EXERCISE 10

Spell each psychology term studied in this unit by having someone dictate the terms to you.

1. _____

2. _____

3. _____

4. _____

5. _____

6. _____

7. _____

8. _____

EXERCISE 11

Fill in the blanks below.

1. _____ is the name of the nursing unit in the hospital that cares for patients with disorders of the nervous system. _____ is the name of the doctor who specializes in this area of medicine.

2. The patient is admitted to the hospital with the admitting diagnosis of stroke or _____ _____. The abbreviation for this term is _____. The patient is paralyzed on the left side of her body. She has _____.

3. A child is diagnosed as having an inflammation of the meninges or _____. The doctor performs a procedure to obtain cerebrospinal fluid for diagnostic study. The procedure is called

_____ _____.

To perform this procedure, the doctor uses a special tray named after the procedure. It is called a

_____ _____ tray.

4. Name four diagnostic procedures that end in the suffix *-gram* that the doctor may order to gather information about the nervous system organs or about their functions:

a. _____

b. _____

c. _____

d. _____

UNIT 5

The Eye and the Ear

Unit Objectives

Upon completion of this unit, you will be able to:

1. Name and locate the parts and accessory structures of the eye and briefly describe the function of each part.
2. Describe how the eye is protected.
3. Trace the pathway of light from the outside environment to the cerebrum.
4. Name and describe the function of the two types of nerve cells located in the retina.
5. Name and locate the parts of the ear.
6. Trace the travel of sound waves from the outside environment to the brain.
7. Describe cataract, glaucoma, retinal detachment, and tinnitus.

▮ THE EYE

The eye (Fig. 23–18) is the organ of vision. The eye receives light waves that are focused on the retina and produces visual nerve impulses that are transmitted to the visual area of the brain by the optic nerve. The eye is divided into three layers: sclera, choroid, and retina.

The eye, a spherical, delicate structure, is protected by the skull bones and its accessory organs; eyelashes (close eyelids when disturbed), eyelids (protect and shade), lacrimal apparatus (glands secrete lubricating tears), and the conjunctiva (protective membrane). The *conjunctiva* is a transparent membrane that lines the upper and lower eyelid and the anterior portion of the eye. It helps protect the eye from harmful bacteria.

The *sclera,* the outer protective layer of the eye, helps maintain the shape of the eyeball and is the site for muscle attachment. We can see the anterior portion of the sclera. It is often referred to as the white of the eye. The *cornea* is the transparent, avascular part of the sclera that lies over the iris of the eye and allows the light rays to enter.

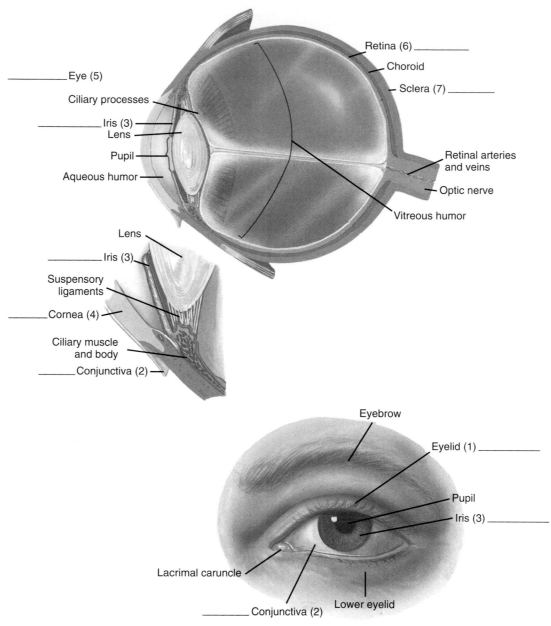

FIGURE 23–18 ▲ The eye.

The middle layer of the eye is called the *choroid*. The choroid contains blood vessels that supply nutrients to the eye. The *iris* and the *ciliary muscle* make up the anterior middle portion of the choroid. The iris, the colored portion of the eye, has an opening in the center called the *pupil*. Muscles of the iris regulate the amount of light entering the eye by dilation and contraction of the pupil.

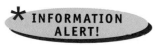

The eye exam of the H&P may include the acronym *PERRLA*, meaning *pupils equal, round, reactive to light and accommodation*.

The *lens*, located directly behind the pupil, focuses light rays on the retina. The ciliary muscle regulates the shape of the lens to make this possible, a process known as *accommodation*.

The inner layer of the eye is called the *retina*. Two different sets of nerve cells, or photoreceptor neurons, called *rods* and *cones*, are responsible for the adaptation to light. The cones are sensitive to bright light, and responsible for color vision. The rods, far more numerous than cones, adapt to provide both peripheral vision and vision in dim light. The rods and cones transmit impulses to the optic nerve. The optic nerve carries these impulses to the vision center in the cerebrum, where they are registered as visual sensations.

The anterior and posterior cavities inside the eyeball are filled with fluid. The small anterior cavity in front of the lens is divided into an anterior and posterior chamber. These chambers are

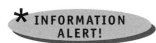

The Pathway of Light Rays

conjunctiva → cornea → aqueous humor → pupil → lens → vitreous humor → retina → optic nerve (converted to nerve impulses) → cerebrum

filled with a watery substance called *aqueous humor,* which is constantly formed and drained. The large posterior cavity behind the lens is filled with a jellylike substance called *vitreous humor,* which remains relatively constant. The functions of these fluids are to maintain the shape of the eyeball with proper intraocular pressure and to assist in bending the light rays to focus on the retina.

Diseases of the Eye

Cataract

Cataracts are the gradual development of cloudiness of the lens of the eyes; they usually occur in both eyes. Most cataracts develop after a person is 50 years of age and are caused by degenerative changes. At first vision is blurred, and if not treated, cataracts eventually lead to loss of eyesight. Treatment is the surgical removal of the lens followed by correction of the visual defects. Two types of surgery used to remove cataracts are the extraction of the entire lens and *phacoemulsification,* which is the use of ultrasonic vibrations to break the lens into pieces, followed by *aspiration,* or sucking out the pieces.

Correction of visual defects includes a lens implant. Following the removal of the cataract, a synthetic lens is inserted into the eye through a corneal incision. Corrective eyeglasses or contact lens may also be used to correct the visual defect caused by cataract extraction.

Glaucoma

Glaucoma is the abnormal increase of intraocular (within the eye) pressure. It is the most preventable cause of blindness and yet is the cause of 15% of all blindness in the United States. The pressure is caused by overproduction of aqueous humor or obstruction of its outflow, causing damage to the retina resulting in blindness.

Two forms of glaucoma exist: chronic and acute. Chronic glaucoma affects vision gradually and may not be diagnosed until after some loss of vision has occurred. The acute form causes severe pain and sudden dimming of vision.

Treatment varies, but glaucoma is often treated with drugs that help reduce the intraocular pressure. The patient has to understand that the medication must be taken for the rest of his or her life.

Retinal Detachment

Retinal detachment is a separation of the retina from the choroid in the back of the eye, allowing vitreous humor to leak between the choroid and the retina. Retinal detachment may be caused by trauma but is often the result of aging. *Photocoagulation, cryosurgery,* and *scleral buckling* are surgical procedures used for treatment.

THE EAR

Two functions of the ear are hearing and equilibrium (sense of balance). The ear is divided into three main parts: the outer ear, the middle ear, and the inner ear (Fig. 23–19).

The Outer Ear

The outer ear is made up of two parts, the pinna, or auricle, and the auditory canal. The *pinna* is the appendage we see on each side of the head. The *auditory canal* is a tube that leads from the outer ear to the middle ear through which sound waves pass.

The Middle Ear

The *tympanic membrane* (eardrum) separates the outer and middle ear. Located just inside the eardrum are three small bones, or *ossicles,* called the *malleus,* the *incus,* and the *stapes.* These three small bones form a chain across the middle ear from the tympanic membrane (eardrum) to the oval window. They transfer vibrations of the eardrum to the inner ear. The middle ear also contains the *eustachian tube,* which leads from the middle ear to the pharynx (throat). The eustachian tube serves to equalize pressure on both sides of the tympanic membrane. Disease-causing bacteria, especially in children, may travel from the throat to the middle ear through the eustachian tube, resulting in middle-ear infection.

The Inner Ear (or Labyrinth)

The *oval window* separates the middle ear from the inner ear. The structure next to the oval window in the inner ear is the *cochlea,* an organ shaped like a snail, with receptors for hearing. It contains special fluids that carry sound vibrations. The inner ear also contains the *semicircular canals.* The cerebellum interprets the impulses from the semicircular canals to maintain balance and equilibrium.

Diseases and Disorders of the Ear

Tinnitus

Tinnitus, a symptom in most disorders of the ear, is described as ringing, buzzing, or roaring noise in the ears. In some patients this noise can be heard by others (objective tinnitus). Common

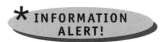

The Passage of Sound Waves Through the Ear

The pathway of sound waves → pinna → auditory canal → tympanic membrane → ossicles (malleus, incus, stapes) → oval window → cochlea → auditory nerve (converted to nerve impulses) → cerebrum

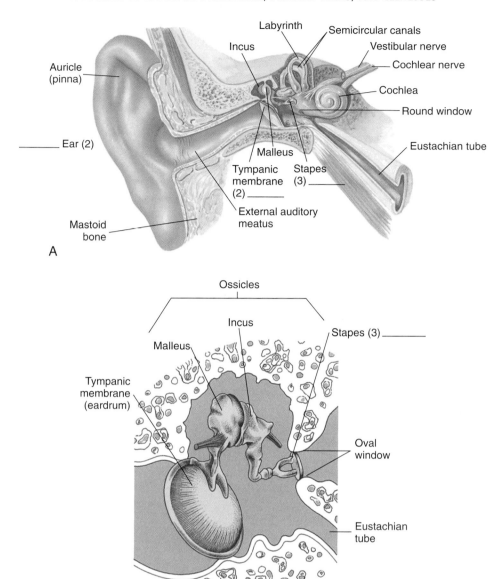

FIGURE 23–19 ▲ *A,* The ear. *B,* Enlarged view of inner ear.

causes of tinnitus include chronic infections, head injuries, prolonged exposure to loud environmental noise, hypertension, and cardiovascular disease. Another common cause of tinnitus is taking drugs that are ototoxic. Ringing in the ears is a very common side effect of aspirin.

Persistent and severe noises in the ear can interfere with the person's ability to carry on normal activities including resting and sleeping. Medical treatment begins with an audiologic and vascular exam to try to determine the underlying cause of the tinnitus. Many cases have been unresponsive to all conventional methods of treatment. One frequent approach to treatment is to try masking the ear noises by providing soft background music. Biofeedback has been marginally effective in cases caused by stress or hysteria. Because the condition is so prevalent, a national association has been established. One of the primary goals of the association is management and study of the condition.

REVIEW QUESTIONS

1. Five body structures that help protect the eye in various ways are:

   a. _____   d. _____

   b. _____   e. _____

   c. _____

2. Explain how sound waves (vibrations) travel from the pinna to the cerebrum (brain).

   _____

   _____

3. Match the terms in Column 1 with the definitions in Column 2.

   Column 1   **Column 2**

   a. choroid   _____ 1. anterior transparent part of the sclera

   b. pupil   _____ 2. the colored portion of the eye

   c. stapes   _____ 3. located directly behind the pupil

   d. retina   _____ 4. outer protective layer of the eye

   e. auditory nerve   _____ 5. the opening in the center of the iris

   f. cornea   _____ 6. inner layer of the eye

   g. cochlea   _____ 7. transmits impulses from the retina to the brain

   h. iris   _____ 8. middle layer of the eye

   i. sclera

   j. lens

   k. optic nerve

4. List in order, beginning with the conjunctiva, the organs of the eye through which the light rays travel to the retina.

   a. _____   d. _____

   b. _____   e. _____

   c. _____   f. _____

5. Name and describe the function of the two types of nerve cells located in the retina.

   a. nerve cell: _____

      function: _____

b. nerve cell: _____

function: _____

6. List the parts of:

a. the outer ear: _____

b. the middle ear: _____

c. the inner ear: _____

7. Describe the clinical presentation of cataracts.

_____

8. The physician's eye-pressure exam for glaucoma will reveal:

_____

9. List six factors that cause tinnitus.

a. _____   d. _____

b. _____   e. _____

c. _____   f. _____

10. List two treatments for tinnitus.

a. _____   b. _____

11. An exam in which retinal detachment is the diagnosis will show:

_____

12. Three surgical procedures used to treat retinal detachment are:

a. _____   c. _____

b. _____

■ MEDICAL TERMINOLOGY RELATING TO THE EYE AND THE EAR

Upon mastery of the medical terminology for this unit, you will be able to:

1. Spell and define the word parts and medical terms for the eye and ear.

2. Given the meaning of a medical condition relating to the eye or ear, build the corresponding medical term with word parts.

3. Analyze the medical terms that are built from word parts that relate to the eye and ear.

4. Given a description of hospital situations in which the health unit coordinator may encounter medical terminology, apply the correct medical terms to the situation involved.

Word Parts

Listed below are the combining forms for this unit. Memorize each combining form. Practice pronouncing each word part aloud.

Word Roots/ Combining Forms	Meaning
Eye	
1. blephar/o (blĕf'-ah-rō)	eyelid
2. conjunctiv/o (kŏn-jŭnk'-tĭv-ō)	conjunctiva (membrane covering the eye and lining of the eyelid)
3. irid/o (ī'-rĭd-ō)	iris (colored portion of the eye)
4. kerat/o (kĕr-ah-tō)	cornea (clear anterior covering of the eye; also means hard)
5. ophthalm/o (ŏf-thal'-mō)	eye
6. retin/o (rĕt'-ĭn-ō)	retina (inner layer of eye)
7. scler/o (sklĕ'-rō)	sclera (white covering of the eye)
Ear	
1. myring/o (mĭ-rĭng'-gō)	tympanic membrane (eardrum)
2. ot/o (ō'-tō)	ear
3. staped/o (stā-pē'-dō)	stapes (in middle ear)

EXERCISE 1

1. Write the combining forms for the eye in the spaces provided on the diagram in Figure 23–18. The number preceding the combining form in the list above matches the number of the body part on the diagram.

2. Write the combining forms for the ear in the spaces provided on the diagram in Figure 23–19. The number preceding the combining form in the list above matches the number of the body part on the diagram.

EXERCISE 2

Define each combining form listed below.

1. retin/o   _____

2. kerat/o   _____

3. scler/o   _____

4. ophthalm/o   _____

5. conjunctiv/o   _____

6. ot/o   _____

7. myring/o   _____

8. blephar/o   _____

9. irid/o   _____

10. staped/o   _____

EXERCISE 3

Write the word roots for each part of the body listed below.

1. *eye*

_____

2. *eyelid*

_____

3. *retina*

_____

4. *ear*

_____

5. *eardrum*

_____

6. *sclera*

_____

7. *conjunctiva*

_____

8. *iris*

_____

9. *cornea*

_____

10. *stapes*

_____

■ MEDICAL TERMS RELATING TO THE EYE AND THE EAR

The following list is made up of medical terms you will need to know for the eye and ear. Exercises following this list will assist you in learning these terms. Practice pronouncing these terms aloud.

General Terms	Meaning
ophthalmologist (ŏf'-thal-mŏl'-ō-jĭst)	one who specializes in the diagnosis and treatment of the eye (doctor)
ophthalmology (ŏf'-thăl-mŏl'-ō-jē)	study of the eye (and its diseases and disorders)
optometrist (ŏp-tŏm'-ĕ-trĭst)	a professional person trained to examine the eyes and prescribe glasses
otorrhea (ō-tō-rē'-ah)	discharge from the ear

Surgical Terms	Meaning
blepharoplasty (blĕf'-ah-rō-plăs-tē)	surgical repair of the eyelid
blepharorrhaphy (blĕf'-ah-rōr'-ah-fē)	suturing of an eyelid
cataract extraction (kăt'-ah-răkt) (ĕk-străk'-shŭn)	removal of the clouded lens of the eye
corneal (kor'-nē-al) transplant	transplantation of a donor cornea into the eye of the recipient
enucleation (ē-nū-klē-ā'-shŭn)	removal of an organ; often used to indicate surgical removal of the eye-ball
iridectomy (ĭr-ĭ-dĕk'-tō-mē)	excision of (a part of) the iris
iridosclerotomy (ĭr-ĭ-dō-sklĕ-rŏt'-ō-mē)	incision into the iris and sclera
keratotomy (kĕr-ah-tot'-ō-mē)	incision into the cornea (radial keratotomy is an operation in which a series of incisions, in spokelike fashion, are made in the cornea; done to correct myopia [nearsightedness])
myringoplasty (mĭ-rĭng'-gō-plăs-tē)	surgical repair of the tympanic membrane
myringotomy (mĭ-rĭng-gŏt'-ō-mē)	incision of the tympanic membrane
ophthalmectomy (ŏf-thal-mĕk'-tō-mē)	excision of the eye
scleroplasty (sklĕ'-rō-plăs-tē)	surgical repair of the sclera
sclerotomy (sklĕ-rŏt'-ō-mē)	incision into the sclera
stapedectomy (stă-pē-dĕk'-tō-mē)	excision of the stapes

Diagnostic Terms	Meaning
cataract (kăt'-ah-răkt)	cloudiness of the lens of the eye
conjunctivitis (kŏn-jŭnk-tī-vī'-tĭs)	inflammation of the conjunctiva (pinkeye)
glaucoma (glaw-kō'-mah)	an eye disease caused by increased pressure within the eye
keratocele (kĕr'-ah-tō-sĕl)	herniation (of a layer) of the cornea
keratoconjunctivitis (kĕr'-ah-tō-kŏn-jŭnk-tĭ-vī'-tĭs)	inflammation of the cornea and conjunctiva
otitis media (ō-tī'-tĭs) (mē'-dē-ah)	inflammation of the middle ear
retinal detachment (rĕt'-ĭn-al) (dē-tăch'-mĕnt)	complete or partial separation of the retina from the choroid
strabismus (străh-bĭz'-mŭs)	a weakness of the muscle of the eye that causes the eye to look in different directions (medical term for crossed eyes)

Terms Relating to Diagnostic Procedures	Meaning
ophthalmoscope (ŏf-thal'-mō-skōp)	instrument used for visual examination of the eye
otoscope (ō'-tō-skōp)	instrument used for visual examination of the ear

EXERCISE ④

Analyze and define each medical term listed below.

1. ophthalmoscope

_____

2. ophthalmologist

_____

3. ophthalmectomy

_____

4. otorrhea

_____

5. otoscope

_____

6. iridosclerotomy

_____

7. *iridectomy*

_____

8. *blepharoplasty*

_____

9. *blepharorrhaphy*

_____

10. *keratoconjunctivitis*

_____

11. *keratocele*

_____

12. *conjunctivitis*

_____

13. *myringotomy*

_____

14. *myringoplasty*

_____

15. *keratotomy*

_____

EXERCISE 5

Build medical terms from each definition listed below.
1. *inflammation of the middle ear*

_____

2. *instrument used for visual examination of the eye*

_____

3. *suturing of the eyelid*

_____

4. *discharge from the ear*

_____

5. *incision into the iris and the sclera*

_____

6. *surgical repair of the sclera*

_____

7. *excision of part of the iris*

_____

8. *herniation of the cornea*

_____

9. *an instrument used for visual examination of the ear*

_____

10. *excision of the eye*

_____

11. *incision of the sclera*

_____

12. *surgical repair of the eyelid*

_____

13. *incision into the tympanic membrane*

_____

14. *surgical repair of the tympanic membrane*

_____

15. *inflammation of the cornea and conjunctiva*

_____

16. *inflammation of the conjunctiva*

_____

17. incision into the cornea

_____

EXERCISE 6

Define each medical term listed below.

1. cataract

_____

2. cataract extraction

_____

3. retinal detachment

_____

4. enucleation of the eye

_____

5. strabismus

_____

6. glaucoma

_____

7. optometrist

_____

8. corneal transplant

_____

EXERCISE 7

Spell each medical term studied in this unit by having someone dictate the terms to you.

1. _____
2. _____
3. _____
4. _____
5. _____

---

6. _____
7. _____
8. _____
9. _____
10. _____
11. _____
12. _____
13. _____
14. _____
15. _____
16. _____
17. _____
18. _____
19. _____
20. _____
21. _____
22. _____
23. _____
24. _____
25. _____
26. _____
27. _____
28. _____

EXERCISE 8

Answer the following questions.

1. Instruments used to examine the eye and ear visually are usually part of the equipment stored at the nurses' station in the hospital. The instrument used to examine the eye is

called a(an) _____ . The instrument used

to examine the ear is called a(an) _____ .

2. Children often develop inflammation of the middle ear, called

_____ _____ .

Children who have had repeated middle-ear infections may

have a build-up of fluid in the middle ear. The doctor may surgically treat this condition by making an incision into the eardrum, known as _____, and inserting tiny tubes.

3. The patient is admitted to the hospital with a diagnosis of cloudiness of the lens of the right eye, or _____. She is scheduled for surgical removal of the diseased lens. The operation is called _____ _____.

4. Two medical words are used to describe surgical removal of the eyeball. They are _____ and _____ .

5. _____ is the medical term for crossed eyes.

UNIT 6

The Cardiovascular and Lymphatic Systems

Outline

Unit Objectives

Upon completion of this unit, you will be able to:

1. Name and describe the functions of the organs of the circulatory system.

2. Name and describe the structures of the heart and describe the circulation of blood through the heart.

3. Name three kinds of blood vessels and briefly describe the function of each.

4. Briefly describe the composition of blood and list and relate the function of the three types of blood cells.

5. Name and describe the functions of the organs of the lymphatic system.

6. Describe two functions of the spleen.

7. Describe coronary artery disease, congestive heart failure, anemia, varicose veins, and acquired immunodeficiency syndrome.

■ THE CARDIOVASCULAR AND LYMPHATIC SYSTEMS

Organs of the Circulatory System

Heart
Blood vessels
Blood

Functions of the Circulatory System

Transportation of nutrients, oxygen, hormones to cells, and removal of wastes
Protection by the white blood cells and antibodies to defend the body against foreign invaders
Regulation of body temperature, fluids, and water volume of cells

All living cells, which are metabolically active structures, need constant nourishment and oxygen for life and the continuous removal of their waste products. The circulatory system provides the vital transportation service that carries nourishment (oxygen, nutrients, and hormones) to the cells of the body and carries the waste away (nitrogenous wastes, carbon dioxide, and heat). Blood is the most frequently examined tissue by clinicians to determine the state of health.

The heart pumps blood to the lungs and the body cells through a network of tubing called *blood vessels.* Blood is the carrying agent for food, oxygen, waste, and other materials needed or produced by cell function.

■ THE HEART

The heart is located in the mediastinum, the cavity between the lungs, situated behind the sternum. It is a four-chambered organ the size of a fist, and it weighs less than a pound. The heart performs the action of pumping the blood through the blood vessels to all parts of the body, circulating it in a one-way movement. The heart is surrounded by the *pericardium,* a loose fitting double-layered sac. Serous membranes of the pericardium secrete a small amount of fluid to prevent irritation as the heart contracts.

Structure of the Heart

The heart wall is made up of three layers. The outer layer of the heart wall, the *epicardium,* is the visceral layer of the pericardium. The thickest, muscular middle layer, is called the *myocardium.* The *endocardium,* the inner lining of the heart, also forms the heart valves.

The heart is divided into four cavities or chambers (Fig. 23–20) through which blood entering the heart travels. Each chamber has a valve (or one-way door) that prevents the blood from flowing backward into its chamber. The *septum* is a partition dividing the heart into a right and left side. Each side is divided by halves into two upper chambers—the *right atrium* and the *left atrium*—and two lower chambers—the *right ventricle* and the *left ventricle.* The left atrium is separated from the left ventricle by the *bicuspid,* or *mitral, valve.* On the right side, the right atrium is separated from the right ventricle by the *tricuspid,* or

atrioventricular (AV) valve. The *semilunar valves* (pulmonary and aortic) are located between the right ventricle and the pulmonary artery and between the left ventricle and the aorta.

Conduction System of the Heart

The regular and coordinated cardiac muscle contraction is conducted by electrical impulses originated within the heart muscle. A normal heartbeat begins with an impulse from the sinoatrial (SA) node to the atrioventricular (AV) node, through the bundle branches, and finally through the Purkinje fibers to effect a complete heart contraction. The rhythm generated by the electrical impulses is measured by the electrocardiogram (EKG). (See Fig. 16–2, page 316, for an EKG.)

■ BLOOD VESSELS

Blood vessels are the tubular structures through which the blood flows to and from the heart to the body parts (Fig. 23–21). There are three major types of blood vessels: arteries, capillaries, and veins.

Arteries carry blood away from the heart, except for the pulmonary artery. The pulmonary artery is the only artery in the body that carries blood with low levels of oxygen and a high concentration of carbon dioxide. All other arteries carry blood high in oxygen concentration from the heart to the body cells. *Arterial walls* are the thickest because they must withstand the pumping force of the heart. Arteries branch into *arterioles,* tiny arteries that connect the arteries to capillaries. The aorta is the largest artery of the body, being approximately 1 inch in diameter. It carries blood away from the left ventricle of the heart.

The *veins* are the vessels that carry blood from the capillary beds back to the heart. Venous blood carries carbon dioxide and other waste products except for the pulmonary veins. They carry blood high in oxygen concentration from the lungs to the heart. The vein walls are thinner than the arterial walls and contain tiny valves to help prevent the backward flow of blood and to keep it moving in one direction. *Venules* are tiny veins that connect the capillaries with the veins. The *superior vena cava* and the *inferior vena cava* are large veins through which the blood returns from the body to the right atrium.

Capillaries are microscopic, thin-walled blood vessels. The exchange of substances takes place between the blood and the body cells while the blood is in the capillaries. The cells take in nutrients and oxygen from the blood and give off waste and carbon dioxide to the blood. The blood carries the waste to the organ that removes it from the body. The capillaries provide the link between the arteries and veins.

Flow of Blood Through the Blood Vessels of the Body

Blood leaves the heart through the aorta. It travels first through the arteries and then through the arterioles to the capillaries, where the exchange of gases, nutrients, and waste takes place. The blood returns from the capillaries by first entering the venules and then flowing through the veins, finally entering the right atrium of the heart through the superior and inferior venae cavae. The superior vena cava returns blood to the heart from the upper part of the body, and the inferior vena cava returns blood to the heart from the lower part of the body.

YOUR HEART AND HOW IT WORKS

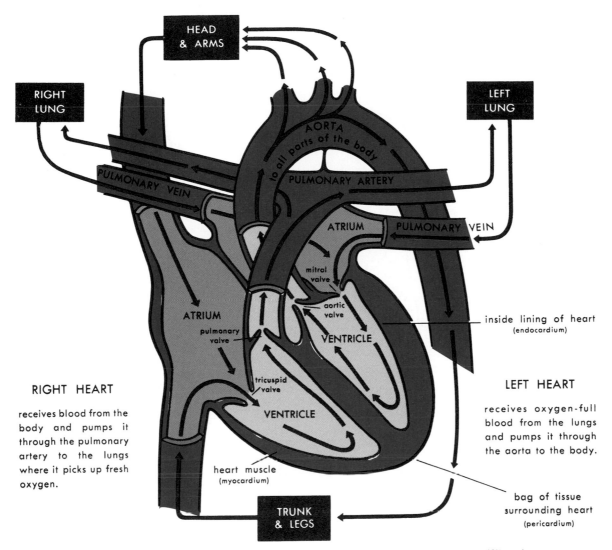

FIGURE 23-20 ▲ The heart. (Courtesy of the American Heart Association and its affiliates.)

Blood Pressure

Blood pressure (BP), measured in milliliters of mercury (mm Hg)—120/70, records the forces created by the circulating blood against the walls of the arteries, veins, and chambers of the heart. The upper number, systolic blood pressure, represents the pressure in the aorta and other large arteries during ventricular contraction. The lower number, diastolic blood pressure, represents the pressure during relaxation of the heart.

■ BLOOD

Blood is the carrying agent of the transportation system. It is a warm, sticky fluid ranging in color from dark bluish-red to bright red, according to the amount of oxygen it is carrying. An adult has approximately 5.7 L (6 qt) of blood.

✱ **INFORMATION ALERT!**

Pathway: Blood saturated with CO_2 returns to the right side of the heart via the inferior and superior vena cava → right atrium → tricuspid valve → right ventricle → pulmonary valve → pulmonary artery → to the lungs → (exchange of CO_2 and O_2 takes place in the lungs) from the lungs saturated with O_2 → pulmonary veins → left atrium → bicuspid valve (mitral valve) → left ventricle → aortic valve → aorta

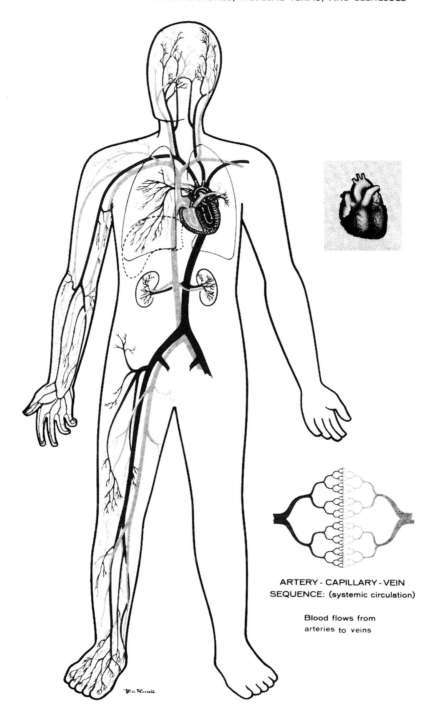

ARTERY - CAPILLARY - VEIN
SEQUENCE: (systemic circulation)

Blood flows from
arteries to veins

FIGURE 23–21 ▲ The blood vessels. (Courtesy of the American Heart Association and its affiliates.)

Function of Blood

The blood has three main functions: transportation, fighting infection, and regulation.

Transportation

The blood carries oxygen from the lungs and nutrients from the digestive tract to the body cells. It carries waste products from the cells, carbon dioxide to the lungs, and other waste (urea) to the kidneys. The blood also transports hormones and other chemicals.

Fighting Infection

Certain blood cells help the body fight disease-causing organisms. White blood cells, or leukocytes, acting as the main line of defense against infection, respond when encountering microbes or toxins.

Regulation

The blood distributes hormones and other chemicals as needed, maintains body temperature by the dilation and constriction of blood vessels in the skin, and maintains the homeostatic balance of fluids necessary for survival.

Blood Composition

Blood is made up of plasma and cells.

Plasma

Plasma is the clear, fluid portion of the blood, in which the blood cells are suspended. Plasma is approximately 90% water and contains over 100 other constituents, such as glucose, fibrinogen, and protein. It makes up approximately 50% of the total amount of the blood. Plasma transports nutrients, waste material, hormones, and so forth, to and from the body cells. Fibrinogen assists in the blood-clotting process.

Blood Cells, or Formed Elements

There are three kinds of *blood cells*, each carrying out certain functions.

Erythrocytes (RBCs) are produced by the red bone marrow. Red bone marrow is found in the flat bones of the body, such as the sternum or the pelvic bones. A *sternal puncture* is a procedure used to obtain bone marrow from the sternum. The bone marrow is then studied to determine its ability to produce RBCs. The function of the RBC is to carry oxygen and carbon dioxide. *Hemoglobin* is the oxygen carrying pigment of the erythrocyte that gives blood its color. The average RBC count is 4.5 to 5 million/mm^3 of blood. Erythrocytes exist approximately 4 months. It is estimated that each erythrocyte travels approximately 700 miles during its lifetime.

Leukocytes (white blood cells) are colorless cells produced by the spleen, bone marrow, and lymph nodes. Their chief function is to fight against pathogenic microorganisms (disease-causing bacteria). The normal white blood cell (WBC) count is 5,000 to 9,000/mm^3 of blood. An elevated blood count may indicate the presence of an infection in the body. Leukocytes last a very short time—approximately 14 hours or less.

Platelets (thrombocytes) are also formed in the red bone marrow. Their prime function is to aid in the clotting of blood. A normal platelet count is about 250,000/mm^3 of blood. Platelets exist for a short time in the bloodstream and are replaced approximately every 4 days.

■ CIRCULATION OF BLOOD THROUGH THE HEART

Blood carrying the waste product carbon dioxide returns from circulating through the body and enters the right atrium of the heart through the superior vena cava and the inferior vena cava. The blood travels through the tricuspid valve to the right ventricle. The right ventricle pumps the blood through the *pulmonary arteries* to the lungs. (The pulmonary artery is the only artery that transports waste-carrying blood.) The blood, while in the lungs, gets rid of the carbon dioxide and takes on oxygen. This exchange changes the appearance of the blood from a bluish-red color to a bright red color. The oxygenated blood returns to the left atrium through the *pulmonary veins*.

The pulmonary vein is the only vein in the body to carry oxygenated blood. The blood passes through the bicuspid valve to the left ventricle. The left ventricle pumps the blood through the aorta and out to the body parts. Refer to Figure 23–20; the arrows indicate the passage of blood through the heart.

■ LYMPHATIC SYSTEM

The lymphatic system consists of the spleen, thymus gland, lymph nodes, a fluid called lymph, and the lymphatic vessels. The two principal functions of the lymphatic system are the maintenance of fluid balance and immunity. Lymphatic vessels collect excessive tissue fluids and return them to the blood circulation.

Spleen

The *spleen*, the largest lymphatic organ, is located in the upper left abdomen and is protected by the lower ribs. Two important functions of the spleen are to destroy old RBCs, bacteria, and germs and to store blood for emergency use. The spleen produces the RBCs in the fetus.

Thymus Gland

The *thymus gland*, one of the primary lymphatic organs, plays an important role in the development of the body's defenses against infections by promoting the maturation of cells that provide immune responses (T lymphocytes).

■ DISEASES AND DISORDERS OF THE CIRCULATORY SYSTEM

Coronary Artery Disease

Coronary artery disease (CAD) is usually caused by occlusion, or narrowing of the arteries due to the build-up of plaque on the arterial walls, a condition called *atherosclerosis. Angina pectoris* is a condition caused by lack of oxygen to the myocardium as a result of atherosclerosis of the coronary arteries. Atherosclerosis can completely block the artery, creating a condition called *coronary occlusion*; or a *thrombus* (blood clot) can develop on segments of the artery containing plaque, causing a blockage, a condition referred to as *coronary thrombosis*. Both conditions may lead to a *myocardial infarction (MI)* (heart attack) because they reduce the flow of blood to the heart, which denies the myocardium the oxygen and nutrients it needs. A symptom of an MI is sudden onset of chest pain, sometimes radiating to the arms. The severity of the heart attack depends on which artery is blocked and to what extent it is blocked.

Coronary artery bypass graft surgery (CABG) may be performed in coronary artery disease to improve the blood supply to the myocardium. This type of surgery consists of using a vein from the leg grafted to the aorta and the clogged coronary artery to form an alternative route for the flow of blood.

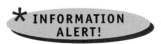
★ INFORMATION ALERT!

Because leukocytes fight incompatible blood cells, it is absolutely essential that patients be typed and cross-matched before receiving blood. Before scientists learned to group blood into types that could be safely given from one person to another, many deaths resulted from incompatible blood transfusions. The blood types are O, A, B, and AB.

Angioplasty, surgical repair of a blood vessel, refers to various techniques such as the use of surgery, lasers, or tiny balloons at the tip of a catheter to repair or replace damaged blood vessels. *Percutaneous transluminal coronary angioplasty (PTCA)* is a cardiac procedure in which fatty plaques in the blood vessels are flattened against the vessel walls by passing a balloon in a catheter through the affected blood vessels. A coronary stent, a wire mesh tube, is commonly placed in the cleared artery to maintain its patency. *Laser angioplasty* makes use of light amplification by stimulated emission of radiation (laser beam) through a fiberoptic probe to open blocked arteries.

Congestive Heart Failure

Congestive heart failure (CHF) occurs when the heart is unable to pump the required amount of blood, resulting in the accumulation of blood in the lungs and liver. CHF develops gradually. Symptoms are fatigue, dyspnea (shortness of breath) and peripheral edema. Diagnostic testing includes chest x-ray, EKG, echocardiogram, angiogram, and blood tests. Treatment includes dietary changes (restricted sodium, fats, cholesterol, fluids) and administration of medications such as angiotensin-converting enzyme (ACE) inhibitors, β blockers, digoxin, and diuretics. Surgical options to correct the underlying cardiac problem include coronary bypass surgery, valve repair or replacement, cardiac resynchronization therapy, and heart transplantation.

Anemia

Anemia is a disorder characterized by an abnormally low level of hemoglobin in the blood or inadequate numbers of RBCs. It may result from decreased RBC production, from increased RBC destruction, or from blood loss. Treatment varies according to the cause. The anemic person becomes easily fatigued. Pallor may also indicate anemia. Sternal puncture to obtain bone marrow for study and blood tests are used to diagnose anemia.

Varicose Veins

Varicose veins are swollen, distended, and knotted veins usually in the superficial veins of the leg. The one-way valves in the veins assist in moving the blood upward to the heart. Standing or sitting for prolonged periods causes the valves to dilate from the

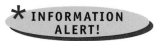

✱ INFORMATION ALERT!

Rh blood groups, a complex system of erythrocyte surface antigens, were first identified in <u>rh</u>esus monkeys in 1940. The presence of even one antigen on the RBC makes a person Rh positive. Rh incompatibility is generally not a problem in the first pregnancy because the mother does not produce the anti–Rh-positive antibodies until after birth. Rh incompatibility may cause problems in subsequent pregnancies, requiring treatment of mother and baby to correct the disorder. Rh negative women carrying Rh positive babies of subsequent pregnancies will form anti-Rh antibodies unless treated with RhoGAM before or shortly after birth.

weight of pooled blood and can result in the valves losing their elasticity. Other causes include pregnancy, obesity, illness, injury, and heredity. Elevation of the leg and elastic stockings are used to reduce blood pooling in the great saphenous vein, the largest superficial vein. A minimally invasive surgery in which the affected veins are pulled out, ambulatory phlebectomy, may be required in more severe cases. Hemorrhoids are internal or external varicose veins in the rectal area.

Acquired Immunodeficiency Syndrome

Acquired immunodeficiency syndrome (AIDS), manifested by the destruction of patients' immune systems, makes its carriers very susceptible to infection. AIDS is caused by the human immunodeficiency virus (HIV), which infects certain white blood cells of the body's immune system and gradually destroys the body's ability to fight infection. Many infected persons develop previously rare types of pneumonia (*Pneumocystis carinii* pneumonia) and a form of skin cancer (Kaposi's sarcoma).

HIV has been isolated from semen and blood and is transmitted by direct or intimate contact involving the mucous membranes or breaks in the skin, across the placenta from mother to fetus, or before or during birth. The sharing of hypodermic needles among IV drug users, blood transfusions, and needle sticks are other ways of becoming infected. The virus cannot penetrate intact skin. AIDS has become one of the deadliest epidemic diseases of modern times and will remain a major global health concern until more definitive treatment is realized.

REVIEW QUESTIONS

1. Label the following diagram of the heart, including the blood vessels through which the blood enters and leaves the heart. Include the following parts:

endocardium	pulmonary artery	right atrium
myocardium	pulmonary vein	left atrium
pericardium	aorta	right ventricle
bicuspid valve	superior vena cava	left ventricle
tricuspid valve	inferior vena cava	

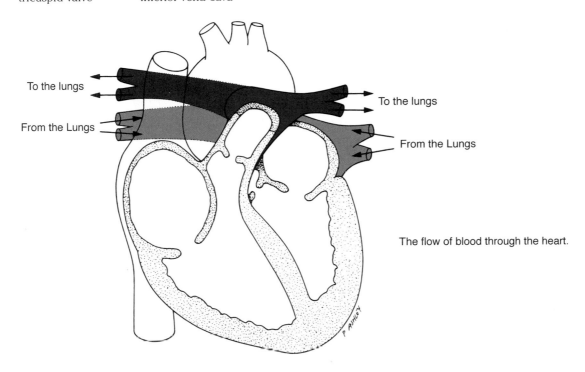

To the lungs

To the lungs

From the Lungs

From the Lungs

The flow of blood through the heart.

2. Using arrows, trace on the same diagram the circulation of blood from the superior and inferior vena cava to the aorta.

3. Blood travels through a network of tubes called blood vessels. Name, in sequence, the types of blood vessels the blood travels through when leaving the heart to reentry, and write the function of each.

   a. _____

   b. _____

   c. _____

   d. _____

   e. _____

4. The fluid portion of the blood is called the _____. Its functions are:

   a. _____

   b. _____

   c. _____

5. List three types of blood cells (formed elements) and briefly describe the function of each.

    a. _____

    b. _____

    c. _____

6. Name the four blood types.

    a. _____

    b. _____

    c. _____

    d. _____

7. Two functions of the spleen are:

    a. _____

    b. _____

8. Match the terms in Column 1 with the phrases in Column 2.

Column 1   **Column 2**

a. anemia   _____ 1. caused by lack of oxygen to the myocardium

b. CHF   _____ 2. the heart is unable to efficiently pump blood

c. CAD   _____ 3. narrowing of arteries

d. coronary thrombosis   _____ 4. below normal level of hemoglobin

e. myocardial infarction   _____ 5. causes occlusion of an artery

f. bypass   _____ 6. surgery for varicose veins

g. angina pectoris   _____ 7. damage to the heart muscle

h. ambulatory phlebectomy   _____ 8. caused by HIV

i. AIDS

■ MEDICAL TERMINOLOGY RELATING TO THE CIRCULATORY SYSTEM

Upon mastery of the medical terminology for this unit, you will be able to:

1. Spell and define the word parts and the medical terms for the circulatory system.

2. Given the meaning of a medical condition relating to the circulatory system, build with word parts the corresponding medical term.

3. Analyze the medical terms that are built from word parts that relate to the circulatory system.

4. Given a list of word parts, identify them as word roots, suffixes, or prefixes.

5. Given descriptions of hospital situations in which the health unit coordinator may encounter medical terminology, apply the correct medical terms to the situation described.

Word Parts

The list below contains the word parts you need to memorize for the circulatory system. The exercises included in this unit will help you with this task. You will continue to use these word parts throughout this course and during your employment. Practice pronouncing each word part aloud.

Word Roots/ Combining Forms — Meaning

Word Root/Combining Form	Meaning
angi/o (ăn′-jē-ō)	blood vessel
aort/o (ā-ōr′-tō)	aorta
arteri/o (ar-tē′-rē-ō)	artery
cardi/o (kar′-dē-ō)	heart
hem/o (hē′-mō); hemat/o (hĕm′-ah-tō)	blood
phleb/o (flĕb′-ō); ven/o (vē′-nō)	vein
splen/o (splē′-nō)	spleen
thromb/o (thrŏm′-bō)	clot

Color Word Roots/ Combining Forms — Meaning

Color Word Root/Combining Form	Meaning
cyan/o (sī′-ah-nō)	blue
erythr/o (ĕ-rĭth′-rō)	red
leuk/o (loo′-kō)	white

Prefixes — Meaning

Prefix	Meaning
brady- (brā-dee)	slow
endo- (ĕn′-dō)	inside
hyper- (hī′-per)	above normal
hypo- (hī′-pō)	below normal
peri- (pĕr′-ē)	surrounding (outer)
tachy- (tăk-kē)	fast, rapid

Suffixes — Meaning

Suffix	Meaning
-emia (ē′-mē-ah) (may also be used as word root)	condition of the blood
-megaly (mĕg′-ah-lē)	enlargement
-pexy (pĕk′-sē)	surgical fixation (suspension)
-sclerosis (sklĕ-rō′-sĭs) (may also be used as word root)	hardening
-stenosis (stĕ-nō′-sĭs) (may also be used as word root)	narrowing

EXERCISE 1

Identify each word part listed here by writing *P* for prefix, *S* for suffix, or *WR* for word root in the space provided. Then define each word part in the space provided. Word parts studied in previous units are also included in this exercise.

Word Part	Type	Meaning
Example: pexy	S	surgical fixation
1. hypo	___	___
2. a, an	___	___
3. hem	___	___
4. spleen	___	___
5. cyt	___	___
6. stenosis	___	___
7. endo	___	___
8. leuk	___	___
9. erythr	___	___
10. angi	___	___
11. cardi	___	___
12. arteri	___	___
13. peri	___	___
14. inter	___	___
15. intra	___	___
16. sclerosis	___	___
17. emia	___	___
18. megaly	___	___
19. phleb	___	___
20. aort	___	___
21. thromb	___	___
22. hyper	___	___
23. tachy	___	___
24. brady	___	___

EXERCISE 2

Write the word parts for the meanings listed on the following page. Identify each word part you write in the answer column. Use *P* for prefix, *S* for suffix, and *WR* for word root or combining form. For review purposes, word parts from previous units are included in this exercise.

Meaning	Type	Word Parts
1. aorta	_____	_____
2. enlargement	_____	_____
3. hardening	_____	_____
4. between	_____	_____
5. artery	_____	_____
6. blood vessel	_____	_____
7. white	_____	_____
8. narrowing	_____	_____
9. spleen	_____	_____
10. without	_____	_____
11. surgical fixation	_____	_____

Meaning	Type	Word Parts
12. inside	_____	_____
13. blood	_____	_____
14. cell	_____	_____
15. below normal	_____	_____
16. red	_____	_____
17. heart	_____	_____
18. surrounding (outer)	_____	_____
19. blood condition	_____	_____
20. vein	_____	_____
21. clot	_____	_____
22. fast, rapid	_____	_____
23. slow	_____	_____

■ MEDICAL TERMS RELATING TO THE CIRCULATORY SYSTEM

The following list is made up of medical terms you will need to know for the circulatory system. Exercises following this list will assist you in learning these terms. Practice the pronunciation of these terms out loud.

General Terms	Meaning
arrhythmia (ah-rĭth′-mē-ah)	variation from a normal rhythm, especially of the heartbeat
aortic (ā-or′-tĭk)	pertaining to the aorta
bradycardia (brā-dy-cār′-dĭă)	condition of slow heart (rate)
cardiac arrest (kar′-dē-ăk) (ah-rĕst′)	sudden and often unexpected stoppage of the heartbeat
cardiologist (kar-dē-ŏl′-ō-jĭst)	one who specializes in the diagnosis and treatment of the heart (doctor)
cardiology (kar-dē-ŏl′-ō-jē)	the study of the heart (and its functions and diseases)
cardiomegaly (kar′-dē-ō-mĕg′-ah-lē)	enlargement of the heart
cardiovascular (kar′-dē-ō-văs′-kū-lar)	pertaining to the heart and blood vessels
coronary (kŏr′-ō-nā-rē)	a term used to describe blood vessels that supply blood to the heart
endocardial (ĕn-dō-kar′-dē-al)	pertaining to within the heart
erythrocyte (ĕ-rĭth′-rō-sīt)	red blood cell (RBC)
hemorrhage (hĕm′-ō-rĭj)	the rapid flow of blood (from a blood vessel)
hypertension (hī-per-tĕn′-shŭn)	high blood pressure
hypotension (hī-pō-tĕn′-shŭn)	low blood pressure
intravenous (ĭn-trah-vē′-nŭs)	within a vein
leukocyte (loo′-kō-sīt)	white blood cell (WBC)
phlebotomy (flĕ-bŏt′-ō-mē)	incision into the vein (to withdraw blood)
splenomegaly (splē-nō-mĕg′-ah-lē)	enlargement of the spleen
tachycardia (tăk-ē-kar′-dē-ah)	condition of rapid heart (rate)
thrombosis (thrŏm-bō′-sĭs)	abnormal formation of a blood clot

Surgical Terms	Meaning
angioplasty (ăn'-jē-ō-plăs-tē)	surgical repair of a blood vessel (Fig. 23–22)
angiorrhaphy (ăn-jē-ōr'-ah-fē)	suturing of a blood vessel
hemorrhoidectomy (hĕm-ō-roi-dĕk'-tō-mē)	excision of hemorrhoids
splenectomy (splĕ-nĕk'-tō-mē)	excision of the spleen
splenopexy (splĕ'-nō-pĕk-sē)	surgical fixation of the spleen

Diagnostic Terms	Meaning
anemia (ah-nē'-mē-ah)	condition of blood without (deficiency in the number of erythrocytes [RBCs])
aneurysm (ăn'-ū-rĭzm)	a dilation of a weak area of the arterial wall
arteriosclerosis (ar-tē'-rē-ō-sclĕ-rō'-sĭs)	abnormal condition of hardening of the arteries
arteriostenosis (ar-tē'-rē-ō-stĕ-nō'-sĭs)	abnormal condition of narrowing of an artery
congestive heart failure (CHF)	inability of the heart to pump sufficient amounts of blood to the body parts
coronary occlusion (kŏr'-ŏ-nā-rē) (ō-kloo'-zhŭn)	the closing off of a coronary artery, which usually results in damage to the heart muscle; commonly referred to as a heart attack
coronary thrombosis (kŏr'-ŏ-nā-rē) (thrŏm-bō'-sĭs)	the blocking of a coronary artery by a blood clot; commonly referred to as a heart attack
edema (ĕ-dē'-mah)	an abnormal accumulation of fluid in the intercellular spaces of the body
embolism (ĕm'-bō-lĭzm)	a floating mass that blocks a vessel
endocarditis (ĕn-dō-kar-dī'-tĭs)	inflammation of the inner (lining) of the heart
hematology (hē-mah-tŏl'-ō-jē)	study of the blood (also, a diagnostic division within a hospital laboratory that performs diagnostic tests on blood components)
hematoma (hē-mah-tō'-mah)	a tumor-like mass formed from blood (in the tissues)
hemophilia (hē-mō-fĭl'-ē-ah)	a congenital disorder characterized by excessive bleeding
hemorrhoid (hĕm'-ōrr-oyd)	enlarged veins in the rectal area
leukemia (loo-kē'-mē-ah)	a type of cancer characterized by rapid abnormal production of white blood cells
myocardial infarction (MI) (mī-ō-kar'-dē-al) (ĭn-fark'-shŭn)	damage to the heart muscle caused by insufficient blood supply to the area; a condition the layperson refers to as a heart attack
pericarditis (pĕr-ĭ-kar-dī'-tĭs)	inflammation of the outer (sac) of the heart (or pericardium)
thrombophlebitis (thrŏm'-bō-flĕ-bī' tĭs)	inflammation of a vein (as the result of a clot)
ventricular fibrillation (VFib)	life-threatening uncoordinated contractions of the ventricles. Immediate application of an electrical shock with a defibrillator is necessary treatment.

Terms Relating to Diagnostic Procedures	Meaning
angiogram (ăn'-jē-ō-grăm)	an x-ray image of a blood vessel (using dye as a contrast medium)
aortogram (ā-ōr'-tō-grăm)	an x-ray image of the aorta (using dye as a contrast medium)
arteriogram (ar-tē'-rē-ō-grăm)	an x-ray image of an artery (using dye as a contrast medium)
cardiac catheterization (kar'-dē-ăk) (kăth'-ĕ-ter-ĭ-zā'-shŭn)	a diagnostic procedure used to visualize the heart to determine the presence of heart disease or heart defects. A long catheter is threaded from a blood vessel to the heart cavities. Dye is used as a contrast medium.
electrocardiogram (EKG) (ē-lĕk'-trō-kar'-dē-ō-grăm)	a record of the electrical activity of the heart
electrocardiograph (ē-lĕk'-trō-kar'-dē-ō-grăf)	an instrument used to record electrical activity of the heart
electrocardiography (ē-lĕk'-trō-kar-dē-ōg'-rah-fē)	the process of recording the electrical activity of the heart
hematocrit (hē'-măt-ō-krĭt)	hematocrit, which means "to separate blood," is a laboratory test that measures the volume percentage of RBCs in whole blood
hemoglobin (hē'-mō-glō'-bĭn)	the oxygen-carrying pigment of the RBCs

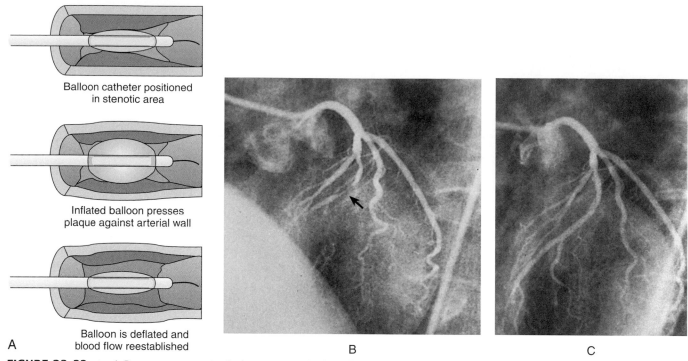

Balloon catheter positioned
in stenotic area

Inflated balloon presses
plaque against arterial wall

Balloon is deflated and
blood flow reestablished

A

B

C

FIGURE 23–22 ▲ *A*, Percutaneous transluminal coronary angioplasty (PTCA). *B*, Coronary artery before PTCA. The arrow indicates stenotic area, estimated at 95% minimum blood flow distal to the lesion. *C*, Coronary arteriogram after PTCA in the same patient. Blood flow is estimated to be 100%.

EXERCISE 3

Analyze and define each medical term listed below.

1. *aortic*

_____

_____

2. *splenomegaly*

_____

_____

3. *hemorrhage*

_____

_____

4. *thrombosis*

_____

_____

5. *leukocyte*

_____

_____

6. *erythrocyte*

_____

_____

7. *cardiologist*

_____

_____

8. *cardiomegaly*

_____

_____

9. *phlebotomy*

_____

_____

10. *angiorrhaphy*

_____

_____

11. *splenectomy*

_____

_____

12. *splenopexy*

_____

_____

13. *endocarditis*

_____

_____

14. *arteriosclerosis*

_____

_____

15. *arteriostenosis*

_____

_____

16. *thrombophlebitis*

_____

_____

17. *hematoma*

_____

_____

18. *hematology*

_____

_____

19. *leukemia*

_____

_____

20. *anemia*

_____

_____

21. *electrocardiogram*

_____

_____

22. *electrocardiograph*

_____

_____

23. *electrocardiography*

_____

_____

24. *angiogram*

_____

_____

25. *arteriogram*

_____

_____

26. *aortogram*

_____

_____

27. *pericarditis*

_____

_____

28. *tachycardia*

_____

_____

29. *bradycardia*

_____

_____

30. *angioplasty*

_____

_____

EXERCISE 4

Using the word elements you have studied in this unit and previous units, build medical terms from each definition listed below.

1. x-ray image of the aorta _____

2. x-ray image of an artery _____

3. x-ray image of a blood vessel _____

4. a record of the electrical activity of the heart _____

5. inflammation of the inner lining of the heart _____

6. hardening of the arteries _____

7. inflammation of a vein due to a blood clot formation _____

8. study of the blood _____

9. study of the heart _____

10. one who specializes in the diagnosis and treatment of the heart _____

11. enlarged heart _____

12. incision into a vein _____

13. excision of the spleen _____

14. surgical fixation of the spleen _____

15. rapid discharge of blood _____

16. white blood cell _____

17. red blood cell _____

18. inflammation of the outer (sac) of the heart _____

EXERCISE 5

Define each medical term listed below.
1. *hematocrit*

_____

2. *hemoglobin*

_____

3. *cardiac arrest*

_____

4. *cardiovascular*

_____

5. *hemorrhoidectomy*

_____

6. *myocardial infarction*

_____

7. *hemorrhoid*

_____

8. *intravenous*

_____

9. *cardiac catheterization*

_____

10. aneurysm

_____

11. embolism

_____

12. hypertension

_____

13. hypotension

_____

14. congestive heart failure

_____

15. coronary

_____

16. edema

_____

17. arrhythmia

_____

18. tachycardia

_____

EXERCISE 6

Spell each medical term studied in this unit by having someone dictate the terms to you.

1. _____

2. _____

3. _____

4. _____

5. _____

6. _____

7. _____

8. _____

9. _____

10. _____

11. _____

12. _____

13. _____

14. _____

15. _____

16. _____

17. _____

18. _____

19. _____

20. _____

21. _____

22. _____

23. _____

24. _____

25. _____

26. _____

27. _____

28. _____

29. _____

30. _____

31. _____

32. _____

33. _____

34. _____

35. _____

36. _____

37. _____

38. _____

39. _____

40. _____

41. _____

42. _____

43. _____

44. _____

45. _____

46. _____

47. _____

48. _____

49. _____

50. _____

51. _____

52. _____

53. _____

EXERCISE 7

Fill in the following blanks with the requested information.

1. _____ is a division within the laboratory that performs diagnostic tests on blood components. _____ and

   _____ are two tests performed in this laboratory division whose results yield RBC information.

2. The coronary care unit (CCU) in the hospital is an intensive care unit set up to care for patients who have had heart attacks. The admitting diagnosis of these patients may be:

   a. _____

   b. _____

   c. _____

3. Below is a list of medical terms. Circle the terms that may be found on the surgical schedule. Underline the part of the word that makes it a surgical procedure.

   cardiology   hemorrhoidectomy

   electroencephalogram   hypertension

   endocarditis   splenectomy

4. A doctor who performs surgery on the heart or blood vessels may be called a _____ surgeon.

5. A patient is having symptoms that indicate a disease or complication involving the circulatory system. The attending doctor is a good practitioner. He wishes the patient to see a heart specialist. He will contact a

   _____.

6. Each hospital has a team of people to call for emergency conditions such as sudden stoppage of the heart or

   _____. This team may be called the

   _____ team.

7. The doctor orders a diagnostic procedure to record the electrical activity of the heart. He or she orders a(n)

   _____. The technician brings a(n)

   _____ (machine) to the patient's bedside to perform this test.

8. The patient is scheduled for an x-ray image of the blood vessels to be visualized by the use of dye as a contrast medium. The patient is scheduled for a(n)

   _____.

9. The patient is scheduled for a diagnostic test that uses dye as a contrast medium to visualize parts of the heart. A long catheter is threaded from a blood vessel to the heart.

   _____ is the name of this test.

10. Below are listed three types of blood cells. Look under "Doctors' Orders for Hematology Studies" on p. 269. Write the name of the laboratory test used to study each cell listed below:

    a. leukocyte _____

    b. erythrocyte _____

    c. platelet _____

11. _____ is the clear, fluid portion of the blood that may be ordered by the doctor to be administered intravenously to the patient.

UNIT 7

The Digestive System

Unit Objectives

Upon completion of this unit, you will be able to:

1. Define the overall functions of the digestive system.
2. Name and describe the functions of the organs of the digestive system.
3. Name the digestive enzymes.
4. Trace the passage of food through the digestive tract.
5. Name the five sphincters of the digestive tract.
6. List the accessory organs to the digestive tract and tell how each contributes to the digestive process.
7. Describe peptic ulcer, diverticular disease, gallstones, and pyloric stenosis.

■ ORGANS OF THE DIGESTIVE SYSTEM

Digestive Tract

Mouth
Pharynx
Digestive sphincter muscles
Esophagus
Stomach
Small intestine
Large intestine

Accessory Organs

Salivary glands
Teeth and tongue
Liver
Gallbladder
Pancreas

The accessory organs play a vital role in the digestive process. Although food does not pass through the salivary glands, liver, gall bladder, or pancreas, these organs provide secretions necessary for the chemical digestion of food.

Functions of the Digestive System

Ingestion: Taking nutrients into the digestive tract through the mouth.
Digestion: The mechanical and chemical breakdown of food for use by the body cells.
Absorption: The transfer of digested food from the small intestine to the bloodstream.
Elimination: The removal of solid waste from the body.

Food passes through a long tubular structure called the *digestive tract* (also called the *alimentary canal* and the *gastrointestinal (GI) tract*, which extends from the mouth to the rectum. Along the way food is prepared for absorption by the organs of the digestive tract and the accessory organs. The waste material—that material that is not transferred to the bloodstream during absorption—is eliminated from the body. Ingestion, digestion, absorption, and elimination are the main functions of the digestive system.

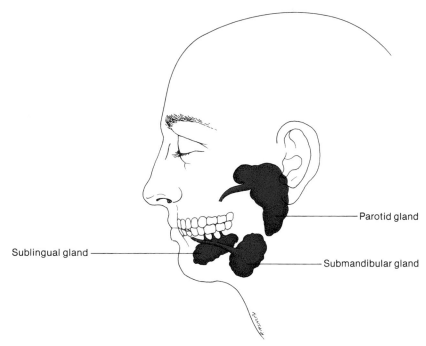

Sublingual gland

Parotid gland

Submandibular gland

FIGURE 23-23 ▲ The salivary glands.

■ THE DIGESTIVE TRACT

Mouth

In the mouth the chewing of food, or *mastication*, starts the mechanical breakdown of food necessary for *metabolism*, the utilization of digested food by body cells. The tongue helps guide the food to the teeth where mechanical digestion begins. The salivary glands (Fig. 23–23) produce saliva that contains the enzyme amylase. This enzyme starts the chemical breakdown of carbohydrates (starches and sugars). The three pairs of salivary glands are:

1. *Parotid,* the largest, located near the ear
2. *Submandibular,* located near the lower jaw
3. *Sublingual,* the smallest, located under the tongue

Each salivary gland has a duct (canal) that opens into the mouth to allow for the flow of saliva.

Pharynx

The *pharynx* (throat) allows for the passage of food from the mouth to the esophagus and is about 5 inches long (12.5 cm). The pharynx is shared with the respiratory tract, because it is also used for the passage of air. The epiglottis, a flexible flap of cartilage, prevents food from entering the respiratory system.

Digestive Sphincter Muscles

Sphincters, circular muscles that close or open a natural body opening, regulate the passage of substances. The arrangement of the circular fibers creates a central opening when relaxed and a closure when they are contracted. There are five sphincter muscles along the digestive tract. These digestive sphincters are called *upper esophageal, lower esophageal (cardiac), pyloric, ileocecal,* and *anal* sphincters.

Esophagus

The *esophagus* is a muscular tube that extends from the pharynx to the stomach. It passes through the thoracic cavity, behind the heart, to the abdominal cavity. The esophagus is approximately 9 inches (22.5 cm) long. Its function is simply the passage of food, which is propelled along by involuntary wavelike movements; this action is called *peristalsis.* The movement of food into and out of the esophagus is regulated by an upper esophageal sphincter and the lower esophageal (cardiac) sphincter, located between the esophagus and the stomach.

Stomach

The stomach is located in the upper left portion of the abdomen, below the diaphragm. It is a container for food during part of the digestive process. Gastric glands located in the mucous membrane lining of the stomach secrete enzymes (lipase and pepsin) and hydrochloric acid. These secretions continue the chemical breakdown of food. The muscles of the stomach are circular, diagonal and longitudinal. This muscular construction of the stomach makes the organ very strong (Fig. 23–24). The function of the stomach is to secrete the enzymes, mix, and churn the food to a liquid consistency. This process of mixing and churning continues the mechanical breakdown of food. When the food is liquefied it is referred to as chyme.

After about 30 minutes the food begins to leave the stomach at 30-minute intervals. It passes through the pyloric sphincter muscle into the duodenum, which is the first part of the small intestine. It takes 2 to 4 hours for the stomach to empty completely.

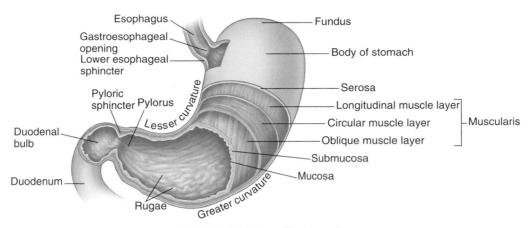

FIGURE 23-24 ▲ The stomach.

Small Intestine

The small intestine, so called because it is smaller in diameter than the large intestine, is approximately 20 feet long. It extends from the stomach to the large intestine (Fig. 23–25). The first part of the small intestine is called the *duodenum*. Two accessory organs, the *pancreas* and the *gallbladder*, secrete into the duodenum through tiny tubes called *ducts*. The pancreas secretes enzymes. The gallbladder secretes bile that has been produced by the liver and stored in the gallbladder. The *jejunum*, followed by

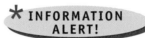

INFORMATION ALERT!

Pathway: Food ingestion → mouth → esophagus → cardiac sphincter → stomach → pyloric sphincter → small intestine (duodenum, jejunum, ileum) → nutrients absorption by the blood and carried to all cells for metabolism waste → ileocecal sphincter → large intestine (cecum, ascending colon, transverse colon, descending colon, sigmoid colon, rectum) → anal sphincter → elimination

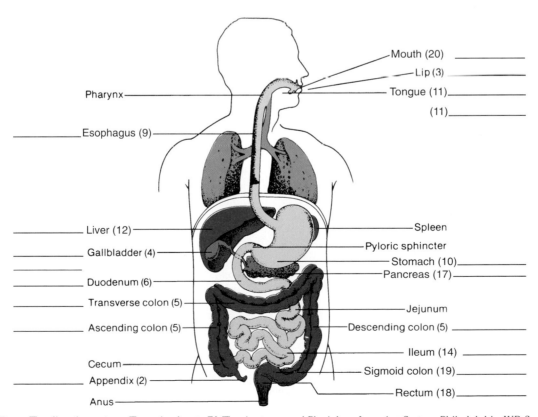

FIGURE 23-25 ▲ The digestive system. (From Applegate EJ: The Anatomy and Physiology Learning System, Philadelphia: W.B. Saunders, 1995, with permission.)

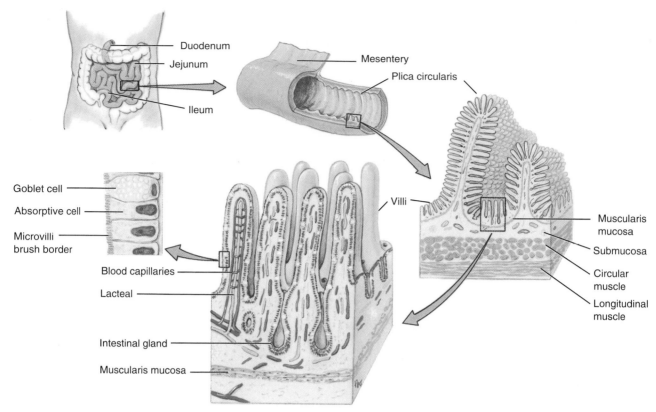

FIGURE 23–26 ▲ Intestinal villi. (From Applegate EJ: The Anatomy and Physiology Learning System, Philadelphia: W.B. Saunders, 1995, with permission.)

the *ileum,* forms the remainder of the small intestine. (The ilium, part of the pelvic bone studied in the musculoskeletal system, has the same pronunciation as ileum. Correct spelling of the word to communicate the proper meaning is absolutely essential.) The mucosal cells located in the lining of the small intestine secrete enzymes that continue the chemical breakdown of food. Some of these enzymes are sucrase, maltase, lipase, peptidase, and lactase. Digestion is completed in the small intestine and absorption takes place here.

Absorption is the passage of the end products of digestion from the small intestine into the bloodstream. The passage of nutrients from the small intestine to the bloodstream is facilitated through the capillary walls of the villi, which have a surface area of approximately 100 square feet. The *villi,* tiny fingerlike projections that line the walls of the small intestine (Fig. 23–26), increase the surface area of the small intestine to make it the main site of digestion and absorption. The blood carries the nutrients to all body cells, where they are used according to need. The process of cell utilization of nutrients is called *metabolism.*

The food substance (waste) that is not absorbed continues to move by peristalsis through the ileocecal sphincter into the large intestine.

Large Intestine

The large intestine is approximately 5 feet long. Peristalsis continues into the large intestine. The large intestine extends from the ileum to the *anus,* the opening at the end of the rectum to the outside. The large intestine is divided into the following parts, listed in sequence extending from the ileum: the *cecum;* the

colon, which is divided into four parts—the ascending colon, the transverse colon, the descending colon, and the sigmoid colon— and the *rectum.* The function of the large intestine is the absorption of water and the elimination of the solid waste products of digestion from the body.

The appendix is a small blind tube attached to the cecum. It has no function.

Accessory Organs: Liver, Gallbladder, and Pancreas

The liver, the largest gland in the body, is located in the upper right portion of the abdominal cavity. Although it has many important functions, we will discuss only one, the production of bile. The liver secretes bile, which aids in the digestion of fats. Bile is stored in the gallbladder, a small sac located under the liver. The gallbladder concentrates the bile by reabsorbing water. When food enters the duodenum from the stomach, the gallbladder is stimulated to contract and release bile into the duodenum.

The pancreas is located behind the stomach. Part of its function is to secrete the enzymes lipase, protease, amylase, and bicarbonate into the duodenum. These enzymes continue the digestion process by chemically breaking down the food particles. The islets of Langerhans are contained in the pancreas. They secrete two hormones—glucagon and insulin—which are released directly into the bloodstream. Insulin is necessary for the metabolism of carbohydrates in the body and decreases blood glucose levels. Glucagon, also instrumental in digestion, increases glucose.

■ DISEASES AND CONDITIONS OF THE DIGESTIVE SYSTEM

Gastritis and Peptic Ulcer Disease

A peptic ulcer is a lesion, or sore, of the mucous membrane of the stomach (gastric ulcer), or duodenum (duodenal ulcer) (Fig. 23–27). A combination of factors causes peptic ulcer disease (PUD), including excessive secretion of gastric enzymes, hydrochloric acid, *Helicobacter pylori*, heredity, and taking certain drugs, especially nonsteroidal antiinflammatory drugs (NSAIDs).

Symptoms include pain 1 to 3 hours after eating, which is usually relieved by eating or taking antacids. Also a gnawing sensation in the epigastric region is experienced. If untreated, bleeding, hemorrhage, or perforation may occur. Perforation allows the contents of the stomach or small intestine to escape into the peritoneal cavity. The GI series, gastroscopy, and gastric analysis are used for diagnosing peptic ulcers. Because symptoms of peptic ulcer are similar to symptoms of stomach or duodenal cancer, early diagnosis is important. Early treatment includes diet control, medication, and if present, eradication of *H. pylori* bacteria with antibiotics. Surgery may be indicated when there is scarring, recurrent bleeding, or perforation.

Diverticular Disease

Diverticular disease is caused by the forming of small pouches, called *diverticula,* on the large intestine wall, generally the colon (Fig. 23–28). There are two forms of diverticular disease: diverticulosis and diverticulitis. In diverticulosis, diverticula are present but for most people cause no symptoms. In diverticulitis, the diverticula are inflamed or infected and may cause obstruction, infection, or hemorrhage.

Symptoms include cramping in the abdomen and muscle spasms. Medical treatment includes eating a high-fiber or re-

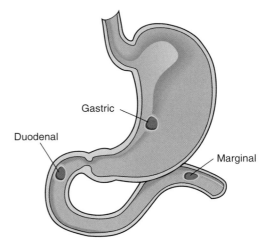

FIGURE 23–27 ▲ Types of ulcers.

stricted diet and taking antibiotics to treat infection. Severe cases may require surgical removal of the involved segment of the intestine and a temporary colostomy (surgical opening between the colon and the body surface).

Cholelithiasis and Choledocholithiasis

Cholelithiasis, or *gallstones,* a common condition affecting 20% of the population over 40 years of age, is more common in women than men (Fig. 23–29). The stones form because of changes in the bile content. Gallstones can lodge in the common bile duct, which leads to the duodenum. This condition is called choledocholithiasis. Pain is caused by pressure building up in the gallbladder.

Symptoms of a typical gallbladder attack include acute abdominal pain after eating a fatty meal. Sometimes the pain is so severe the patient may seek emergency treatment. Other symptoms are digestive disturbances, such as belching and flatulence.

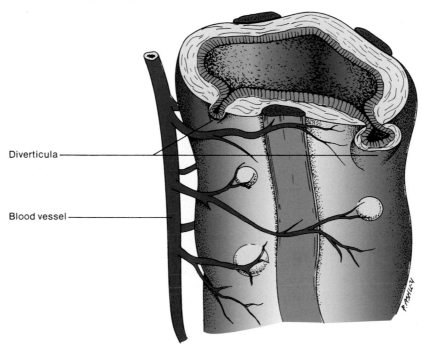

FIGURE 23–28 ▲ Diverticula.

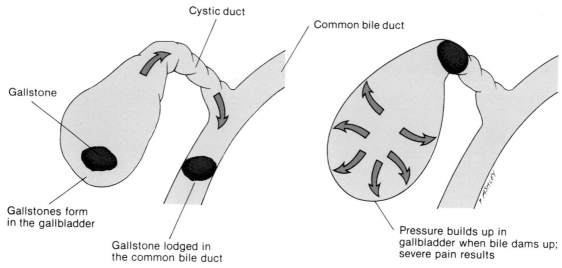

Cystic duct

Common bile duct

Gallstone

Gallstones form in the gallbladder

Gallstone lodged in the common bile duct

Pressure builds up in gallbladder when bile dams up; severe pain results

FIGURE 23–29 ▲ Gallstones.

A cholecystogram or abdominal ultrasound is used for diagnosing gallstones. Treatment includes laparoscopic cholecystectomy and choledocholithotomy.

Pyloric Stenosis

Pyloric stenosis is an obstruction caused by narrowing of the pyloric sphincter muscle. The condition may be congenital or acquired. In adults the condition is most often caused by peptic ulceration or tumors that may be cancerous. Symptoms include vomiting that becomes progressively more frequent and forceful. Infants with pyloric stenosis may at first be diagnosed with failure to thrive. Adults will experience a gradual weight loss.

Diagnosis is confirmed by an upper gastrointestinal examination using barium as a contrast medium. Treatment is usually surgical. In infants a formula that is thickened with cereal may be enough to stretch out the sphincter muscle if the stenosis is not severe.

REVIEW QUESTIONS

1. Define:

   a. ingestion _____

   b. digestion _____

   c. absorption _____

   d. elimination _____

2. Describe the overall function of the digestive system.

   _____

   _____

3. Beginning with the mouth, list in order the organs that food passes through during ingestion, digestion, and elimination. Include the names of the parts of the small intestine, large intestine, and the sphincter muscles.

   _____

   _____

   _____

4. List the digestive enzymes, the organs that secrete the digestive enzymes, and the digestive organ in which they perform their functions.

Name of Digestive Enzyme	Organ of Secretion	Organ of Function
a. _____	_____	_____
b. _____	_____	_____
c. _____	_____	_____
d. _____	_____	_____
e. _____	_____	_____

5. Name the six accessory organs of digestion.

a. _____   d. _____

b. _____   e. _____

c. _____   f. _____

6. A narrowing of the opening between the stomach and the small intestine is called:

_____

7. Describe the function of the following organs in the digestive process:

a. mouth _____

b. stomach _____

c. small intestine _____

d. large intestine _____

e. gallbladder _____

8. Match the terms in Column 1 with the definitions in Column 2.

Column 1	Column 2
a. diverticulitis	_____ 1. lesion of the mucous membrane of the stomach
b. cholelithiasis	_____ 2. inflamed diverticula
c. cholecystectomy	_____ 3. stones in the gallbladder
d. diverticulosis	_____ 4. stone in the common bile duct
e. peptic ulcer	_____ 5. diverticula with no symptoms
f. choledocholithiasis	

■ MEDICAL TERMINOLOGY RELATING TO THE DIGESTIVE SYSTEM

Upon mastery of the medical terminology for this unit, you will be able to:

1. Spell and define the word parts and medical terms for the digestive system.

2. Given the meaning of a medical condition relating to the digestive tract, build with word parts the corresponding medical terms.

3. Given a list of medical terms, identify those that are surgical procedures and those that are diagnostic studies.

4. Compare the three *-tomy* suffixes.

5. Analyze and define medical terms, built from word parts that relate to the digestive system.

6. Given a description of hospital situations in which the health unit coordinator may encounter medical terminology, apply the correct medical terms to the situations described.

Word Parts

The list below contains the word parts you need to memorize for the digestive system. The exercises included in this unit will help you with this task. You will continue to use these word parts throughout this course and during your employment. Practice pronouncing each part aloud.

Word Roots/Combining Forms	Meaning
1. abdomin/o (ăb-dŏm′-ĭ-nō)	abdomen
2. appendic/o (ăp-ĕn-dĕk′-ō)	appendix
3. cheil/o (kī′-lō)	lip
4. chol/o (kō′-lō) or chol/e (kō′-lē)	bile, gall
5. col/o (kō′-lō)	colon
6. cyst/o (sĭs′-tō)	bladder (urinary unless otherwise used)
7. duoden/o (doo-ō-dē′-nō)	duodenum
8. enter/o (ĕn′-ter-ō)	intestine
9. esophag/o (ĕ-sŏf′-ah-gō)	esophagus
10. gastr/o (găs′-trō)	stomach
11. gloss/o (glŏss′-ō); lingu/o (lĭng′-gwō)	tongue
12. hepat/o (hĕp′-a-tō)	liver
13. herni/o (her′-nē-ō)	protrusion of a body part
14. ile/o (ĭl′ĕ-ō)	ileum
15. lapar/o (lăp′-ah-rō)	abdomen
16. lith/o (lĭth′-ō)	stone or calculus
17. pancreat/o (păn′-krē-ă-tō)	pancreas
18. proct/o (prŏk′-tō)	rectum
19. sigmoid/o (sĭg′-moy-dō)	sigmoid colon (part of the colon)
20. stomat/o (stō′-mah-tō)	mouth

Suffixes	Meaning
-iasis (ī′-ah-sĭs)	condition of
-stomy (ŏs′-tō-mē)	creation of an artificial opening into

-tomy Suffixes

You are already familiar with two *-tomy* suffixes that are used to describe surgical procedures. They are *-tomy*, which means incision into a part of the body, and *-ectomy*, which means surgical removal of a part of the body. The third *-tomy* suffix you will study in this unit is *-stomy*, which describes a surgical procedure performed to create an artificial opening into a part of the body. For example, in the medical term *colostomy* (col/o is the combining form for colon), a portion of the colon is attached to the surface of the abdomen, which creates an artificial opening between the colon and the abdominal surface (Fig. 23–30). This artificial opening is used for the passage of stools.

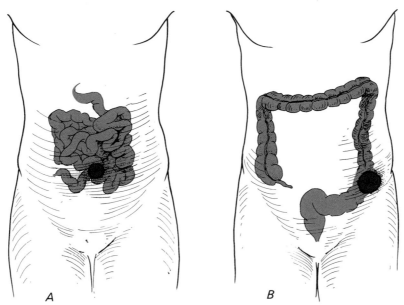

FIGURE 23–30 ▲ *A*, Ileostomy. *B*, Colostomy. (From LaFleur M: Exploring Medical Language, 5th ed. St. Louis: Mosby, 2002, p. 399.)

EXERCISE 1

Write the combining forms for the digestive system in the spaces provided on the diagram in Figure 23–25 (page 521). The number preceding the combining form in the preceding list matches the number of the body part in the diagram.

EXERCISE 2

Define the word parts listed below. Indicate the word parts that are suffixes by writing *S* after each in the space provided.

Word Parts	Definition	Suffix?
1. stomat		
2. gloss		
3. gastr		
4. proct		
5. pancreat		
6. enter		
7. hepat		
8. cheil		
9. esophag		

10. iasis   _____   _____

11. chol   _____   _____

12. cyst   _____   _____

13. duoden   _____   _____

14. col   _____   _____

15. ile   _____   _____

16. abdomin   _____   _____

17. appendic   _____   _____

18. lapar   _____   _____

19. lith   _____   _____

20. stomy   _____   _____

21. herni   _____   _____

22. sigmoid   _____   _____

EXERCISE 3

Define the three -*tomy* suffixes. Build a medical term using each suffix and write the meaning of each term you have built.

1. -*tomy*

_____

2. -*ectomy*

_____

3. -*stomy*

_____

■ MEDICAL TERMS RELATING TO THE DIGESTIVE SYSTEM

The following is a list made up of medical terms you will need to know for the digestive system. Exercises following this list will assist you in learning these terms. Practice pronouncing each term aloud.

General Terms	Meaning
abdominal (ăb-dŏm'-ĭn-al)	pertaining to the abdomen
diarrhea (dī'-ah-rē'-ah)	frequent discharge of watery stool
duodenal (doo-ō-dē'-nal)	pertaining to the duodenum
dysentery (dĭs'-ĕn-tĕr-ē)	condition of bad or painful intestines accompanied by diarrhea
glossoplegia (glŏss-ō-plē'-jē-ah)	paralysis of the tongue
hepatoma (hĕp-ah-tō'-mah)	a tumor of the liver
hepatomegaly (hĕp'-ah-tō-mĕg'-ah-lē)	enlargement of the liver
hernia (her'-nē-ah)	an abnormal protrusion of a body part through the containing structure
jaundice (jawn'-dĭs)	yellowness of the skin and eyes; a symptom of hepatitis
pancreatic (păn-krē-ăt'-ĭk)	pertaining to the pancreas
proctorrhea (prŏk-tō-rē'-ah)	excessive discharge from the rectum
stomatogastric (stō'-mah-tō-găs'-trĭk)	pertaining to the mouth and stomach
sublingual (sŭb-lĭng'-gwal)	pertaining to under the tongue
ulcer (ŭl'-ser)	a sore of the skin or mucous membrane

Surgical Terms	Meaning
abdominal herniorrhaphy (ăb-dŏm'-ĭn-al) (her-nē-ōr'-ah-fē)	suturing of a weak spot or opening in the abdominal wall to prevent protrusion of organs
appendectomy (ăp-ĕn-dĕk'-tō-mē)	excision of the appendix
cheiloplasty (kī'-lō-plăs-tē)	surgical repair of the lip
cholecystectomy (kō-lē-sĭs-tĕk'-tō-mē) Note: e is used as the combining vowel between the word roots *chol* and *cyst*	excision of the gallbladder
colectomy (kō-lĕk'-tō-mē)	excision of the colon
colostomy (kō-lŏs'-tō-mē)	creation of an artificial opening into the colon; a portion of the colon is attached to the surface of the abdomen for the passage of stools
esophagoenterostomy (ē-sŏf'-ah-gō-ĕn-ter-ŏs'-tō-mē)	creation of an artificial opening between the esophagus and the intestine
gastrectomy (găs-trĕk'-tō-mē); pyloroplasty (pī-lōr'-ō-plăs-tē); and vagotomy (vă-gŏt'-ō-mē)	a surgical procedure performed for treatment of ulcers; gastrectomy is the removal of the stomach; pyloroplasty is the plastic repair of the pyloric sphincter, located at the lower end of the stomach; vagotomy is the incision into the vagus nerve, performed to reduce the amount of gastric juices in the stomach
gastric bypass—malabsorptive	surgical procedure for obesity in which a small pouch is created at the top of the stomach to restrict food intake.
gastrostomy (găs-trŏs'-tō-mē)	creation of an artificial opening into the stomach (for feeding purposes)
glossorrhaphy (glŏ-sŏr'-ah-fē)	suturing of the tongue
herniorrhaphy (her-nē-ōr'-ah-fē)	surgical repair of a hernia (suturing of the containing structure, e.g., the abdominal wall)
ileostomy (ĭl-ē-ŏs'-tō-mē)	creation of artificial opening into the ileum; a portion of the ileum is attached to the surface of the abdomen for passage of stools
laparotomy (lăp-ah-rŏt'-ō-mē)	incision into the abdominal wall

Diagnostic Terms	Meaning
appendicitis (ah-pĕn-dĭ-sī'-tĭs)	inflammation of the appendix
cholecystitis (kō-lē-sĭs-tī'-tĭs)	inflammation of the gallbladder
cholelithiasis (kō-lē-lĭ-thī'-ah-sĭs) Note: e is used as the combining vowel between the word roots *chol* and *lith*	a condition of gallstones
Crohn's (krōnz) disease	chronic inflammatory disease that can affect any part of the bowel, most often the lower small intestine
diverticulitis (dī-ver-tĭk-ū-lī'-tĭs)	inflammation of the diverticula (small pouches in the intestinal wall)
duodenal ulcer (dū-ō-dē'-nal) (ŭl'-sĕr)	ulcer (sore open area) in the duodenum
gastric ulcer (găs'-trĭk) (ŭl'-ser)	ulcer pertaining to the stomach

Diagnostic Terms (cont'd)	Meaning
gastritis (găs-trī′-tĭs)	inflammation of the stomach
hepatitis (hĕp-ah-tī′-tĭs)	inflammation of the liver
ileitis (ĭl-ē-ī′-tĭs)	inflammation of the ileum
infectious hepatitis (ĭn-fĕk′-shŭs) (hĕp-ah-tī′-tĭs)	inflammation of the liver (caused by a virus)
pancreatitis (păn-krē-ah-tī′-tĭs)	inflammation of the pancreas
stomatitis (stŏ-mah-tī′-tĭs)	inflammation of the mouth
ulcerative colitis (ul′-sĕ-rā-tĭv) (kō-lī′-tĭs)	inflammation of the colon with the formation of ulcers

Terms Related to Diagnostic Procedures	Meaning
abdominocentesis (ăb-dŏm′-ĭ-nō-sĕn-tē′-sĭs)	aspiration of fluid from the abdominal cavity
barium enema (BE) (bă′-rē-ŭm) (ĕn′-ĕ-mah)	x-ray of the colon (fasting x-ray); barium is used as the contrast medium
cholangiogram (kō-lăn′-jē-ŏ-grăm)	x-ray image of the bile ducts (fasting x-ray), usually done after a cholecystectomy; dye is the contrast medium
cholecystogram (kō-lē-sĭs′-tō-grăm)	x-ray image of the gallbladder (fasting x-ray), also known as a GB series; dye is used as the contrast medium
colonoscopy (kō-lŏn-ŏs′-kō-pē)	visual examination of the colon
colonoscope (kō-lŏn′-ō-skōp)	instrument used for visual examination of the colon
esophagogastroduodenoscopy (EGD) (ĕ-sŏf′-ah-gō-doo-odd-ĕn-ŏs′-kō-pē)	visual examination of the esophagus, stomach, and duodenum
esophagoscope (ĕ-sŏf′-ah-gō-skōp)	instrument used for the visual examination of the esophagus
esophagoscopy (ĕ-sŏf′-ah-gŏs′-kō-pē)	visual examination of the esophagus
gastroscope (găs′-trō-skōp)	instrument used for the visual examination of the stomach
gastroscopy (găs-trŏs′-kō-pē)	visual examination of the stomach
proctoscope (prŏk′-tō-skōp)	instrument used for the visual examination of the rectum
proctoscopy (prŏk-tŏs′-kō-pē)	visual examination of the rectum
sigmoidoscopy (sĭg-mol-dŏs′-kŏ-pē)	visual examination of the sigmoid colon
upper gastrointestinal (UGI) (găs′-trō-ĭn-tĕs′-tĭ-nal)	x-ray of the esophagus and the stomach (fasting x-ray); barium is used as the contrast medium; UGI with small-bowel follow-through is an x-ray of the stomach and small intestines

EXERCISE 4

Analyze and define the terms listed below.

1. glossoplegia

2. appendectomy

3. cholecystectomy

4. gastrostomy

5. hepatomegaly

6. ileostomy

7. pyloroplasty

8. protorrhea

9. cholecystitis

10. gastritis

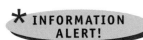

Scope It Out

Modern medical advances and surgical innovation have paved the way for a growing number of minimally invasive surgeries. From appendectomies and blepharoplasty (cosmetic repair of eyelids) to cardiac and foot surgery, the thin, flexible tube with a small video camera and a light on the end is able to penetrate organs, joints, and cavities; diagnose and correct various conditions; and record the episode at the same time. Local or general anesthesia may be used during the procedure. Frequently, conscious sedation is administered, using a combination of sedatives and pain relievers to achieve an altered state of consciousness. Typically, most endoscopies are performed on an outpatient basis.

The expanding use of the fiberoptic endoscope beyond the digestive system is responsible for smaller incisions, shorter recovery time, and lower medical costs. Nearly all specialties are making use of endoscopy as a more efficient means of diagnostic and therapeutic intervention.

The endoscope, an instrument used for visual examination within a hollow organ or body cavity, is introduced through a small incision. Through a separate small incision, tiny folding surgical instruments are introduced (e.g., forceps, scissors, brushes, snares, and baskets for tissue excision) and manipulated within the tissue.

Arthroscopy: Visual examination of joints for diagnosis and treatment.

Bronchoscopy: Examination of the trachea and lung's bronchial trees to diagnose abscesses, bronchitis, carcinoma, tumors, tuberculosis, alveolitis, infection, inflammation.

Colonoscopy: Examination of the inside of the colon and large intestine to detect polyps, tumors, ulceration, inflammation, colitis diverticula, Crohn's disease, and discovery and removal of foreign bodies.

Colposcopy: Direct visualization of the vagina and cervix to detect cancer, inflammation, and other conditions.

Cystoscopy: Examination of the bladder, urethra, urinary tract, ureteral orifices, and prostate (men) with insertion of the endoscope through the urethra.

Esophagogastroduodenoscopy (EGD): Visual examination of the upper gastrointestinal (GI) tract (also referred to as gastroscopy) to diagnose hemorrhage, hiatal hernia, inflammation of the esophagus, and gastric ulcers.

Endoscopic biopsy: Removal of tissue specimens for pathologic examination and analysis.

Endoscopic laser foraminoplasty: With the use of an endoscope and a laser to create an opening through the foramen (itself an opening) into the epidural space, the endoscopic surgeon can visualize the nerves in the spinal column to repair ruptured or herniated discs.

Endoscopic retrograde cholangiopancreatography (ERCP): Makes use of the endoscope for radiographic examination with contrast medium introduced through a catheter. The endoscopist will visualize the liver's biliary tree, the gallbladder, the pancreatic duct, and other nearby anatomy to check for stones, obstructions, and disease. Fluoroscopic x-ray images are taken to show any abnormality or blockage. If disease is detected, it can sometimes be treated at the same time or biopsy can be performed to test for cancer or other pathological conditions. ERCP may reveal biliary cirrhosis, cancer of the bile ducts, pancreatic cysts, pseudocysts, pancreatic tumors, chronic pancreatitis, and gallbladder stones.

Gastroscopy: Examination of the lining of the esophagus, stomach, and duodenum. Gastroscopy is often used to diagnose ulcers and other sources of bleeding and to guide the biopsy of suspect GI cancers.

Hysteroscopy: Visual examination of the uterus.

Laparoscopy: Visual examination of the abdominal cavity: stomach, liver, and other abdominal organs including the female reproductive organs (e.g., the fallopian tubes, uterus, and ovaries).

- Laparoscopic adrenalectomy
- Laparoscopic appendectomy
- Laparoscopic choledochoscopy and choledocholithotomy
- Laparoscopic cholecystectomy
- Laparoscopic tubal ligation

Laryngoscopy: Visual examination of the larynx (voice box).

Proctoscopy, proctosigmoidoscopy, sigmoidoscopy: Visual examination of the rectum and sigmoid colon.

Thoracoscopy: Visual examination of the thorax (chest: pleura [sac that covers the lungs], pleural spaces, mediastinum, and pericardium).

---

11. sublingual

_____

12. ileitis

_____

13. cholecystogram

_____

14. sigmoidoscopy

_____

15. gastrectomy

_____

16. gastroscopy

_____

17. gastroscope

_____

18. colitis

_____

19. hepatitis

_____

20. colostomy

_____

21. herniorrhaphy

_____

22. colonoscope

_____

23. colonoscopy

_____

24. esophagogastroduodenoscopy

_____

EXERCISE 5

Using the word parts studied in this unit and previous units, build medical terms from the definitions listed below. Also, identify which are surgical procedures by writing *S* in the space provided, and which are diagnostic studies by writing *D* in the space provided. Underline the word part that indicates that the word is a surgical procedure or a diagnostic study. (Note: Some words in the list will not fall into either of these categories.)

Examples: gastr<u>ectomy</u>   S
          gastro<u>scopy</u>   D

 1. inflammation of the mouth

 2. inflammation of the gallbladder

 3. a condition of gallstones

 4. x-ray image of the gallbladder

 5. excision of the gallbladder

 6. inflammation of the pancreas

 7. instrument used for visual examination of the rectum

 8. visual examination of the rectum

 9. aspiration of fluid from the abdominal cavity

10. creation of an artificial opening into the colon

11. creation of an artificial opening into the ileum

12. visual examination of the esophagus

13. instrument used for visual examination of the stomach

14. creation of an artificial opening between the esophagus and the intestines

15. inflammation of the stomach

16. suturing of the tongue

17. surgical repair of the lip

18. excision of the colon

19. paralysis of the tongue

20. pertaining to the mouth and stomach

21. pertaining to under the tongue

22. discharge from the rectum

23. enlargement of the liver

24. tumor of the liver

25. pertaining to the pancreas

26. inflammation of the appendix

27. surgical removal of the appendix

28. visual examination of the colon

29. instrument used for visual examination of the colon

30. visual examination of the esophagus, stomach, and duodenum

EXERCISE 6

Define the following medical terms:

1. *dysentery*

2. *upper gastrointestinal (UGI)*

3. *barium enema*

4. *cholecystogram*

5. jaundice

_____

6. ulcerative colitis

_____

7. gastric ulcer

_____

8. Crohn's disease

_____

EXERCISE 7

Spell each medical term studied in this unit by having someone dictate the terms to you.

1. _____
2. _____
3. _____
4. _____
5. _____
6. _____
7. _____
8. _____
9. _____
10. _____
11. _____
12. _____
13. _____
14. _____
15. _____
16. _____
17. _____
18. _____

19. _____
20. _____
21. _____
22. _____
23. _____
24. _____
25. _____
26. _____
27. _____
28. _____
29. _____
30. _____
31. _____
32. _____
33. _____
34. _____
35. _____
36. _____
37. _____
38. _____
39. _____
40. _____
41. _____
42. _____
43. _____
44. _____
45. _____
46. _____
47. _____
48. _____
49. _____

50. _____

51. _____

52. _____

53. _____

54. _____

55. _____

56. _____

57. _____

58. _____

59. _____

EXERCISE 8

Answer the following questions.

1. A surgical procedure to make an artificial opening from the small intestine to the abdomen is listed on the surgery schedule. Circle the correct surgical term for this procedure and explain your choice:
   a. iliostomy
   b. ileostomy
   c. ileotomy

   _____

   _____

2. A patient enters the hospital with a diagnosis of gallstones. The admitting diagnosis in medical terms will be

   _____ . The doctor orders a diagnostic study to visualize the gallbladder to determine the presence of disease or gallstones. He or she orders a

   _____ . The result of the diagnostic study indicates surgery for the removal of the gallbladder. The medical term for this operation

   is _____ .

3. The doctor orders a medication to be administered under the patient's tongue. _____ is the word written on the doctors' order sheet to indicate this.

4. List three visual examinations the doctor may order on the digestive tract and name the instrument used for each examination.

   a. _____

   b. _____

   c. _____

5. A patient enters the hospital with an admitting diagnosis of abdominal pain. The doctor orders two x-rays, one of the stomach and small intestine, and one of the colon. He or she orders a _____ and a

   _____ . Surgery is indicated. The doctor plans to remove the stomach, repair the pyloric sphincter, and make an incision into the vagus nerve. The medical terms used to describe the surgery are:

   a. _____

   b. _____

   c. _____

6. The following surgical procedures are listed on the surgical schedule, and you are preparing consent forms for them. Circle the terms that are spelled incorrectly, and correctly spell the misspelled terms in the space provided.

   a. laportotomy _____

   b. appendectomy _____

   c. herniorraphy _____

   d. collectomy _____

   e. gastrostomy _____

UNIT 8

The Respiratory System

Unit Objectives

Upon completion of this unit, you will be able to:

1. Describe the overall function of the respiratory system.

2. Name and locate the organs of the respiratory system and tell the function of each.

3. Compare internal respiration with external respiration.

4. Describe the pathway of air from the outside to the capillary blood in the lungs.

5. Describe pneumothorax, hemothorax, pulmonary embolism, and chronic obstructive pulmonary disease (COPD).

■ THE RESPIRATORY SYSTEM

Organs of the Respiratory System

Nose
Pharynx
Larynx
Trachea
Bronchi
Lungs

Division of the Respiratory System

The upper respiratory system refers to the nose, nasal cavities, sinuses, pharynx, and larynx. The lower respiratory system refers to the trachea, bronchi, alveoli, and lungs (Fig. 23–31).

Function of the Respiratory System

The function of the respiratory system is to exchange gases. Oxygen is taken into the body and carbon dioxide is removed. This process is referred to as *respiration*. The respiratory system also helps to regulate the acid–base balance and produce vocal sounds.

Respiration

External respiration, or breathing, is the exchange of gases between the lungs and the blood. Oxygen is inhaled into the lungs and passes through the capillary wall into the blood to be carried to the blood cells. Carbon dioxide passes out of the capillary blood to the lungs to be exhaled to the outside environment.

The exchange of gases also takes place within the body between the blood in the capillaries and individual body cells. This is called *internal respiration*. The body cells take on the oxygen from the blood and at the same time give off carbon dioxide to the blood to be transported back to the lungs, where it is exhaled from the body.

The Nose

Air enters the respiratory system through the nose. The nose is divided into a right and left nostril by a partition called the *nasal septum*. The nose prepares the air for the body by (1) warming and moistening the air, (2) removing pathogenic microorganisms, and (3) removing foreign particles, such as dust, from the air. Tiny, hairlike growths in the nose called *cilia* trap and move the foreign particles toward the outside and away from delicate lung tissue. Particles too large to be handled by the *cilia* produce a sneeze or cough, which forcibly expels the foreign particles.

The Pharynx

Both air and food travel through the *pharynx* (throat). The food passes from the pharynx to the esophagus, while the air passes from the pharynx into the larynx, which is located anterior to the esophagus.

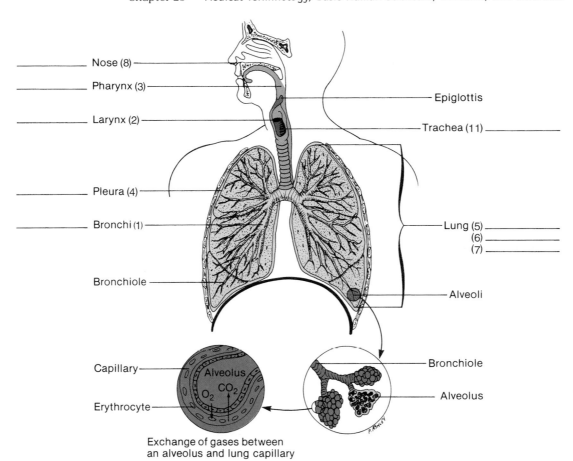

Nose (8)
Pharynx (3)
Larynx (2)
Pleura (4)
Bronchi (1)
Bronchiole
Epiglottis
Trachea (11)
Lung (5)
(6)
(7)
Alveoli

Capillary
Alveolus
O_2 CO_2
Erythrocyte

Bronchiole
Alveolus

Exchange of gases between
an alveolus and lung capillary

FIGURE 23–31 ▲ The respiratory system.

The Larynx

The *larynx* (voice box) is a tubular structure located below the pharynx. As mentioned earlier, the pharynx is a passageway for both food and air. A flap of cartilage, called the *epiglottis*, automatically covers the larynx during the act of swallowing to prevent the food from passing from the pharynx into the larynx. The larynx contains the *vocal cords*. As the air is exhaled past the vocal cords, the vibration of the cords produces sound.

The Trachea

The *trachea* (windpipe), a vertical tube 4 to 5 inches (10 to 12.5 cm) long, extends from the larynx to the bronchi. A series of C-shaped cartilage rings prevents the trachea from collapsing. The function of the trachea is the passage of air.

Bronchi

Behind the heart, close to the center of the chest, the trachea branches into two tubes: one leading to the right lung and the other leading to the left lung. These tubes are called *bronchi* (singular: *bronchus*). The function of the bronchi is the passage of air.

The Lungs

The lungs are cone-shaped organs located in the thoracic cavity. The right lung is the larger of the two and is divided into three lobes. The left lung is divided into two lobes. After the bronchus enters the lung, it divides into smaller tubes and continues to subdivide into even smaller tubes called *bronchioles*. At the end of each bronchiole is a grapelike cluster of air sacs called *alveoli*

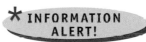

✱ **INFORMATION ALERT!**

Pathway: air → nose → pharynx → larynx → trachea → bronchi → bronchioles → alveoli where the exchange of carbon dioxide and oxygen takes place.

(singular: *alveolus*). The walls of the alveoli are single celled, which allows for the exchange of gases to take place between the alveoli and the capillaries. The *pleura* is a double sac that surrounds each lung and lines the walls of the thoracic cavity. The *visceral pleura* lines the outer surface of the lungs, whereas the *parietal pleura* covers the chest wall. The small amount of fluid within the sacs allows the lungs to expand and contract without friction.

■ CONDITIONS OF THE RESPIRATORY SYSTEM

Pneumothorax and Hemothorax

Pneumothorax

Pneumothorax is the collection of air or gas in the pleural cavity, resulting in a collapsed lung, or *atelectasis* (Fig. 23–32). It may be caused by a chest wound, or it may be a spontaneous collapse

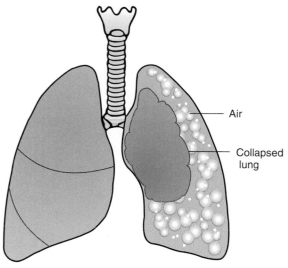

FIGURE 23–32 ▲ Pneumothorax.

due to lung disease. The pleural cavity is airtight, with negative pressure. As air enters the pleural cavity it creates pressure against the lung, causing it to collapse.

Symptoms include sudden sharp chest pain, shortness of breath, cyanosis, and stopping of normal chest movements on the affected side. Treatment ranges from observation and supplemental oxygen for an uncomplicated pneumothorax to a thoracentesis to remove the air or gas from the cavity and a thoracotomy, with the insertion of chest tubes. The tubes are connected to an underwater drainage system with suction and remain in place until air is no longer expelled from the pleural space.

Hemothorax

A *hemothorax* is the collection of blood in the pleural cavity; it is usually caused by chest trauma. Symptoms include chest pain, shortness of breath, respiratory failure, tachycardia, and anxiety.

Treatment includes stabilizing the patient, stopping the bleeding, insertion of a chest tube to evacuate the blood and air from the pleural space, and reexpanding the lung.

Pulmonary Embolism (PE)

Pulmonary embolism is the most common complication in hospitalized patients. It strikes 6 million adults a year, causing 100,000 deaths. Pulmonary embolism is usually caused by a blood clot that has been dislodged from a leg or pelvic vein, *deep vein thrombosis* (DVT), that blocks a pulmonary artery. Symptoms are cough, dyspnea (difficulty in breathing), chest pain, cyanosis (blue tinge to the skin), tachycardia, and shock. It is difficult to distinguish from pneumonia and myocardial infarction. Chest x-ray, pulmonary arteriography, arterial blood gases, and lung perfusion scans coupled with a lung ventilation scan are used to diagnose pulmonary embolism. Treatment includes thrombolytic, anticoagulant, and oxygen therapy.

Chronic Obstructive Pulmonary Disease (COPD)

Chronic obstructive pulmonary disease (COPD) is the persistent obstruction of bronchial air flow. This chronic condition of the respiratory system is the second leading cause of hospital admissions in this country. COPD is actually a group of respiratory diseases, of which bronchitis, asthma, and emphysema are the most common.

COPD is attributed to cigarette smoking, environmental pollution, occupational hazards, and chronic infections. Symptoms include shortness of breath, chronic cough, wheezing, increased sputum production, and fatigability upon even mild exertion. Symptoms are progressive and lung damage is irreversible. There is no known cure. Treatment focuses on maintaining the remaining lung function and relieving symptoms as much as possible.

REVIEW QUESTIONS

1. In external respiration the blood in the capillaries takes on _____ and gives off

   _____ to the lungs.

2. In internal respiration the body cells take on _____ from the blood in the capillaries and at the

   same time give off _____ to the blood in the capillaries to be transported to the lungs.

3. List in sequence the organs through which the air from the outside travels to the blood in the capillaries of the lung.

    a. _____   e. _____

    b. _____   f. _____

    c. _____   g. _____

    d. _____

4. _____ is a passageway for both food and air. _____ is a cartilage flap that prevents food from entering the larynx.

5. List three things that happen to the inhaled air in the nose.

    a. _____

    b. _____

    c. _____

6. The vocal cords are located in the _____ .

7. Describe the lungs.

    _____

    _____

8. a. Blood in the pleural cavity is called _____ .

    b. Air in the pleural cavity is called _____ .

    c. A collapsed lung is known as _____ .

    d. A thrombus blocking a pulmonary artery is called _____ _____ .

9. In _____ _____ _____ _____ , symptoms are progressive and lung damage is irreversible.

10. List four factors that cause COPD.

    a. _____

    b. _____

    c. _____

    d. _____

■ MEDICAL TERMINOLOGY RELATING TO THE RESPIRATORY SYSTEM

Upon mastery of the medical terminology for this unit, you will be able to:

1. Spell and define the terms related to the respiratory tract.

2. Given the meaning of a medical condition relating to the respiratory system, build with word parts the corresponding medical term.

3. Analyze and define medical terms that are built from word parts that relate to the respiratory system.

4. State the meaning of the abbreviations used in this unit.

5. Given a description of a hospital situation in which the health unit coordinator may encounter medical terminology, apply the correct medical term to the situation described.

Word Parts

The list below contains the word parts you need to memorize for the body respiratory system. The exercises included in this unit will help you with this task. You will continue to use these word parts throughout the course and during your employment. Practice pronouncing each word part aloud.

Combining Forms	Meaning
1. bronch/o (brŏn'-kō)	bronchus (s.); bronchi (pl.)
2. laryng/o (lah-rĭng'-gō)	larynx (voice box)
3. pharyng/o (fah-rĭng'-gō)	pharynx (throat)
4. pleur/o (ploo'-rō)	pleura
5. pneum/o (nū'-mō)	lung (also means air)
6. pneumon/o (nū-mŏn'-ō)	lung
7. pulmon/o (pŭl'-mŏ-nō)	lung
8. rhin/o (rī'-nō)	nose
9. thorac/o (thŏ'-rah-kō)	chest
10. tonsill/o (tŏn'-sĭl-ō) (Note: the word root for tonsil has a double *l*)	tonsil
11. trache/o (trā'-kē-ō)	trachea (windpipe)

Prefix	Meaning
dys- (dĭs)	difficult, labored, painful, abnormal

Suffix	Meaning
-pnea (nē'-ah)	respiration, breathing

EXERCISE 1

Write the combining forms for the respiratory system in the spaces provided on the diagram in Figure 23–31. The number preceding the combining form in the list above matches the number of the body part on the diagram.

EXERCISE 2

Write the combining forms (and suffix) for each term listed below.

1. lung

  a. _____

  b. _____

  c. _____

2. pharynx

  _____

3. larynx

  _____

4. trachea

  _____

5. tonsil

  _____

6. bronchus

  _____

7. pleura

  _____

8. nose

  _____

9. breathing

  _____

10. chest

  _____

■ MEDICAL TERMS RELATING TO THE RESPIRATORY SYSTEM

The following list is made up of medical terms you will need to know for the respiratory system. Exercises following this list will assist you in learning these terms. Practice the pronunciation of these terms aloud.

General Terms	Meaning
adenoids (ăd′-ĕn-oyds)	tissue in the nasopharynx
apnea (ăp′-nē-ah)	without breathing (temporary stoppage of breathing)
bronchotracheal (brŏn-kō-trā′-kē-al)	pertaining to the bronchi and trachea
dyspnea (dĭsp-nē′-ah)	difficulty in breathing
endotracheal (ĕn-dō-trā′-kē-al)	pertaining to within the trachea
pharyngocele (fah-rĭng′-gō-sēl)	(an abnormal) protrusion in the pharynx
pharyngoplegia (fah-rĭng-gō-plē′-jē-ah)	paralysis of the pharynx
pulmonary (pŭl′-mŏ-nĕr-ē)	pertaining to the lungs
thoracentesis (thō-rah-sĕn-tē′-sĭs)	surgical puncture and drainage of fluid from the chest (cavity for diagnostic or therapeutic purposes)
thoracic (thō-răs′-ĭk)	pertaining to the chest
thoracocentesis (thō′-rah-kō-sĕn-tē′-sĭs)	surgical puncture and drainage of fluid from the chest (cavity for diagnostic or therapeutic purposes [the same as thoracentesis])
tracheoesophageal (trā′-kē-ō-ĕ-sŏf-ah-jē′-al)	pertaining to the trachea and esophagus

Surgical Terms	Meaning
adenoidectomy (ăd′-ĕ-noy-dĕk′-tō-mē)	surgical removal of the adenoids
laryngectomy (lar-ĭn-jĕk′-tō-mē)	excision of the larynx
lobectomy (lō-bĕk′-tō-mē)	excision of a lobe (of a lung—may also refer to the brain or liver)
pleuropexy (ploo′-rō-pĕk′-sē)	surgical fixation of the pleura
pneumonectomy (nū-mŏ-nĕk′-tō-mē)	excision of the lung (may be total or partial removal of a lung)
rhinoplasty (rhī-nō-plăs′-tē)	surgical repair of the nose
thoracotomy (thō-rah-kŏt′-ō-mē)	incision into the chest cavity
tonsillectomy (tŏn-sĭl-lĕk′-tō-mē)	surgical removal of the tonsils
tracheostomy (trā-kē-ŏs′-tō-mē)	artificial opening into the trachea (through the neck)

Diagnostic Terms	Meaning
adenoiditis (ăd′-ĕ-noy-dī-tĭs)	inflammation of the adenoids
asthma (ăz′-mah)	chronic disease characterized by periodic attacks of dyspnea, wheezing, and coughing
bronchitis (brŏn-kī′-tĭs)	inflammation of the bronchi
chronic obstructive pulmonary disease (COPD)	chronic obstruction of the airway that results from emphysema, asthma, or chronic bronchitis
emphysema (ĕm-fĭ-sē′-mah)	degenerative disease characterized by destructive changes in the walls of the alveoli, resulting in loss of elasticity to the lungs
laryngitis (lar-ĭn-jī′-tĭs)	inflammation of the larynx
pharyngitis (fah-rĕn-jī′-tĭs)	inflammation of the pharynx
pleuritis (ploo-rī′-tĭs); pleurisy (ploo′-rĕ-sē)	inflammation of the pleura
pneumonia (nū-mōn′-nē-ah)	inflammation or infection of the lung
pneumonitis (nū-mō-nī′-tĭs)	
pneumothorax (noo-mō-thor-ăks)	air in the pleural cavity causes the lung to collapse
tuberculosis (TB) (too-ber′kū-lō′-sĭs)	chronic infectious, inflammatory disease that commonly affects the lungs
rhinopharyngitis (rī′-nō-făr-ĭn-jī′-tĭs)	inflammation of the nose and throat

Diagnostic Terms—cont'd	Meaning
rhinorrhagia (rī-nō-rā'-jē-ah)	bleeding from the nose, also called epistaxis
tonsillitis (tŏn-sĭ-lī'-tĭs)	inflammation of the tonsils
upper respiratory infection (URI) (rĕ-spī'-rah-tō-rē)	infection of pharynx, larynx, or bronchi

Terms Related to Diagnostic Procedures	Meaning
bronchogram (brŏn'-kō-grăm)	x-ray of the bronchi and lung (with the use of a contrast medium)
bronchoscope (brŏn'-kō-skōp)	instrument used to visually examine the bronchi
bronchoscopy (brŏn-kŏs'-kō-pē)	visual examination of the bronchi
laryngoscope (lăr-rĭng'-gō-skōp)	instrument for visual examination of the larynx

EXERCISE 3

Analyze and define each medical term listed below.

1. dyspnea

_____

2. pharyngocele

_____

3. apnea

_____

4. bronchotracheal

_____

5. tracheoesophageal

_____

6. endotracheal

_____

7. pharyngoplegia

_____

8. rhinopharyngitis

_____

9. rhinorrhagia

_____

10. bronchoscope

_____

11. bronchoscopy

_____

EXERCISE 4

Using the word parts studied in this unit and previous units, build medical terms from each definition listed below.

1. inflammation of the bronchi _____

2. inflammation of the larynx _____

3. artificial opening into the trachea _____

4. excision of a lung _____

5. excision of a lobe (of the lung) _____

6. surgical fixation of the pleura _____

7. surgical repair of the nose _____

8. incision into the chest cavity _____

9. surgical puncture and drainage of the chest cavity _____

10. inflammation of the tonsils _____

11. inflammation of the adenoids _____

EXERCISE 5

Complete the spelling of each medical term listed below.

Medical Term	Meaning
1. pn _ _ _ othor _ _	air in the pleural cavity causing the lungs to collapse

2. em _ _ _ se _ _   disease of the alveoli of the lung

3. _ _ _ umon _ _   an inflammation or infection of the lung

4. pleuro _ _ _ _   surgical fixation of the pleura

5. phar _ _ _ itis   inflammation of the pharynx

EXERCISE 6

Write the meaning of each abbreviation listed below.
1. COPD

2. URI

3. PE

EXERCISE 7

Define each medical term listed below.
1. adenoids

2. lobectomy

3. emphysema

4. pneumonia

5. upper respiratory infection

6. apnea

7. dyspnea

8. pharyngocele

9. laryngectomy

10. pneumothorax

11. rhinorrhagia

12. bronchogram

13. laryngoscope

14. asthma

15. chronic obstructive pulmonary disease

16. tuberculosis

EXERCISE 8

Spell each term studied in this unit by having someone dictate the terms to you.

1.

2.

3.

4. _____

5. _____

6. _____

7. _____

8. _____

9. _____

10. _____

11. _____

12. _____

13. _____

14. _____

15. _____

16. _____

17. _____

18. _____

19. _____

20. _____

21. _____

22. _____

23. _____

24. _____

25. _____

26. _____

27. _____

28. _____

29. _____

30. _____

31. _____

32. _____

33. _____

34. _____

35. _____

36. _____

37. _____

38. _____

39. _____

40. _____

41. _____

42. _____

EXERCISE 9

Answer the following questions.

1. The patient was admitted to the hospital with the diagnosis of hemothorax. The doctor is planning to perform a procedure on the patient to remove fluid from the chest cavity by surgical puncture. This procedure is called a

   _____ .

2. A patient suddenly stops breathing. During this emergency the doctor may perform the following procedure to assure the opening of the air passageway. The doctor uses a

   _____ (an instrument for visual exami-

   nation of the larynx) to insert a (an) _____ (pertaining to within the trachea) tube. These are two items of equipment that may be used during an emergency. You may be asked to locate these items for the nursing staff or doctor. Upon assignment to a nursing unit, locate and be able to identify this equipment.

3. The patient is having difficulty breathing. The doctor per-

   forms a procedure called _____ (artificial opening into the trachea) to facilitate breathing. A tube is inserted into the trachea to prevent it from collapsing. It has the same name as the procedure. It is called

   a (an) _____ tube. A tray, which has the same name as the procedure, called a (an)

   _____, is used by the nursing staff to care for the patient. A patient with a tracheostomy may have difficulty talking; therefore, the health unit coordinator should not use the intercom to communicate with this patient.

4. The patient is scheduled for a visual examination of the

   bronchus, called a _____ .

_____ is the instrument the doctor uses to perform the examination.

5. The patient is admitted to the hospital with a (an)

_____ (a collapsed lung). The patient is having difficulty breathing; the medical term for this is

_____ . The doctor treats this condition by making a surgical incision into the chest wall,

called a (an) _____ , for the purpose of inserting tubes. A tray, which has the same name as the

procedure, a (an) _____ tray, is obtained from the central service department for the doctor's use.

6. T & A is the abbreviation for excision of the tonsils, called

_____ and excision of the adenoids,

called _____ .

UNIT 9

The Urinary System and the Male Reproductive System

Outline

Unit Objectives
The Urinary System
Organs of the Urinary System
Function of the Urinary System
The Kidneys
The Ureters
The Urinary Bladder
Urethra
The Male Reproductive System
Organs of the Male Reproductive System
Functions of the Male Reproductive System
The Testes
Production of Sperm
The Prostate Gland
Diseases and Conditions of the Urinary System and the Male Reproductive System
Pyelonephritis
Renal Calculi
Tumors of the Prostate Gland
Review Questions
Medical Terminology Relating to the Urinary System and the Male Reproductive System
Word Parts
Exercise 1
Exercise 2

Medical Terms Relating to the Urinary System and the Male Reproductive System
Exercise 3
Exercise 4
Exercise 5
Exercise 6
Exercise 7
Exercise 8

Unit Objectives

Upon completion of this unit, you will be able to:

1. Describe the overall functions of the urinary system and the male reproductive system.

2. Name the organs of the urinary system and tell the function of each organ.

3. Name the components of urine.

4. Name the organs of the male reproductive system and describe the function of each organ.

5. Describe the passageway of sperm from the testes to the outside of the body.

6. State the location and describe the function of the seminal vesicle glands and the prostate gland.

7. Describe pyelonephritis, renal calculi, and tumors of the prostate gland.

■ THE URINARY SYSTEM

Organs of the Urinary System

Kidneys (2)
Ureters (2)
Bladder (1)
Urethra (1)

Function of the Urinary System

The functions of the urinary system are to monitor and regulate extracellular fluids and to remove waste products from the blood and excrete it from the body. While toxic substances are also eliminated through the skin, lungs, and intestines, the urinary system is a major contributor to homeostasis in the body by maintaining the proper balance of water, electrolytes, and pH of body fluids. The urinary system may also be referred to as the excretory system.

The Kidneys

The kidneys are two fist-sized, bean-shaped organs located in the lumbar region on either side of the spine, posterior to the abdominal cavity. The primary functions of the kidneys are to remove waste from the blood, balance the water and elec-

trolytes in the body by removing and retaining water, and assist in RBC production by releasing erythropoietin (eh-RITH-ro-POY-eh-tin). Nephrons, the basic functional unit of the kidney, begin removing waste and water as the blood flows into the kidney through the renal artery. Each kidney contains about one million nephrons. At the entrance of each nephron is a cluster of capillaries called the glomerulus (pl. glomeruli) where the process of filtering the blood begins. The antidiuretic hormone (ADH) released by the posterior pituitary gland (neurohypophysis) stimulates the production of urine containing soluble waste. When there is a danger of dehydration the posterior pituitary gland will decrease the amount of ADH that is released. The nephrons will continue to remove waste but the fluid portion of urine will decrease. Voided urine is more concentrated and in smaller amounts. This process maintains the fluid balance in the body. Diuretics, commonly prescribed for edema, hypertension, and congestive heart failure are chemicals that serve to increase the rate of urinary output. After the urine is produced, it drains into a space in the kidney called the renal pelvis. From the renal pelvis the urine is transported to the bladder by the ureters.

The Ureters

The ureters are tubes that provide the drainage system for urine from the renal pelvis of each kidney to the bladder (Fig. 23–33). They are small in diameter and are approximately 10 to 12 inches

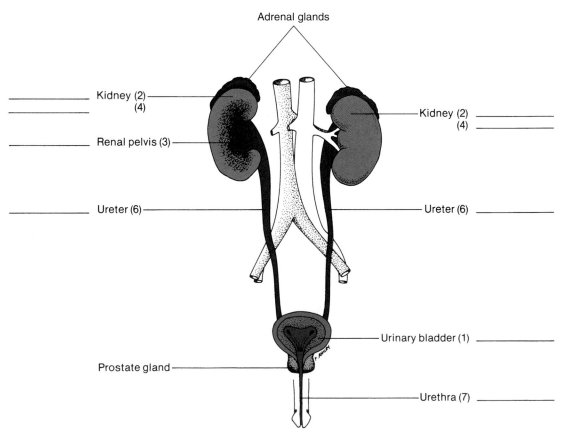

FIGURE 23–33 ▲ The male urinary system.

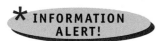
INFORMATION ALERT!

Production and pathway of urine: Blood flows via the renal artery into the nephrons of the kidneys where filtering of the blood takes place and urine is produced → renal pelvis → ureter → bladder → urethra → outside

(25 to 30 cm) long. They extend from the renal pelvis of the kidney and enter the posterior portion of the bladder.

The ureters have muscular walls that contract to keep the urine moving toward the bladder. A backup of urine into the kidney is prevented by a flap fold of mucous membrane at the entrance of the ureters into the bladder.

The Urinary Bladder

The urinary bladder is a hollow muscular bag located in the pelvic cavity. The bladder is a temporary reservoir for the urine it receives from the ureters. The need to urinate, or void, is stimulated by the distention of the bladder as it fills with urine.

The Urethra

The urethra is the tube through which the urine passes from the bladder to the outside of the body. The female urethra is approximately 1 to 2 inches (3.75 cm) long, and the male urethra, which is also a part of the male reproductive system (also carries seminal fluid at the time of ejaculation), is approximately 8 inches (20 cm) long.

Urine

Urine is a straw-colored fluid that is approximately 95% water and 5% waste material (urea, uric acid, creatinine, and ammonia). The daily amount of urine produced by the kidneys is about 1500 mL.

◼ THE MALE REPRODUCTIVE SYSTEM

Organs of the Male Reproductive System (Fig. 23–34)

Testes
Scrotum
Vas deferens
Urethra
Seminal vesicles
Prostate
Penis

Functions of the Male Reproductive System

The functions of the male reproductive system are to produce and eject the male reproductive cell (sperm, or spermatozoa) and to secrete the hormone testosterone.

The Testes

The testes (singular: testis), or testicles, are a pair of egg-shaped organs located outside the body, suspended in a sac called the scrotum. They are the main sex glands of the male. The func-

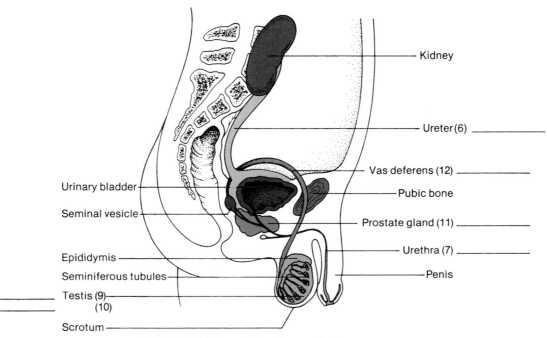

FIGURE 23–34 ▲ The male reproductive system.

tion of the testes is to produce sperm (sex cells) and testosterone (hormone). Testosterone is responsible for the development of the male secondary sex characteristics, such as beard and deep voice, and for the function of certain reproductive organs.

Production of Sperm

Sperm is produced in coiled tubes, located inside the testes, called seminiferous tubules. The sperm passes on to a tiny 20-foot tube called the epididymis, located in the scrotum. The sperm is stored in the epididymis for a short time, during which it matures and becomes motile (able to move by itself). The sperm then travels through a pair of tubes about 2 feet long called the vas deferens. The vas deferens carries the sperm to the urethra. The urethra connects with both the bladder and the vas deferens and passes through the penis to the outside. It is a passageway for both semen and urine. The seminal vesicles are glands located near the bladder that open into the vas deferens just prior to its joining with the urethra. The seminal vesicles produce a secretion that nourishes the sperm. This secretion makes up much of the volume of semen (sperm plus secretions). The junction of the vas deferens and the urethra is surrounded by a gland called the prostate gland.

The Prostate Gland

The prostate gland secretes a fluid that aids in the motility of the sperm. The prostate gland also aids in ejaculation (the expulsion of semen from the male urethra). Each ejaculation contains an average of 200 million sperm. Erection (stiffening) of the penis, produced by an increased blood supply to the spongelike tissue of the penis, allows for deposit of the sperm in the female vagina during ejaculation. A fold of skin called the prepuce, or foreskin, covers the tip of the penis; this is often removed shortly after birth by the surgical procedure of circumcision.

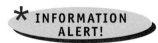
＊ INFORMATION ALERT!

The passageway of sperm: from the seminiferous tubules (production) → epididymis (sperm mature and become motile) → vas deferens (passageway) → seminal vesicles (add nourishing secretions) → prostate (add motility secretions) → urethra (passageway) → to the outside.

■ DISEASES AND CONDITIONS OF THE URINARY SYSTEM AND THE MALE REPRODUCTIVE SYSTEM

Pyelonephritis

Pyelonephritis is the infection of the renal pelvis and the kidney caused by bacterial invasion of the urinary tract. Typically the infection spreads from the bladder to the urethra to the kidneys. Three stages of the disease process are: pyelitis—inflammation of the renal pelvis; pyelonephritis—inflammation of the renal pelvis and kidney; and pyonephrosis—collection of pus in the renal pelvis. As the disease progresses, the name changes. Symptoms include dysuria (pain during urination), nocturia (excessive urination at night), hematuria (blood in the urine), and dysuria (burning on urination). Urinalysis and culture and sensitivity of bacterial specimens from the urine are used to diagnose the condition. Treatment includes antibiotic therapy.

Renal Calculi

Renal calculi, or kidney stones, usually form in the renal pelvis, where they may remain, or they may enter the ureter and cause obstruction. Back pain or renal colic, resulting from the obstruction, is usually the key symptom. Kidney, ureter, and bladder x-ray image (KUB); intravenous pyelogram (IVP); and kidney ultrasonography are used in diagnosing renal calculi. Treatment is to promote normal passage of the stone. Extracorporeal shock wave lithotripsy (ESWL), the crushing of kidney stones by laser beams, is replacing the need for surgery. Endoscopy is also used to remove small calculi from the lower part of the ureters. If indicated, a stone may be removed through a small incision in the skin (percutaneous nephrolithotomy).

Tumors of the Prostate Gland

Tumors of the prostate gland may be either malignant (cancer of the prostate) or benign (benign prostatic hyperplasia). Often the growth is not diagnosed until it is large enough to obstruct urinary outflow. Treatment of choice is surgical removal of the tumor. A radical, or perineal, prostatectomy is the excision of the entire gland and its capsule through an incision in the perineum. Suprapubic prostatectomy is removal of the prostate gland through an incision in the abdomen and the bladder. Retropubic prostatectomy is the surgical removal of the prostate gland through an incision in the abdomen, but the bladder is not excised. Transurethral prostatic resection is the removal of a portion of the prostate gland through the urethra. There is no surgical incision.

REVIEW QUESTIONS

1. _____ is an organ used by both the urinary system and the male reproductive system.

2. Describe the function of the urinary system.

   _____

   _____

3. The basic functional unit of the kidney is the _____ . Its primary functions are:

   _____

   _____

   _____

4. Describe the flow of urine from the renal pelvis of the kidney to the outside of the body.

   _____

   _____

5. Urine is made up of 95% _____ and 5% _____.

6. The amount of water removed from the blood is determined by the amount of _____ that is released

   by the _____ .

7. Two functions of the testicles are:

   a. _____

   b. _____

8. Trace the travel of the sperm from the testicles to the outside of the body. Indicate which glands add secretions to the sperm along the passageway.

   _____

   _____

9. Match the terms in Column 1 with the phrases in Column 2.

Column 1

a. nephrotripsy

b. pyelonephritis

c. renal calculi

d. hydrolithotripsy

e. benign prostatic hyperplasia

f. perineal prostatectomy

g. lithotripsy

Column 2

_____ 1. kidney stone

_____ 2. growth that may obstruct urinary outflow

_____ 3. infection of the renal pelvis and kidney

_____ 4. crushing of a kidney stone

■ MEDICAL TERMINOLOGY RELATING TO THE URINARY SYSTEM AND THE MALE REPRODUCTIVE SYSTEM

Upon mastery of the medical terminology for this unit, you will be able to:

1. Correctly spell and define the terms related to the urinary system and the male reproductive system.

2. Given the meaning of a medical condition relating to the urinary system and the male reproductive system, build with word parts the correct corresponding medical term.

3. Analyze and define medical terms built from word parts that relate to the urinary system and the male reproductive system.

4. Write the meaning of each abbreviation used in this unit.

5. Given a description of a hospital situation in which the health unit coordinator may encounter medical terminology, apply the correct medical terms to the situation described.

Word Parts

The list below contains the word parts you need to memorize for the urinary system and the male reproductive system. The exercises included in this unit will help you with this task. You will continue to use these word parts throughout the course and during employment. Practice pronouncing each word part aloud.

Urinary System

Word Roots/ Combining Forms	Meaning
1. cyst/o (sĭs'-tō)	bladder, sac
2. nephr/o (nĕf'-rō)	kidney
3. pyel/o (pī'-ĕ-lō)	renal pelvis
4. ren/o (rē'-nō)	kidney
5. ur/o (ū'-rō)	urine, urinary tract
6. ureter/o (ū-rē'-ter-ō)	ureter
7. urethr/o (ū-rē'-thrō)	urethra
8. urin/o (ū'-rĭ-nō)	urine (urinary tract, urination)

Male Reproductive System

Word Roots/ Combining Forms	Meaning
9. orchi/o (or'-kē-ō)	testicle, testis
10. orchid/o (or'-kĭ-dō)	testicle, testis
11. prostat/o (prŏs'-tăt-ō)	prostate
12. vas/o (vās'-ō)	vessel, duct

EXERCISE 1

a. Write the combining forms for the urinary system in the spaces provided on the diagram in Figure 23–33 (p. 546). The number preceding the combining form in the list above matches the number of the body part on the diagram.

b. Write the combining forms for the male reproductive system in the spaces provided on the diagram in Figure 23–34 (p. 547). The number preceding the combining form in the list above matches the number of the body part on the diagram.

EXERCISE 2

Write the combining forms for each term listed below.

1. urine, urinary tract

_____

_____

2. renal pelvis

_____

3. kidney

_____

_____

4. ureter

_____

5. bladder

_____

_____

6. testicle

_____

_____

7. vessel, duct

_____

8. urethra

_____

9. prostate

_____

■ MEDICAL TERMS RELATING TO THE URINARY SYSTEM AND THE MALE REPRODUCTIVE SYSTEM

The following list is made up of medical terms you will need to know for the urinary system and the male reproductive system. Exercises following this list will assist you in learning these terms. Practice pronouncing each term aloud.

General Terms	Meaning
hematuria (hēm-ah-tū′-rē-ah)	blood in the urine
scrotum (scrō′-tŭm)	the skin-covered sac that contains the testes and their accessory organs
urethral (ū-rē′-thral)	pertaining to the urethra
urinary (ū′-rĭ-nër-ē)	pertaining to urine
urinary catheterization (kăth′-ĕ-ter-ĭ-zā′-shŭn)	insertion of a sterile tube through the urethra into the bladder to remove urine
urination (ū-rĭ-nā′-shŭn)	passage of urine from the body, also called micturition
urologist (ū-rŏl′-ō-jĭst)	one who specializes in the diagnosis and treatment of (diseases) of the urinary tract (doctor)
urology (ū-rŏl′-ō-jē)	study of the urinary tract (the branch of medicine that deals with the diagnosis and treatment of diseases of the male and female urinary tract and of the male reproductive organs)
void (voyd)	to pass urine or feces from the body (generally used with reference to passing urine from the bladder to the outside of the body)

Surgical Terms	Meaning
circumcision (sur′-kŭm-sĭzh′-ŭn)	surgical removal of the foreskin of the penis
nephrectomy (nĕ-frĕk′-tō-mē)	excision of the kidney
nephrolithotomy (nĕf′-rō-lĭ-thŏt′-ō-mē)	incision into the kidney (to remove a stone)
nephropexy (nĕf′-rō-pĕk-sē)	surgical fixation of a kidney
orchiectomy (ōr-kē-ĕk′-tō-mē)	excision of (one or both) testes
prostatectomy (prŏs-tah-tĕk′-tō-mē)	surgical removal of the prostate gland
transurethral resection of the prostate gland (TURP) (trăns-ū-rē′-thral) (rē-sĕk′-shŭn)	removal of a portion of the prostate through the urethra by resecting the abnormal tissue in successive pieces
ureterolithotomy (ū-rē′-ter-ō-lĭ-thŏt′-ō-mē)	incision into the ureter to (remove) a stone
urethroplasty (ū-rē′-thrō-plăs′-tē)	surgical repair of the urethra
urethrorrhaphy (ū-rē-thrōr′-ah-fē)	suturing of a urethral tear
vasectomy (vah-sĕk′-tō-mē)	excision of a duct (vas deferens or a portion of the vas deferens; produces sterility in the male)

Diagnostic Terms	Meaning
cystitis (sĭs-tī′-tĭs)	inflammation of the bladder
cystocele (sĭs′-tō-sēl)	herniation of the urinary bladder
hydrocele (hī′-drō-sēl)	scrotal swelling caused by the collection of fluid in the membrane covering the testes
nephritis (nĕ-frī′-tĭs)	inflammation of the kidney
nephrolithiasis (nĕf′-rō-lĭ-thī′-ah-sĭs)	a kidney stone
pyelonephritis (pī′-ĕ-lō-nĕ-frī′-tĭs)	inflammation of the renal pelvis and kidney
renal calculus (rē′-nal) (kăl′-cū-lŭs)	a kidney stone
uremia (ū-rē′-mē-ah)	urine in the blood (caused by inability of the kidneys to filter out waste products from the blood)
ureteralgia (ū-rē-ter-al′-jē-ah)	pain in the ureter

Terms Relating to Diagnostic Procedures	Meaning
blood urea nitrogen (BUN)	laboratory test performed on a blood sample to determine kidney function
creatinine (Cr)	laboratory test usually performed with the BUN to determine kidney function
cystogram (sĭs′-tō-grăm)	x-ray image of the (urinary) bladder; dye is used as a contrast medium
cystoscopy (sĭs-tŏs′-kō-pē)	visual examination of the bladder; usually performed in the operating room so the patient may be anesthetized
intravenous pyelogram (IVP) (ĭn-trah-vē′-nŭs) (pī′-ĕ′-lō-grăm)	x-ray image of the kidney, especially the renal pelvis and ureters; contrast medium is used
kidneys, ureters, and bladder (KUB)	x-ray image of the kidneys, ureters, and bladder
urinalysis (UA) (ū-rĭ-năl′-ĭ-sĭs)	a laboratory test to analyze several constituents of urine to assist in the diagnosis of disease

EXERCISE 3

Analyze and define each medical term listed below.

1. uremia

_____

2. urologist

_____

3. nephrolithotomy

_____

4. prostatectomy

_____

5. nephritis

_____

6. urology

_____

7. orchiectomy

_____

8. nephrolithiasis

_____

9. cystocele

_____

10. cystoscopy

11. nephrectomy

_____

12. nephropexy

_____

13. pyelonephritis

_____

14. ureteralgia

_____

15. urethral

_____

16. ureterolithotomy

_____

17. cystitis

_____

18. urethroplasty

_____

19. urethrorrhaphy

_____

EXERCISE 4

Using the word parts studied so far, build medical terms from each definition listed below.

1. visual examination of the urinary bladder

_____

2. inflammation of the kidney

_____

3. excision of the kidney

_____

4. a doctor who specializes in urology

_____

5. blood in the urine

_____

6. urine in the blood

_____

7. suturing of a urethral tear

_____

8. excision of a duct (vas deferens or a portion of it)

_____

9. excision of the prostate gland

_____

10. pain in the ureter

_____

11. herniation of the bladder

_____

12. x-ray image of the bladder

_____

13. inflammation of the kidney and the renal pelvis

_____

14. incision into the kidney to remove a stone

_____

15. surgical repair of the urethra

_____

16. surgical fixation of a kidney

17. *branch of medicine that deals with the male and female urinary systems and male reproductive system*

_____

18. *excision of the testes*

_____

EXERCISE 5

Define each medical term listed below.

1. *urinalysis*

_____

2. *renal calculus*

_____

3. *hydrocele*

_____

4. *transurethral resection*

_____

5. *circumcision*

_____

6. *urinary*

_____

7. *urination*

_____

EXERCISE 6

Write the meaning of each abbreviation listed below.
1. *IVP*

_____

2. *KUB*

_____

3. *BUN*

_____

4. *TUR*

_____

5. *BPH*

_____

6. *UA*

_____

EXERCISE 7

Spell each medical term studied in this unit by having someone dictate the terms to you.

1. _____
2. _____
3. _____
4. _____
5. _____
6. _____
7. _____
8. _____
9. _____
10. _____
11. _____
12. _____
13. _____
14. _____
15. _____

16. _____

17. _____

18. _____

19. _____

20. _____

21. _____

22. _____

23. _____

24. _____

25. _____

26. _____

27. _____

28. _____

29. _____

30. _____

31. _____

32. _____

33. _____

34. _____

35. _____

36. _____

EXERCISE 8

Answer the following questions.

1. The patient is unable to void. The doctor writes an order to pass a sterile tube through the urethra into the bladder to remove the urine. This procedure is called a(an)

_____. The doctor wants a sample of this urine sent to the lab to be analyzed. He or she writes

an order for a (an) _____.

2. The patient is admitted to the hospital with a diagnosis of

inflammation of the bladder, or _____ .

3. The doctor orders an image of the kidneys, ureters, and urinary bladder. The abbreviation for this x-ray procedure is

_____. He or she also ordered a blood test to determine kidney function. He or she may

have ordered a _____. The abbreviation

tion for this test is _____.

4. The doctor writes an order on the patient's chart for a consultation with a doctor who specializes in the treatment of diseases of the urinary tract and male reproductive system;

this specialist is called a(an) _____.

5. The patient is scheduled for the operating room for a procedure to visualize the urinary bladder. The procedure is

called _____. The patient may be scheduled for this procedure in the operating room

because _____.

UNIT 10

The Female Reproductive System

Unit Objectives

Upon completion of this unit, you will be able to:

1. Describe the primary functions of the female reproductive system.

2. Name the organs of the female reproductive system and describe the function of each organ.

3. Locate the perineum relative to nearby anatomic structures.

4. Name and describe the functions of two hormones produced by the ovaries.

5. Describe endometriosis, ectopic pregnancy, and pelvic inflammatory disease.

■ THE FEMALE REPRODUCTIVE SYSTEM

Organs of the Female Reproductive System (Fig. 23–35)

Uterus (1)
Ovaries (2)
Fallopian tubes (2)
Vagina (1)
External genitalia
Mammary and Bartholin's glands

The reproductive organs do not mature and begin performing the reproductive functions until about the age of 11. The maturing of the reproductive organs is called puberty.

Functions of the Female Reproductive System

The functions of the female reproductive system are to produce the female reproductive cell (ovum), to produce hormones, and to provide for conception and pregnancy.

The Uterus

The uterus is a thick, muscular, pear-shaped organ located in the pelvic cavity between the rectum and the urinary bladder. Three layers make up the uterus: the outer perimetrium, the middle myometrium, and the inner endometrium. In pregnancy, the uterus functions to contain and nourish the unborn child. The rhythmic myometrial contractions during labor assist in the birthing process. The uterus also plays a role in menstruation as the endometrium disintegrates and sloughs off if a fertilized egg is not implanted. The upper rounded region of the uterus is called the fundus. The wide, central portion of the uterus is the body and the lower, narrow end that extends into the vagina is called the cervix.

The Ovaries

The ovaries, a pair of small oval-shaped organs located in the pelvic cavity, produce the female reproductive cell called the ovum (plural: ova). At birth, the female has nearly 1 million ova in the ovaries for which approximately 300,000 remain during the reproductive lifetime. At puberty the ovaries in response to the follicle-stimulating hormone (FSH) will release a mature ova about every 28 days. This process is called ovulation and it occurs about halfway through the menstrual cycle.

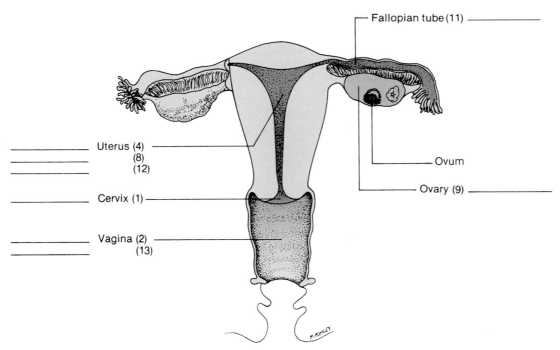

FIGURE 23-35 ▲ The female reproductive system.

The ovaries, also called female endocrine glands, produce two hormones, estrogen and progesterone. Estrogen is responsible for the development of the female reproductive organs and the development of the female secondary sex characteristics, such as breasts and pubic hair. The hormone progesterone plays a part in the menstrual cycle by helping to maintain the lining of the uterus for conception, and in pregnancy.

The Fallopian Tubes

A pair of tubes, each approximately 5 inches (12.5 cm) long, called the fallopian tubes, provide a passageway for the ovum from the ovaries to the uterus. The fallopian tubes are not connected to the ovaries; however, after ovulation the ovum is swept into one of the fallopian tubes, which are connected to the uterus. Fertilization, the union of the sperm and the ovum, usually takes place in the fallopian tube. It takes approximately 5 days for the ovum to pass through the fallopian tube to the uterus.

The Vagina

The vagina is a muscular tube about 3 inches long that connects the uterus to the outside of the body (Fig. 23–36). The outside opening of the vagina is between the rectum (posterior) and the urethra (anterior) of the pelvic floor. The vagina receives the penis during sexual intercourse and is the lower part of the birth canal through which the newborn baby passes from the uterus to the outside of the body. Bartholin's glands (or greater vestibular glands), mucus-producing glands at the external opening of the vagina, secrete lubricating substances.

The Perineum

The pelvic floor of both the male and female is called the perineum. However, this term is most frequently used to describe the area between the vaginal opening and the anus of the female.

Mammary Glands

The mammary glands, specialized organs of milk production, are located within the breasts. Each adult mammary gland contains 15 to 20 glandular lobes. During pregnancy, estrogen and progesterone stimulate development of the mammary glands. The hormone prolactin initiates milk production after birth.

External Reproductive Structures

The vulva (a collective term for the external genitalia) consists of the labia majora and labia minora, the two folds of adipose tissue surrounding the vagina, as well as the vestibule, the recess formed by the labia minora. The clitoris, a small erectile structure, is located anterior to the urethra.

■ DISEASES AND CONDITIONS OF THE FEMALE REPRODUCTIVE SYSTEM

Endometriosis

Endometriosis is a condition in which endometrial tissue (lining of the uterus) is found outside of the uterus, especially in the pelvic area, but it can appear anywhere in the body (Fig. 23–37). The misplaced endometrial tissue undergoes changes, including

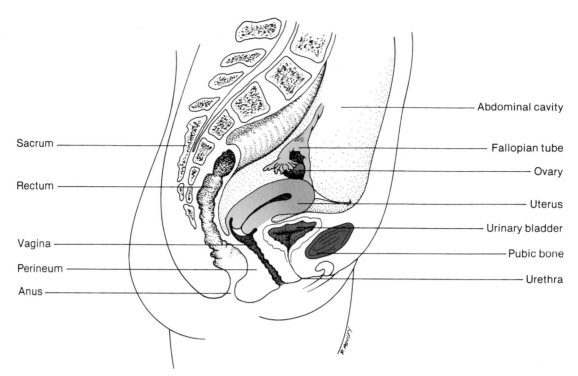

Sacrum

Rectum

Vagina

Perineum

Anus

Abdominal cavity

Fallopian tube

Ovary

Uterus

Urinary bladder

Pubic bone

Urethra

FIGURE 23–36 ▲ Lateral view of the female reproductive system.

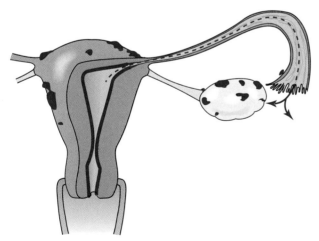

FIGURE 23–37 ▲ Endometriosis.

dometriosis. Endometrial ablation may be performed to suppress ovarian function and to halt the growth of endometrial tissue growth. Conservative surgery may be the removal of cysts or lysis (freeing) of adhesions. For severe cases and for those women not wanting to bear children, a total hysterectomy and bilateral salpingo-oophorectomy is recommended (Fig. 23–38).

Pelvic Inflammatory Disease

Pelvic inflammatory disease (PID) is any infection of the female pelvic organs; it is mostly caused by bacterial infection. Early diagnosis and treatment prevent damage to the reproductive organs. If untreated, PID can lead to infertility and to other severe medical complications. Symptoms include vaginal discharge, abdominal pain, and fever. Treatment includes antibiotic therapy.

Ectopic Pregnancy

In an ectopic (tubal) pregnancy, the fertilized ovum is implanted outside of the uterus; over 90% implant in the fallopian tubes. The fetus may grow large enough to rupture the tube, creating a life-threatening situation. Symptoms of a ruptured fallopian tube include severe abdominal pain on one side and vaginal bleeding. Treatment is surgical repair or removal of the fallopian tube and removal of the products of conception.

bleeding, during menstruation. Symptoms include dysmenorrhea (painful menstruation), causing constant pain in the vagina and lower abdomen. The cause is unknown.

Treatment varies according to the severity of the disease and according to the age and childbearing desires of the patient. Hormonal treatment may be recommended for milder forms of en-

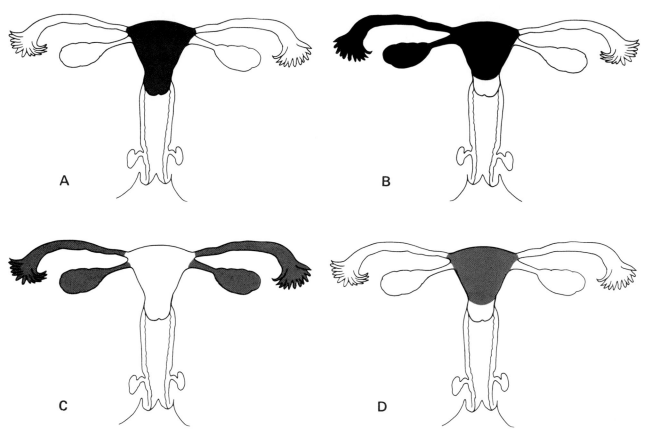

A   B

C   D

FIGURE 23–38 ▲ *A*, Total hysterectomy. *B*, Hysterosalpingo-oophorectomy. *C*, Bilateral salpingo-oophorectomy. *D*, Subtotal hysterectomy.

REVIEW
QUESTIONS

1. _____ and _____ are the names of two hormones produced by the ovaries.

   _____ is the hormone responsible for the secondary sex characteristics and aids in the development of the female reproductive organs.

2. Fertilization usually takes place in the _____.

3. The _____ is the lower portion of the uterus, which extends into the vagina.

4. Describe the primary functions of the female reproductive system.

   _____

   _____

5. List the internal organs of the female reproductive system and write a line or two about the function of each organ.

   a. _____

   b. _____

c. _____

d. _____

6. An ovum begins maturing in response to the _____.

7. An infection of the female pelvic organs that, if left untreated, can lead to infertility is called _____.

8. A pregnancy occurring outside the uterus is called a(n) _____.

9. A condition in which endometrial tissue is found outside the uterus is called _____.

■ MEDICAL TERMINOLOGY RELATING TO THE FEMALE REPRODUCTIVE SYSTEM

Upon mastery of the medical terminology for this unit, you will be able to:

1. Spell and define the terms related to the female reproductive system.

2. Given the meaning of a medical condition relating to the female reproductive system, build with word parts the correct corresponding medical terms.

3. Analyze and define medical terms that are built from word parts related to the female reproductive system.

4. Define terms related to pregnancy, childbirth, and the newborn.

5. Given a description of a hospital situation in which the health unit coordinator may encounter medical terminology, apply the correct medical term to the situation described.

Word Parts

The list below contains the word parts you need to learn for the female reproductive system. The exercises included in this unit will help you with this task. You will continue to use these word parts throughout the course and during employment. Practice pronouncing each word part aloud.

Word Roots/ Combining Forms   Meaning

1. cervic/o (sĕr'-vĭ-ko)   cervix (the necklike portion of the uterus)
2. colp/o (kŏl'-pō)   vagina
3. gynec/o (gī'-nĕ-kō, jĭn'-ĕ-kō)   woman
4. hyster/o (hĭs'-ter-ō)   uterus (womb)
5. mamm/o (măm'-mō)   breast
6. mast/o (măs'-tō)   breast
7. men/o (mĕn'-ō)   menstruation
8. metr/o (mĕ'-trō)   uterus (womb)

9. oophor/o (ō-ŏf'-ō-rō)   ovary
10. perine/o (pĕr-ĭ-nē'-ō)   perineum (the pelvic floor); in the female, the area between the vaginal opening and the anus, and in the male, the region between the scrotum and the anus
11. salping/o (săl-pĭng'-gō)   fallopian or uterine tube
12. uter/o (ū'-tĕr-ō)   uterus (womb)
13. vagin/o (văj'-ĭ-nō)   vagina

EXERCISE ❶

Write the combining forms for the female reproductive system in the spaces provided on the diagram in Figure 23–35 (p. 557). The number preceding the combining forms in the list above matches the number of the body part on the diagram.

EXERCISE ❷

Write the combining form for each of the following.

1. menstruation   _____

2. woman   _____

3. vagina   _____

4. perineum   _____

5. fallopian or uterine tube   _____

6. ovary   _____

7. uterus   _____

8. cervix   _____

9. breast   _____

■ MEDICAL TERMS RELATING TO THE FEMALE REPRODUCTIVE SYSTEM

The list below contains the medical terms you need to memorize for the female reproductive system. The exercises included in this unit will help you with this task. You will continue to use these medical terms throughout the course and during your employment. Practice pronouncing each term aloud.

General Terms	Meaning
gynecologist (gī-nĕ-kŏl′-ō-jĭst, jĭn-ĕ-kŏl′-ō-jĭst)	specialist in the diagnosis and treatment of women (doctor)
gynecology (gī-nĕ-kŏl′-ō-jē, jĭn-ĕ-kŏl′-ō-jē)	study of women (the branch of medicine dealing with diseases and disorders of the female reproductive system)
menopause (mĕn′-ō-pawz)	the period during which the menstrual cycle slows down and eventually stops
menstrual (mĕn′-stroo-ăl)	pertaining to menstruation
menstruation (mĕn-stroo-ā′-shŭn)	discharge of blood and tissue from the uterus, normally occurring every 28 days
ovum (ō′-vŭm) (s.); ova (ō′-vă) (pl.)	female reproductive cell; may be referred to as the female reproductive egg
ureterovaginal (ū-rē′-ter-ō-văj′-ĭ-nal)	pertaining to the ureter and vagina
uterine (ū′-ter-ĭn)	pertaining to the uterus
vaginal (văj′-ĭ-nal)	pertaining to the vagina
vaginoperineal (văj-ĭ-nō-pĕr-ĭ-nē′-al)	pertaining to the vagina and perineum

Surgical Terms	Meaning
cervicectomy (sĕr-vĭ-sĕk′-tō-mē)	excision of the cervix
colporrhaphy (kōl-por′-ah-fē)	suturing of the vagina
dilation and curettage (D&C) (dī-la′-shŭn) (kū-rĕ-tăhzh′)	surgical procedure to dilate the cervix scrape the inner walls of the uterus (endometrium) for diagnostic and therapeutic purposes
hysterectomy (hĭs-tĕ-rĕk′-tō-mē)	surgical removal of the uterus
hysterosalpingo-oophorectomy (hĭs′-ter-ō-săl-pĭng′-gō-ō-ŏf-ō-rĕk′-tō-mē)	excision of the uterus, fallopian tubes, and ovaries
mammoplasty (măm′-ō-plăs-tē)	surgical repair of the breast(s) to enlarge (augmentation) or reduce (reduction) in size or to reconstruct after surgical removal of a tumor
mastectomy (măs-tĕk′-tō-mē)	surgical removal of a breast
oophorectomy (ō-ŏf-ō-rĕk′-tō-mē)	excision of an ovary; if both ovaries are removed, it is referred to as a bilateral oophorectomy

Surgical Terms	Meaning
endometrial ablation (en-dō mē′ trē al ab-lā′ shun)	use of laser to destroy endometrium in abnormal uterine bleeding
perineoplasty (pĕr-ĭ-nē′-ō-plăs-tē)	surgical repair of the perineum
perineorrhaphy (pĕr′-ĭ-nē-ōr′-ah-fē)	suturing of the perineum
salpingo-oophorectomy (săl-pĭng′-gō-ō-ŏf-o-rĕk′-tō-mē)	excision of a fallopian tube and an ovary
salpingopexy (săl-pĭng′-gō-pĕk-sē)	surgical fixation of a fallopian tube

Diagnostic Terms	Meaning
amenorrhea (ā-mĕn-ō-rē′-ah)	without menstrual discharge
cervicitis (ser-vĭ-sī′-tĭs)	inflammation of the cervix
dysmenorrhea (dĭs-mĕn-ō-rē′-ah)	painful menstrual discharge
menometrorrhagia (mĕn-ō-mĕt-rō-rā′-jē-ah)	rapid flow of blood from the uterus at menstruation (and in between menstrual periods)

Diagnostic Terms—cont'd	Meaning
metrorrhagia (mĕ-trō-rā'-jē-ah)	rapid flow of blood from the uterus (bleeding at irregular intervals other than that associated with menstruation)
metrorrhea (mĕ-trō-rē'-ah)	(abnormal) uterine discharge
oophoritis (ō-ŏf-ō-rī'-tĭs)	inflammation of an ovary
salpingitis (săl-pĭn-jī'-tĭs)	inflammation of a fallopian tube
salpingocele (săl-pĭng'-gō-sēl)	herniation of the fallopian tube

Terms Relating to Diagnostic Procedures	Meaning
cervical Pap smear	a laboratory test used to detect cancerous cells; commonly performed to detect cancer of the cervix and uterus
colposcope (kŏl'-pō-skōp)	an instrument used for visual examination of the vagina (and cervix)
colposcopy (kŏl-pŏs'-kō-pē)	visual examination of the vagina (and cervix)
hysterosalpingogram (hĭs'-ter-ō-săl-pĭng'-gō-grăm)	x-ray image of the uterus and fallopian tubes
mammogram (măm'-ō-grăm)	x-ray image of the breast
vaginal speculum (spĕk'-ū-lŭm)	instrument used for expanding the vagina to allow for visual examination of the vagina and cervix

EXERCISE 3

Analyze and define the following medical terms:

1. gynecology

_____

2. colporrhaphy

_____

3. oophorectomy

_____

4. oophoritis

_____

5. salpingo-oophorectomy

_____

6. salpingopexy

_____

7. hysterectomy

_____

8. dysmenorrhea

_____

9. colposcope

_____

10. mammoplasty

_____

11. amenorrhea

_____

12. mammogram

_____

13. hysterosalpingogram

_____

14. colposcopy

_____

EXERCISE 4

Using the word parts you have studied, build medical terms from each definition listed below.

1. *excision of the ovary*

   _____

2. *study of women (branch of medicine dealing with diseases of the reproductive organs of women)*

   _____

3. *surgical fixation of a fallopian tube*

   _____

4. *inflammation of an ovary*

   _____

5. *an instrument used for visual examination of the vagina*

   _____

6. *(abnormal) uterine discharge*

   _____

7. *excision of the cervix*

   _____

8. *excision of the uterus, ovaries, and fallopian tubes*

   _____

9. *herniation of a fallopian tube*

   _____

10. *pertaining to the ureter and vagina*

    _____

11. *inflammation of the cervix*

    _____

12. *excision of the uterus*

    _____

13. *suture of the vagina*

    _____

14. *surgical repair of the perineum*

    _____

15. *pertaining to the vagina*

    _____

16. *surgical removal of a breast*

    _____

17. *excision of a fallopian tube and ovary*

    _____

18. *painful menstruation*

    _____

19. *x-ray image of the uterus and fallopian tubes*

    _____

20. *without menstrual discharge*

    _____

21. *x-ray image of the breast*

    _____

22. *surgical repair of the breast*

    _____

23. *visual examination of the vagina (and cervix)*

    _____

EXERCISE 5

Define the following medical terms:

1. gynecologist

_____

2. uterine

_____

3. vaginal speculum

_____

4. menometrorrhagia

_____

5. dilation and curettage

_____

6. ovum

_____

EXERCISE 6

A surgery schedule lists all the operations to be performed in the hospital on a given day. Information on a surgery schedule includes the patient's name, the operation, and the surgeon. In the sample below, identify the terms spelled incorrectly in the operations listed. Spell the term correctly in the space provided.

Patient Name	Surgery	Doctor
a. Ms. Wallace	dilation and curretage	Dr. Lewis
	_____	
b. Ms. Kelly	histero-solpingo-oopherectomy	Dr. Robinowitz
	_____	
c. Ms. Thomas	periniplasty	Dr. Cohen
	_____	
d. Ms. Clark	colporhaphy	Dr. Jacobson
	_____	
e. Ms. Cohen	salpangpexy	Dr. Sheets
	_____	

EXERCISE 7

Spell each medical term studied in this unit by having someone dictate the terms to you.

1. _____
2. _____
3. _____
4. _____
5. _____
6. _____
7. _____
8. _____
9. _____
10. _____
11. _____
12. _____
13. _____
14. _____
15. _____
16. _____

17. _____

18. _____

19. _____

20. _____

21. _____

22. _____

23. _____

24. _____

25. _____

26. _____

27. _____

28. _____

29. _____

30. _____

31. _____

32. _____

33. _____

34. _____

35. _____

36. _____

37. _____

38. _____

■ TERMS RELATING TO OBSTETRICS

Below is a list of common terms used in the field of obstetrics and their definitions.

Obstetric Terms	Meaning
abortion (ah-bor′-shŭn)	termination of pregnancy before the fetus is capable of survival out of the uterus; may be spontaneous or therapeutic abortion
amniotic fluid (ăm-nē-ŏt′-ĭk)	fluid that surrounds the fetus
cesarean section (sē-sā′-rē-ăn)	incision into the uterus through the abdominal wall to deliver the fetus
congenital (kŏn-jĕn′-ĭ-tal)	term to describe a condition that exists at birth
ectopic pregnancy (ĕk-tŏp′-ĭk)	the fertilized ovum is implanted outside of the uterus
fetus (fē′-tŭs)	the unborn child in the uterus from the third month of development to birth
natal (nā′-tal)	pertaining to birth
neonatal (nē′-ō-nā′-tal)	pertaining to the first 4 weeks after birth
obstetrician (ŏb-stĕ-trĭsh′-ăn)	a doctor who practices obstetrics
obstetrics (ŏb-stĕt′-rĭ-ks)	branch of medicine that deals with pregnancy and childbirth
placenta (plah-sĕn-tah) (afterbirth)	a spongy structure developed during pregnancy through which the unborn child is nourished
postnatal (pōst-nā′-tal)	pertaining to after birth
prenatal (prē-nā′-tal)	pertaining to before birth

EXERCISE 8

Match the word in Column 1 with its meaning in Column 2.

Column 1

a. congenital

b. abortion

c. fetus

d. postnatal

e. natal

f. prenatal

g. obstetrics

h. ectopic pregnancy

Column 2

_____ 1. occurring before birth

_____ 2. present at birth

_____ 3. early termination of pregnancy

_____ 4. unborn child

_____ 5. a branch of medicine

_____ 6. pregnancy outside the uterus

_____ 7. occurring after birth

_____ 8. birth

EXERCISE 9

Define each term listed below.

1. obstetrician

_____

2. placenta

_____

3. amniotic fluid

_____

4. cesarean section

_____

EXERCISE 10

Answer the following questions.

1. In a large hospital there is usually a nursing unit for patients who are hospitalized for surgery of the female reproductive tract. This unit is called _____ . A separate nursing unit is used for delivery and care of the newborn and for care of the mothers. This unit is called

   _____.

2. The doctor plans to perform a pelvic examination of a female patient. The _____ is the instrument she or he uses to expand the vagina. During the pelvic examination the doctor plans to remove some cells from the cervix to be studied for the presence of cancer. The cells are sent to the laboratory for a

   _____ test.

UNIT 11

The Endocrine System

Outline

Unit Objectives
The Endocrine System
    Primary Organs of the Endocrine System
    Functions of the Endocrine System
    The Pituitary Gland
    The Thyroid Gland
    The Parathyroid Glands
    Pancreas
    The Adrenal Glands
    Sex Glands
Diseases of the Endocrine System
    Diabetes Mellitus (Type I or Type II)
    Graves' Disease
Review Questions
Medical Terminology Relating to the Endocrine System
    Word Parts
    Exercise 1

Medical Terms Relating to the Endocrine System
    Exercise 2
    Exercise 3
    Exercise 4
    Exercise 5
    Exercise 6
Web Sites of Interest

Unit Objectives

Upon completion of this unit, you will be able to:

1. Describe the overall function of the endocrine system.
2. Name the glands of the endocrine system and describe the hormones produced by each gland and the function of each of the hormones.
3. Compare endocrine glands with exocrine glands.
4. Describe diabetes mellitus and Graves' disease.

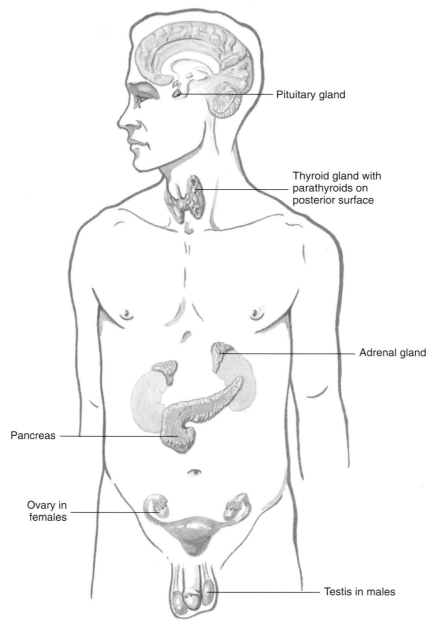

FIGURE 23–39 ▲ Primary organs of the endocrine system.

■ THE ENDOCRINE SYSTEM

Primary Organs of the Endocrine System (Fig. 23–39)

Hypothalamus
Pituitary
Thyroid gland
Parathyroid gland
Pancreas (Islets of Langerhans)
Adrenal glands
Ovaries (female) and Testes (male)

Functions of the Endocrine System

The functions of the endocrine system are much the same as those of the nervous system—communication, integration, and control; however, endocrine functions are carried out in a much different manner. They both use chemicals (hormones and neurotransmitters), but neurotransmitters act immediately and are short-lived, while the effects of the endocrine system hormones are further reaching and longer lasting. The organs of the endocrine system are the endocrine glands, which produce controlling substances called hormones. Endocrine, or ductless, glands do not have tubes to carry their secretions to other parts of the body; endocrine secretions go directly into the bloodstream, which carries them to other parts of the body. In contrast to the endocrine glands, the exocrine glands of the body have tubes to carry their secretions from the producing gland to other parts or organs of the body. For example, the saliva produced by the parotid gland (an exocrine gland) flows from the parotid gland through a tube into the mouth. Some nonendocrine organs such as the heart, lungs, kidneys, liver, and placenta also produce and release hormones.

The Pituitary Gland

The pituitary gland, often referred to as the master gland, has a master of its own! Although the pituitary gland produces hormones that stimulate the functions of other endocrine glands, it is the hypothalamus of the brain that directly regulates the secretory activity of the pituitary gland. The pituitary gland, attached to the hypothalamus, is a pea-sized gland located in the cranial cavity at the base of the brain. The pituitary gland is divided into two lobes: the anterior and the posterior.

The anterior lobe, or adenohypophysis produces the following five hormones:

1. *Adrenocorticotropic hormone (ACTH)*, which stimulates the action of part of the adrenal gland.
2. *Thyroid stimulating hormone (TSH)*, which stimulates the action of the thyroid gland.
3. *Growth hormone (GH)*, which promotes body growth.
4. *Prolactin (PRL)*, which stimulates and sustains milk production in lactating females. Prolactin has no known effect in males.
5. *Gonadotropins*, which stimulate the growth and maintenance of the gonads (ovaries [F] and testes [M]). Follicle-stimulating hormone (FSH) stimulates follicles in ovaries (F) and seminiferous tubes (M) and luteinizing hormone (LH) stimulates ovulation (F) and production of male sex cell (spermatogenesis).

The posterior lobe, or neurohypophysis, produces two hormones:

1. *Antidiuretic hormone (ADH)*, which stimulates reabsorption of water by the kidney.
2. *Oxytocin*, which stimulates uterine contractions while a female is in labor.

The Thyroid Gland

The thyroid gland, shaped like a butterfly, is located in the lower neck on the front and sides of the trachea. It produces the hormone thyroxine, which maintains metabolism of the body cells. Iodine is necessary in the body for the production of thyroxine by the thyroid gland, which is critical for normal growth and development.

The Parathyroid Glands

The parathyroid glands are four small bodies located posterior to the thyroid gland. They produce parathyroid hormone, which regulates the amount of calcium in the blood.

Pancreas

The pancreas functions as both an exocrine gland and endocrine gland. The endocrine component, the islets of Langerhans, are microscopic bunches of cells scattered throughout the pancreas (refer to Unit 7 of this chapter). They secrete the hormones insulin and glucagon, which are necessary for the metabolism of carbohydrates in the body. Glucagon works with insulin to regulate blood glucose levels.

The Adrenal Glands

The adrenal glands, situated on top of each kidney, are divided into two parts: the adrenal cortex (outer part) and the adrenal medulla (inner part). The adrenal cortex produces three steroid hormones: mineralocorticoids, glucocorticoids, and androgens. Mineralocorticoids regulate electrolyte balance, essential to normal body function and to life itself. Cortisol and cortisone are two glucocorticoids that influence protein, sugar, and fat metabolism. Cortisone, because of its antiinflammatory effect, is used therapeutically for treatment of various ailments. During physical or emotional stress, cortisol secretions increase to assist with the body's response. Androgens are hormones that are responsible for the masculinizing effect in males. Testosterone produced by the testes has the same masculinizing effect and is discussed further in Unit 9, The Urinary System and the Male Reproductive System.

The adrenal medulla produces two hormones, epinephrine (or adrenaline) and norepinephrine, that help the body to respond to emergency or stressful situations by increasing the function of vital organs (heartbeat and respiration), raising blood pressure, and providing extra nourishment for the voluntary muscles so they can perform an extra amount of work.

Sex Glands

The ovaries of the female and the testes of the male are endocrine glands. Ovaries are described in Unit 10, and the testes are discussed in Unit 9.

▪ DISEASES OF THE ENDOCRINE SYSTEM

Diabetes Mellitus (Type I or Type II)

Diabetes mellitus, one of the most common endocrine disorders, results in the inability of the body to store and use carbohydrates in the usual manner. Contributing factors are the inability of the islets of Langerhans to produce enough insulin, increase in the rate that the body uses the insulin, increase in the rate of insulin storage in the body, or drop in the efficiency of the use of insulin. In type I, the beta cells of the pancreatic islets are destroyed and the patient must take regular injections of insulin. In type II, the body is unable to respond to its insulin normally. Patients tend to be overweight, a factor believed responsible for the characteristic insulin resistance. Individuals with type II diabetes control their blood sugar level with diet, exercise, oral hypoglycemics, and insulin injections.

Symptoms of diabetes mellitus are polyuria, an increase in urine output; polyphagia, an increase in appetite; polydipsia, an increase in thirst; glycosuria, an elevation of sugar in the urine; and hyperglycemia, an elevation of sugar in the blood.

Diagnostic studies include urinalysis, fasting blood sugar, and hemoglobin A1C. Treatment depends on the severity of the disease. Mild diabetes can be controlled by a diet that usually contains limited amounts of sugar, carbohydrates, and fats. Some patients may need to take oral hypoglycemics in concert with their diet modifications. Moderate to severe diabetes may require insulin therapy. Too much glucose in the blood may cause a condition called diabetic coma, whereas too much insulin in the blood may cause a condition called insulin shock.

Graves' Disease

Graves' disease, a form of hyperthyroidism, causes overproduction of thyroxine, an increase in the size of the thyroid gland (goiter), and many changes in the other systems. Accompanying symptoms include intolerance to heat, nervousness, loss of weight, and goiter. The cause of Graves' disease is unknown, but it is five times more common in women than in men. It usually occurs between the ages of 20 and 40 years. T_3 and T_4 uptake tests and a thyroid scan may be used to diagnose Graves' disease. Treatment includes prescribing antithyroid drugs, radioactive iodine, and performing a subtotal thyroidectomy.

REVIEW QUESTIONS

1. _____ is necessary in the body for the production of thyroxine.

2. Indicate the hormones produced by each endocrine gland by writing the number of the hormone listed in Column 2 by the name of the endocrine gland listed in Column 1. You may want to write more than one number in each space.

Column 1

_____ a. parathyroid hormone
_____ b. GH
_____ c. TSH
_____ d. FSH
_____ e. oxytocin
_____ f. ACTH
_____ g. cortisone
_____ h. epinephrine
_____ i. insulin
_____ j. PRL
_____ k. thyroxine
_____ l. ADH

Column 2

1. anterior pituitary gland
2. adrenal cortex gland
3. thyroid gland
4. posterior pituitary gland
5. parathyroid gland
6. islets of Langerhans
7. adrenal medulla gland

3. Explain why the pituitary gland is sometimes referred to as the master gland. Explain the role of the hypothalamus in the secretion of the pituitary.

4. What is the overall function of the endocrine system?

5. Insulin is secreted by the _____ located throughout the _____ .

6. What is the function of insulin in the body?

    _____

7. Describe the symptoms of diabetes mellitus.

    a. _____

    b. _____

    c. _____

    d. _____

    e. _____

8. Graves' disease is a form of _____ .

MEDICAL TERMINOLOGY RELATING TO THE ENDOCRINE SYSTEM

Upon mastery of the medical terminology for this unit, you will be able to:

1. Spell and define the terms related to the endocrine system.

2. Given the meaning of a medical condition relating to the endocrine system, build with word parts the correct corresponding medical terms.

3. Given a description of a hospital situation in which the health unit coordinator may encounter medical terminology, apply the correct medical terms to the situation described.

Word Parts

The list below contains the word parts you need to memorize for the endocrine system. The exercises included in this unit will help you with this task. You will continue to use these word parts throughout the course and during employment. Practice pronouncing each word part aloud.

Word Roots/Combining Forms

Word Roots/Combining Forms	Meaning
aden/o (ăd'-ĕ-nō)	gland
adren/o (ah-drē'-nō)	adrenal
adrenal/o (ah-drē'-nal-ō)	adrenal
parathyroid/o (păr-ah-thī'-roy-dō)	parathyroid
thyr/o (thī'-rō)	thyroid
thyroid/o (thī'-roy-dō)	thyroid

EXERCISE 1

Write the combining forms for each medical term listed below.

1. gland   _____

2. thyroid   _____

                            _____

3. adrenal   _____

                            _____

4. parathyroid   _____

MEDICAL TERMS RELATING TO THE ENDOCRINE SYSTEM

The following list is made up of medical terms you will need to know for the endocrine system. Exercises following this list will assist you in learning these terms. Practice pronouncing each term aloud.

General Terms	Meaning
adenitis (ăd-ĕ-nīi'-tĭs)	inflammation of a gland
adenoid (ăd'-ĕ-noyd)	resembling a gland (adenoids: glandular tissue located in the nasopharynx)
adenoma (ăd-ĕ-nō'-mah)	a tumor of glandular tissue
adenosis (ăd-ĕ-nō'-sĭs)	abnormal condition of a gland
adrenal (ah-drē'-nal)	adrenal gland located near the kidney
adrenalitis (ah-drē-năl-ī'-tĭs)	inflammation of the adrenal gland
gland	a secretory organ that produces hormones or other substances
hormones	chemical messengers produced by the endocrine system
secretion (sē-krē'-shŭn)	a substance produced by a gland

Surgical Terms	Meaning
parathyroidectomy (păr'-ah-th-ī-roy-dĕk'-tō-mē)	excision of the parathyroid gland
thyroidectomy (th-ī-roy-dĕk'-tō-mē)	surgical removal of the thyroid gland

Diagnostic Terms	Meaning
Addison's disease (ăd'-i-sŭnz)	disease caused by lack of production of hormones by the adrenal gland
Cushing's disease (koosh'ĭngz)	a disorder caused by overproduction of certain hormones by the adrenal cortex
diabetes insipidus (dī-ah-bē'-tĭs) (ĭn-sĭp'-ĭ-dĭs)	disease caused by inadequate antidiuretic hormone production by the posterior lobe of the pituitary gland
diabetes mellitus (DM) (dī-ah-bē'-tĭs) (mĭl-ī'-tĭs)	disease that results in the inability of the body to store and use carbohydrates in the usual manner. It may be caused by inadequate production of insulin by the islets of Langerhans
hyperthyroidism (hī-per-thī'-roy-dĭzm)	excessive production of thyroxin and often an enlarged thyroid gland (goiter); also called Graves' disease or exophthalmic goiter
hypothyroidism (hī-pō-thī'-roy-dĭzm)	condition of underproduction of thyroxin by the thyroid gland

Terms Relating to Diagnostic Procedures	Meaning
blood glucose monitoring	method of monitoring the patient's glucose level by using a finger stick to obtain blood; performed by nursing staff
fasting blood sugar (FBS)	laboratory test to determine the amount of glucose in the blood after patient has fasted for 8–10 hours; may be used to diagnose and/or monitor diabetes mellitus
hemoglobin A1C (Hb A$_{1C}$)	laboratory test performed to more precisely determine the control of diabetes. Test result shows the percentage of glycated (or glycosylated) hemoglobin in the blood. Excess glucose in the bloodstream, which usually occurs when diabetes is poorly controlled, binds (or glycates) with hemoglobin molecules in the RBCs
protein-bound iodine	laboratory test performed on a sample of blood to determine thyroid activity
T$_3$, T$_4$, and T$_7$ uptake	studies performed on a blood sample that use nuclear substances to determine the function of the thyroid gland
thyroid scan	diagnostic study for thyroid gland function

EXERCISE 2

Using the word parts studied in this unit and previous units, build medical terms from each definition listed below.

1. inflammation of a gland _____

2. surgical removal of the thyroid gland _____

3. surgical removal of the parathyroid gland _____

4. resembling a gland _____

5. tumor of glandular tissue _____

6. abnormal condition of a gland _____

7. inflammation of the adrenal gland _____

EXERCISE 3

The following are conditions caused by oversecretion or undersecretion of endocrine glands. In the space provided write the name of the gland involved with the condition.

1. diabetes mellitus _____

2. hyperthyroidism _____

3. Addison's disease _____

4. hypothyroidism _____

5. Cushing's disease _____

6. diabetes insipidus _____

EXERCISE 4

Complete the following words:

1. dia _ _ t _ _   ins _ p _ d _ _

2. Ad _ _ _ on's dis _ _ se

3. Cu _ _ ing's dis _ _ se

4. h _ poth _ _ oid _ _ m

5. sec _ _ ti _ ns

EXERCISE 5

Spell each term studied in this unit by having someone dictate the terms to you.

1. _____
2. _____
3. _____
4. _____
5. _____
6. _____
7. _____
8. _____

9. _____
10. _____
11. _____
12. _____
13. _____
14. _____
15. _____
16. _____
17. _____
18. _____
19. _____
20. _____
21. _____
22. _____
23. _____

EXERCISE 6

Answer the following questions.

1. The patient is admitted to the hospital with a possible diagnosis of _____ , caused by an inadequate amount of insulin in the body. Insulin is produced by the _____ . The doctor may order any of these three laboratory tests: _____, _____, or _____, to assist in diagnosing the patient's condition. He or she also orders _____ to be performed by the nursing staff to determine the patient's glucose level.

2. If the patient is suffering from an insufficiency of a certain hormone in the body, the doctor may order a hormonal medication to be given to the patient to make up for the deficiency. The following is a list of hormonal medications. Indicate which endocrine gland should secrete each hormone.

   a. ACTH _____

   b. cortisone _____

c. insulin _____

d. epinephrine _____

e. Premarin (estrogen) _____

f. testosterone _____

g. thyroid preparation _____

3. The patient is admitted to the hospital with a diagnosis of a thyroid condition. List three tests the doctor may order to gather information about the patient's thyroid function.

a. _____

b. _____

c. _____

■ WEB SITES OF INTEREST

http://www.merck.com/pubs/mmanual_home/contents.html
http://www.americanheart.org
http://www.niddk.nih.gov/health
http://www.nlm.nih.gov
http://www.nimh.nih.gov
http://www.epilepsyfoundation.org
http://www.lungusa.org
http://www.cancer.org
http://www.kidney.org

Word Parts

Each word element present in Chapter 23 is noted in **bold text** along with its meaning and the unit of Chapter 23 in which it is found. Additional word parts you may encounter in your medical work are provided in normal text and instead of unit number, a sample medical term incorporating the word part is provided.

Word Element	Meaning	Unit Number (or Sample Medical Term)	Word Element	Meaning	Unit Number (or Sample Medical Term)
a	**without**	1	**-cele**	**herniation, protrusion**	4
abdomin/o	**abdomen**	7	**-centesis**	**surgical puncture to aspirate fluid**	4
acou/o	hearing	*acoumeter*			
acr/o	extremities, height	*acromegaly*	**cerebell/o**	**cerebellum**	4
aden/o	**gland**	11	**cerebr/o**	**cerebrum**	4
adren/o	**adrenal**	11	**cervic/o**	**cervix**	10
adrenal/o	**adrenal**	11	**cheil/o**	**lip**	7
-ac	pertaining to	*cardiac*	cholangi/o	bile duct	*cholangioma*
-al	**pertaining to**	2	**chol/e,**	**bile, gall**	7
-algia	**pain**	3	**chol/o**		
amnion/o	amnion, amniotic fluid	*amnionitis*	choledoch/o	common bile duct	*choledocholithiasis*
an-	**without**	1			
angi/o	**blood vessel**	6	**chondr/o**	**cartilage**	3
aort/o	**aorta**	6	**clavic/o**	**clavicle**	3
-apheresis	removal	*plasmapheresis*	**clavicul/o**	**clavicle**	3
appendic/o	**appendix**	7	-coccus	berry-shaped (form of bacterium)	*staphylococcus*
-ar	**pertaining to**	3			
arteri/o	**artery**	6	**col/o**	**colon**	7
arthr/o	**joint**	3	**colp/o**	**vagina**	10
-ary	pertaining to	*pulmonary*	**conjunctiv/o**	**conjunctiva**	5
-asthenia	weakness	*myasthenia*	**cost/o**	**rib**	3
atel/o	imperfect, incomplete	*atelectasis*	**crani/o**	**cranium**	3
ather/o	yellowish, fatty plaque	*atherosclerosis*	crypt/o	hidden	*onychocryptosis*
-atresia	absence of normal body opening, occlusion	*hysteratresia*	**cutane/o**	**skin**	2
			cyan/o	**blue**	6
aut/o	self	*autopsy*	**cyst/o**	**bladder, sac**	7, 9
balan/o	glans penis	*balanitis*	-cyte	cell	*erythrocyte*
bi-	two	*bilateral*	**cyt/o**	**cell**	1, 2
blephar/o	**eyelid**	5	**derm/o**	**skin**	2
brady-	**slow**	6	**dermat/o**	**skin**	2
bronch/o	**bronchus**	8	diverticul/o	diverticulum	*diverticulosis, diverticulitis*
cancer/o	**cancer**	2			
carcin/o	**cancer**	2	**duoden/o**	**duodenum**	7
cardi/o	**heart**	2	**dys-**	**difficult, labored, painful, abnormal**	8
caud/o	tail or down	*caudal*			

Word Element	Meaning	Unit Number (or Sample Medical Term)	Word Element	Meaning	Unit Number (or Sample Medical Term)
ech/o	sound	*echocardiogram*	**leuk/o**	**white**	6
-ectasis	expansion	*atelectasis*	**lingu/o**	**tongue**	7
-ectomy	**excision, surgical removal**	1, 3	**lip/o**	**fat**	2
electr/o	**electricity, electrical activity**	1, 3	**lith/o**	**stone, calculus**	7
-emia	**condition of the blood**	6	**-logist**	**one who specializes in the diagnosis and treatment of**	2
encephal/o	**brain**	4	**-logy**	**study of**	2
endo-	**within**	6	-lysis	loosening, dissolution, separating	*urinalysis*
enter/o	**intestine**	7	-malacia	softening	*chondromalacia*
epididym/o	epididymis	*epididymitis*	**mamm/o**	**breast**	10
episi/o	vulva	*episiotomy*	**mast/o**	**breast**	10
epitheli/o	**epithelium**	2	**-megaly**	**enlargement**	6
erythr/o	**red**	6	melan/o	black	*melanoma*
esophag/o	**esophagus**	7	**men/o**	**menstruation**	10
eti/o	cause (of disease)	etiology	**mening/o**	**meninges**	4
femor/o	**femur**	3	**menisc/o**	**meniscus**	3
fibr/o	fiber	*fibromyalgia*	meta-	after, beyond, change	*metastasis*
gastr/o	**stomach**	7	-meter	instrument used to measure	*spirometer*
-genic	**producing, originating, causing**	2	**metr/o**	**uterus**	10
gloss/o	**tongue**	7	-metry	measurement	*pelvimetry*
-gram	**record, x-ray image**	3	myc/o	fungus	*onychomycosis*
-graph	**instrument used to record**	3	**my/o**	**muscle**	3
-graphy	**process of recording, x-ray imaging**	3	**myel/o**	**spinal cord, bone marrow**	4
gravid/o	pregnancy	*gravida*	**myring/o**	**tympanic membrane**	5
gynec/o	**woman**	10	nat/o	birth	*prenatal*
hem/o	**blood**	6	natr/o	sodium	*hyponatremia*
hemat/o	**blood**	6	necr/o	death (cells, body)	*necrosis*
hepat/o	**liver**	7	**nephr/o**	**kidney**	9
herni/o	**protrusion of a body part**	7	neo-	new	*neonatal*
hist/o	**tissue**	2	**neur/o**	**nerve**	4
humer/o	**humerus**	3	noct/i	night	*nocturia*
hyper-	**above normal**	6	-odynia	pain	*cardiodynia*
hypo-	**below normal**	6	**-oid**	**resembling**	2
hyster/o	**uterus**	10	olig/o	scanty, few	*oliguria*
-ial	pertaining to	*endometrial*	**-oma**	**tumor**	2
-iasis	**condition of**	7	**onc/o**	**cancer**	2
-iatrist	specialist, physician	*physiatrist*	onych/o	nail	*onychomalacia*
iatr/o	physician, treatment	*iatrogenic*	**oophor/o**	**ovary**	10
-ic	**pertaining to**	3	**ophthalm/o**	**eye**	5
-ior	pertaining to	*posterior*	-opsy	to view	*biopsy*
ile/o	**ileum**	7	**orchi/o**	**testicle, testis**	9
inter-	between	*intervertebral*	**orchid/o**	**testicle, testis**	9
intra-	**within**	1	organ/o	organ	*organic*
irid/o	**iris**	5	**-osis**	**abnormal condition**	3
isch/o	deficiency, blockage	*ischemia*	**oste/o**	**bone**	3
-itis	**inflammation**	3	**ot/o**	**ear**	5
kal/i	potassium	*hyperkalemia*	-oxia	oxygen	*hypoxia*
kerat/o	**cornea**	5	**-ous**	**pertaining to**	2
labyrinth/o	labyrinth	*labyrinthitis*	**pancreat/o**	**pancreas**	7
lact/o	milk	*lactorrhea*	**para-thyroid/o**	**parathyroid**	11
lamin/o	**lamina**	3	part/o	give birth to, labor, childbirth	*parturition*
lapar/o	**abdomen**	7	**patell/o**	**patella**	3
laryng/o	**larynx**	8	**path/o**	**disease**	2
lei/o	smooth	*leiomyosarcoma*	-pathy	disease	*neuropathy*
			peri-	**surrounding (outer)**	6

Word Element	Meaning	Unit Number (or Sample Medical Term)	Word Element	Meaning	Unit Number (or Sample Medical Term)
perine/o	perineum	10	-scopy	visual examination	3
-pexy	surgical fixation	6	sigmoid/o	sigmoid colon	7
-phagia	swallowing	dysphagia	-sis	state of	diagnosis
phalang/o	phalange	3	son/o	sound	sonogram
pharyng/o	pharynx	8	somat/o	body	psychosomatic
phas/o	speech	4	-spasm	involuntary muscle contraction	bronchospasm
phleb/o	vein	6			
-phobia	fear of	claustrophobia	spin/o	spine	4
phot/o	light	photophobia	splen/o	spleen	6
-plasty	surgical repair	3	staped/o	stapes	5
-plegia	paralysis, stroke	4	staphyl/o	grape-like clusters	staphylococcus
pleur/o	pleura	8	-stasis	control, stop, standing	metastasis
-pnea	respiration breathing	8	-stenosis	narrowing	6
pneum/o	air, lung	8	stern/o	sternum	3
pneumon/o	lung	8	stomat/o	mouth	7
-poiesis	formation	hematopoiesis	-stomy	creation of an artificial opening	7
poli/o	gray matter	4			
prim/i	first	primigravida	strepto-coccus	twisted chains	streptococcus
proct/o	rectum	7			
prostat/o	prostate	9	sub-	under, below	1
psych/o	mind	4	supra-	above	suprascapular
-ptosis	drooping, sagging, prolapse	nephroptosis	tachy-	fast, rapid	6
puerper/o	childbirth	peurperal	thorac/o	chest	8
pulmon/o	lung	8	-thorax	chest	pneumothorax
pyel/o	renal pelvis	9	thromb/o	clot	6
pylor/o	pylorus, pyloric sphincter	pyloroplasty	thyr/o	thyroid	11
quadr/i	four	quadriplegia	thyroid/o	thyroid	11
radic/o, radicul/o, rhiz/o	nerve root	radiculitis	tom/o	cut, section	tomogram
			-tomy	surgical incision or to cut into	3
ren/o	kidney	9	tonsill/o	tonsil	8
retin/o	retina	5	trache/o	trachea	8
rhabd/o	rod-shaped, striated	rhabdomyolysis	trans-	through, across, beyond	1
rhin/o	nose	8	trich/o	hair	2
-rrhagia	rapid flow of blood	4	-trophy	development, nourishment	3
-rrhaphy	surgical repair	4			
-rrhea	excessive discharge, flow	4	ungu/o	nail	2
-rrhexis	rupture	hysterorrhexis	ur/o	urine, urinary tract	9
salping/o	fallopian or uterine tube	10	ureter/o	ureter	9
sarc/o	connective tissue, flesh	2	urethr/o	urethra	9
-sarcoma	malignant tumor	rhabdomyo-sarcoma	uria-	urine, urination	albuminuria
			urin/o	urine	9
scapul/o	scapula	3	uter/o	uterus	10
scler/o	sclera, hard	5	vagin/o	vagina	10
-sclerosis	hardening	6	vas/o	vessel, duct	9
-scope	instrument used for visual examination	3	ven/o	vein	6
			vertebr/o	vertebra	3
-scopic	pertaining to visual examination	arthroscopic	viscer/o	internal organs	2

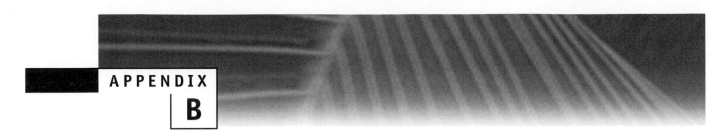

Abbreviations

The following is a list of alphabetized abbreviations used frequently in doctors' orders. Most of the abbreviations related to specific departments, such as laboratory and diagnostic imaging, are not included here. For those, please refer to the chapters concerning those departments.

Abbreviation	Meaning	Abbreviation	Meaning
>	greater than	ARC	AIDS-related complex
<	less than	AROM	active range of motion
↑	increase or above	ASA	acetylsalicylic acid (aspirin)
/	per or by	ASAP	as soon as possible
Δ	change	as tol	as tolerated
@	at	ax	axillary
↓	decrease or below	BAER or AER	brain stem auditory response
°	degree or hour	BE	barium enema
A	apical	bid	twice a day
AA	active assisted	bili	bilirubin
ā	before	BiPap	bi-level positive airway pressure
āā	of each	BiW, biw	twice a week
AAROM	active-assistive range of motion	BKA	below-the-knee amputation
Ab	antibody	B/L	bilateral
abd	abdominal	BLE	both lower extremities
ABG	arterial blood gases	BM	bowel movement
ABR	absolute bed rest	BMP	basic metabolic panel
ac	before meals	BP	blood pressure
ACL	anterior cruciate ligament (ACL) repair	BR	bed rest
ADA	American Diabetic Association	BRP	bathroom privileges
ADL	activity(ies) of daily living	BS	blood sugar
ad lib	as desired	BSC	bedside commode
A-drive	floppy drive	BUE	both upper extremities
AE	antiembolism	BUN	blood urea nitrogen
AFB	acid-fast bacillus	Bx	biopsy
Ag	antigen	c̄	with
AIDS	acquired immunodeficiency syndrome	C	Celsius
AKA	above-the-knee amputation	CA	cancer
AM	morning	Ca or Ca⁺	calcium
AMA	against medical advice	CABG	coronary artery bypass graft
amb	ambulate	CAD	coronary artery disease
AMO	against medical orders	cal	calorie
amp	ampule	cap	capsule
A&O	alert and oriented	CT	computed axial tomography
AP	anteroposterior	cath	catheterize
appt	appointment	CBC	complete blood cell count
APS	adult protective services	CBG	capillary blood gases

Abbreviation	Meaning
CBI	continuous bladder irrigation
CBR	continuous bed rest
cc or cm³	cubic centimeter
CCU	coronary care unit
CDC	Centers for Disease Control
C-drive	hard drive stored inside the computer
CEO	chief executive officer
CFO	chief financial officer
CHF	congestive heart failure
CHO	carbohydrate
chol	cholesterol
CHUC	certified health unit coordinator
CI	clinical indications
cl	clear
CMP	comprehensive metabolic panel
CMS	circulation, motion, sensation
CMV	cytomegalovirus
CNA	certified nursing assistant
c/o	complained of
CO₂	carbon dioxide
COA or C of A	conditions of admission
comp or cmpd	compound
con't	continue
COO	chief operating officer
COPD	chronic obstructive pulmonary disease
CP	cold packs
CPAP	continuous positive airway pressure
CPM	continuous passive motion
CPR	cardiopulmonary resuscitation
CPS	child protective services
CPT	chest physical therapy
CPU	central processing unit
CPZ	Compazine
CQI	continuous quality improvement
C&S	culture and sensitivity
CSF	cerebral spinal fluid
CT	computed tomography
Cx	culture
CXR	chest x-ray
CVA	cerebrovascular accident
CVC	central venous catheter
CVICU	cardiovascular intensive critical care unit
CVP	central venous pressure
CXR	chest x-ray
DAT	diet as tolerated
	direct antiglobulin test
D/C or DC	discontinue
	discharge
Diff	differential
Dig	digoxin
Disch	discharge
D/LR	dextrose in lactated Ringer's solution
DME	durable medical equipment
DNR	do not resuscitate
D/NS	dextrose in normal saline
DO	doctor of osteopathy
dr or ʒ	dram
DRG	diagnosis-related group
D/RL	dextrose in Ringer's lactate
DSS	dioctyl sodium sulfosuccinate (Colace)

Abbreviation	Meaning
DSU	day surgery unit
D/W	dextrose in water
DW	distilled water
D₅W	5% dextrose in water
D₁₀W	10% dextrose in water
DX	diagnosis
EBV	Epstein-Barr virus
EC	enteric coated
ECF	extended care facility
ECG or EKG	electrocardiogram
EchoEG	echoencephalogram
ED	emergency department
EEG	electroencephalogram
EGD	esophagogastroduodenoscopy
elix	elixir
EMG	electromyogram
ENG	electronystagmography
EPC	electronic pain control
EPS	electrophysiological study
ER	emergency room
ERCP	endoscopic retrograde cholangiopancreatography
ES	electrical stimulation
ESR	erythrocyte sedimentation rate
ESRD	end-stage renal disease
ET	endotracheal tube
ETS	elevated toilet seat
F	Fahrenheit
FBS	fasting blood sugar
Fe	iron
FF	force fluids
FFP	fresh frozen plasma
fib	fibrinogen
FS	full strength
	frozen section
5-FU	5-fluorouracil
F/U	follow-up
FWB	full weight bearing
FWW	front wheel walker
Fx, fx	fracture
G, gm, g	gram
GB	gallbladder
GI	gastrointestinal
gluc	glucose
gr	grain
GTT	glucose tolerance test
gtt(s)	drop(s)
Gyn	gynecology
h, hr, hrs	hour/s
h or (H)	hypodermic
HA	heated aerosol
H/A	headache
HBₛAg	hepatitis B surface antigen
HBOT	hyperbaric O₂ therapy
HBV	hepatitis B virus
HCG	human chorionic gonadotropin
hct	hematocrit
HCTZ	hydrochlorothiazide
HCV	hepatitis C virus
HD	hemodialysis

Abbreviation	Meaning
HDL	high-density lipoprotein
hgb	hemoglobin
H&H	hemoglobin and hematocrit
HIPAA	Health Insurance Portability and Accountability Act
HIV	human immunodeficiency virus
HL or heplock	heparin lock
HMO	health maintenance organization
HNP	herniated nucleus pulposus
HO	house officer
h/o	history of
H_2O	water
H_2O_2	hydrogen peroxide
HOB	head of bed
H&P	history and physical
HP	hot packs
hs	bedtime
HUC	health unit coordinator
	health unit clerk
HUS	health unit secretary
Hx	history
ICD	implantable cardioverter defibrillator
	International Classification of Diseases
ICU	Intensive Care Unit
ID labels	identification labels
IM	intramuscular
I&O	intake and output
IPG	impedance plethysmography
IPPB	intermittent positive pressure breathing
irrig	irrigate
IS	incentive spirometry
ISOM	isometric
IV	intravenous
IVF	intravenous fluids
IVP	intravenous pyelogram
IVPB	intravenous piggyback
IVU	intravenous urogram
JCAHO	Joint Commission on the Accreditation of Healthcare Organizations
K or K^+	potassium
KCl	potassium chloride
kg	kilogram
KO	keep open
KUB	kidney, ureter, bladder
L	liter
lat	lateral
lb, #	pound(s)
L&D	labor and delivery
LDL	low-density lipoprotein
LE	lower extremities
liq	liquid
LLE	left lower extremity
LLL	left lower lobe
LLQ	left lower quadrant
L/min	liters per minute
LOC	laxative of choice
	leave on chart
	level of consciousness
	loss of consciousness
LP	lumbar puncture

Abbreviation	Meaning
LPN	licensed practical nurse
LR	lactated Ringer's solution
L&S	liver and spleen
LS	lumbosacral
Lt or Ⓛ	left
LTC	long-term care
LUE	left upper extremity
LUL	left upper lobe
LUQ	left upper quadrant
lytes or e-lytes	electrolytes
MAR	medication administration records
MD	doctor of medicine
MDI	metered dose inhaler
Med	medical
mEq	milliequivalent
μg, mcg	microgram
mg	milligram
Mg or Mg^+	magnesium
$MgSO$	magnesium sulfate
MI	myocardial infarction
MICU	medical intensive care unit
min	minute
mL	milliliter
MN	midnight
MOM	Milk of Magnesia
MR	may repeat
MRI	magnetic resonance imaging
MSO^4 or MS	morphine sulfate
MSSU	medical short-stay unit
Na or Na^+	sodium
NAHUC	National Association of Health Unit Coordinators
NAS	no added salt
NCS	nerve conduction studies
nec	necessary
Neuro	neurology
NG	nasogastric
NICU	neonatal intensive care unit
NINP	no information, no publication
NKA	no known allergies
NKDA	no known drug allergies
NKFA	no known food allergies
NKMA	no known medication allergies
noc	night
non rep	do not repeat
NP	nasopharynx
NPO	nothing by mouth
NS	normal saline
NSA	no salt added
NTG	nitroglycerin
N/V	nausea and vomiting
NVS or neuro ✓s	neurological vital signs or checks
NWB	non–weight-bearing
O_2	oxygen
OB	obstetrics
OBS	observation
OCG	oral cholecystogram
OD	right eye
OOB	out of bed

Abbreviation	Meaning
O&P	ova and parasites
OPS	outpatient surgery
OR	operating room
ORE	oil retention enema
ORIF	open reduction, internal fixation
Ortho	orthopedics
OS	left eye
OSA	obstructive sleep apnea
OSHA	Occupational Safety and Health Administration
OSMO	osmolality
OT	occupational therapy
OU	both eyes
oz	ounce
$\bar{p}$	after
P	pulse
PA	posteroanterior
PACU	postanesthesia care unit
PAP	prostatic acid phosphatase
PAS	pulsatile antiembolism stockings
PBZ	pyribenzamine
PC	personal computer
	packed cells
pc	after meals
PCA	patient-controlled analgesia
PCN	penicillin
PCT	patient care technician
PCXR	portable chest x-ray
PD	peritoneal dialysis
PDR	*Physicians' Desk Reference*
Peds	pediatrics
PEG	percutaneous endoscopic gastrostomy
PEEP	positive end-expiratory pressure
PEP	positive expiratory pressure
PET	positron emission tomography
PHI	protected health information reference
PICC	peripherally inserted central catheter
PICU	pediatric intensive care unit
PID	pelvic inflammatory disease
PM	evening, night
po	by mouth or postoperative
POCT or PCT	point-of-care testing performed on the nursing unit
PO day	postoperative day
Post-op, post-op	after surgery
PP	postpartum
pp	postprandial (after meals)
	postprandial
P&PD	percussion and postural drainage
PPE	personal protective equipment
PPO	preferred provider organization
pr	per rectum
Pre-op, pre-op	before surgery
prn	whenever necessary
PROM	passive range of motion
PSA	patient support associate
	prostatic specific antigen
Psych	psychiatry
PT	physical therapy
	prothrombin time

Abbreviation	Meaning
Pt	patient
PTA	physical therapy assistant
PTHC or PTC	percutaneous transhepatic cholangiography
PTCA	percutaneous transluminal coronary angioplasty
PTT or APTT	partial thromboplastin time or activated partial thromboplastin time
PWB	partial weight bearing
q	every
qd	daily
qh	every hour or fill in hour
qid	four times a day
qod	every other day
R	rectal
RA	room air
RBC	red blood cells
RBS	random blood sugar
RD	registered dietitian
RDW	red cell distribution width
reg	regular
RL	Ringer's lactate
RLE	right lower extremity
RLL	right lower lobe
RLQ	right lower quadrant
R&M	routine and microscopic
RML	right middle lobe
RN	registered nurse
R/O	rule out
ROM	range of motion
Rout	routine
RPR	rapid plasma reagin
RR	recovery room
	respiratory rate
RSV	respiratory syncytial virus
RT	respiratory therapist
Rt	routine
rt or Ⓡ	right
RUE	right upper extremity
RUL	right upper lobe
RUQ	right upper quadrant
Rx	take (treatment, medication, etc.)
$\bar{s}$	without
$\bar{\bar{ss}}$	semis (one-half)
SAD	save a day
SaO_2 or O_2 sats	oxygen saturation
SBFT	small-bowel follow-through
SBU	small business unit
SC, sq, or sub-q	subcutaneous
SDS	same-day surgery
SEP	somatosensory evoked potential
SHUC	student health unit coordinator
SICU	surgical intensive care unit
SL	sublingual
SNAT	suspected non-accidental trauma
SNF	skilled nursing facility
SO_4	sulfate
SOB	shortness of breath
sol'n	solution
SOS	if needed (one dose only)
SSE	soap suds enema

Abbreviation	Meaning
SSU	short-stay unit
st	straight
stat	immediately
STM	soft tissue massage
subling, SL	sublingual (under the tongue)
supp	suppository
Surg	surgery
SVN	small volume nebulizer
syr	syrup
T_3, T_4, T_7	thyroid tests
T&A	tonsillectomy and adenoidectomy
tab	tablet
TAH	total abdominal hysterectomy
TB	tuberculosis
TBD	to be done
TBT	template bleeding time
T&C or T & x-match	type and crossmatch
TCDB	turn, cough, and deep breathe
TCT or TT	thrombin clotting time or thrombin time
TDWB	touchdown weight bearing
TED	antiembolism stockings
temp	temperature
TENS	transcutaneous electrical nerve stimulation
THR or THA	total hip replacement/total hip arthroplasty
TIA	transient ischemic attack
TICU	trauma intensive care unit
tid	three times a day
tinct or tr	tincture
TKO	to keep open
TKR or TKA	total knee replacement/total knee arthroplasty
TPN	total parenteral nutrition
TPR	temperature, pulse, respiration
TRA	to run at

Abbreviation	Meaning
T&S	type and screen
TSH	thyroid-stimulating hormone
T/stat	timed stat
TT	tilt table
TTWB	toe-touch weight bearing
TUR	transurethral resection
TWE	tap water enema
Tx	traction or treatment
U	unit
UA or U/A	urinalysis
UCR	usual, customary, and reasonable
UD	unit dose
UGI	upper gastrointestinal
ung	unguent (ointment)
US	ultrasound
USN	ultrasonic nebulizer
VAD	venous access device
VDRL	Venereal Disease Research Laboratories
VDT	video display terminal
VEP	visual evoked potential
vib & perc	vibration and percussion
VMA	vanillylmandelic acid
VNS	visiting nurse service
VS	vital signs
WA or W/A	while awake
WBAT	weight bearing as tolerated
WBC	white blood cell
wk	week
WNL	within normal limits
WP	whirlpool
wt	weight
www	World Wide Web
x-match	crossmatch
Zn	zinc

The National Association of Health Unit Coordinators Standards of Practice*

A *standard of practice* is a statement of guidelines serving as a model of performance by which practitioners shall conduct their actions.

These standards are set forth to obtain the best possible service from practitioners to provide the organization and competency needed to coordinate the health unit in an exemplary fashion, enabling better care of the patient.

The National Association of Health Unit Coordinators (NAHUC) has formulated standards of practice fundamental enough to encompass all health units. NAHUC recognizes that these standards cannot be permanent. They will need to be evaluated and revised to keep pace with the advancement of technology and the health unit's changing objectives and functions.

Purposes

The purpose of the NAHUC standards is to specify guidelines for health unit coordinators to follow. These standards have as their objectives:

1. To define the realm of the health unit coordinator in the health care system.
2. To specify the primary responsibilities of the health unit coordinator in the nonclinical area of health care.

Basic Assumptions

The NAHUC standards for health unit coordinators are based on these assumptions:

1. Health unit coordinators provide the nondirect patient care or nonclinical functions for health services.
2. Standards for these services are established by the consensus of health unit coordinators and educators, and health care agencies.
3. Health unit coordinators accept basic responsiblity for their competency through individual growth, continued education, and certification.
4. Health unit coordinators are responsive to the changing needs of health care.

---

*Modified from National Association of Health Unit Coordinators, Standards of Practice, 1981, with permission.

Criteria for Statements of Standards

A standard is used as a model for the action of practitioners. Criteria used in establishing the NAHUC standards for health unit coordinators are:

1. A standard is established by an authority, in this instance, the National Association of Health Unit Coordinators.
2. A standard is founded on appropriate knowledge.
3. A standard is broad in scope, relevant, attainable, and definitive.
4. A standard is subject to continued evaluation and revision.

Standards of Practice for Health Unit Coordinators

Standard 1—Education

Health unit coordinators shall be prepared through appropriate education and training programs for their responsibility in the provision of nondirect patient care and nonclinical services.

Guidelines

Education shall be set forth by adopted NAHUC educational standards.

Standard 2—Policy and Procedure

Written standards of health unit coordinator practice and related policies and procedures shall define and describe the scope and conduct of nonclinical service provided by the health unit coordinator staff. These standards, policies, and procedures shall be reviewed annually and revised as necessary. They shall be dated to indicate the last review, signed by the responsible authority, and implemented.

Guidelines

1. Polices shall include a criteria-based job description.
2. Personnel policies will be included.
3. Policies will include the philosophy and objectives of the health unit organization.
4. Operational and nonclinical policies and procedures will be included.

Standard 3—Standards of Performance

Written evaluation of health unit coordinators shall be criteria-based and related to the standards of performance as defined by the health care organization.

Guidelines

1. Standards of performance shall delineate functions, responsibility, qualifications, and accountability, reflecting autonomy of practice.
2. Standards of performance shall be reviewed and evaluated at least annually or as needed to reflect current job requirements.
3. Evaluations shall be available to health unit coordinators.

Standard 4—Communication

The health unit coordinator shall appropriately integrate with the nursing and medical staff, other hospital staff, and vistors that contribute to patient care and well-being.

Guidelines

1. The health unit shall have a written organizational plan that defines authority, accountability, and communication.
2. The organization shall ensure that health unit coordinator service functions are fulfilled.
3. Health unit coordinators' meetings shall be no fewer than six times a year to define problems and propose solutions and follow-up evaluations. A record shall be maintained documenting the monitoring and evaluation of these meetings.

Standard 5—Professionalism and Ethics

The health unit coordinator shall take all possible steps to provide the optimal achievable quality of nondirect patient care and nonclinical services and to maintain the optimal professional and ethical conduct and practices of its members.

Guidelines

1. The health unit coordinator shall participate in staff development.
2. He or she shall perform services according to approved policies.
3. The unit coordinator shall attend all required meetings.
4. He or she shall augment knowledge with pertinent new knowledge.
5. The health unit coordinator shall maintain current competence.

Standard 6—Leadership

The health unit coordinator service shall be organized to meet and maintain established standards of nonclinical services.

Guidelines

1. The service shall be directed by a qualified individual with appropriate education, experience, and knowledge of health unit coordinator services.
2. It shall provide leadership and guidance to the health unit coordinator.
3. The service shall have the responsibility and authority to ensure:
   a. hospital policy and procedures are met
   b. hospital goals and objectives are met
   c. all responsible steps are taken to provide optimal achievable quality of nondirect patient care and nonclinical functions.
4. It is desirable that the health unit coordinator leader have an associate degree in health service management.

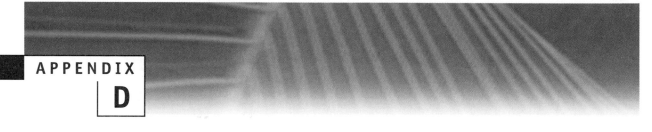

Task and Knowledge Statements from National Association of Health Unit Coordinators Job Analysis Study, 1996

Task Statements

Check charts for orders that need to be transcribed
Clarify questionable orders
Prioritize orders
Process orders according to priority
Enter orders on a Kardex
Interpret medical symbols/abbreviations
Initiate critical pathway protocols
Notify nursing staff of new orders
Notify and document consulting physicians of consult requests
Request services from ancillary departments
Request patient information from external facilities
Schedule diagnostic tests and procedures
Follow test preparation procedures
Enter orders onto a medication administration record
Indicate on the order sheet that each order has been processed
Sign off orders (e.g., signature, title, date, and time)
Flag charts for cosignature
Process daily diagnostic tests and procedures
Process nursing treatment orders
Label and assemble patient charts upon admission
Obtain patient information prior to admission
Assign beds to patients coming into the unit
Inform nursing staff of patient admissions, transfers, discharges, and returning surgical patients
Assemble necessary forms for patients being transferred to an external facility
Prepare patient charts for transfer to other units
Notify appropriate departments and individuals when patients are discharged (i.e., home, expired, AMA, transferred, etc.)
Disassemble patient charts, put in appropriate order, and send to medical records office upon expiration or discharge
Schedule follow-up appointments
Maintain a supply of chart forms
Maintain stock of patient care supplies and equipment
Maintain stock of clerical and desk supplies
Arrange for maintenance and repair of equipment
Maintain a hazard-free environment
Report unit activities to oncoming shift
Maintain patient census logs
Maintain patient charts by thinning and adding forms as needed
File forms and reports
Graph and chart information onto appropriate forms

Maintain patient census board
Prepare surgical charts
Process postoperative charts
Perform quality assurance activities on charts (i.e., verify chart forms are filed/labeled correctly, all orders transcribed, etc.)
Participate in emergency and disaster plans
Participate in response to cardiac or respiratory arrests (i.e., page codes, call physicians, etc.)
Orient new staff members to the unit
Process patient charges
Receive diagnostic test results
Notify physicians of diagnostic test results
Report diagnostic test results to nursing staff
Communicate facility policies to visitors, patients, and staff (i.e., visiting hours, no smoking, etc.)
Screen telephone calls and visitor requests for patient information to protect patient confidentiality
Restrict access to patient information (i.e., charts, computer)
Greet patients, physicians, visitors, and facility staff who arrive on the unit
Transport patient specimens, supplies, and medications
Respond to patient, physician, visitor, and facility staff requests and complaints
Communicate with patients and staff via intercom
Send and receive documents via fax machine
Duplicate documents using copy machine
Maintain computer census (i.e., ADT functions)
Retrieve diagnostic results from computer
Follow established computer downtime procedures
Contact personnel via paging system
Answer unit telephone calls
Enter orders via computer
Generate reports using computer
Participate in department, staff, or health unit coordinator meetings
Review facility-specific publications, memos, policies, etc.

Knowledge Statements

Knowledge of the components of a physician's order
Knowledge of the use of flagging a chart for indicating there are orders to be transcribed
Knowledge of the need to frequently check charts for new orders

Knowledge of the procedures for the transcription of orders

Knowledge of prioritization of medical conditions or situations

Knowledge of the definition of terms regarding priorities

Knowledge of problem-solving techniques

Knowledge of the methods used in problem identification

Knowledge of the roles and functions of the health care staff

Knowledge of basic medical terminology

Knowledge of basic medical symbols

Knowledge of basic medical abbreviations

Knowledge of how to handle stat orders

Knowledge of the proper response time for processing stat orders

Knowledge of the purpose of documentation

Knowledge of placement of forms and reports in a chart

Knowledge of times for diagnostic tests and medication deliveries

Knowledge of how to handle routine orders

Knowledge of the proper response time for processing orders

Knowledge of the procedures used to process orders that are outside routine time frames

Knowledge of the operating hours of ancillary departments

Knowledge of the procedures to follow to obtain services from ancillary departments

Knowledge of procedures used to order services, diagnostics, and medications

Knowledge of military time conversions

Knowledge of the names and functions of ancillary departments

Knowledge of the various methods used to communicate orders

Knowledge of documentation methods

Knowledge of medical staff privileges

Knowledge of when to use references

Knowledge of routine times diagnostic tests are performed

Knowledge of how to use references

Knowledge of the location of standard chart forms in the patient record

Knowledge of the methods used to enter into and retrieve information from the order entry computer screen

Knowledge of basic computer terminology

Knowledge of types of medical equipment

Knowledge of pertinent information needed prior to admission

Knowledge of the use of telephone equipment

Knowledge of the techniques used in telephone communication

Knowledge of the purpose of different forms

Knowledge of basic diagnostic terms

Knowledge of the methods used to obtain blood and blood products

Knowledge of the equivalencies between apothecary and metric dosages

Knowledge of dosages of common medications

Knowledge of the components of the Kardex

Knowledge of the components of a medication administration record

Knowledge of the components of a medication order

Knowledge of generic and trade names for common medications

Knowledge of the classifications of medications

Knowledge of procedures for renewal of medication orders

Knowledge of policies and procedures for amount of stock to be kept on the unit

Knowledge of policies and procedures for ordering replacement stock

Knowledge of procedures for proper and safe storage of unit supplies and equipment

Knowledge of policies and procedures for maintenance and repair of equipment

Knowledge of procedures for proper and safe storage of medications

Knowledge of facility's policies regarding transporting and handling of medications

Knowledge of safe and unsafe work conditions

Knowledge of infection control policies and procedures

Knowledge of the policies and procedures used to ensure the safety of staff, patients, and visitors on the unit

Knowledge of professional demeanor

Knowledge of the effects of power outages on telephone use

Knowledge of the methods used to respond to emergency telephone calls

Knowledge of the use of the patient intercom system

Knowledge of the techniques used in intercom communication

Knowledge of patient placement procedures

Knowledge of the circumstances under which the intercom should be used

Knowledge of the definition of confidentiality

Knowledge of patient's rights

Knowledge of circumstances that constitute breaches of confidentiality

Knowledge of policies and procedures regarding confidentiality

Knowledge of the standards of practice and code of ethics for health unit coordinating

Knowledge of verbal and nonverbal communication techniques

Knowledge of the components of a patient census log

Knowledge of the purpose of a census log

Knowledge of the classification of patient acuity

Knowledge of the purposes of compiling patient and unit statistics

Knowledge of the tools used to determine patient acuity

Knowledge of the purpose of the chart maintenance

Knowledge of procedures for maintaining charts

Knowledge of the methods used to organize information

Knowledge of the methods used to place forms and reports in a logical order

Knowledge of the methods used to stamp, label, or identify the patient's chart

Knowledge of the proper use of office equipment

Knowledge of the function of the patient census board

Knowledge of bed assignment methods

Knowledge of the normal and abnormal values for common diagnostic tests

Knowledge of the policies and procedures for discontinuing all preoperative orders postoperatively

Knowledge of importance of discontinuing all preoperative orders postoperatively

Knowledge of the process used to transcribe orders for transfusion of blood and blood products

Knowledge of the process used to transcribe orders for total parenteral nutrition/hyperalimentation

Knowledge of quality assurance policies and procedures

Knowledge of policies and procedures regarding emergency and disaster plans

Knowledge of the procedures for cardiac monitoring

Knowledge of policies and procedures for posting informational materials

Knowledge of the procedures for orienting new personnel

Knowledge of the methods used to evaluate the competency of orientees

Knowledge of the methods used to ensure unit's accountability regarding patient charges

Knowledge of the methods used to indicate the services and supplies used by each patient

Knowledge of services provided by outside vendors and agencies

Knowledge of the unit coordinator's responsiblity to participate in job-related training

Knowledge of the importance of keeping abreast of job-related changes

Knowledge of the different types of diagnostic tests

Knowledge of procedures to obtain services and supplies from outside sources

Knowledge of patient chart locations on the unit

Knowledge of routes of common medications

Knowledge of stop dates of common medications

Knowledge of chain of communication for clarification of orders

Knowledge of conflicting patient conditions and procedures

Knowledge of the location of general information on the Kardex

Knowledge of the term "critical pathway"

Knowledge of general diagnoses and pathways

Knowledge of coordination of services from multiple ancillary departments

Knowledge of the definition of stop dates

Knowledge of the use of paging system

Knowledge of information retrieval system

Knowledge of the purpose of processing patient charges

Knowledge of the policies and procedures for processing patient charges

Knowledge of pertinent information to request services from ancillary departments

Knowledge of reviewing standing orders

Knowledge of pertinent information to schedule follow-up appointments

Knowledge of pertinent information necessary to maintain patient census log

Knowledge of pertinent information necessary to maintain patient census board

Knowledge of pertinent information when preparing a surgical chart

Knowledge of pertinent information to process postoperative chart

Knowledge of pertinent information to participate in emergency and disaster plans

Knowledge of pertinent information to participate in arrest situations

Knowledge of pertinent information used to orient new staff members

Knowledge of pertinent information in diagnostic test results

Knowledge of pertinent information that needs to be communicated to patients, staff, and visitors

Knowledge of universal precautions

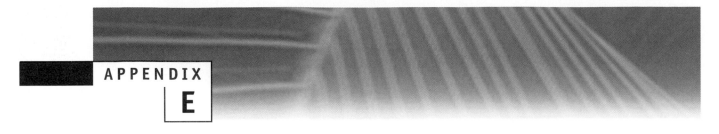

National Association of Health Unit Coordinators: Code of Ethics

This code of ethics is to serve as a guide by which health unit coordinators may evaluate their professional conduct as it relates to patients, colleagues, and other members of the health care profession. This code of ethics shall be subject to monitoring, interpretation, and periodic revision by the association's board of directors.

Therefore, in the practice of our profession, we the members of the National Association of Health Unit Coordinators accept the following principles:

Principle One

All members shall conduct themselves in such a manner as to gain the respect and confidence of the patients, health care personnel, and the community, as well as respecting the human dignity of each individual.

Principle Two

All members shall protect the patients' rights, including the right to privacy.

Principle Three

All members shall strive to achieve and maintain a high level of competency.

Principle Four

All members shall strive to improve their knowledge and skills by participating in educational and professional activities and sharing the benefits of their attainments with their colleagues.

Principle Five

Unethical and illegal professional activities shall be reported to the appropriate authorities.

A Comprehensive List of Laboratory Studies and Blood Components

*The divisions indicated on this chart would be those found in a large hospital. Many hospitals combine bacteriology and virology into the microbiology department. Space has been left at the end of each alphabetical section so that you can insert new tests as they are developed.

Procedure	Abbreviation	Laboratory Division	Specimen
ABO grouping (complete blood type)		Blood bank	Blood
Acetoacetic acid		Urinalysis	Urine
Acetone		Chemistry	Blood or urine
*Acid-fast culture	Culture for AFB (acid-fast bacilli)	Bacteriology	Sputum and tubercular lesions
*Acid-fast stain		Bacteriology	Sputum and tubercular lesions
Acid phosphatase	acid p'tase	Chemistry	Blood
Activated clotting time	ACT	Hematology/POCT	Blood
Activated partial thromboplastin time	APTT	Hematology	Blood
Addis count		Urinalysis	Urine
Adrenaline and noradrenaline (see epinephrine and norepinephrine)			
Adrenocorticotropic hormone	ACTH	Chemistry	Blood
Alanine aminotransferase	ALT	Chemistry	Blood
Albumin	Alb.	Chemistry	Blood or urine
Albumin/globulin ratio	A/G ratio	Chemistry	Blood
Alcohol (ethanol)		Chemistry	Blood
Aldolase		Chemistry	Blood
Aldosterone		Chemistry	Blood or urine
Alkaline phosphatase	ALP	Chemistry	Blood
Alkaline phosphatase isoenzymes		Chemistry	Blood
α_1-Antitrypsin		Chemistry	Blood
α_1-Fetoprotein		Chemistry	Blood
17 α-Hydroxyprogesterone		Chemistry	Urine
Amino acids, fractionated		Chemistry	Urine
Ammonia	NH_3	Chemistry	Blood
Amniotic fluid		Chemistry	Amniotic fluid
Amoeba (ova and parasites)	O&P	Parasitology	Stool
Amphotericin level		Chemistry	Blood
Amylase		Chemistry	Blood or urine
Androstenedione		Chemistry	Urine
Angiotensin-converting enzyme	ACE	Chemistry	Blood
Ankylosing spondylitis (see HLA B27 typing)			

*POCT, point of care testing. Some laboratory testing on blood, urine and stool may be performed on the nursing unit.

Procedure	Abbreviation	Laboratory Division	Specimen
Antideoxyribonuclease	DNA	Serology	Blood
Antidiuretic hormone	ADH	Chemistry	Blood
Antigen blood group (factor VIII)		Serology	Blood
Antimicrobial serum assay		Bacteriology	Blood
Antimony		Chemistry	Urine
Antinuclear antibody	ANA	Serology	Blood
Antistreptolysin O	ASO titer	Serology	Blood
Antithyroglobulin antibody		Serology	Blood
Arsenic, quantitative		Chemistry	Urine
Ascorbic acid		Chemistry	Blood
Aspartate aminotransferase	AST	Chemistry	Blood
Barbiturates		Toxicology	Blood or urine
Basic metabolic panel	BMP	Chemistry	Blood
Bence Jones proteins	BJP	Chemistry	Urine
Beta natriuretic peptide	BNP	Chemistry	Blood
β-Hemolytic strep culture		Bacteriology	Nose or throat culture
β$_2$-Microglobulin		Chemistry	Blood
Bile		Urinalysis/chemistry	Urine or stool
Bilirubin (total and direct)	bili	Chemistry	Blood
Biopsy	bx	Pathology	All specimens
Bleeding time		Hematology	Blood
Blood culture		Bacteriology	Blood
Blood sugar (BS) (glucose random)	RBS	Chemistry	Blood
Blood survey of coagulation defects		Hematology	Blood
Blood type (ABO and Rh)		Blood bank	Blood
Blood type and crossmatch	T&C, T&X-match	Blood bank	Blood
Blood urea nitrogen	BUN	Chemistry	Blood
Blood volume (Cr 51)		Chemistry	Blood
Blood volume (Risa)		Chemistry	Blood
Bone marrow examination		Hematology	Bone marrow
Bromide		Chemistry	Blood
Bromsulphalein	BSP	Chemistry	Blood
Bronchial smear—Gram stain		Bacteriology	Bronchial smear
Brucella abortus		Serology	Blood
Buccal smear—sex chromosomes		Cytology	Buccal smear
Calcitonin		Chemistry	Blood
Calcium	Ca or Ca+	Chemistry	Blood or urine
Calcium ionized		Chemistry	Blood
Capillary fragility		Hematology	Blood
Carbon dioxide	CO$_2$	Chemistry	Blood
Carbon monoxide	CO	Chemistry	Blood
Carboxyhemoglobin		Chemistry	Blood
Carcinoembryonic antigen	CEA	Serology	Blood
Cardiac enzymes	(CPK, LDH, SGOT)	Chemistry	Blood
Carotene		Chemistry	Blood
Catecholamines (blood)		Chemistry	Blood
Catecholamines (urine)		Chemistry	Urine
Cell indices	RBC indices	Hematology	Blood
Cerebrospinal fluid tests	CSF	Tests may be ordered from all divisions	Cerebrospinal fluid
Ceruloplasmin (see ferroxidase)			
Cervical and vaginal smear	(Pap test)	Cytology	Cells from cervix and vagina
Chlamydia culture		Bacteriology	Swabs from specified areas
Chlamydia serology		Serology	Blood
Choral hydrate		Chemistry	Blood
Chloramphenicol level		Chemistry	Blood
Chloride	Cl	Chemistry	Blood, CSF, sweat, and urine
Cholesterol	Chol	Chemistry	Blood

Procedure	Abbreviation	Laboratory Division	Specimen
Cholinesterase		Chemistry	Blood
Chorionic gonadotropin (serum)	HCG	Chemistry	Blood serum
Chorionic gonadotropin (urine)	HCG	Urinalysis	Urine
Chorionic gonadotropin (24-hour urine)	HCG	Chemistry	Urine-24-hour
Chromium 51 (blood volume)		Hematology	Blood
Chromosome study (buccal smear)		Cytology	Buccal smear
Chromosome study		Chemistry	Blood—tissue
Citric acid		Chemistry	Urine
Clot retraction		Hematology	Blood
Clotting time (coagulation time)	Coag. time or Lee-White	Hematology	Blood
CMV(cytomegalovirus) culture	CMV culture	Bacteriology	Blood or urine
CMV (cytomegalovirus) inclusions	CMV inclusions	Bacteriology	Blood or urine
CMV (cytomegalovirus) serology	CMV serology	Serology	Blood
Coagulation profile (platelets, APTT, prothrombin time, and bleeding time)		Hematology	Blood
Coagulation time, clotting time, thrombin clotting time, thrombin time	Coag. time, TCT, TT	Hematology	Blood
Cocci culture (fungus)		Bacteriology	Sputum
Coccidioides, complement fixation		Serology	Blood
Coccidioides, precipitin		Serology	Blood
Coccidioidomycosis—CSF titer		Serology	Cerebrospinal fluid
Cold agglutinins		Serology	Blood
Colloidal gold curve		Serology	Cerebrospinal fluid
Colony count		Bacteriology	Body fluids
Complement	C_3	Chemistry	Blood
Complete blood count	CBC	Hematology	Blood
Complete urinalysis	UA	Urinalysis	Urine
Comprehensive metabolic panel	CMP	Chemistry	Blood
Coombs' test—direct/indirect		Blood bank	Blood
Copper		Chemistry	Blood
Coproporphyrins		Chemistry	Urine
Cord blood (grouping, Rh, and direct Coombs')		Blood bank	Blood
Corticosterone		Chemistry	Blood or urine
Cortisol (compound F)		Chemistry	Blood or urine
Cortisol (compound S)		Chemistry	Blood or urine
C-reactive protein	CRP	Serology	Blood
Creatine		Chemistry	Blood
Creatinine		Chemistry	Blood
Creatinine clearance	CC, creat cl or cr cl	Chemistry	Blood and urine
Creatine phosphokinase	CPK or CK	Chemistry	Blood
Creatinine urine		Chemistry	Urine
Cryptococcus stain (India ink)		Microbiology	Cerebrospinal fluid
Culture and sensitivity	C&S	Bacteriology	Any body fluid
Cyanocobalamin (see Schilling test)			
Cystine		Chemistry	Urine
Cytology smears		Cytology	Any body cells
Cytotoxic antibodies		Blood bank	Blood
Dehydroepiandrosterone	DHEA	Chemistry	Blood or urine
Deoxycorticosterone		Chemistry	Blood or urine
11-Deoxycortisols (compound S)		Chemistry	Blood or urine
Diacetic acid (see acetoacetic acid)			
Differential cell count	Diff.	Hematology	Blood
Digitoxin level		Chemistry	Blood
Digoxin level		Chemistry	Blood
Dihydrotestosterone	DHT	Chemistry	Blood
Dilantin level		Chemistry	Blood
Direct Coombs' (direct antiglobulin) test	DAT	Blood bank	Blood

Procedure	Abbreviation	Laboratory Division	Specimen
Drug screen		Chemistry	Blood or urine
d-Xylose		Chemistry	Blood or urine
Electrolytes	Lytes-E'lytes	Chemistry/POCT	Blood
Electrophoresis, Hb		Chemistry	Blood
Electrophoresis, Immuno.		Chemistry	Blood
Electrophoresis, Lipids		Chemistry	Blood
Electrophoresis, Lipoprotein		Chemistry	Blood
Electrophoresis, Protein	Protein ELP	Chemistry	Blood
Enterovirus	Virology	Stool	
Eosinophils		Hematology	Blood
Epinephrine and norepinephrine (catecholamines)		Chemistry	Urine
Epstein-Barr virus	EBV	Serology	Chemistry
Erythrocyte sedimentation rate	ESR	Hematology	Blood
Esophageal cytology		Cytology	Cells from esophagus
17β-Estradiol (E_2)		Chemistry	Urine
Estrogen receptor assay		Chemistry	Urine
Estrogens, E_1, E_2 (estrone, 17β-estradiol)		Chemistry	Urine
Ethyl alcohol, blood		Chemistry	Blood
Euglobulin clot lysis		Hematology	Blood
Factor assay (specify factor)		Hematology	Blood
Factor identifying test		Hematology	Blood
Fasting blood sugar (glucose, fasting)	FBS	Chemistry	Blood
Febrile agglutinins		Serology	Blood
Fecal fat, quantitative		Chemistry	Stool
Ferroxidase		Chemistry	Blood
Fibrin split products screen	FSP	Hematology	Blood
Fibrindex		Hematology	Blood
Fibrinogen level		Hematology	Blood
Fibrinolysin		Hematology	Blood
Fluorescent treponemal antibody	FTA	Serology	Blood
Folate (folic acid)		Chemistry	Blood
Follicle-stimulating hormone	FSH	Chemistry	Urine (24-hour)
Fractionated alkaline phosphatase		Chemistry	Blood
Free fatty acids	FFA	Chemistry	Blood
Free thyroxine index	T_7	Chemistry	Blood
Fresh frozen plasma	FFP	Blood bank	Blood
Frozen cells		Blood bank	Blood
Frozen section	FS	Pathology	Any body tissue
Fungus culture		Bacteriology	Body specimen
Fungus serology		Serology	Blood
Fungus smear		Cytology	Body specimen
Galactose, qualitative		Urinalysis	Urine
Gallium		Chemistry	Urine
Gastric analysis		Chemistry or GI lab	Gastric fluid
Gastric cytology		Cytology	Gastric fluid
Gastric washings (TB/AFB)		Bacteriology	Gastric fluid
Gastrin		Chemistry	Blood
Gentamicin level		Toxicology	Blood
γ-Globulin (serum)		Chemistry	Blood
Globulin (total protein & albumin)		Chemistry	Blood
Glucose		Chemistry/urinalysis/POCT	Blood or urine
Glucose (CSF)		Chemistry	Cerebrospinal fluid
Glucose, fasting	FBS	Chemistry	Blood
Glucose, 2-hour postprandial	2 h PP BS	Chemistry	Blood
Glucose, random	BS	Chemistry	Blood
Glucose tolerance test	GTT	Chemistry	Blood or urine
γ-Glutamyl transpeptidase	GGT	Chemistry	Blood
Glycosylated hemoglobin	HbA_{1c} GHB, GHB	Chemistry	Blood

Procedure	Abbreviation	Laboratory Division	Specimen
Gram stain (smear)		Bacteriology	Any body fluid
Growth hormone	GH or HGH	Chemistry	Blood
Guaiac		Urinalysis/feces/POCT	Urine or stool
Guthrie test (serum phenylalanine)	PKU	Chemistry	Blood
Hanging drop prep (*Trichomonas*)		Bacteriology	Vaginal smear
Haptoglobins		Chemistry	Blood
Heavy metals		Chemistry	Urine
Helicobacter pylori	CLO test	Serology/POCT	Biopsy specimen
Hematocrit	Hct, Crit	Hematology/POCT	Blood
Hemoglobin	Hgb	Hematology/POCT	Blood
Hemoglobin & Hematocrit	H & H	Hematology/POCT	Blood
Hemoglobin electrophoresis		Chemistry	Blood
Hemogram		Hematology	Blood
Hemosiderin		Chemistry	Urine
Hepatitis A antibody	anti-HAV	Serology	Blood
Hepatitis B core antibody	anti-HB_cAg	Serology	Blood
Hepatitis B surface antigen	HB_sAg	Serology	Blood
Hepatitis B surface antibody	anti-HB_sAg	Serology	Blood
Hepatitis screen (acute)		Serology	Blood
Herpes serology		Serology/microbiology	Blood
Herpes smear		Microbiology	Smear of specified area
Heterophil antibodies screen		Serology	Blood
High-density lipoproteins	HDL	Chemistry	Blood
Histoplasma, culture		Bacteriology	Sputum
Histoplasma, serology		Serology	Blood
HLA B27 typing		Blood bank	Blood
Homovanillic acid	HVA	Chemistry	Urine
Human chorionic gonadotropin	HCG	Chemistry/POCT	Blood
Human immunodeficiency virus screen	$HIVB_{24}AG$	Serology	Blood
Human placental lactogen	HPL	Chemistry	Urine
Hydroxybutyrate dehydrogenase	HBD	Chemistry	Blood
17-Hydroxycorticosteroids		Chemistry	Urine
5-Hydroxyindoleacetic acid	5-HIAA	Chemistry	Blood or urine
17-Hydroxysteroids (see 17-hydroxycortico-steroids)			
Icterus index		Chemistry	Blood
Immunodiffusion		Chemistry	Blood
Immunoelectrophoresis	IEP	Chemistry	Blood
Immunoglobulin A	IgA	Chemistry	Blood
Immunoglobulin E	IgE	Chemistry	Blood
Immunoglobulin G	IgG	Chemistry	Blood
Immunoglobulin M	IgM	Chemistry	Blood
Immunologic pregnancy test	HCG	Urinalysis	Urine (morning specimen)
India ink test		Bacteriology	Cerebrospinal fluid
Indices, red blood cells	RBC indices	Hematology	Blood
Indirect Coombs'		Blood bank	Blood
Insulin tolerance test	ITT	Chemistry	Blood
Iodine uptake	^{131}I	Chemistry	Blood
Iontophoresis (sweat electrolytes)		Chemistry	Sweat
Iron	Fe	Chemistry	Blood
Iron-binding capacity	IBC	Chemistry	Blood
Isocitrate dehydrogenase	ICD	Chemistry	Blood
Isoenzymes (Isozymes)	CK-MB	Chemistry	Blood
Isoenzymes (Isozymes)	CPK or CK	Chemistry	Blood
Isoenzymes (Isozymes)	LDH	Chemistry	Blood
Ivy bleeding time	Bl. time	Hematology	Blood
17-Ketogenic steroids	17 KGS	Chemistry	Blood or urine
Ketones (acetone)		Urinalysis or chemistry	Urine or blood
K&L chains (Bence Jones proteins)		Chemistry	Urine
Lactate (lactic acid)		Chemistry	Blood

Procedure	Abbreviation	Laboratory Division	Specimen
Lactate dehydrogenase	LDH	Chemistry	Blood or cerebrospinal fluid
Lactate dehydrogenase isoenzymes	LDH Iso.	Chemistry	Blood
Lactose tolerance test		Chemistry or GI lab	Blood
Lead		Chemistry	Blood or urine
LE cell prep (see lupus erythematosus)			
Lee-White coagulation time	Coag. time or Lee-White	Hematology	Blood
Legionella culture (Legionnaires' disease)		Microbiology	Bronchial washing
Legionella serology		Serology/microbiology	Blood
Leptospira culture		Bacteriology	Urine
Leucine aminopeptidase (also called cytosol aminopeptidase)	LAP	Chemistry	Blood or urine
Leukocyte alkaline phosphatase		Hematology	Blood
Leukocyte count (see white blood cell count)			
Librium level (chlordiazepoxide)		Chemistry	Blood
Lipase		Chemistry	Blood
Lipid phenotype		Chemistry	Blood
Lipoprotein electrophoresis		Chemistry	Blood
Lithium level	Li	Chemistry	Blood
Low-density lipoproteins	LDH	Chemistry	Blood
Lupus erythematosus	LE cell prep.	Hematology	Blood
Luteinizing hormone	LH	Chemistry	Blood
Luteinizing hormone-releasing factor	LHRF	Chemistry	Blood
Macroglobulin		Chemistry	Blood
Magnesium	Mg or Mg$^+$	Chemistry	Blood
Melanin		Urinalysis or chemistry	Urine
Mercury	Hg	Chemistry	Urine
Metanephrine		Chemistry	Urine
Methemoglobin		Chemistry	Blood
Microglobulin β_2 (see β_2-microglobulin)			
Mixed lymphocyte culture		Serology	Blood
Monospot (see heterophil antibodies screen)			
Myoglobin		Chemistry	Urine
Nasopharyngeal culture	N-P culture	Bacteriology	Nose swab
Neutral fat (lipid profile fractionation)		Chemistry or GI lab	Blood
5'-Nucleotidase		Chemistry	Blood
Occult blood		Urinalysis/microbiology POCT	Urine or stool
17-OH corticosteroids (see 17-hydroxycorticosteroids)			
Orinase tolerance test		Chemistry	Blood
Osmolality		Chemistry	Blood or urine
Osmotic fragility, RBCs		Hematology	Blood
Ova and parasites	O&P	Parasitology	Stool
Packed cell volume (see hematocrit)			
Pancreatic cytology		Cytology	Pancreatic fluid
Pap smears and stains		Cytology	Many body areas, such as cervix and stomach
Parasites, schistosomes		Parasitology	Stool or urine
Parathyroid A&B		Chemistry	Blood
Parathyroid hormone	PTH	Chemistry	Blood
Partial thromboplastin time	PTT	Hematology	Blood
Peak & Trough Level (many drugs)		Toxicology	Blood
Peritoneal fluid smear		Cytology	Peritoneal fluid
pH		Chemistry/POCT	Blood, urine, or stool
Phenobarbital level		Chemistry	Blood
Phenolsulfonphthalein	PSP	Chemistry	Urine
Phenothiazine level		Chemistry	Blood or urine
Phenylalanine (see Guthrie test)			
Phospholipids		Chemistry or GI lab	Blood

Procedure	Abbreviation	Laboratory Division	Specimen
Phosphorus	PO$_4$	Chemistry	Blood or urine
Phosphatase, acid (see acid phosphatase)			
Phosphatase, alkaline (see alkaline phosphatase)			
Pinworm		Parasitology	Scotch tape prep.
Pituitary gonadotropin	FSH	Chemistry	Blood
Placental lactogen, human	HPL	Chemistry	Urine
Plasma cortisol		Chemistry	Blood
Plasma osmolality		Chemistry	Blood
Platelet adhesion study		Hematology	Blood
Platelet aggregation		Hematology	Blood
Platelet concentrate		Blood bank	Blood
Platelet count	Plts or Plt ct	Hematology	Blood
Porphobilinogen		Chemistry	Urine
Porphyrins		Chemistry	Urine
Porter-Silber chromogens (see 17-hydroxycorticosteroids)			
Potassium	K	Chemistry	Blood or urine
Pregnanediol		Chemistry	Urine
Pregnanetriol		Chemistry	Urine
Progesterone		Chemistry	Blood or urine
Prolactin		Chemistry	Blood
Pronestyl level (procainamide)		Chemistry	Blood
Prostate specific antigen	PSA	Chemistry	Blood
Prostatic acid phosphatase	PAP	Chemistry	Blood
Protein (cerebrospinal fluid)		Chemistry	Cerebrospinal fluid
Protein (urine)		Urinalysis	Urine
Protein-bound iodine	PBI	Chemistry	Blood
Protein electrophoresis		Chemistry	Blood
Protein, total		Chemistry	Blood
Proteus Ox-19		Serology	Blood
Prothrombin time	PT, pro-time	Hematology	Blood
Quantitative urine culture (colony count)		Bacteriology	Urine
Quinidine level		Chemistry	Urine
Rapid plasma reagin	RPR	Serology	Blood
Red blood cells	RBC	Hematology	Blood
Red cell distribution width	RDW	Hematology	Blood
Red cell fragility		Hematology	Blood
Red cell indices	RBC indices	Hematology	Blood
Red cell morphology	RBC morph.	Hematology	Blood
Red cell survival		Chemistry	Blood
Renin		Chemistry	Blood
Respiratory virus		Virology	Blood
Reticulocyte count	Retics	Hematology	Blood
RH factor		Blood bank	Blood
RH globulin work-up		Blood bank	Blood
Rheumatoid factor	RA	Serology	Blood
Rubella antibody		Serology	Blood
Rubella, culture		Bacteriology	Blood
Rubeola, culture		Bacteriology	Blood
Salicylate level		Chemistry	Blood or urine
Schilling test		Chemistry	Urine
Secretin		Chemistry	Duodenal secretions
Secretin with pancreatic cytology		Cytology or GI lab	Duodenal secretions
Sedrate (see erythrocyte sedimentation rate)			
Semen		Urinalysis	Semen
Serotonin, serum		Chemistry	Blood
Serotonin, urine	5-HIAA	Chemistry	Urine
Serum glutamic-oxaloacetic transaminase	SGOT	Chemistry	Blood or cerebrospinal fluid
Serum glutamic-pyruvic transaminase	SGPT	Chemistry	Blood

Procedure	Abbreviation	Laboratory Division	Specimen
Serum protein electrophoresis	SPE	Chemistry	Blood
Sickle cell prep		Hematology	Blood
Sodium	Na	Chemistry	Blood, urine, or sweat
Sputum, culture		Bacteriology	Sputum
Stool, culture		Bacteriology	Stool
Stool for ova and parasites	O&P	Microbiology	Stool
Strychnine		Chemistry	Urine
Sulfa level		Chemistry	Blood
Sweat chloride		Chemistry	Sweat
Sweat electrolytes (Na & Cl)		Chemistry	Sweat
Tegretol level (carbamazepine)		Toxicology	Blood or urine
Template bleeding time	TBT	Hematology	Blood
Testosterone		Chemistry	Blood
Theophylline level		Toxicology	Blood
Thrombin clotting time	TCT	Hematology	Blood
Thromboplastin time, activated partial (see activated partial thromboplastin time)			
Thyroid antibody titer	TAT	Serology	Blood
Thyroid-binding globulin	TBG	Chemistry	Blood
Thyroid globulin antibody		Serology	Blood
Thyroid-stimulating hormone	TSH	Chemistry	Blood
Thyroxine	T_4	Chemistry	Blood
Tobramycin level		Toxicology	Blood
Total iron binding capacity	TIBC	Chemistry	Blood
Total lipids		Chemistry or GI lab	Blood
Total protein	TP	Chemistry	Blood, urine, or cerebrospinal fluid
Toxicology screen		Toxicology	Blood, urine, or gastric contents
Toxoplasma		Serology	Blood
Triglycerides		Chemistry	Blood
Triiodothyronine resin uptake	T_3	Chemistry	Blood
Troponin		Chemistry	Blood
Tuberculosis culture		Bacteriology	Sputum, urine, or cerebrospinal fluid
Type & x-match		Blood Bank	Blood
Type & screen	T & S	Blood Bank	Blood
Typhoid o & h		Bacteriology	Blood
Urea clearance		Chemistry	Blood or urine
Urea nitrogen		BUN	Chemistry
Uric acid		Chemistry	Blood or urine
Urinalysis	UA	Urinalysis	Urine
Urine reflex		Urinalysis/microbiology	Urine
Urobilinogen		Urinalysis/chemistry	Urine or stool
Uroporphyrins		Chemistry	Urine
Vaginal smear		Cytology	Vaginal smear
Vanillylmandelic acid	VMA	Chemistry	Urine
Venereal Disease Research Laboratories	VDRL	Serology	Blood
Vitamin B_{12} (see Schilling test)			
Washed cells		Blood bank	Blood
White blood cell count	WBC	Hematology	Blood
Whole blood		Blood bank	Blood
Wound culture		Bacteriology	Any wound

Glossary

The following is a list of terms provided in the vocabulary lists at the beginning of chapters 1 through 22. After each definition is the number of the chapter in which the term is introduced.

Accountability   Taking responsibility for your actions, being answerable to someone for something you have done (6)

Accreditation   Recognition that a health care organization has met an official standard (2)

Active Exercise   Exercise performed by the patient without assistance as instructed by the physical therapist (17)

Activities of Daily Living   Tasks that enable individuals to meet basic needs (eating, bathing, etc.) (17)

Activity Order   Doctors' order that defines the type and amount of activity a hospitalized patient may have (10)

Acuity   Level of care a patient would require based on his or her medical condition, used to evaluate staffing needs (3)

Acute Care   Short-term care for serious illness or trauma (2)

Admission Day Surgery   Surgery for which the patient enters the hospital the day of surgery; it may be called same-day surgery or AM admission (19)

Admission Orders   Written instructions by the doctor for the care and treatment of the patient upon entry into the hospital (19)

Admission Packet   A preassembled packet of standard chart forms to be used on the admission of a patient to the nursing unit (8)

Admission Service Agreement or Conditions of Admission Agreement   A form signed upon the patient's admission that sets forth the general services that the hospital will provide; it may also be called the conditions of admission, contract for services, or treatment consent (19)

Admixture   The result of adding a medication to a container of intravenous solution (13)

Advance Directives   Documents that indicate a patient's wishes in the event that the patient becomes incapacitated (19)

Aerosol   Liquid suspension of particles in a gas stream for inhalation purposes (17)

Afebrile   Without fever (10)

Ageism   Discrimination on grounds of age (5)

Aggressive   A behavioral style in which a person attempts to be the dominant force in an interaction (5)

Airborne Precautions/Isolation   Required use of mask and ventilated room, in conjunction with standard precautions (22)

Allergy   An acquired, abnormal immune response to a substance that does not normally cause a reaction; could include medications, food, tape, and many other substances. (8)

Allergy Identification Bracelet   A plastic band with a cardboard insert on which allergy information is printed or a red plastic band that has allergy information written directly on it, which the patient wears throughout the hospitalization (8, 19)

Allergy Information   Information obtained from the patient concerning his or her sensitivity to medications and/or food (19)

Allergy Labels   Labels affixed to the front cover of a patient's chart that indicate a patient's allergies (8)

Amniocentesis   A needle puncture into the uterine cavity to remove amniotic fluid, the liquid that surrounds the unborn baby (14)

Ampoule (Ampule)   Small glass vial sealed to keep contents sterile, used for subcutaneous, intramuscular, and intravenous medications (13)

Antibody   An immunoglobulin (protein) produced by the body that reacts with and neutralizes an antigen (usually a foreign substance) (14)

Antigen   Any substance that induces an immune response (14)

Apical Rate   Heart rate obtained from the apex of the heart (10)

Apnea   The cessation of breathing (16)

Apothecary System   Ancient system of weight and volume measurements used to measure drugs and solutions (13)

Assertive   A behavioral style in which a person stands up for his or her own rights and feelings without violating the rights and feelings of others (5)

Assignment Sheet   A form completed at the beginning of each work shift that indicates the nursing staff member(s) assigned to each patient on that nursing unit (3)

Assistant Nurse Manager   A registered nurse who assists the nurse manager in coordinating the activities on the nursing unit (3)

Attending Physician   The term applied to a physician who admits and is responsible for a hospital patient (2)

Attitude   A manner of thought or feeling that can be seen expressed in a person's behavior (6)

Autologous Blood   The patient's own blood donated previously for transfusion as needed by the patient; also called auto-transfusion (11)

Automatic Stop Date   Date on which specific categories of medications must be discontinued unless renewed by the physician (13)

Autonomy   Independent—personal liberty (6)

Autopsy   An examination of a body after death; it may be performed to determine the cause of death or for medical research (20)

Axillary Temperature   The temperature reading obtained by placing the thermometer in the patient's axilla (armpit) (10)

Bedside Commode   A chair or wheelchair with an open seat, used at the bedside by the patient for the passage of urine and stool (10)

Behavior   What people do and say (6)

Binder   A cloth or elastic bandage usually used for abdominal or chest support (11)

Biopsy   Tissue removed from a living body for examination (14)

Blood Gases A diagnostic study to determine the exchange of gases in the blood (16)

Blood Pressure The measure of the pressure of blood against the walls of the blood vessels (10)

Blood Transfusion Consent A patient's written permission to receive or refuse blood or blood products (19)

Bolus Concentrated dose of medication or fluid, frequently given intravenously (13)

Bowel Movement The passage of stool (21)

Brainstorming A structured group activity that allows three to ten people to tap into the creativity of the group to identify new ideas. Typically in quality improvement, the technique is used to identify probable causes and possible solutions of quality problems (7)

Broken Record Assertive skill, wherein a person repeats his or her position over and over again (5)

Calorie A measurement of energy generated in the body by the heat produced after food is eaten (11)

Capitation A payment method whereby the provider of care receives a set dollar amount per patient regardless of services rendered (2)

Capsule Gelatinous single-dose container in which a drug is enclosed to prevent the patient from tasting the drug (13)

Cardiac Arrest The patient's heart contractions are absent or insufficient to produce a pulse or blood pressure; may also be referred to as code arrest (22)

Cardiac Monitor Monitor of heart function, providing visual and audible record of heartbeat (16)

Cardiac Monitor Technician One who monitors patient heart rhythms and notifies RN of rhythm changes (additional training required) often done in conjunction with health unit coordinator responsibilities on a telemetry unit (1, 16)

Cardiopulmonary Resuscitation (CPR) The basic life-saving procedure of artificial ventilation and chest compressions done in the event of a cardiac arrest (all health care workers are required to be certified in CPR) (7)

Career Ladder A pathway of upward mobility (1)

C-Arm A mobile fluoroscopy unit used in surgery or at the bedside (15)

Case Manager A health care professional and expert in managed care who assists patients in assessing health and social service systems to assure that all required services are obtained; also coordinates care with doctor and insurance companies (2)

Catheterization Insertion of a catheter into a body cavity or organ to inject or remove fluid (11)

Cell Phone Wireless phone, which may be carried by some hospital personnel and doctors (4)

Celsius A scale used to measure temperature in which the freezing point of water is 0° and the boiling point is 100° (formerly called Centigrade) (21)

Census A list of all occupied and unoccupied hospital beds (7, 19)

Census Sheet A daily listing of all patient activity (admissions, discharges, transfers and deaths) within the hospital; may also be called the admissions, discharges, and transfers sheet (ADT) (20)

Census Worksheet A list of patient's names with room and bed number located on a nursing unit with blank spaces next to each name. May be used by the health unit coordinator to record patient activities. Also called a patient information sheet or patient activity sheet (7)

Centers for Disease Control Division of the U.S. Public Health Service that investigates and controls diseases that have epidemic potential (22)

Central Line Catheter or Central Venous Catheter (CVC) Large catheter that provides access to the veins and/or to the heart to measure pressures. The catheter is threaded through to the superior vena cava or right atrium used for the administration of intravenous therapy (13)

Central Service Department Charge Slip A form that is initiated to charge a discharged patient for any items that were not charged to them at the time of use (7)

Central Service Department Credit Slip A form that is used to credit a patient for items found in the room unused after patient's discharge or if it is found that a patient was mistakenly charged for an item not used for that patient (7)

Central Service Department Discrepancy Report A list of items that are missing from nursing unit patient supply cupboard or closet that were not charged to a patient; it is sent to the nursing unit from the central service department each day (8)

Certification The process of testifying to or endorsing that a person has met certain standards (1)

Certified Health Unit Coordinator (CHUC) A health unit coordinator who has successfully passed the national certification examination sponsored by the National Association of Health Unit Coordinators (NAHUC) (1)

Certified Nursing Assistant A health care giver who performs basic nursing tasks and has been certified by passing a required certification examination (3)

Change-of-Shift Report The communication process between shifts, in which the nursing personnel going "off duty" report the nursing unit activities to the personnel coming "on duty" (health unit coordinators may give reports to each other or may listen to the nurse's report) (7)

Chief Executive Officer The individual directly in charge of a hospital who is responsible to the governing board (2)

Chronic Care Care for long-duration illnesses such as diabetes or emphysema (2)

Clean Catch A method of obtaining a urine specimen using a special cleansing technique; also called a midstream urine (14)

Clinical Indications Notations recorded when ordering diagnostic imaging to indicate the reason for doing the procedure (15)

Clinical Pathways A method of outlining a patient's path of treatment for a specific diagnosis, procedure, or symptom (3)

Clinical Tasks Tasks performed at the bedside or in direct contact with the patient (1)

Code Blue A term used in hospitals to announce when a patient stops breathing or his or her heart stops beating, or both) (7)

Code of Ethics A set of standards for behavior based on values (6)

Code or Crash Cart A cart stocked by the nursing and pharmacy staff with emergency medication, advanced breathing supplies, intravenous solutions and appropriate tubing, needles, a heart monitor and defibrillator, an oxygen tank, and a suction machine (used when a patient stops breathing or his or her heart stops beating, or both) (7)

Communicable Disease A disease that may be transmitted from one person to another (22)

Communication   The process of transmitting feelings, images, and ideas from the mind of one person to the mind of another person for the purpose of obtaining a response (5)

Community Health   The emphasis on prevention and early detection of disease for members of a community (2)

Computed Tomography   A radiographic process of creating computerized images (scans) of body organs in horizontal slices (referred to as a CT scan) (15)

Computer   An electronic machine capable of accepting, processing, and retrieving information (4)

Computer Terminal   A computer terminal is made up of three components: a keyboard, a viewing screen, and a printer (4)

Confidentiality   Keeping private any confidential information, either spoken or written (6)

Conflict   Emotional disturbance—people's striving for their own preferred outcome, which, if attained, prevents others from achieving their preferred outcome (5)

Consultation Order   A request by the patient's attending doctor for the opinion of a second doctor with respect to diagnosis and treatment of the patient (18)

Continuous Quality Improvement (CQI)   The practice of continuously improving quality at each level of each department of every function of the health care organization (also called total quality management [TQM]) (7)

Contrast Media   Substances (solids, liquids, or gases) used in diagnostic imaging procedures that permit the radiologist to distinguish between the different body densities; they may be injected, swallowed, or introduced by rectum or vagina (15)

Copy Machine   A machine used for making copies of typed or written materials (4)

Coroner's Case   A death that occurs due to sudden, violent, or unexplained circumstances or a patient that expires during first 24 hours after admission to the hospital (20)

Crisis Stress   A profound effect experienced by individuals, resulting from common, uncontrollable, often-unpredictable life experiences (death, divorce, illness, etc.) (7)

Cultural Differences   Factors such as age, gender, race, socioeconomic status, etc. (5)

Culturally Sensitive Care   Care that involves understanding and being sensitive to patient's cultural background (5)

Culture   A set of values, beliefs, and traditions that are held by a specific social group (5)

Culture and Sensitivity   The growth of microorganisms in a special media (culture), followed by a test to determine the antibiotic to which they best respond (sensitivity) (14)

Cursor   A flashing indicator that lets the computer user know the area on the viewing screen that will receive the information (4)

Custodial Care   Care and services of a nonmedical nature, which consist of feeding, bathing, watching, and protecting the patient (20)

Cytology   The study of cells (14)

Daily Laboratory Tests   Tests that are ordered once by the doctor but are carried out every day until the doctor discontinues the order (14)

Daily TPRs   Taking each patient's temperature, pulse, and respiration at (a) certain time(s) each day (21)

Damages   Monetary compensation awarded by a court for an injury caused by the act of another (6)

Decoding   The process of translating symbols received from the sender to determine the message (5)

Defendant   The person against whom a civil or criminal action is brought (6)

Deposition   Pretrial statement of a witness under oath, taken in question-and-answer form, as it would be in court, with opportunity given to the adversary to be present to cross-examine (6)

Dialysis   The removal of wastes in the blood usually excreted by the kidneys (17)

Diet Manual   Hospitals are required to have an up-to-date diet manual that has been jointly approved by the medical and dietary staffs. The manual must be available in the dietary office and on all nursing units (12)

Diet Order   A doctor's order that states the type and amount of food and liquids the patient may receive (12)

Differential   Identification of the types of white cells found in the blood (14)

Dipstick Urine   The visual examination of urine using a special chemically treated stick (14)

Direct Admission   A patient who was not scheduled to be admitted and is admitted from the doctor's office, clinic, or emergency room (19)

Director of Nurses   A registered nurse in charge of nursing services (may be called director of patient services, nursing administrator, or vice president of nursing services) (3)

Disaster Procedure   A planned procedure that is carried out by hospital personnel when a large number of persons have been injured (22)

Discharge Order   A doctor's order that states the patient may leave the hospital. A doctor's order is necessary for a patient to be discharged from the hospital (18)

Discharge Planning   Centralized, coordinated, multidisciplinary process that ensures that the patient has a plan for continuing care after leaving the hospital (20)

Discrimination   Seeing a difference; prejudicial treatment of a person (6)

Doctor   A person licensed to practice medicine (1)

Doctors' Orders   The health care a doctor prescribes in writing for a hospitalized patient (1)

Doctors' Roster   Alphabetical listing of names, telephone numbers, and directory telephone numbers of physicians on staff (most hospitals have made this available on computer as well) (4)

Donor-Specific or Donor-Directed Blood   Blood donated by relatives or friends of the patient to be used for transfusion as needed (11)

Downtime Requisition   A requisition (paper order form) used to process information when the computer is not available for use (4)

Dumbwaiter   A mechanical device for transporting food or supplies from one hospital floor to another (4)

Echoencephalogram (EchoEg)   A graphic recording that indicates (by sound waves) the position of the brain within the skull (16)

Egg-Crate Mattress   A foam-rubber mattress (11)

Elective Surgery   Surgery, which is not emergency or mandatory and can be planned at a time of convenience (19)

Electrocardiogram (EKG or ECG)   A graphic recording produced by the electric impulses of the heart (16)

Electroencephalogram (EEG)   A graphic recording of the electric impulses of the brain (16)

Electrolytes   A group of tests done in chemistry, which usually includes sodium, potassium, chloride, and carbon dioxide (14)

Electromyogram (EMG) A record of muscle contraction produced by electrical stimulation (16)

Electrophysiological Study (EPS) An invasive measure of electrical activity (16)

Elitism Discrimination based on social/economic class (5)

E-mail (electronic mail) A method of sending and receiving messages to anyone with an e-mail address via the computer (4)

Emergency Admission An admission necessitated by accident or a medical emergency; such an admission is processed through the emergency department (19)

Empathy Capacity for participating in and understanding the feelings or ideas of another (6)

Encoding Translating mental images, feelings, and ideas into symbols to communicate them to the receiver (5)

Endoscopy The visualization of a body cavity or hollow organ by means of an endoscope. Gastrointestinal (GI) studies are also performed in the endoscopy department (16)

Enema The introduction of fluid and/or medication into the rectum and sigmoid colon (11)

Enteral Feeding Set Includes equipment needed to infuse tube feeding; includes plastic bag for feeding solution and may be ordered with or without a pump (12)

Enteral Nutrition The provision of liquid formulas into the GI tract by tube or orally (12)

Epidemiology The study of the occurrence, distribution, and causes of health and disease in humans; the specialist is called an epidemiologist (22)

Ergonomics A branch of ecology concerned with human factors in the design and operation of machines and the physical environment (7)

Erythrocyte A red blood cell (14)

Esteem Needs A person's need for self-respect and for the respect of others (5)

Ethics Behavior that is based on values (beliefs); how we make judgments in regard to right and wrong (6)

Ethnocentrism The inability to accept other cultures, or an assumption of cultural superiority (5)

Evidence All the means by which any alleged matter of fact, the truth of which is submitted to investigation at trial, is established or disproved; evidence includes the testimony of witnesses, and the introduction of records, documents, exhibits, objects, or any other substantiating matter offered for the purpose of inducing belief in the party's contention by the judge or jury (6)

Expert Witness A witness having special knowledge of the subject about which he or she is to testify; the knowledge must generally be such as is not normally possessed by the average person (6)

Expiration A death (20)

Extended Care Facility A medical facility caring for patients requiring expert nursing care or custodial care (20)

Extravasation Leakage of fluid into tissue surrounding a vein (13)

Extubation Removal of a previously inserted tube (as in an endotracheal tube) (17)

Facesheet A form initiated by the admitting department included in the inpatient medical record that contains personal and demographic information, usually computer generated at the time of admission (may also be called the information sheet or front sheet) (19)

Fahrenheit A scale used to measure temperature in which 32° is the freezing point of water and 212° is the boiling point (21)

Fasting No solid foods by mouth and no fluids containing nourishment (i.e., sugar or milk) (14)

Fax Machine A telecommunication device that transmits copies of written material over a telephone wire from one site to another (4)

Febrile Elevated body temperature (fever) (10)

Feedback Response to a message (5)

Fidelity Doing what one promises (6)

Flagging A method used by the doctor to notify the nursing staff that she or he has written a new set of orders (9)

Fluoroscopy The observation of deep body structures made visible by use of a viewing screen instead of film; a contrast medium is required for this procedure (15)

Fogging Assertive Skill Skill in which a person responds to a criticism by making noncommittal statements that cannot be argued against (5)

Foley Catheter A type of indwelling retention catheter (11)

Food Allergy A negative physical reaction to a particular food involving the immune system (people with food allergies must avoid the offending foods) (12)

Food Intolerance A more common problem than food allergies involving digestion (people with food intolerances can eat some of the offending food without suffering symptoms) (12)

Fowler's Position A semi-sitting position (10)

Gastric Suction Used to remove gastric contents (11)

Gastrointestinal Study A diagnostic study related to the gastrointestinal system (16)

Gastrostomy Feeding Feeding by means of a tube inserted into the stomach through an artificial opening in the abdominal wall (12)

Gavage Feeding by means of a tube inserted into the stomach, duodenum, or jejunum, through the nose, or an opening in the abdominal wall, also called tube feeding (12)

GI Study A diagnostic study related to the gastrointestinal system (16)

Governing Board A group of community citizens at the head of the hospital organizational structure (2)

Guaiac A method of testing stool and urine using guaiac as a reagent for hidden (occult) blood (may also be called a hemoccult slide test) (14)

Harris Flush or Return Flow Enema A mild colonic irrigation that helps expel flatus (11)

Health Maintenance Organization An organization that has management responsibility for providing comprehensive health care services on a prepayment basis to voluntarily enrolled persons within a designated population (2)

Health Records Number The number assigned to the patient on or before admission; it is used for records identification and is used for all subsequent admissions to that hospital (may also be called medical records number) (19)

Health Unit Coordinator (HUC) The nursing team member who performs the non-clinical patient care tasks for the nursing unit (may also be called unit clerk or unit secretary) (1)

Hemovac A disposable suction device (evacuator unit) that is connected to a drain inserted into or close to a surgical wound (11)

Heparin Lock A vascular access device (also called intermittent infusion device) placed on a peripheral intravenous catheter when used intermittently (11)

Hepatitis B Virus (HBV) An infectious bloodborne disease that is a major occupational hazard for health care workers (22)

Holter monitor   A portable device that records the heart's electrical activity and produces a continuous ECG tracing over a specified period (16)

Home Health   Equipment and services provided to patient in home to provide comfort and care (2)

Hospice   Supportive care for terminally ill patients and their families (2)

Hospital Departments   Divisions within the hospital that specialize in services, such as the dietary department, which plans and prepares meals for patients, employees, and visitors (1)

Hospitalist   A full-time, acute care specialist whose focus is exclusively on hospitalized patients (2)

Hostile Environment   A sexually oriented atmosphere or pattern of behavior that is determined to be sexual harassment (6)

Human Immunodeficiency Virus (HIV)   The virus that causes acquired immune deficiency syndrome (AIDS) (22)

Hydrotherapy   Treatment with water (17)

Hyperbaric Oxygen Therapy (HBOT)   A treatment that involves breathing 100% oxygen while in an enclosed system pressurized to greater than one atmosphere (sea level) (17)

Hypertonic   Concentrated salt solution (>0.9%) (17)

Hypnotics   Drugs that reduce pain or induce sleep, can include sedatives, analgesics, and anesthetics (13)

Hypotonic   Dilute salt solution (0.9%) (17)

Implied Contract   A nonexplicit agreement that impacts some aspect of the employment relationship (6)

Incident   An episode that does not normally occur within the regular hospital routine (22)

Incontinence   Inability of the body to control the elimination of urine and/or feces (11)

Independent Transcription   The health unit coordinator assumes full responsibility for transcription of doctors' orders; cosignature by the nurse is not required (1)

Induced Sputum Specimen   A sputum specimen obtained by performing a respiratory treatment to loosen lung secretions (17)

Indwelling (Retention) Catheter   A catheter that remains in the bladder for a longer period until a patient is able to void completely and voluntarily or as long as hourly accurate measurements are needed (11)

Infiltrate   To strain through or pass into a substance or space (13)

Informed Consent   A doctrine that states that before a patient is asked to consent to a risky or invasive diagnostic or treatment procedure he or she is entitled to receive certain information: (1) a description of the procedure, (2) any alternatives to it and their risks, (3) the risks of death or serious bodily disability from the procedure, (4) the probable results of the procedure, including any problems of recuperation and time of recuperation anticipated, and (5) anything else that is generally disclosed to patients asked to consent to the procedure (6, 19)

Infusion Pump   A device used to regulate flow or rate of intravenous fluid. It is commonly called an IV pump (11)

Ingestion   The taking in of food by mouth (12)

Inpatient   A patient who has been admitted to a health care facility at least overnight for treatment and care (2, 8)

Intake and Output   The measurement of the patient's fluid intake and output (10)

Integrated Delivery Networks   Health care organizations merged into systems that can provide all needed health care services under one corporate umbrella (2)

Intermittent (Straight) Catheter   A single-use catheter that is introduced long enough to drain the bladder (5 to 10 minutes) and then removed (11)

Intervention   Synonymous with treatment (17)

Intramuscular (IM) Injection   Injection of a medication into a muscle (13)

Intravenous (IV)   Administered directly into a vein (13)

Intravenous Hyperalimentation or Total Parenteral Nutrition (TPN)   Method used to administer calories, proteins, vitamins, and other nutrients into the bloodstream of a patient who is unable to eat. Must be infused into the superior vena cava through a central line catheter—not given through a peripheral IV catheter (13)

Intravenous Infusion   The administration of fluid through a vein (11)

Intubation   Insertion and placement of a tube (within the trachea may be endotracheal or tracheostomy) (17)

Invasive Cardiac Study   A method of studying the heart by making an entry into the body, such as by placing a cardiac catheter into a blood vessel (16)

Invasive Procedure   A procedure in which the body cavity is entered by use of a tube, needle, device, or even ionizing radiation (16)

Irrigation   Washing out of a body cavity, organ, or wound (11)

Isolation   The placement of a patient apart from other patients insofar as movement and social contact are concerned, for the purpose of preventing the spread of infection (22)

Isometric   Of equal dimensions. Holding ends of contracting muscle fixed so that contraction produces increased tension at a constant overall length (17)

IV Push (IVP)   Method of giving concentrated doses of medication directly into the vein (13)

Jackson-Pratt (JP)   A disposable suction device (evacuator unit) that is connected to a drain inserted into or close to a surgical wound (11)

Kangaroo Pump   A brand name of a feeding pump used to administer tube feeding (12)

Kardex File   A portable file that contains and organizes by room number the Kardex forms for each patient on the nursing unit (9)

Kardex Form   A form that the health unit coordinator records doctors' orders on to be used by the nursing staff for a quick reference of the patient's current orders (9)

Kardexing   The process of recording and updating doctors' orders on the Kardex form (many hospitals have eliminated the paper Kardex form in favor of entering all patient orders into the computer) (9)

Keyboard   A computer component used to type information into the computer (4)

K-Pad   An electric device used for heat application (also called a K-thermia pad, aquathermia pad, or aquamatic pad) (11)

Label Printer   A machine that prints patient labels—located near the health unit coordinator's area (4)

Liability   The condition of being responsible either for damages resulting from an injurious act or from discharging an obligation or debt (6)

Licensed Practical Nurse   A graduate of a 1-year school of nursing who is licensed in the state in which he or she is practicing He or she gives direct patient care and functions under the directions of the registered nurse (1, 3)

Living Will A declaration made by the patient to family, medical staff, and all concerned with the patient's care stating what is to be done in the event of a terminal illness; it directs the withholding or withdrawing of life-sustaining procedures (19)

Love and Belonging Needs A person's need to have affectionate relationships with people and to have a place in a group (5)

Lozenge Medicated tablet or disk that dissolves in the mouth (13)

Lumbar Puncture A procedure used to remove cerebrospinal fluid from the spinal canal (14)

Magnetic Resonance Imaging A technique used to produce computer images (scans) of the interior of the body using magnetic fields (15)

Managed Care The use of a planned and systematic approach to providing health care, with the goal of offering quality care at the lowest possible cost (2)

Material Safety Data Sheet (MSDS) A basic hazard communication tool that gives details on chemical dangers and safety procedures (22)

Medicaid A federal and state program that provides medical assistance for the indigent (2)

Medical Emergency An emergency that is life threatening (22)

Medical Malpractice Professional negligence of a health care professional; failure to meet a professional standard of care resulting in harm to another; for example, failure to provide "good and accepted medical care" (6)

Medicare Government insurance—enacted in 1965 for individuals over the age of 65, any person with a disability who has received social security for 2 years (some disabilities are covered immediately) (2)

Medication Administration Record (MAR) List of medications that each individual patient is currently taking; it is used by the nurse to administer the medications (13)

Medication Nurse Registered nurse or licensed practical nurse who administers medications to patients (13)

Menu A list of options that is projected on the viewing screen of the computer (4)

Merger The combining of individual physician practices and small, stand alone hospitals into larger networks (2)

Message Images, feelings, and ideas transmitted from one person to another (5)

Metric System A system of weights and measures based on multiples of 10 (13)

Microfilm A film containing a greatly reduced photo image of printed or graphic matter (18)

Modem A device that enables a computer to send and receive data over regular phone lines (4)

Name Alert A method of alerting staff when two or more patients with the same or similarly spelled last names are located on a nursing unit (8)

Narcolepsy A chronic ailment consisting of recurrent attacks of drowsiness and sleep during daytime (16)

Narcotic Controlled drug that relieves pain or produces sleep (13)

Nasogastric Tube (NG Tube) A tube that is inserted through the nose into the stomach (11)

Nebulizer A gas-driven device that produces an aerosol (17)

Negative Assertion An assertive skill in which a person verbally accepts the fact that they have made an error without letting it reflect on their worth as a human being (5)

Negative Inquiry An assertive skill in which a person requests further clarification of a criticism to get to the real issue (5)

Negligence Failure to satisfactorily perform one's legal duty, such that another person incurs some injury (6)

Nerve Conduction Studies (NCS) Measures how well individual nerves can transmit electrical signals (often performed with an electromyogram) (16)

Neurologic Vital Signs (Neurochecks) The measurement of the function of the body's neurologic system; includes checking pupils of the eyes, verbal response, and so forth (10)

Nonassertive A behavioral style in which a person allows others to dictate her or his self-worth (5)

Non-clinical Tasks Tasks performed away from the bedside (1)

Noninvasive Cardiac Study A method of studying the heart without entering the body to perform the procedure (16)

Noninvasive Procedure A procedure that does not require entering the body, including puncturing the skin (16)

Nonverbal Communication Communication that is not written or spoken but creates a message between two or more people by use of eye contact, body language, symbolic and facial expression (5)

Nosocomial Infection An infection that is acquired from within the health care facility (22)

Nuclear Medicine A technique that uses radioactive materials to determine function capacity of an organ (15)

Nurse Manager A registered nurse who assists the director of nursing in carrying out administrative responsibilities and is in charge of one or more nursing units (may also be called unit manager, clinical manager, or patient care manager) (3)

Nurses' Station The desk area of a nursing unit (1)

Nursing Observation Order A doctors' order that requests the nursing staff to observe and record certain patient signs and symptoms (10)

Nursing Service Department The hospital department responsible for ensuring the physical and emotional care of the hospitalized patients (3)

Nursing Team A group of nursing staff members who care for patients on a nursing unit (1)

Nursing Unit Administration A division within the hospital responsible for non-clinical patient care (3)

Nursing Unit An area within the hospital with equipment and nursing personnel to care for a given number of patients (may also be referred to as a wing, floor, pod, strategic business unit, ward, or station) (1)

Nutrients Substances derived from food, which are utilized by body cells; for example, carbohydrates, fats, proteins, vitamins, minerals, and water (12)

Observation Patient A patient who is assigned to a bed on the nursing unit to receive care for a period of less than 24 hours; may also be referred to as a medical short stay or ambulatory patient (19)

Obstructive Sleep Apnea (OSA) The cessation of breathing during sleep (16)

Occult Blood Blood that is undetectable to the eye (14)

Occupational Safety and Health Administration (OSHA) A U.S. governmental regulatory agency concerned with the health and safety of workers (22)

Old Record The patient's record from previous admissions stored in the health records department that may be retrieved for review when a patient is admitted to the emergency room, nursing unit, or outpatient department (older microfilmed records may also be requested by patient's doctor) (8)

"On Call" Medication Medications prescribed by the doctor to be given prior to the diagnostic imaging procedure; the department notifies the nursing unit of the time the medication is to be administered to the patient (15)

One-Time or Short-Series Order A doctors' order that is executed according to the qualifying phrase, and then is automatically discontinued (9)

Oral By mouth (13)

Oral Temperature The temperature reading obtained by placing the thermometer in the patient's mouth under the tongue (10)

Ordering The process of requesting diagnostic procedures, treatments, or supplies from hospital departments other than nursing (9)

Organ Donation Donating or giving one's organs and/or tissues after death; one may designate specific organs (i.e., only cornea) or any needed organs (20)

Organ Procurement The process of removing donated organs; it may be referred to as harvesting (20)

Orthostatic Vital Signs The measurement of blood pressure and pulse rate first in supine (lying), then in sitting, and finally in standing position (11)

Outpatient A patient receiving care by a health care facility but not admitted to or staying overnight (8)

Pacemaker An electronic device, either temporary or permanent, that regulates the pace of the heart when the heart is incapable of doing it (16)

Pap Smear A test performed to detect cancerous cells in the female genital tract; the Pap staining method can also study body secretions, excretions, and tissue scrapings (14)

Paracentesis A surgical puncture and drainage of a body cavity (14)

Paraphrase Repeating messages in your own words to clarify their meaning (5)

Parenteral Routes Nonoral methods for giving fluids or medications (i.e., injections or intravenously) (13)

Passive Exercise Exercise in which the patient is submissive and the physical therapist moves the patient's limbs (17)

Patency A term indicating that there are no clots at the tip of the needle or catheter and that the needle tip or catheter is not against the vein wall (open) (11)

Pathogenic Microorganisms Disease-carrying organisms too small to be seen with the naked eye (22)

Pathology The study of body changes caused by disease (14)

Patient A person receiving health care, including preventive, promotion, acute, chronic, and all other services in the continuum of care (1)

Patient Account Number A number assigned to the patient to access insurance information, usually a unique number is assigned each time the patient is admitted to the hospital (19)

Patient Call System Intercom A device used to communicate between the nurses' station patient rooms on the nursing unit (4)

Patient Care Conference A meeting that will include the doctor or doctors caring for the patient, the primary nurses, the case manager or social worker, and other care givers involved with the patient's care (20)

Patient-Controlled Analgesia (PCA) Medications administered intravenously by means of a special infusion pump controlled by the patient within order ranges written by the doctor (13)

Patient Identification Bracelet A plastic band with a patient identification label affixed to it, which is worn by the patient throughout their hospitalization. In the obstetrics department, the mother and baby would have the same identification label affixed to their ID bracelets (19)

Patient Identification Labels Labels containing individual patient information to identify patient records (8)

Patient Support Associate Job description as well as title varies among hospitals—may include some patient admitting responsibilities, coding or stocking nursing units (3)

Pedal Pulse The pulse rate obtained on the top of the foot (10)

Penrose Drain A drain that that is inserted into or close to a surgical wound and may lie under a dressing, extend through a dressing, or be connected to a drainage bag or a suction device (11)

Percutaneous Endoscopic Gastrostomy (PEG) Insertion of a tube through the abdominal wall into the stomach using endoscopic guidance (12)

Perennial Stress The wear and tear of day-to-day living with the feeling that one is a square peg trying to fit in a round hole (7,8)

Perioperative Services A department of the hospital that provides care before (preoperative), during (intraoperative), and after (postoperative) surgery. It encompasses total care of the patient during the surgical experience (3)

Peripheral Intravenous Catheter A catheter that begins and ends in the extremities of the body; used for the administration of intravenous therapy (11)

Philosophy Principles; underlying conduct (6)

Physiologic Needs A person's physical needs, such as the need for food and water (5)

Piggyback A method by which drugs are usually administered intravenously in 50 to 100 mL of fluid (13)

Plaintiff The person who brings a lawsuit against another (6)

Plasma The fluid portion of the blood in which the cells are suspended; it contains a clotting factor called fibrinogen (14)

Plethysmography The recording of the changes in the size of a part as altered by the circulation of blood in it (16)

Pneumatic Hose Stockings that promote circulation by sequentially compressing the legs from ankle upward, promoting venous return (also called sequential compression devices) (11)

Pneumatic Tube System A system in which air pressure transports tubes carrying supplies, requisitions, or *some* lab specimens from one hospital unit or department to another (4)

Pocket Pager A small electronic device that when activated by dialing a series of telephone numbers delivers a message to the carrier of the pager (4)

Policy and Procedure Manual A handbook with such information as guidelines for practice, hospital regulations, and job descriptions for hospital personnel (1)

Portable X-ray An x-ray taken by a mobile x-ray machine, which is moved to the patient's bedside (15)

Position An alignment of the body on the x-ray table favorable for taking the best view of the part of the body to be imaged (15)

Positioning Order A doctor's order that requests that the patient be placed in a specified body position (10)

Positive Pressure Pressure greater than atmospheric pressure (17)

Postmortem   After death (a postmortem examination is the same as an autopsy) (20)

Postoperative Orders   Orders written immediately after surgery. Postoperative orders cancel preoperative orders (19)

Postprandial   After eating (14)

Power of Attorney for Health Care   The patient appoints a person (called a proxy or agent) to make health care decisions should the patient be unable to do so (19)

Preadmit   The process of obtaining information and partially preparing admitting forms prior to the patient's arrival at the health care facility (19)

Preoperative Health Unit Coordinator Checklist   A checklist used by the health unit coordinator to ensure that the patient's chart is ready for surgery (19)

Preoperative Nursing Checklist   A checklist used to ensure the chart and the patient are properly prepared for surgery (19)

Preoperative Orders   Orders written by the doctor before surgery to prepare the patient for the surgical procedure (19)

Primary Care Nursing   One nurse provides total care to assigned patients (3)

Primary Care Physician   Sometimes referred to as the gatekeepers, these general practitioners are the first physicians to see a patient for an illness (2)

Principles   Basic truths; moral code of conduct (6)

Proactive   To take action prior to an event, to use the power, freedom, and ability to choose responses to whatever happens to us, based on our values (circumstances do not control us, we control them) (7)

Proprietary   For profit (2)

Protective Care   Another term for isolation (22)

Pulse Deficit   The difference between the radial pulse and the apical heartbeat (21)

Pulse Oximetry   A noninvasive method to measure the oxygen saturation of arterial blood (10)

Pulse Rate   The number of times per minute the heartbeat is felt through the walls of the artery (10)

Quid Pro Quo   (Latin) Involves making conditions of employment (hiring, promotion, retention) contingent on the victim providing sexual favors (6)

Radial Pulse   Pulse rate obtained on the wrist (10)

Radiopaque Catheter   A catheter coated with a substance that does not allow the passage of x-rays, thus allowing the movement of the catheter to be followed on the viewing screen (16)

Random Specimen   A body fluid sample that can be collected at any time (14)

Range of Motion   The range on which a joint can move (17)

Reactive   To take action or respond after an event happens; circumstances are often in control (7,8)

Receiver   The person receiving the message (5)

Recertification   A process for certified health unit coordinators to exhibit continued personal, professional growth, and current competency to practice in the field (1)

Rectal Temperature   The temperature reading obtained by placing the thermometer in the patient's rectum (10)

Rectal Tube   A plastic or rubber tube designed for insertion into the rectum; when written as a doctor's order, "rectal tube" means the insertion of a rectal tube into the rectum to remove gas and relieve distension (11)

Reduction   The correction of a deformity in a bone fracture or dislocation (17)

Reference Range   Range of normal values for a laboratory test result (14)

Registered Dietitian (RD)   One who has completed an educational program, served an internship, and passed an examination sponsored by the American Dietetic Association (12)

Registered Nurse   A graduate of a 2- or 4-year college-based school of nursing or a 3-year diploma, hospital-based program, who is licensed in the state in which he or she is practicing. He or she may give direct patient care or supervise patient care given by others (3)

Registrar   The admitting personnel who registers a patient to the hospital (19)

Registration   The process of entering personal information into the hospital information system to enroll a person as a hospital patient and create a patient record; patients may be registered as inpatients, outpatients, or observation patients (19)

Regular Diet   A diet that consists of all foods, designed to provide good nutrition (12)

Release of Remains   A signed consent that authorizes a specific funeral home or agency to remove the deceased from a health care facility (20)

Requisition   The form used to order diagnostic procedures, treatments, or supplies from hospital departments other than nursing when the computer is down (also called a down-time requisition) (9)

Resident   A graduate of a medical school who is gaining experience in a hospital (2)

Resistive Exercise   Exercise using opposition. A T-band or water provides resistance for patient exercises (17)

Respect   Holding a person in esteem or honor; having appreciation and regard for another (6)

Respiration Rate   The number of times a patient breathes per minute (10)

Respiratory Arrest   When the patient ceases to breathe or when respirations are so depressed that the blood cannot receive sufficient oxygen and therefore the body cells die (may also be referred to as code arrest) (22)

Respondeat Superior   (Latin) "Let the master answer." Legal doctrine that imposes liability upon the employer. Note: The employee is also liable for his own actions (6)

Restraints   Devices used to control patients exhibiting dangerous behavior or to protect the patient (11)

Retaliation   Revenge; payback (6)

Reverse Isolation   A precautionary measure taken to prevent a patient with low resistance to disease from becoming infected (22)

Rhythm Strip   A cardiac study that demonstrates the waveform produced by electric impulses from the electrocardiogram (16)

Risk Management   A department in the hospital that addresses the prevention and containment of liability regarding patient care incidents (22)

Routine Preparation   The standard preparation suggested by the radiologist to prepare the patient for a diagnostic imaging study (15)

Scan   An image produced using a moving detector or a sweeping beam (scans are produced by computed tomography magnetic resonance imaging and ultrasonography) (15)

Scheduled Admission   A patient admission planned in advance; it may be urgent or elective (19)

Scope of Practice   A legal description of what a specific health professional may and may not do (6)

Self-Actualization Need   The need to maximize one's potential (5)

Self Esteem   Confidence and respect for one-self (5)

Sender   The person transmitting the message (5)

Serology   The study of blood serum or other body fluids for immune bodies, which are the body's defense when disease occurs (14)

Serum   Plasma from which fibrinogen, a clotting factor, has been removed (14)

Set of Doctors' Orders   An entry of doctors' orders made at one time on the doctors' order sheet, dated, notated for time, and signed by the doctor; may include one or more orders (9)

Sexual Harassment   Unwanted, unwelcome behavior; sexual in nature (6)

Sheepskin   A pad made out of lamb's wool or synthetic material; used to prevent pressure sores (used primarily in long-term care) (11)

Shift Manager   A registered nurse who is responsible for one or more units during his or her assigned shift (may also be called nursing coordinator) (3)

Shredder   A machine located in most nursing stations that shreds confidential material (chart forms that have a patient's label affixed with patient name, room number, patient account number, medical record number, etc. that do not have any documentation on them) (4)

Signing-Off   A process of recording data (date, time, name, and status), on the doctors' order sheet to indicate the completion of transcription of a set of doctors' orders (9)

Sitz Bath   Application of warm water to the pelvic area (11)

Skin Tests   Tests in which the reactive materials are placed on the skin or just beneath the skin to determine the presence of certain antibodies within the body (13)

Spirometry   A study to measure the body's lung capacity and function (16)

Split or Thinned Chart   Portions of the patient's current chart that are removed when the chart becomes so full that it is unmanageable (8)

Sputum   The mucous secretion from lungs, bronchi, or trachea (14)

Staff Development   The department responsible for both orientations of new employees and continuing education of employed nursing service personnel (may also be called educational services) (3)

Standard Chart Forms   Patient chart forms that are included in all inpatients charts (8)

Standard of Care   The legal duty one owes to another according to the circumstances of a particular case; it is the care that a reasonable and prudent person would have exercised in the given situation (6)

Standard Precautions   The creation of a barrier between the health care worker and the patient's blood and body fluids (may also be called universal precautions) (22)

Standard Supply List   A computerized or written record of the amount of each item that the nursing unit currently needs to last until the next supply order date. (Separate lists are found taped inside cabinet doors, supply drawers and on code or crash cart.) (7)

Standing Order   A doctor's order that remains in effect and is executed as ordered until the doctor discontinues or changes it (9)

Standing PRN Order   Same as a standing order, except that it is executed according to the patient's needs (9)

Stat Order   A doctors' order that is to be executed immediately, then automatically discontinued (9)

Statute   A law passed by the legislature and signed by the governor at the state level and the president at the federal level (6)

Statute of Limitations   The time within which a plaintiff must bring a civil suit; the limit varies depending upon the type of suit, and it is set by the various state legislatures (6)

Stereotyping   The assumption that all members of a culture or ethnic group act alike (generalizations that may be inaccurate) (5)

Sternal Puncture   The procedure to remove bone marrow from the breastbone cavity for diagnostic purposes; also called a bone marrow biopsy (14)

Stool   The body wastes from the digestive tract that are discharged from the body through the anus (21)

Stress   A physical, chemical, or emotional factor that causes bodily or mental tension and may be a factor in disease causation (7)

Stuffing Charts   Placing extra chart forms in patients' charts on a nursing unit so they will be available when needed (8)

Subculture   Sub-groups within a culture; people with a distinct identity but who have certain ethnic, occupational, or physical characteristics found in a larger culture (5)

Subcutaneous (SQ) Injection   Injection of a small amount of a medication under the skin into fatty or connective tissue (13)

Supplemental Chart Forms   Patient chart forms used only when specific conditions or events dictate their use (8)

Supply Needs Sheet   A sheet of paper used by all the nursing unit personnel to jot down items that need reordering (7)

Suppository   Medicated substance mixed in a solid base that melts when placed in a body opening; suppositories are commonly used in the rectum, vagina, or urethra (13)

Surfing the Web   Using different web sites on the internet to locate information (2)

Surgery Consent   A patient's written permission for an operation or invasive procedure (19)

Surgery Schedule   A list of all the surgeries to be performed on a particular day; the schedule may be printed from the computer or sent to the nursing unit by the admitting department (19)

Suspension   Fine-particle drug suspended in liquid (13)

Symbols   Notations written in black or red ink on the doctors' order sheet to indicate completion of a step of the transcription procedure (9)

Tablet   Solid dosage of a drug in a disk form (13)

Tact   Use of discretion regarding feelings of others (6)

Team Leader   A registered nurse who is in charge of a nursing team (may also be called pod leader) (3)

Team Nursing   Consists of a charge nurse, two to three team leaders with four to five team members working under the supervision of each team leader (3)

Ted Hose   A brand name for antiembolism (A-E) hose (11)

Telemetry   The transmission of data electronically to a distant location (16)

Telephoned Orders   Orders for a patient telephoned to a health care facility by the doctor (9)

Temperature   The quantity of body heat, measured in degrees—either Fahrenheit or Celsius (10)

Terminal Illness   An illness ending in death (20)

Therapeutic Diet   A regular diet with modifications or restrictions (also called a special diet) (12)

Thoracentesis   A needle puncture into the pleural space in the chest cavity to remove pleural fluid for diagnostic or therapeutic reasons (14)

Tissue Typing   Identification of tissue types to predict acceptance or rejection of tissue and organ transplants (14)

Titer   The quantity of substance needed to react with a given amount of another substance—used to detect and quantify antibody levels (14)

Titrate   To adjust the amount of treatment to maintain a specific physiologic response (17)

Topical   Direct application of medication to the skin, eye, ear, or other parts of the body (13)

Tort   A wrong against another person or his property that is not a crime but for which the law provides a remedy (6)

Total Parenteral Nutrition (TPN)   The provision of all necessary nutrients via veins (discussed in detail in Chapter 13)

Tower   The system unit of the computer, which houses internal components (4)

Traction   A mechanical pull to part of the body to maintain alignment and facilitate healing; traction may be static (continuous) or intermittent (17)

Transcription   A process used to communicate the doctors' orders to the nursing staff and other hospital departments; computers or handwritten requisitions are used (1)

Transfer Order   A doctor's order that requests a patient to be transferred to another hospital room (18)

Tube Feeding   Administration of liquids into the stomach, duodenum, or jejunum through a tube (12)

Tuberculosis (TB)   A disease caused by *Mycobacterium tuberculosis,* an airborne pathogen (22)

Tympanic Membrane Temperature   The temperature reading obtained by placing an aural (ear) thermometer in the patient's ear (10)

Type and Crossmatch   The patient's blood is typed, then tested for compatibility with blood from a donor of the same blood type and Rh factor (14)

Type and Screen   The patient's blood type and Rh factor are determined, and a general antibody screen is performed (14)

Ultrasonography   A technique that uses high-frequency sound waves to create an image (scan) of body organs (may also be referred to as sonography or echography) (15)

Unit Dose   Any premixed or prespecified dose; often administered with SVN or IPPB treatments (17)

Urinalysis   The physical, chemical, and microscopic examination of the urine (14)

Urinary Catheter   A tube used for removing urine or injecting fluids into the bladder (11)

Urine Reflex   Urine is tested; if certain parameters are met, a culture will be performed (14)

Urine Residual   The amount of urine left in the bladder after voiding (11)

Valuables Envelope   A container for storing the patient's jewelry, money, and other valuables, which are placed in the hospital safe for safekeeping (19)

Value Clarification   Examination of our value system (6)

Values   Personal belief about worth of principal, standard, or quality; what one holds as most important (6)

Venipuncture   Needle puncture of a vein (11)

Verbal Communication   The use of language or the actual words spoken (5)

Viewing Screen   A computer component that displays information; it resembles a television, and it may also be called a monitor or a video display terminal (VDT) (4)

Vital Signs   Measurements of body functions including temperature, pulse, respiration, and blood pressure (10)

Voice Paging System   The system on which the hospital telephone operator pages a message to a doctor or makes other announcements; the system reaches all hospital areas (only used when absolutely necessary to keep noise level down) (4)

Void   To empty, especially the urinary bladder (11)

Voluntary   Not for profit (2)

Walla Roo   A chart rack located on the wall outside of a patient's room which stores the patient's chart and when unlocked forms a shelf to write upon (8)

Web Address   (URL—uniform resource locator). Keywords that when entered after http//www. on the Internet will take user to specified location referred to as a website (2)

Work Ethics   Moral values regarding work (6)

Workable Compromise   Dealing with a conflict in such a way that the solution is satisfactory to all parties (5)

CHAPTER 1

Exercise 1

1. CHUC
2. HUC
3. SHUC
4. Pt

Exercise 2

1. certified health unit coordinator
2. health unit coordinator
3. student health unit coordinator
4. patient

Review Questions

1. a. clinical
   b. non-clinical
   c. non-clinical
   d. clinical
   e. non-clinical
   f. clinical
   g. non-clinical
2. a. 1940; implementation of health unit coordinating at Montefiore Hospital in Pittsburgh, Pennsylvania
   b. 1966; one of the first educational programs was implemented in a vocational school in Minneapolis, Minnesota
   c. 1980; the National Association of Health Unit Coordinators was established in Phoenix, Arizona
   d. 1983; first offering of the Health Unit Coordinator Certification Examination by NAHUC
3. a. any three of the following:
      communicate all new doctors' orders to the patient's nurse
      maintain the patient's chart
      perform the non-clinical tasks for patient admission, transfer, and discharge
      prepare the patient's chart for surgery
      handle all telephone communication for the nurses' station
   b. any three of the following:
      transcribe the doctors' orders
      place and receive doctor's telephone calls to and from the doctor's office
      provide information to the physician regarding procedures
      obtain the patient's chart and procedure equipment
   c. any three of the following:
      schedule diagnostic procedures, treatments, and services
      request services from maintenance and other service departments
      work with the admitting department with patient admission, transfer, and discharge
      order the supplies for the nursing unit
   d. any three of the following:
      advise visitors of patient location
      provide information on location of bathroom, visitors lounge, cafeteria, etc

inform visitors of visiting rules and special precautions regarding their visit to a patient's room
receive telephone calls from the patient's relatives and friends regarding patient condition
handle visitor complaints
4. a process used to communicate the doctors' orders to the nursing staff and other hospital departments
5. The health unit coordinator assumes full responsibility for transcription of doctors' orders; co-signature of nurse is not needed.
6. any three of the following:
   professional representation
   format to share ideas and challenges
   national networking
   national directory
   opportunity to develop leadership skills
7. any three of the following:
   increased credibility
   gain a broader perspective of health unit coordinating (not just your own specialty)
   increased mobility, geographically and/or vertically
   peer and public recognition and respect
   improved self-image
8. a. health unit coordinating
   b. health unit management
   c. health service management
   d. health service administration
9. Policy and Procedure Manual

CHAPTER 2

Exercise 1

1. CEO	11. HO	21. PPO
2. CFO	12. JCAHO	22. Psych
3. COO	13. LTC	23. RR
4. DSU	14. MD	24. SAD
5. DO	15. Neuro	25. SDS
6. DRG	16. OB	26. SNF
7. ECF	17. OR	27. Surg
8. ED	18. Ortho	28. UCR
9. ER	19. PACU	29. www
10. HMO	20. Peds	

Exercise 2

1. chief executive officer
2. chief financial officer
3. chief operating officer
4. day surgery unit
5. doctor of osteopathy
6. diagnosis related groups
7. extended care facility
8. emergency department
9. emergency room
10. health maintenance organization
11. house officer

12. Joint Commission on Accreditation of Healthcare Organizations
13. long-term care
14. medical doctor
15. neurology
16. obstetrics
17. operating room
18. orthopedics
19. postanesthesia care unit
20. pediatrics
21. preferred provider organization
22. psychiatry
23. recovery room
24. save a day
25. same day surgery
26. skilled nursing facility
27. surgical
28. usual, customary, and reasonable
29. World Wide Web

Review Questions

1. the care and treatment of the sick
2. a. education of physicians and other health care personnel
   b. research
   c. prevention of disease
   d. local health center
3. attending physician
4. resident
5. a. the type of patient service offered
   b. ownership of the hospital
   c. type of accreditation the hospital has been given
6. 1. j   6. a   11. i
   2. m   7. k   12. f
   3. l   8. b   13. d
   4. n   9. e   14. h
   5. g   10. c
7. 1. i   5. l   9. f
   2. g   6. a   10. h
   3. j   7. c   11. e
   4. b   8. k   12. d
8. a. business office
   b. admitting department
   c. pathology, or clinical laboratory
   d. diagnostic imaging
   e. radiation therapy, or radiation oncology
   f. pharmacy
   g. physical therapy
   h. occupational therapy
   i. respiratory care
   j. dietary department
   k. endoscopy department
   l. gastroenterology, or GI laboratory
   m. cardiovascular studies department
   n. neurodiagnostics department
   o. health records, or medical records, department
   p. central service department
   q. outpatient department, or clinic
   r. social service department
   s. home care department
   t. housekeeping, or environmental services
   u. materials management, or purchasing department
   v. pastoral care or chaplain
   w. maintenance department
   x. laundry
   y. communications department
   z. security department
   aa. hospital information systems

9. accreditation
10. a. CPR
    b. infectious disease control
    c. fire and safety
    d. universal precautions
11. the governing board
12. chief executive officer (CEO)
13. any 3 of the following:
    internet
    newspaper classified advertisements
    job placement/career counselors
    employment agencies
    health care facility bulletin boards
    networking with professionals in the field
    instructors
    health care hotlines
    library resources
14. managed care / advocate
15. a. short-term care for serious illnesses or for trauma
    b. the combining of individual practices and small stand alone hospitals
    c. for profit
    d. Health Maintenance Organization – an organization that has management responsibility for providing comprehensive health care services on a prepayment basis
    e. uniform resource locator (Web address)
    f. a per member, monthly payment to a provider that covers contracted health care services and is paid in advance of its delivery
16. hospice
17. home health agency
18. to provide quality care for the lowest possible cost
19. hospital insurance
20. medical insurance (premium and deductible)
21. a. secondary
    b. primary
    c. tertiary
    d. primary
22. worker's compensation

CHAPTER 3

Exercise 1

1. CCU   8. Med   15. Psych
2. CNA   9. MICU   16. RN
3. CVICU   10. Neuro   17. SICU
4. Gyn   11. NICU   18. SSU
5. ICU   12. Ortho   19. TICU
6. L & D   13. PICU
7. LPN   14. PSA

Exercise 2

1. coronary care unit
2. certified nursing assistant
3. cardiovascular intensive care unit
4. gynecology
5. intensive care unit
6. labor and delivery
7. licensed practical nurse
8. medical
9. medical intensive care unit
10. neurology
11. neonatal intensive care unit
12. orthopedics

13. pediatric intensive care unit
14. patient support associate
15. psychology
16. registered nurse
17. surgical intensive care unit
18. short stay unit
19. trauma intensive care unit

Review Questions

1. 1. e   6. b   11. a
   2. c   7. h   12. l
   3. d   8. m   13. f
   4. n   9. j   14. k
   5. g   10. i
2. responsible for ensuring the physical and emotional care of the hospitalized patient
3. any three of the following:
   Nurse or clinical manager: assists the director of nursing in carrying out administrative responsibilities and is usually in charge of one or more nursing units
   Assistant nurse manager: assists the nurse manager in coordinating the activities of the nursing units
   Registered nurse: may give direct patient care or supervise patient care given by others
   Licensed practical nurse: gives direct patient care – functions under the direction of the RN
   Certified nursing assistant: a health care provider who performs basic nursing tasks such as bathing and seeding patients
4. a. pre-operative area: area in the hospital where patients are prepared for surgery
   b. intra-operative care: operating room—area in the hospital where surgery is performed
   c. post-operative: postanesthesia care—area in the hospital where patients are cared for immediately after surgery until they have recovered from the effects of the anesthesia
5. A patient who is critically ill in need of constant specialized nursing care would be admitted to ICU and would be transferred to a step-down unit when their condition improved.
6. In the primary nursing care delivery model, one RN provides total care to assigned patients, whereas in the team nursing model, a team leader who is an RN and team members provide care for the patients.
7. acuity
8. staff development
9. care that involves all departments that deal with the patient working together on the nursing unit to provide care
10. a. Registered Nurse
    b. Licensed Practical Nurse
    c. Certified Nursing Assistant
11. used as a method of outlining a patient's path of treatment for a specific diagnosis, procedure, or symptom

CHAPTER 4

Exercise 1

1. A Drive
2. C Drive
3. CPU
4. PC
5. VDT

Exercise 2

1. floppy drive
2. hard drive stored inside the computer
3. central processing unit
4. personal computer
5. video display terminal

Review Questions

1. a. speak slowly and distinctly
   b. give first and last name of patient and/or doctor and spell last name
   c. state number slowly and repeat
   d. leave your name and number and repeat both
2. a. answer the telephone promptly (before the third ring)
   b. identify yourself properly by stating your location, name and status
   c. speak into the telephone
   d. give the caller your undivided attention
   e. speak clearly and distinctly
   f. be courteous at all times
   g. when you cannot answer a question, tell the caller that you will get someone who can answer the question; do not say, "I don't know"
   h. if it is necessary to step away or answer another call, place the caller on hold after getting his or her permission
3. a. who the message is for
   b. the caller's name
   c. date and time of the call
   d. purpose of the call
   e. phone number to call if a return call is expected
   f. your name
4. a. a list of options projected on the viewing screen
   b. made up of three components: Keyboard, viewing screen, and printer
   c. a flashing indicator that lets the user know the area on the screen that will receive the information
   d. a computer component that displays information
   e. alphabetical listing of names, telephone numbers, and directory of telephone numbers of physicians on staff
   f. a requisition (paper order form) used to process information when the computer is not available for use
   g. a machine located in most nursing stations that shreds confidential material
   h. a system by which air pressure transports tubes carrying supplies, requisitions, or messages from one hospital unit or department to another
   i. a machine that prints patient labels – located near the health unit coordinator's area
5. a. to locate information or a person
   b. to answer other telephone lines
   c. to protect patient confidentiality (caller will not hear conversations)
6. Have the chart handy so you may look for facts that you may be asked. Write down the facts you wish to discuss.
7. posts material in an attractive manner and keeps the posted material current; when material has been read and initialed by nursing personnel, the health unit coordinator removes material and places on the nurse manager's desk
8. (Example) 4 East, Sally Jones, health unit coordinator.
9. A. (d.)
   B. (c.)
   C. (d)
10. a. access patient information
    b. order diagnostic tests and equipment
    c. enter discharges and transfers

11. True
12. E-mail is electronic mail and a method of sending and receiving messages to anyone with an e-mail address via the computer.
13. a. Do not use for personal messages or to send inappropriate material such as jokes.
    b. Send or respond to necessary person or department only, refrain from sending to all or using "reply all" unless necessary.
14. a. sending personal messages or jokes
    b. sending or responding to everyone when not necessary or requested
15. Many hospital personnel use the fax machine located in the nurses station—using the re-dial option may send the document or doctors' orders you are faxing to a different location, possibly violating patient confidentiality.

CHAPTER 5

Exercise 1

1. a	5. d	9. a
2. b	6. d	10. b
3. b	7. d	
4. c	8. c	

Exercise 2

1. AS	7. AS	13. AS
2. AG	8. AG	14. AG
3. NA	9. AG	15. AS
4. NA	10. AS	16. AS
5. AS	11. AG	
6. AG	12. NA	

Exercise 3

Answers will vary. Below are examples of responses for each behavior:
1. Assertive: "It upset me when you threw the chart down in front of me and left without giving me a chance to respond."
   Nonassertive: Be upset and say nothing.
   Aggressive: "This is a 24-hour facility, what I don't get done, you can do!"
2. Assertive: "I understand that you would prefer someone who is accustomed to working in pediatrics. I may need a little assistance, and will do my best to get the job done." *(Fogging)*
   Nonassertive: "I'm sorry; I know I'm not qualified to work in pediatrics."
   Aggressive: "You're lucky to have me, if you don't want me to be here, I'll leave."
3. Assertive: "You're right, I did miss that order, I will order it right now." *(Negative assertion)*
   Nonassertive: "I'm sorry; I'm so stupid! What should I do now?"
   Aggressive: "Well, maybe if you gave me a little more help, I wouldn't be missing orders!"
4. Assertive: "Only relatives may visit the patient, on the instructions of the physician". Repeat as necessary. *(Broken record)*
   Nonassertive: "I don't think you're supposed to visit, but maybe just this once we could sneak you in."
   Aggressive: "You are not allowed to visit; I don't care who you are!"
5. Assertive: "I was not aware that you felt this way. What about my work is sloppy?" *(Negative Inquiry)*
   Nonassertive: "I've always been sloppy. It's just the way I am. I'm sorry."
   Aggressive: "I'm a lot neater than most of the other people around here!"
6. Assertive: "I know it must seem that nothing is done right here, however, most things are done very well. I'll call you as soon as I receive the results."

Nonassertive: "I'm sorry; I should have called earlier and had them ready for you when you came in."
Aggressive: "You don't understand how hectic it is around here. You doctors always think everyone else is incompetent!"

Review Questions

1. Answers will vary.
2. a. the person transmitting the message
   b. images, feelings, and ideas transmitted from one person to another
   c. the person receiving the message
   d. response to the message
   e. process of sender translating mental images, feelings, and ideas into symbols in order to communicate them to the receiver
   f. process of receiver translating the verbal and non-verbal symbols to determine the meaning of the message
3. a. sender
   b. message
   c. receiver
   d. feedback
4. Answers will vary.
5. a. poor choice of words
   b. contradiction of verbal and non-verbal language used
6. a. poor listening skills
   b. poor feedback skills
7. any three of the following:
   clothing
   hair
   jewelry
   body art
   cosmetics
   automobile
   house
   perfume or cologne
8. any three of the following:
   posture
   ambulation
   touching
   personal distance
   eye contact
   breathing
   hand gestures
   facial expressions
9. a. 55%
   b. 38%
   c. 7%
10. a. unsuccessful encoding by sender
    b. unsuccessful decoding by receiver
11. a. unsuccessful decoding: The nurse was not aware of the patient's cultural background (see Table 5–1, p. 65).
    b. unsuccessful encoding: Joe was disrespectful in using the term, honey and also used medical terms that Mrs. Fredrick didn't understand. Mrs. Fredrick by crying was expressing both her esteem and safety and security needs.
    c. unsuccessful decoding: Sue was distracted and failed to listen for the page.
    d. unsuccessful decoding: Cindi was stereotyping Mr. Potter based on his status and personal hygiene.
12. Answers will vary.
13. Answers will vary.
14. a. safety and security need: Responding with "Cancer?" lets the patient to further discuss his or her fears. A response such as "Don't worry about it" shuts off further communication from patients.
    b. physiological need: Any nonverbal or verbal response that communicates to the patient that you understand the urgency of the request and you will follow through immediately.

c. esteem need: Give constructive feedback such as,"You have good leadership skills, I hope you are elected" as opposed to destructive feedback such as "What do you want to do that for, you are busy enough already."

d. beloning and love need: Give feedback that encourages the patient to expound on the subject. Avoid disagreeing by using phrases such as,"Oh come now, you are not that old."

e. self-esteem need: Give descriptive feedback such as,"I liked your opening remarks" rather than "You did okay."

f. safety and security need: Avoid such responses, as "It won't hurt." Acknowledge the fear that is being expressed. *Note:* Telling a child that it won't hurt will destroy his or her trust. Sometimes a child life representative will demonstrate a painful procedure on a teddy bear to ease a child's fear.

g. esteem nced: Give descriptive rather than evaluative feedback. Avoid saying,"I think you are doing a great job here. Why do you want to leave?" A phrase such as,"Looking for something else?" encourages further communication.

h. safety and security need: An appropriate response includes reassurance to the patient that his integrity is not being questioned.

15. Answers will vary.

16. a. non-assertive
    b. aggresive
    c. assertive

17. a. a skill that allows you to say no over and over again without raising your voice or getting irritated or angry.
    b. a skill that allows you to accept manipulative criticism and anxiety-producing statements by offering no resistance and by using a non-committal reply.
    c. a skill that allows you to accept your errors and faults without becoming defensive or resorting to anger.
    d. a skill that allows you to actively prompt criticism in order to use the information, or if manipulative, to exhaust it.

18. Any four of the following:
    always identify yourself by nursing unit, name, and status
    avoid putting the person on hold
    listen to what the caller is saying
    write down what the caller is saying
    acknowledge the anger
    do not allow the caller to become abusive

19. a. the inability to accept other cultures, or an assumption of cultural superiority
    b. a judgment or opinion made without adequate knowledge
    c. subgroups within a culture; people with a distinct identity but who have certain ethnic, occupational or physical characteristics found in a larger culture
    d. the group whose values prevail within a society
    e. the assumption that all members of a culture or ethnic group act alike

CHAPTER 6

Exercise 1

1. APS	3. NINP	5. HIPAA
2. CPS	4. SNAT	6. PHI

Exercise 2

1. Adult Protective Services
2. Child Protectve Services
3. no information, no publication
4. suspected non-accidental trauma
5. HIPAA
6. PHI

Exercise 3

Personal answers required; answers will vary.

Review Questions

1. any four of the following:
   philosophy and standards of the organization
   leadership style of supervisors
   how meaningful or important the work is to the person
   how challenging the work is for the person
   how the person fits in with co-workers
   personal characteristics of worker; abilities, interests, aptitudes, values, and expectations

2. Answers will vary. *Example:* A patient is admitted with complications of alcoholism, the health unit coordinator's religion prohibits drinking

3. any six of the following:
   dependability
   accountability
   consideration
   cheerfulness
   empathy
   trustworthiness
   respectfulness
   courtesy
   tactfulness
   conscientiousness
   honesty
   cooperation
   attitude

4. To protect patients' health information. The privacy Rule mandates that patients be provided with a copy of privacy practices when treated in a doctor's office or admitted to a health care facility.

5. Information about the patient that includes demographic information which may identify the individual and relates to their past, present or future physical or mental health condition and related health care services.

6. Answers will vary. *Examples:*
   a. It wouldn't be appropriate to discuss this information, especially in the cafeteria.
   b. Walk over to the two members, say "Excuse me," and change the subject. After the wife is out of hearing distance, explain that their discussion could be overheard.
   c. "I appreciate your concern, but I can't discuss her diagnosis or condition with you. I will let the nurse know that you have observed that she hasn't eaten today."
   d. You would ask him to hold while you transfer him to the nurse in charge.
   e. You would deny knowledge of the patient; if he became insistent or rude, you would ask him to hold while you transferred him to the nurse in charge.
   f. "It would be inappropriate for me to discuss anything that happened at work outside the workplace."
   g. Advise her that you can't discuss any patient with her and suggest that she could visit or call her friend in the hospital.

7. any two of the following:
   do not discuss patient information
   conduct conversations with other health personnel outside of the hearing distance of the patients and visitors.
   do not discuss medical treatment with the patient or relatives
   do not discuss general patient information
   do not discuss hospital incidents away from the nursing unit
   refer all telephone calls from reporters, police personnel, legal agencies, and so forth to the nurse manager.

8. any three of the following:
   follow the hospital policy for duplicating portions of the patient's chart
   control access to the patient's chart
   ask outside agency personnel for picture identification
   control transportation of the patient's chart
9. Your professional appearance will earn trust, respect, and confidence of your employer, coworkers, patients, and others.
10. a. *quid pro quo*
    b. a hostile working place
11. advise the person to stop, and explain that you do not like or welcome his or her behavior
12. call security immediately
13. a. to provide feedback
    b. to make compensation decisions
14. keep a diary of accomplishments, classes taken, and in-services attended during the evaluation process
15. 1. b   3. a   5. d
    2. e   4. f   6. c
16. 1. d   4. c   7. a
    2. i   5. f   8. e
    3. g   6. h
17. a. false: Even though as a health unit coordinator you may be certified but not licensed, you are responsible for your errors.
    b. false: Only authorized personnel should be allowed to read a patients' chart
    c. false: You should work within your scope or practice
18. a. confidentiality
    b. nonmaleficence
    c. autonomy
    d. beneficence (one may answer *nonmaleficence*, but the distinction is that *beneficence* is the prevention of harm, whereas *nonmaleficence* indicates that one will not inflict harm)
    e. veracity
19. a. more efficient patient care
    b. greater satisfaction for the patient, the patient's physician, and the health care organization
20. Answers will vary.

CHAPTER 7

Exercise 1

1. CPR
2. CQI

Exercise 2

1. cardiopulmonary resuscitation
2. Continuous Quality Improvement

Exercise 3

Answers will vary.

Review Questions

1. a. management of the nursing unit supplies and equipment
   b. management of the activities at the nurses' station
   c. management related to the performance of tasks
   d. management of time
   e. management of stress

2. a. Often it is the health unit coordinator's responsibility to take inventory using the standard supply list and to order supplies. The supply need list would also be used when ordering supplies.
   b. The health unit coordinator also may have the responsibility to make sure equipment stored on the nursing unit is in working order and is returned to appropriate storage place.
   c. It is the health unit coordinator's responsibility to keep unit manuals up to date by adding new materials sent to the nursing unit and to make sure that manuals and text books remain on the nursing unit.
   d. It is the responsibility of the health unit coordinator to report and request repair of any maintenance problems regarding the nursing unit (including heating, cooling, plumbing, electrical problems, etc.).
   e. The health unit coordinator enters the order for patients' rental equipment and would report and request repair for any equipment in need of repair.
   f. The health unit coordinator must know where the emergency equipment is kept, and order supplies and replacements as requested.

3. Answers will vary. Examples of acceptable answers follow:
   a patient has a DNR order
   a patient is out on a 2-hour pass
   a patient is going to surgery (note time)
   a patient is in recovery
   no visitors for room 423
   no phone calls for a patient
   a patient has an NINP order

4. The information would be recorded next to the patient's name on the unit census work sheet.

5. Health personnel, doctors, and visitors are constantly asking the health unit coordinator the whereabouts of patients and/or patients' charts. By maintaining the census worksheet you can find the answer at a glance.

6. a. communicate pertinent information to visitors
   b. respond to visitors' questions and requests
   c. initially handle visitors' complaints, and locate the patient's nurse when necessary.

7. a. listen carefully and attentively to what the person is saying
   b. ask pertinent objective questions and gather as many facts as possible.
   c. respond to the complaint accordingly.

8. a. orders involving a patient in a medical crisis take priority over all other tasks
   b. transcribing stat orders
   c. answering the nursing unit telephone (preferably prior to third ring).

9. a. call the code (1)
   b. answer the ringing telephone (2)
   c. check the surgical charts for the necessary reports (3)
   d. process the two discharge orders (4)
   e. order the chest x-ray for today (5)
   f. retrieve objects from the pneumatic tube system (6)

10. a. plan for rush periods
    b. plan a schedule for the routine health unit coordinator tasks
    c. group activities. Save time by grouping activities together
    d. complete one task before beginning another
    e. know your job and perform your job
    f. take the breaks assigned to you
    g. avoid unnecessary conversation
    h. delegate tasks to volunteers

11. a. a computerized or written record of the amount of each item that the nursing unit currently needs to last until the next supply order date.
    b. a list of patients' names with room and bed numbers located on a nursing unit with blank spaces next to each name (may be printed form a computer menu). This sheet may be used by the

health unit coordinator to record patient activities (some hospitals may use a patient information sheet or a patient activity sheet to record patient activity).

  c. the communication process between shifts, in which the nursing personnel going off duty report the nursing unit activities to the personnel coming on duty

  d. a form that is used to credit a patient for items found in the room unused after the patient's discharge, or for items charged to the patient but not used for him or her

  e. a form that is initiated to charge a discharged patient for any items that were not charged to him or her at the time of use.

12. a. Listen to Mrs. Frances with understanding and empathy, tell her that you will ask her husband's nurse to come talk to her. Document what Mrs. Frances said, and advise her husband's nurse of what was said prior to him or her going in to speak to Mrs. Frances.

  b. Advise the visitor of the rules and if she persists in taking the child to Mr. Blair's room, ask the patient's nurse to speak to her (there may be extenuating circumstances that you are unaware of).

  c. Go in the room and ask that only two visitors be in the room at one time or suggest (if possible) that they all go out to the waiting room or to the cafeteria.

  d. Ask the nurse manager if it could be moved to a more convenient place. She or he may want to bring it to a health unit coordinator meeting for discussion.

  e. Suggest that you would be glad to help her in any other way, but you are not trained or legally covered by your job description to assist patients in going to the restroom.

13. Any of the following (in detail) would be examples of information that you would communicate during shift report:

a patient is out on a pass

there were new admissions and the orders are done

there are pending discharges

an NINP order

a patient is scheduled for surgery

a patient is in the recovery room and will be returning to the unit

14. Answers will vary. Examples of acceptable answers follow:

  a. You receive a telephone message for Mary to call the pharmacy at her convenience. Rather than waste time trying to locate Mary, record this information on the note pad.

  b. You need to call the doctor's office and you are unable to complete the call because the line is busy; record the task on the note pad, along with the doctor's telephone number and other pertinent data so that you will have it available when you are able to place the call.

15. a. Ask for assistance when necessary.

  b. When returning to the nursing unit from a break, if you see that several charts are lying about; open each chart and check for new orders—place charts in the chart rack that do not have new orders—read all of the new orders, notify the patient's nurse of any stats and provide him or her with a copy of the orders, fax, or send copies to the pharmacy, then proceed to transcribe all other orders one chart at a time.

  c. Always complete a set of orders that you have started transcribing prior to taking a break.

  d. Follow the ten steps of transcription outlined in Chapter 9 and never sign off on orders until you are sure that you have completed each step.

16. the study of work for the purpose of making the workplace more comfortable and to improve both health and productivity.

17. a. acute, which consist of fractures, crushing, or low back strain injuries

  b. cumulative, which occur over time due to repetitive motion activity.

18. any of the following:

The computer terminal should be located where it will reduce awkward head and neck postures—position the terminals so that you must look slightly downward to look at the middle of the screen—the preferred viewing distance is 18 to 24 inches (Fig. 7–9, p. 104).

Adjust your chair so that you sit straight yet in a relaxed position, with a backrest supporting the small of your back and your feet flat on the floor.

Adjust your chair back to a slightly backward position and extend your legs out slightly so there are no sharp angles that cause pressure to be placed on your hip or knee joints as you work.

Your wrists should be straight as you type with forearms level and elbows close to your body—reduce bending of the wrists by moving the entire arm.

Use a computer wrist pad.

Eliminate situations that would require constant bending over to complete your tasks.

Shift your weight in your chair frequently.

Use proper body mechanics when lifting—don't bend over with legs straight or twist while lifting and avoid trying to lift above shoulder level.

Take frequent mini-stretches of your neck (lean your head down in each direction for a 5-second count).

Stand, walk, and stretch your back and legs at least every hour. These small breaks in position help avoid neuromuscular strain and alleviate the tension of job stress.

Remain drug free, eat a balanced diet, exercise, and get proper rest to be at your best performance level.

19. a. perennial stress: the wear and tear of day to day living with the feeling that one is a square peg trying to fit in a round hole: examples: traffic, difficult relationships, etc.

  b. crisis stress: common, uncontrollable, often unpredictable life experiences that have a profound effect on individuals: examples: death, divorce, illness, etc.

20. any five of the following:

effective time management

realizing that the nurses, doctors, and other health care workers may be working under a lot of stress, and that their expressions of frustration should not be taken personally—be empathetic and understanding.

saying "no" tactfully when asked to do additional work if you truly don't have time

asking for help when you need it

keeping your sense of humor—humor is a great stress reliever as long as it is timely and appropriate

taking your scheduled breaks.

21. to continuously improve quality at every level of every department of every function of the health care organization.

22. any four of the following:

The telephone should be within easy reach.

Frequently used forms should be stored within reaching distance.

Charts should be located in an area where they can be easily reached.

The label printer should be in close proximity.

The fax machine should be in close proximity.

The unit reference books and manuals should be kept within reach distance.

The unit shredder should be in close proximity.

23. You would read all new orders, notify the patient's nurse of any stats and provide him or her with a copy of the orders, send or fax all pharmacy copies, and then proceed to transcribe all other orders, one chart at a time.

CHAPTER 8

Exercise 1

1. Hx
2. NKA
3. C of A
4. ID labels
5. H & P
6. MAR
7. NKMA
8. NKDA
9. NKFA

Exercise 2

1. conditions of admission
2. identification labels
3. no known food allergies
4. medication administration record
5. no known allergies
6. no known drug allergies
7. history and physical
8. history
9. no known medication allergies

Review Questions

1. in-patient
2. a. Place all charts in proper sequence (usually according to room number) in the chart rack when they are not in use.
   b. Place new chart forms in each patient's chart before the immediate need arises. In many health care facilities, this is referred to as "stuffing the chart." Label each chart form with the patient's ID label before placing it in the chart. New chart forms are placed on top of old chart forms for easy access. The new forms may be folded in half to show the old form has not been completely used.
   c. Place diagnostic reports in the correct patient's chart behind the correct divider. Match the patient's name on the report with the patient's name on the front of the chart. (Don't depend on room numbers as patients are often transferred to another room.)
      Review the patients' charts frequently for new orders (always check each chart for new orders prior to returning them to the chart rack).
   d. Properly label the patient's chart so that it can easily be located at all times.
      Check each chart to be sure all the forms are labeled with the correct patient's name. Chart forms should be in the proper sequence.
   e. Check the chart frequently for patient information forms or face sheets. Usually five copies are maintained in the chart. Physicians may remove copies for billing purposes. The health unit coordinator may print additional copies of the face sheet from the computer or may order them from admitting.
   f. Assist physicians or other professionals in locating the patient's chart.
3. a. The physicians' order form is the form on which the doctor requests the care and treatment procedures for the patient.
   b. The graphic record is a graphic representation of the patient's vital signs (temperature, pulse, respiration, and blood pressure) for a given number of days.
   c. The physicians' progress record is a form on which the physician records the patient's progress during the period of hospitalization.
   d. The history and physical form is a chart form that is usually dictated by the patient's doctor, hospitalist or resident The hospital medical transcription department types the dictated report and sends it to the nursing unit to be placed in the patient's chart. It is used to record the medical history and the present symptomatic history of the patient. A review of all body systems or physical assessment of the patient is also recorded.

   e. Nurses' progress notes is a standard chart form that is used to outline the patient's care and treatment and to record the treatment, progress and activities of the patient.
   f. Medication administration record (MAR) is a standard chart form that is used to record all medications given by nursing personnel.
4. a. The face sheet or information form contains information about the patient, such as name, address, telephone number, name of employer, the admission diagnosis, health care insurance policy information, and next of kin.
   b. The service agreement (conditions of admission) form is signed by the patient in the admitting department and then sent to the unit to be placed in the patient's chart. The form provides legal permission to the hospital/ doctor to treat the patient and also serves as a financial agreement.
   c. The advanced directive checklist is a chart form that documents that the patients were informed of their choice to declare their health care decisions.
5. a. supplemental patient chart forms are additional to the standard patient chart forms and are added to the patients' charts according to their specific care and treatment.
   b.–c. *Examples:* any of the following:
      clinical pathway form
      anticoagulant record
      diabetic record
      consultation form
      operating room records
      therapy records
      parenteral fluid or infusion record
      frequent vital signs record
      consent forms
6. a. means of communication
   b. planning patient care
   c. research
   d. educational purposes
   e. legal document
   f. history of patient illnesses, care, treatment, and outcomes
7. outpatient
8. admission packet
9. a. Draw (in black ink) one single line through the error. Record "mistaken entry" with the date, time, your first initial, last name, and status in a blank area near (directly above or next to) the error
   b. Chart forms that are affixed with the wrong or incorrect ID label may be shredded if no notations have been made on them. If the chart form has notations on it, the chart form cannot be shredded. Draw an X with a black ink pen through the incorrect label and write "mistaken entry" with the date, time, your first initial, last name and status above the incorrect label. Affix the correct patient ID label on the form next to the incorrect label (do not place correct label over incorrect label). It is also permissible to hand print the patient information in black ink next to the incorrect label that you have drawn an *X* through.
10. 1530
11. 11:45 PM
12. a. placing extra chart forms in patients' charts on a nursing unit so they will be available when needed
    b. portions of the patient's current chart that are removed when the chart becomes so full that it is unmanageable
    c. preprinted labels containing individual patient information to identify patient records
    d. a method of alerting staff when two or more patients with the same or similarly spelled last names are located on a nursing unit
    e. labels affixed to the front cover of a patient's chart that indicate a patient's allergies

f. the patient's record from previous admissions stored in the health records department that may be retrieved for review when a patient is admitted to the emergency room, nursing unit or outpatient department (may also be requested by patient's doctor)

g. a chart rack located on the wall outside of a patient's room which stores the patient's chart and when unlocked forms a shelf to write upon

13. a. Affix the patient's ID label to the form. Some physicians may have preprinted consent forms for certain procedures or surgeries.

b. Write in black ink the first and last names of the doctor who is to perform the surgery or procedure.

c. All medical terminology should be spelled correctly and all information written legibly.

d. Write in black ink the surgery or procedure to be performed exactly as the physician wrote it on the physician's order sheet except write out abbreviations.

e. Do not record the date and time. The person obtaining the patient's signature will complete this.

14. a. release of side rails

b. refusal to permit blood transfusion

c. consent form for human immunodeficiency virus

d. consent to receive blood transfusion

CHAPTER 9

Review Questions

1. Symbols are placed on the doctors' order sheet to indicate completion of the task.

2. Answers will vary. *Example:* 0/00/00 0925 Mary Smith/CHUC

3. a. read the complete set of doctors' orders

b. send or fax the pharmacy copy of the doctors' order sheet to the pharmacy department

c. complete stat orders

d. place telephone calls as necessary to complete doctors' orders

e. select the patient's name from the census on the computer screen or collect all necessary forms

f. order diagnostic tests, treatments, and supplies

g. kardex all doctors' orders except medication orders

h. write medication orders on MAR

i. recheck your performance of each step for accuracy and thoroughness

j. sign-off the completed set of doctors' orders

4. It is a legal document. *Note:* The color of ink used would be in accordance with hospital policy.

5. a. after the step of transcription is completed to document completion of that step

6. a. the absence of symbols

b. absence of sign-off

7. to communicate new orders to the nursing staff and to update the patient's profile

8. New doctors' orders may involve changing or discontinuing an existing order. Information not subject to change, such as the patient's name, is usually recorded in black ink, and allergies are always recorded in red ink.

9. a. Ordering is the process of inputting the doctors' orders into the computer or of copying the doctors' order onto a requisition. Whichever method is used, the purpose of ordering is to forward the doctors' orders to the various hospital departments that will execute the order.

b. Kardexing is the process of recording all new doctors' orders onto the patient's Kardex form.

c. A requisition is a form used to order diagnostic procedures, treatments, or supplies from hospital departments other than nursing

when the computer is down (also called a *down-time requisition*).

d. Flagging is a method used by the doctor to notify the nursing staff that she or he has written a new set of orders.

10. a. the line directly below the doctors' signature.

b. so there is not a space left and another order can not be added after sign-off

11. Accuracy in transcribing doctors' orders is essential to avoid errors that may cause harm to a patient.

12. a. ord (or computer order number)

b. M

c. K

d. *(Example)* called Mary 1035
PCS or PC Faxed 1035 (with time and your initials recorded)
(Example) notified Nancy 1050

13. Ordering is the sixth step of transcription—unless the order is written to be done stat.

14. a. activity

b. diet

c. vital sign frequency

d. treatment

e. diagnostic studies

15. a. standing: In effect and given routinely until discontinued or changed by the doctor.

b. standing PRN: In effect and given as needed by the patient until automatically discontinued or changed by the doctor.

c. one-time or short-series: In effect for one time or a short period, automatically discontinued when the order has been completed.

d. stat: Given immediately, then automatically discontinued.

16. a. short-order series

b. standing prn

c. one time—stat

d. standing

e. standing

f. short-order series

17. The doctor will write *stat*—"now" is also usually considered equivalent to *stat*.

18. a. Read and understand each word of doctors' orders. If in doubt, check with a patient's nurse or the doctor. Use symbols and write the symbol after you have completed each step of transcription. When new orders are recorded at the top of the doctors' order sheet, check the previous order sheet to see if these orders are continued from the previous page. If the set of orders finish near the bottom of the doctors' order sheet, cross through the remaining space with diagonal lines. Record the sign off information on the line directly below the doctor's signature to avoid leaving space in which future orders could be written and missed. Check for new orders before returning a chart from the counter or elsewhere to the chart rack.

b. When in doubt about the correct interpretation of doctors' orders, always check with the patient's nurse or the doctor.

c. Compare the patient's name and the hospital number on the patient's ID label you have placed on the order requisition form and/or selected on the computer screen with the same information on the patient's chart cover. Never select computer labels by the patient's room number only.

d. Compare the patient's name and the doctor's name on Kardex form with the same information on the label on the patient's chart cover. Do not use the information on the doctors' order sheet. It may have the wrong information on it. Never select by using room number alone. If the patient has been transferred the room number printed on the patient ID label on the chart forms may no longer be correct.

e. When you cannot read an order because of the doctor's handwriting, refer to the progress record form on the patient's chart. The orders are often recorded on this form also, and reading this information may assist you in interpreting the orders on the physicians' order form. If the order remains unclear, ask the doctor who wrote it for clarification. Don't waste time asking others. They may be guessing also. If a doctor has a reputation for poor handwriting, ask him or her to wait while you read the orders so you can clarify orders that you can't read.

19. a. Make sure you have the correct chart. Check both the chart spine and the patient ID label on the doctor's order sheet.
    b. Begin recording the orders directly below the last entry on the doctor's order sheet (sign-off of last set of orders). In other words, do not leave a space between your entry and the last entry.
    c. Record the orders in ink.
    d. Record the date and time.
    e. Record each order as the doctor states it. Do not hesitate to ask questions if you do not understand what is being said.
    f. Read the entire set of orders back to the physician.
    g. Sign the orders as shown in Figure 9–3.

CHAPTER 10

Exercise 1

1. CBR	16. qd	31. ax
2. c̄	17. tid	32. TPR
3. A & O	18. q hr	33. P
4. qid	19. temp	34. h, hr, hrs
5. °	20. as tol	35. prn
6. BP	21. rt or Ⓡ	36. NVS or neuro ✓s
7. q	22. lt or Ⓛ	37. ↓
8. amb	23. D/C or DC	38. HOB
9. ABR	24. VS	39. BSC
10. ↑	25. I & O	40. q 4 hr or q4°
11. BRP	26. OOB	41. CMS
12. RR	27. min	42. SOB
13. ad-lib	28. wt	43. CVP
14. qod	29. BR	44. Rout
15. bid	30. R	

Exercise 2

1. left	24. absolute bed rest
2. right	25. temperature
3. discontinue or discharge	26. as tolerated
4. vital signs	27. intake and output
5. blood pressure	28. every
6. three times a day	29. pulse
7. complete bed rest	30. axillary or axilla
8. with	31. rectal
9. temperature, pulse and respiration	32. as necessary
10. bed rest	33. respiratory rate
11. minute	34. every four hours
12. bathroom privileges	35. hour, hours
13. as desired	36. neurologic vital signs or neurologic checks
14. increase, above, or elevate	37. decrease, below, or lower
15. out of bed	38. routine
16. alert and oriented	39. shortness of breath
17. weight	40. head of bed
18. ambulate	41. bedside commode
19. every other day	42. circulation, motion, and sensation
20. every day	43. central venous pressure
21. two times a day	44. routine
22. four times a day	
23. every hour	

Review Questions

1. a. periodic observations by the nurse (ordered by the doctor) of the patient's condition; these observations are referred to as signs and symptoms.
   b. patient activity orders refer to the amount of walking, sitting, and so forth that the patient may do in a given period during his or her hospital stay.
   c. patient positioning is often determined by the nursing staff; however, the doctor may want the patient to remain in a special body position to maintain body alignment, promote comfort, and facilitate body functions.
   d. measurements of body functions, including temperature, pulse, respiration, and blood pressure
   e. the quantity of body heat, measured in degrees—either Fahrenheit or Celsius
      i. the temperature reading obtained by placing the thermometer in the patient's mouth under the tongue
      ii. the temperature reading obtained by placing the thermometer in the patient's rectum
      iii. the temperature reading obtained by placing the thermometer in the patient's axilla (armpit)
      iv. the temperature reading obtained by placing an aural (ear) thermometer in the patient's ear
   f. a noninvasive method to measure the oxygen saturation of arterial blood
   g. elevated body temperature (fever)
   h. without fever
2. a. complete bed rest
   b. bed rest with bathroom privileges when alert and oriented
   c. weight every other day
   d. vital signs four times a day
   e. temperature, pulse and respiration and blood pressure three times a day
   f. elevate head of bed twenty degrees
   g. check dressing as necessary
   h. temperature rectal or axillary only
   i. neurologic vital signs every two hours
   j. intake and output every shift
   k. out of bed as desired
   l. up as tolerated
   m. temperature, pulse, respiration and blood pressure every four hours
   n. ambulate today
   o. discontinue vital signs
   p. elevate head of bed thirty degrees
   q. may use bedside commode
   r. log roll every two hours
   s. check circulation, motion and sensation toes left foot
   t. central venous pressure every three hours
   u. call me if patient complains of shortness of breath

CHAPTER 11

Exercise 1

1. SSE	16. IV	31. con't
2. KO	17. cath	32. CBI
3. MR	18. LR	33. TKO
4. sol'n	19. st	34. mL
5. nec	20. cc	35. IVF
6. cm	21. $\bar{p}$	36. ETS
7. TWE	22. abd	37. PICC
8. NG	23. TCDB	38. VAD
9. NS	24. min	39. CVC
10. D/LR	25. gtts	40. D_5W
11. hs	26. Δ	41. $D_{10}W$
12. DW	27. ASAP	42. B/L
13. @	28. /	43. HL or hep lock
14. ORE	29. H_2O_2	44. SCD
15. irrig	30. ac	

Exercise 2

1. 1000 milliliter lactated Ringers at 125 cubic centimeters per hour, then discontinue
2. Soap suds enema hour of sleep (bedtime) may repeat times one
3. Give ore retention enema follow $\bar{c}$ tap water enema if necessary
4. Irrigate catheter three times a day $\bar{c}$ normal saline solution
5. 1000 cubic centimeters five percent dextrose in 0.9 normal saline at to keep open
6. Insert nasogastric tube
7. Turn, cough, deep breath every two hours
8. Change intravenous tubing as soon as possible
9. Please obtain elevated toilet seat for patient
10. Start intravenous fluids of ten percent dextrose in water at one hundred twenty cubic centimeters per hour
11. Insert heparin lock
12. Shave bilateral inguinal groin area
13. Apply sequential compression device

Review Questions

1. any five of the following:
   Fleets enema
   rectal tube
   irrigation trays
   urinary catheter trays
   IV solutions
   IV catheters and needles
   IV tubing
   suction catheters and tubing
   sterile gloves
   exam gloves
   masks
   syringes and needles
   disposable suture removal kits
   dressings
      abdominal pads
      Telfa pads
      gauze pads in various sizes
      Kling
      Vaseline gauze
      tape (various types)
   alcohol pads
   glycerin swabs
   irrigation solutions, etc. (could vary among hospitals)

2. any five of the following:
   alternating pressure pad
   egg-crate mattress
   Ted hose
   pneumatic Hose
   colostomy kit
   stomal bags
   elastic abdominal binder
   foot board
   foot cradle
   feeding pump and tubing
   IV infusion pump
   hypothermia machine
   K-pad
   restraints
   adult disposable diapers
   sitz bath, disposable
   sterile trays
      tracheostomy tray
      bone marrow tray
      paracentesis tray
      lumbar puncture (spinal tap) tray
      thoracentesis tray
      central line tray, etc (could vary among hospitals)

3. any three of the following:
   Harris flush
   oil retention
   soap suds enema
   tap water enema
   Fleets

4. a. indwelling (retention catheter)—stays in place
   b. intermittent (straight) catheter—a single use catheter that is removed after bladder is drained

5. a. amount
   b. solution
   c. rate

6. a. Hemovac
   b. Jackson Pratt (JP)

7. a. peripherally
   b. central line

8. Any two of the following:
   dextrose in lactated Ringers
   D_5LR
   $D_{10}LR$
   0.9 NS (*Note:* There are many more answers that would be acceptable)

9. The laboratory would discard the blood and the patient would need to have his or her blood redrawn, causing additional discomfort and delaying treatment

10. Any two of the following:
    K-pad
    hot compresses
    warm soaks
    sitz bath

11. Any two of the following:
    alcohol sponge bath
    ice bag
    hypothermia machine

12. a. a vascular access device (also called intermittent infusion device) placed on a peripheral intravenous catheter when used intermittently
    b. a disposable suction device (evacuator unit) that is connected to a drain inserted into or close to a surgical wound
    c. a disposable suction device (evacuator unit) that is connected to a drain inserted into or close to a surgical wound
    d. the patient's own blood donated previously for transfusion as needed by the patient; also called autotransfusion

e. blood donated by relatives or friends of the patient to be used for transfusion as needed

f. insertion of a catheter into a body cavity or organ to inject or remove fluid

g. a drain that that is inserted into or close to a surgical wound and may lie under a dressing, extend through a dressing, or be connected to a drainage bag or a suction device

h. a catheter is threaded through to the superior vena cava or right atrium used for the administration of intravenous therapy

i. a type of commercial blood glucose monitor used to check the glucose level of blood.

13. The amount of urine left in the bladder after voiding

14. a. to discontinue a daily charge to the patient
b. so the item can be cleaned and prepared for another patient's use

15. return the unit of packed cells to the blood bank for proper storage (after confirming this with the nurse)

16. make two trips to pick each unit up separately or ask another person to pick up one unit while you pick up the other

17. The central service department (CSD) distributes the supplies used for nursing procedures.

18. a. true
b. false
c. false
d. true
e. true

19. a. Have the IV team insert a PICC
b. Cont IVF alternate 1000cc of LR c̄ 1000cc of D₅W @ 125 cc/hr via CVC
c. Insert NG tube and connect to low gastric suction

CHAPTER 12

Exercise 1

1. Na or Na⁺
2. MN
3. NPO
4. reg
5. cl
6. cal
7. ADA
8. liq
9. chol
10. DAT
11. FF
12. CHO
13. NSA
14. FS
15. PEG
16. NAS
17. RD
18. K or K+

Exercise 2

1. sodium
2. nothing by mouth
3. regular
4. midnight
5. liquid
6. calorie
7. no salt added
8. American Diabetic Association
9. diet as tolerated
10. clear
11. cholesterol
12. carbohydrate
13. force fluids
14. full strength
15. percutaneous endoscopic gastrostomy
16. no added salt
17. registered dietitian
18. potassium

Review Questions

1. a. NPO p̄ MN
b. cl liq breakfast, then NPO
c. 1000cal ADA diet
d. low chol diet
e. DAT
f. reg dict
g. low Na diet
h. NSA

2. a. a regular diet with modifications or restrictions
b. a diet that consists of all foods, designed to provide good nutrition
c. administration of liquids into the stomach, duodenum, or jejunum, through a tube
d. patient can not have any thing to eat or drink not even water

3. a. continuous
b. bolus
c. cyclic

4. a. standard
b. therapeutic
c. therapeutic
d. standard
e. therapeutic
f. standard
g. therapeutic
h. therapeutic

5. a. regular
b. soft
c. full liquid
d. clear liquid
(*Note:* Variations such as mechanical soft or pureed may also be ordered for DAT.)

6. The personnel working in the dietary department do not know what the patient could tolerate.

7. a. The patient is scheduled for surgery.
b. The patient is scheduled for a diagnostic procedure, test or examination.

8. Any three of the following:
Isocal HN
Deliver 2.0
Ultracal HN Plus
Jevity
Pulmocare
Boost High Nitrogen
Boost Plus Respalor
Megnacal (*Note:* many more are on the market)

9. No: 2.5 gm Na would be a modification to the soft diet and is not a diet change.

10. No: Limit fluids to 1200 cc/day is a modification to the regular diet and is not a diet change.

11. Yes: All dietary orders need to be sent to the dietary department.

12. The patient's food is prepared by the dietary department and if a patient eats a food that he or she is truly allergic to, it could cause discomfort or in some cases anaphylactic shock

CHAPTER 13

Exercise 1

1. L
2. ASA
3. stat
4. cap
5. tab
6. MOM
7. U
8. OD
9. mg
10. KCL
11. G, gm, or g
12. OU
13. mL
14. mEq
15. pc
16. ung
17. WA
18. N/V
19. gr
20. IM
21. subling or SL
22. tinct or tr
23. PO
24. oz
25. OS
26. amp
27. dr or ℨ
28. supp
29. NTG
30. SC, sq, or sub-q
31. μg or mcg
32. noc
33. syr
34. IVPB
35. ac
36. PCN
37. pr
38. TPN
39. PCA
40. cc
41. IVP
42. LOC
43. MS or MSO₄
44. PRN

Exercise 2

1. potassium chloride
2. oculus sinister (left eye)
3. ampule
4. syrup
5. dram
6. night
7. microgram
8. ounce
9. subcutaneous
10. immediately
11. ante cibum (before meals)
12. millequivalent
13. post cibum (after meals)
14. unguent (ointment)
15. milliliter (same as cc)
16. per os (by mouth)
17. tincture
18. intramuscular
19. grain
20. milligram
21. suppository
22. gram
23. oculus unitas (both eyes)
24. nausea & vomiting
25. while awake
26. nitroglycerin
27. acetylsalicylic acid (aspirin)
28. capsule
29. tablet
30. milk of magnesia
31. liter
32. unit
33. oculus dexter (right eye)
34. sublingual (under tongue)
35. intravenous piggyback
36. penicillin
37. total parenteral nutrition
38. patient-controlled analgesia
39. per rectum
40. cubic centimeter
41. *pro re nata* (as needed)
42. laxative of choice
43. intravenous push
44. morphine sulfate

Exercise 3

1. intramuscular, as needed
2. gram, intravenous piggyback
3. milligram, by mouth,
4. drops, both eyes
5. milligram, sublingual, as needed
6. milk of magnesia, cubic centimeters, as needed
7. units
8. aspirin, milligram, by mouth, per rectum
9. total parenteral nutrition, cubic centimeters
10. before meals

Exercise 4

Answers found by using the *Physicians' Desk Reference*

Exercise 5

1. gr ii
2. 5cc
3. 4 dr
4. 0.5 g
5. gr iss
6. 500 mg
7. gr xv
8. 1 L
9. 1000 g
10. gr 1/6
11. gr 1/150

Exercise 6

1. a. name of the drug
   b. dosage
   c. routes of administration
   d. frequency of administration
   e. qualifying phrase

2.
a.	Compazine	10 mg	IM	stat	
	1	2	3	4	
b.	Ativan	.05 mg	IV	q 6 h prn	anxiety
	1	2	3	4	5
c.	Xanax	.05 mg	po	qid	
	1	2	3	4	
d.	Ambien	5 mg	po	hs prn	
	1	2	3	4	
e.	Lomotil	ī	PO	after each loose stool	
	1	2	3	4	
f.	Percodan tabs	1–2	po	q 4h prn	severe pain
	1	2	3	4	5
g.	Lente insulin	25 U	sq	qd	
	1	2	3	4	
h.	Amoxicillin	500 mg	po	q 8 h	
	1	2	3	4	
i.	Compazine	5 mg	IM	q6 h prn	N/V
	1	2	3	4	5
j.	Tigan supp	200 mg	pr	now	
	1	2	3	4	

Exercise 7

1. Tylenol 500 mg q 4 hr po for pain
2. Ampicillin 250 mg po qid
3. Penicillin 1,600,000 U IM q 12 hr
4. Donnatal elixir 5 mL po 3 tid ac
5. Neo-Synephrine ophthalmic 10% gtts ii OD bid
6. Benadryl 50 mg po stat
7. Equanil 400 mg po bid & hs
8. Coumadin 5 mg po qd

Exercise 8

1. lower blood sugar
2. thin blood—prevent clots from forming in the blood
3. treat a variety of infections; category includes antibiotic, antifungal, and antiviral drugs
4. decrease acid production (digestive system)
5. used to treat cancer
6. to cause relaxation and reduce restlessness without causing sleep
7. used to induce sleep
8. replace or regulate glandular secretions from glands
9. replace potassium
10. to relieve pain
11. assist in drying secretions (respiratory system)
12. to lower cholesterol
13. correct abnormal cardiac beats
14. used to relieve pain caused when the heart muscle does not get enough oxygen and nutrients to meet the demand
15. used to lower blood pressure
16. cause a quick decrease in circulating fluid volume, causing a decrease in pressure demand on the heart
17. used to treat constipation by stimulate a bowel movement, soften the stool for easier passage, or may be a fiber supplement to increase and maintain normal bowel function
18. to treat nausea and vomiting
19. to treat shock and to lower blood pressure

Review Questions

1. a. a medication order that remains in effect and is executed as ordered until the doctor discontinues or changes it
   b. same as a standing medication order, except that it is executed according to the patient's needs
   c. a medication order that is executed immediately, then automatically discontinued
   d. a medication order executed according to the qualifying phrase, then automatically discontinued

e. a medication order executed according to the qualifying phrase, then automatically discontinued

f. a method of infusing a concentrated dose of medication over 1-5 minutes

g. an injection of a medication given directly into a muscle

h. a medication given by mouth

i. a date on which specific categories of medications must be discontinued unless renewed by the doctor

j. a method of administering calories, proteins, vitamins, and other nutrients directly into the bloodstream

k. allows the patient to self-administer small doses of narcotics intravenously. A special IV infusion pump is used

l. pertains to within a vein

m. direct application of medication to the skin, eye, ear, or other parts of the body

n. a route of administration for nutrition that is used for short-term therapy that is usually less than two weeks in length

o. a method of intermittent infusion of medication that has been diluted in 50 – 100 cc of a commercially prepared solution and infused over 30 – 60 minutes through an established IV line

2. a. *Physicians' Desk Reference* (PDR)
   b. *The American Hospital Formulary* (*Note:* nursing drug handbooks are also used)

3. a. name of the drug
   b. dosage
   c. routes of administration
   d. frequency of administration
   e. qualifying phrases

4. a. oral/sublingual
   b. inhalation
   c. topical
   d. parenteral

5. a. Apothecary system
   b. Metric system

6. a. right drug
   b. right dose
   c. right time
   d. right route
   e. right patient

7. a. narcotic
   b. nonnarcotic analgesic
   c. nonnarcotic analgesic
   d. sedative/hypnotic
   e. narcotic
   f. narcotic
   g. analgesic with narcotic
   h. analgesic with narcotic
   i. sedative/hypnotic
   j. antihistamine
   k. antianxiety drug
   l. antidiabetic drug
   m. antibiotic
   n. antibiotic
   o. drug used to treat asthma and related conditions (respiratory)

   p. antianxiety drug
   q. anticonvulsant
   r. antibiotic
   s. anticoagulant
   t. antidysrhythmic (cardiovascular)
   u. potassium replacement
   v. antiemetic
   w. diuretic
   x. antianginal (cardiovascular)
   y. anticoagulant
   z. potassium replacement

8. 1. f
   2. i
   3. d
   4. j
   5. b
   6. h
   7. k
   8. e
   9. g
   10. l
   11. a
   12. c

CHAPTER 14

Exercise 1

1. FBS
2. O & P
3. Hgb
4. ESR
5. K
6. AFB
7. RBC
8. PP
9. CSF
10. Fe
11. C & S
12. T & X-match or T & C
13. CBC
14. PAP
15. GTT
16. PC
17. PT
18. Ua or U/A
19. ALP or alk phos
20. HB_5Ag
21. FS
22. HIV
23. Mg or Mg+

24. HCG
25. WNL
26. PTT or APIT
27. T_3, T_4, T_7
28. TSH
29. S & A
30. Ag
31. BMP
32. CMV
33. PO_2
34. T & S
35. Ab
36. Cx
37. RSV
38. CMP
39. Lytes
40. Bx
41. POCT or PCT
42. PCV
43. RBS or BS
44. VDRL
45. Retics
46. PSA
47. Diff

48. WBC
49. PO_4 or phos
50. TIBC
51. Hct
52. LP
53. Na
54. NP
55. H & H
56. CO_2
57. ANA
58. HDL
59. BUN
60. Ca
61. CC, creat cl, or cr cl
62. Cl
63. CEA
64. T/Stat
65. LDL
66. ADH
67. CPK or CK
68. EBV
69. pH
70. RDW

Exercise 2

1. fasting blood sugar
2. ova and parasites
3. hemoglobin
4. erythrocyte sedimentation rate or sedimentation rate
5. potassium
6. acid-fast bacilli
7. red blood cells
8. postprandial
9. cerebrospinal fluid
10. iron
11. culture and sensitivity
12. type and crossmatch
13. complete blood cell count
14. prostatic acid phosphatase
15. glucose tolerance test
16. packed cells
17. prothrombin time
18. urinalysis
19. alkaline phosphatase
20. hepatitis B surface antigen
21. frozen section
22. human immunodeficiency virus
23. magnesium
24. human chorionic gonadotropin
25. within normal limits
26. partial thromboplastin time or activated partial thromboplastin time
27. thyroid tests
28. thyroid-stimulating hormone
29. sugar and acetone
30. antigen

31. basic metabolic chemistry panel
32. cytomegalovirus
33. partial pressure of oxygen
34. type and screen
35. antibody
36. culture
37. respiratory syncytial virus
38. comprehensive metabolic chemistry panel
39. electrolytes
40. biopsy
41. point-of-care testing
42. packed cell volume
43. random blood sugar or blood sugar
44. Venereal Disease Research Laboratories
45. reticulocytes
46. prostatic specific antigen
47. differential
48. white blood cell count
49. phosphorus
50. total iron-binding capacity
55. hematocrit
52. lumbar puncture
53. sodium
54. nasopharynx
55. hemoglobin and hematocrit
56. carbon dioxide
57. antinuclear antibody
58. high-density lipoproteins
59. blood urea nitrogen
60. calcium
61. creatinine clearance

62. chloride
63. carcinoembryonic antigen
64. timed stat
65. low-density lipoproteins
66. antidiuretic hormone

67. creatine phosphokinase or creatine kinase
68. Epstein-Barr virus
69. hydrogen ion concentration
70. red cell distribution width

Review Questions

1. a. diagnostic
   b. evaluation of treatment prescribed
2. a. Microbiology studies specimens to determine disease causing organisms.
   b. Chemistry performs tests related to chemical reactions occurring in living organisms.
   c. Hematology performs tests related to the physical properties of blood
3. a. voided
   b. clean catch (or midstream)
   c. catheterization
4. a. blood
   b. urine
   c. sputum
   d. stool
   e. spinal fluid
   Note: Other specimens include eye/ear drainage, wound drainage, bone marrow, plural fluid, biopsies, etc.
5. Notify the laboratory by phone or verbally notify the appropriate nursing personnel on the unit. When calling the laboratory, supply the name of the patient, nursing unit, room number, and the test ordered. Enter the order into the computer immediately if the laboratory is going to draw the specimen. The order is entered when the specimen is collected if drawn by nursing personnel on the unit.
6. Ask the nurse to notify you of the time the patient has finished eating and order the blood to be drawn T/Stat 2 hours after the patient finished eating.
7. A stat laboratory order must be done immediately. A routine laboratory order can be performed at the next scheduled laboratory draw or when the nursing personnel can draw the blood.
8. any five of the following:
   lumbar puncture; also called *spinal tap*
   sternal puncture; also called *bone marrow biopsy*
   abdominal paracentesis
   thoracentesis
   amniocentesis
   biopsy of a part of the body
9. Type and cross-match
10. Check to see that specimen is correctly labeled. Call transport or take the specimen yourself as soon as possible. Do not send specimens that were collected by an invasive procedure (cerebral spinal fluid, cavity fluid, biopsies, etc.) by the tube system.
11. a. sodium (Na)
    b. potassium (K)
    c. chlorides (Cl)
    d. carbon dioxide (CO_2)
12. a. CPK or CK
    b. LDH
    c. AST (SGOT)
13. list any six from Appendix F that have "Chemistry" listed in the "Laboratory Division" column
14. list any six from Appendix F that have "Hematology" listed in the "Laboratory Division" column
15. list any six from Appendix F that are marked with an asterisk
16. Fasting means that the patient's breakfast is held until the test is completed. The patient may have water or other non-nutritional drinks. NPO means no food or liquid by mouth.

17. a. a tissue removed from a living body for examination
    b. a method of obtaining a urine specimen
    c. no solid food or nutritional fluids
    d. a procedure to remove cerebral spinal fluid from the spinal cord
    e. a method of obtaining a urine specimen (same as clean catch)
    f. blood that is undetectable to the eye
    g. after eating
    h. a mucus secretion from the lungs
    i. a procedure to remove bone marrow from the sternum
    j. the physical, chemical, and microscopic examination of urine
    k. a specimen obtained by urinating
    l. the visual examination of urine using a special commercially treated stick
18. a. chemistry
    b. microbiology
    c. chemistry
    d. hematology
    e. chemistry
    f. hematology
    g. blood bank
    h. hematology
    i. serology
    j. chemistry
    k. serology
    l. microbiology
    m. hematology
    n. chemistry
    o. chemistry
    p. hematology
    q. hematology
    r. chemistry
    s. hematology
    t. chemistry
    u. blood bank
    v. blood bank
    w. chemistry
    x. microbiology
    y. chemistry
    z. chemistry
19. any three of the following:
    amikacin
    cyclosporine
    digoxin
    Dilantin
    gentamicin
    kanamycin
    tobramycin
    vancomycin
20. Read the laboratory values you have recorded back to the person in the laboratory
21. a. CBC & lytes q am
    b. H & H stat
    c. T & X-match 6 u pc – hold for surgery in am
    d. sputum spec for C & S for AFB
    e. LP for CSF tube #1: prot & glu; Tube #2 Cx for CMV & fungus; Tube #3 AFB stain
    f. CMP in am

CHAPTER 15

Exercise 1

1. IVP (also called IVU)
2. RLQ
3. KUB
4. BE
5. PA
6. UGI
7. lat
8. LS
9. LUQ
10. AP
11. GI
12. RUQ
13. CT
14. LLQ
15. GB
16. MRI
17. SBFT
18. CXR
19. DSA
20. PCXR
21. PTC or PTHC
22. Fx
23. h/o
24. F/U
25. CI
26. IVU (also called IVP)
27. US
28. R/O
29. PET
30. L&S

Exercise 2

1. barium enema
2. lumbosacral
3. kidneys, ureters, and bladder
4. ultrasound
5. right lower quadrant, left upper quadrant
6. intravenous urogram and upper gastrointestinal

7. computed tomography
8. gastrointestinal
9. posteroanterior, lateral
10. magnetic resonance imaging
11. portable chest x-ray
12. upper gastrointestinal (x-ray), small bowel follow through

Review Questions

1. a. posteroanterior
   b. lateral
   c. barium enema
   d. intravenous pyelogram
   e. intravenous urogram
   f. anteroposterior
   g. kidneys, ureters, and bladder
   h. computed tomography
   i. lumbosacral
   j. upper gastrointestinal
   k. gallbladder
   l. right upper quadrand
   m. rule out
   n. magnetic resonance imaging
   o. liver and spleen
   p. small bowel follow-through
   q. ultrasound
   r. left lower quadrant
   s. chest x-ray
   t. digital subtraction angiography
   u. portable chest x-ray
   v. clinical indications
   w. percutaneous transhepatic cholangiography
   x. positron emission tomography
   y. fracture
2. contrast media
3. portable or mobile x-ray
4. fluoroscopy
5. magnetic resonance imaging
6. ultrasonography
7. routine preparation
8. on-call medications
9. a. anteroposterior (AP)
   b. posteroanterior (PA)
   c. lateral (lat)
   d. oblique
   e. decubitus
10. IVU, GB, BE, UGI
11. List may include any of the x-rays found in the list of doctors' or-ders for special x-ray procedures, or you may supply your own list.
12. a. bone scan (total or regional)
    b. gallium scan (total or regional)
    c. lung ventilation/perfusion studies
    d. thyroid uptake and scan
    e. MUGA scan (cardiac)
    f. DISIDA scan (formerly PIPIDA scan)
    g. PET scan
    (*Note:* Your instructor may supply you with the name of addi-tional studies performed in nuclear medicine.)
13.

	Preparation	Consent
a.	no	no
b.	yes	no
c.	no	yes
d.	no	yes
e.	no	no
f.	yes	no
g.	no	yes
h.	no	no
i.	yes	no
j.	no	yes
k.	yes	no
l.	no	no
m.	yes	no
n.	no	yes
o.	no	no

(Some answers may vary among hospitals.)

14. a. x-ray of LS spine, CI:fx
    b. PA and lat CXR, CI: pneumonia
    c. UGI x-ray, and IVU, GB series, and BE CI: abd. mass
    d. Neither the procedure or the clinical indication can be abbreviated
    e. MRI of the rt. shoulder, CI: rotator cuff injury
15. a. is receiving intravenous fluids
    b. has a seizure disorder
    c. is receiving oxygen
    d. needs isolation precautions
    e. does not speak English
    f. is a diabetic
    g. is sight- or hearing-impaired

CHAPTER 16

Exercise 1

1. EEG
2. EKG or ECG
3. EMG
4. RA
5. LOC
6. IPG
7. ABG
8. CBG
9. EchoEG
10. ERCP
11. EGD
12. EPS
13. ICD
14. NCS
15. OSA
16. BAER
17. ENG
18. SEP
19. VEP

Exercise 2

1. arterial blood gases
2. electrocardiogram
3. electroencephalogram
4. electrocardiogram
5. leave on chart
6. electromyogram
7. room air
8. impedance plethysmography
9. echoencephalogram
10. esophagogastroduodenoscopy
11. endoscopic retrograde cholangiopancreatography
12. electrophysiological study
13. implantable cardiac defibrillator
14. capillary blood gases
15. nerve conduction studies
16. obstructive sleep apnea
17. brainstem auditory evoked response
18. electronystagmography
19. somatosensory evoked potential
20. visual evoked potential

Review Questions

1. a. electromyogram
   b. electrocardiogram
   c. arterial blood gases, room air
   d. electrocardiogram, leave on chart
   e. electroencephalogram
   f. capillary blood gases
2. any two of the following:
   EKG or ECG
   echocardiogram
   transesophageal electrocardiogram
   cardiac or Holter monitor
   exercise electrocardiogram

3. any two of the following:
   cardiac catheterization
   Swan-Ganz catheter insertion
   Thallium, Sestamibi, and Persantine/sestamibi stress tests
4. any four of the following:
   nitroglycerin
   quinidine
   lidocaine
   Lanoxin or digoxin (there are more)
5. a. pacemaker
   b. implantable cardioverter defibrillator (ICD)
6. Any six of the following

Procedure	Organ(s) studied
anoscopy	anal canal
bronchoscopy	bronchi
colonoscopy	large intestines
cholangiopancreatography (ERCP)	biliary and pancreatic ducts
esophagogastroduodenoscopy (EGD)	gastrointestinal tract
proctoscopy	rectum
sigmoidoscopy	sigmoid colon

7. a. performs studies to assess a patient's sleep patterns to determine nature and severity of insomnia, reveal presence of obstructive sleep apnea and severity of condition and to assist in the diagnosis of narcolepsy.
   b. performs diagnostic tests to determine lung function and also performs treatments to treat respiratory disease and conditions.
   c. may include several tests related to the function of the nervous system (brain and spinal cord)
   d. carry out procedures related to the performance of the heart and the vascular system
8. a. Lovenox
   b. heparin
   c. Coumadin (warfarin) (there are more)
9. a. a diagnostic study related to the gastrointestinal system
   b. a cardiac study that demonstrates the waveform produced by electric impulses from one lead
   c. a catheter coated with a substance that does not allow the passage of x-rays, thus allowing the movement of the catheter to be followed on the viewing screen
   d. a portable device that records the heart's electrical activity and produces a continuous ECG tracing over a specified time
10. any four of the following:
    gastric analysis
    Hollander test for vagotomy
    esophageal manometry/motility and reflux
    biliary drainage
    secretin test
    lactose tolerance test
    qualitative fecal fat
11. 1. c   7. a   13. b
    2. d   8. a   14. a
    3. d   9. a   15. a
    4. b   10. a   16. b
    5. c   11. d   17. c
    6. b   12. a   18. a
12. a. IPG this a.m.
    b. EKG (or ECG) now
    c. ERCP tomorrow a.m.
    d. ABG on O_2 @ 2L/M

CHAPTER 17

Exercise 1

1. LUL
2. OT
3. PT
4. L/Min
5. O_2
6. IPPB
7. RUL
8. ROM
9. RLL
10. ADL
11. EMG
12. RML
13. USN
14. SVN
15. LLL
16. lbs #
17. NWB
18. WP
19. HP
20. TENS
21. EPC
22. ES
23. CPM
24. IS
25. MDI
26. CPT
27. AA
28. BiW
29. AKA
30. STM
31. LE
32. HD
33. THR, THA
34. ORIF
35. Tx
36. TT
37. ISOM
38. BKA
39. ET
40. HA
41. PEP
42. P & PD
43. SaO or O_2 Sats
44. UD
45. >
46. TKR, TKA
47. <
48. CP
49. CPR
50. HBOT
51. BiPAP
52. CPAP
53. BUE
54. BLE
55. RUE
56. LUE
57. RLE
58. LLE
59. PTA
60. RT
61. PROM
62. WBAT
63. FWW

Exercise 2

1. oxygen
2. left upper lobe
3. right lower lobe
4. occupational therapy or occupational therapist
5. physical therapy or physical therapy
6. electromyogram
7. activities of daily living
8. pounds
9. right upper lobe
10. right middle lobe
11. non weight bearing
12. range of motion
13. liters per minute
14. small volume nebulizer
15. left lower lobe
16. intermittent positive pressure breathing
17. ultrasonic nebulizer
18. hot packs
19. whirlpool
20. continuous passive motion
21. electrical stimulation
22. electronic pain control
23. transcutaneous electrical nerve stimulation
24. incentive spirometry
25. chest physiotherapy
26. metered dose inhaler
27. open reduction, internal fixation
28. tilt table
29. oxygen saturation
30. above the knee amputation
31. unit dose
32. heated aerosol
33. isometric
34. lower extremities
35. soft tissue massage
36. hemodialysis
37. traction
38. percussion and postural drainage
39. greater than
40. total knee replacement/arthroplasty
41. total hip replacement/arthroplasty
42. endotracheal tube
43. peritoneal dialysis
44. less than
45. twice a week
46. positive expiratory pressure
47. cold packs
48. active assisted
49. cardiopulmonary resuscitation
50. hyperbaric oxygen therapy
51. bi-level positive airway pressure
52. continuous positive airway pressure
53. both upper extremities
54. both lower extremities
55. right upper extremity
56. left upper extremity
57. right lower extremity
58. left lower extremity
59. physical therapist assistant
60. respiratory therapist
61. passive range of motion
62. weight bearing as tolerated
63. front wheel walker

Review Questions

1. a. The respiratory department performs treatments ordered by the doctor that are related to the respiratory system. Diagnostic tests performed by the respiratory department are discussed in Chapter 16.
   b. Physical therapy is the division within the hospital that treats patients to improve and restore their functional mobility by methods such as gait training, exercise, water therapy, and heat and ice treatments.
   c. Occupational therapy is the department within the hospital that works toward rehabilitation of patients, in conjunction with other health team members, to return the patient to the greatest possible independence.
2. a. skeletal
   b. skin
3. a. aligns the ends of a fracture by pulling the limb into a straight position
   b. controls muscle spasm
   c. relieves pain
   d. takes the pressure off the bone ends by relaxing the muscle.
4. The overhead frame and trapeze are used by the patient for assistance in moving while in bed.
5. a. respiratory care
   b. nursing
   c. respiratory care
   d. physical therapy
   e. respiratory care
   f. respiratory care
   g. respiratory care
   h. occupational therapy
   i. nursing
   j. nursing
   k. physical therapy
   l. nursing
   m. physical therapy
   n. physical therapy
   o. respiratory care
   p. physical therapy
   q. respiratory care
6. the removal of wastes in the blood usually excreted by the kidneys
7. a. hemodialysis
   b. peritoneal dialysis

CHAPTER 18

Exercise 1

1. appt
2. disch
3. DME
4. do not resuscitate
5. wk
6. Rx
7. NINP

Exercise 2

1. appointment
2. discharge
3. durable medical equipment
4. do not resuscitate
5. week
6. take (treatment, medication, etc.)
7. no information, no publication

Review Questions

1. a. a doctor's order requesting that a patient be transferred to another hospital room, unit or facility
   b. a doctor's order stating that the patient may leave the hospital
   c. a request by the patient's attending physician for the opinion of a second physician with respect to diagnosis and treatment of the patient
2. a. hospital name
   b. patient's name and age
   c. patient's location (unit and room number)
   d. name of the doctor requesting the consultation
   e. patient's diagnosis

f. urgency of consultation and any additional information provided in the order
g. patient's insurance information located on the patient's face sheet
3. a. a different type of room accommodation (e.g., a private room) is desired
   b. more intense nursing care (regular unit to ICU) or less intense nursing care (ICU to regular unit) is called for
   c. the patient's condition requires that he or she be placed in an isolation room
4. a. arrange with the pharmacy for medications the patient is taking
   b. note on the census when the patient leaves and returns
   c. cancel meals for the length of the absence
   d. cancel any hospital treatments for the length of the absence
   e. arrange for any special equipment that the patient may need
   f. provide the nurse with a temporary absence release to have the patient sign
5. any two of the following
   access and prioritize the patient's needs
   identify and coordinate available resources
   arrange for home care
   arrange admission to a long-term care facility
   arrange for hospice care
6. social services
7. a. financial assistance for patients
   b. transportation home
   c. arrangement of meals for families staying at hospital or for patients for home after discharge
   d. support for abuse victims (call protective services if necessary)
   e. assistance in planning custodial care
   f. arrangement of home-bound teacher or in hospital teacher
   g. evaluation of home care providers
   h. arrangement of living assistance for families of patients when necessary
8. No: DNR must be a written doctor's order to be legal.

CHAPTER 19

Exercise 1

1. H & P
2. MSSU
3. post-op
4. OBS
5. DX
6. HX
7. NKA
8. pre-op
9. OPS
10. SSU

Exercise 2

1. outpatient surgery
2. before surgery
3. no known allergies
4. history
5. diagnosis
6. observation
7. after surgery
8. medical short stay unit
9. history and physical
10. short stay unit

Review Questions

1. 1. c
   2. d
   3. a
   4. b
   5. e
2. a. the number assigned to the patient on or prior to admission; used for records identification and used for all subsequent admissions to that hospital
   b. plastic band with a patient identification label affixed to it; worn by the patient throughout his or her hospitalization.

c. checklist used to ensure that the chart and the patients are properly prepared for surgery.
d. list of all the surgeries to be performed on a particular day; the schedule may be printed from the computer or sent to the nursing unit by the admitting department.
e. a number assigned to the patient to access insurance information; usually a unique number is assigned each time the patient is admitted to the hospital.
f. container for storing the patient's jewelry, money, and other valuables, which are placed in the hospital safe for safekeeping.
g. orders written by the doctor before surgery to prepare the patient for the surgical procedure.
h. orders written immediately after surgery. Postoperative orders cancel preoperative orders.
i. information obtained from the patient concerning his or her sensitivity to medications and/or food.
j. a form initiated in the admitting department that is included in the inpatient medical record containing personal and demographic information, usually computer generated at the time of admission (may also be called the information sheet).
k. a checklist used by the health unit coordinator to ensure that the patient's chart is ready for surgery.
l. surgery that is not emergency or mandatory and can be planned at a time of convenience.
m. plastic band with a cardboard insert on which allergy information is printed, or a red plastic band that has allergy information written directly on it; worn by the patient throughout the hospitalization.
n. the process of obtaining information and partially preparing admitting forms prior to the patient's arrival at the health care facility.
o. the process of entering personal information into the hospital information system to enroll a person as a hospital patient and create a patient record; patients may be registered as inpatients, outpatients, or observation patients.

3. any six of the following:
admitting diagnosis
diet
activity
diagnostic orders
medications—usually medications are needed for the patient's disease condition, for sleeping, and/or for pain
treatment orders
request for old records
patient care category or code status (*Note:* The patient care category or code status may be indicated on the patient's admission orders, and refers to the patient's wishes regarding resuscitation. Code status may be written as *full code, modified support,* or *do not resuscitate.* The physician must follow any state-specific statute and the hospital's policies and procedures before writing a DNR order.

4. a. admission service agreement
b. face or front sheet
c. patient identification bracelet
(Advanced directives may or may not be sent to the unit by the registration staff)

5. (See Procedure 19–1, page 378)
6. (See Procedure 19–2, page 381)
7. any five of the following:
current history and physical record (H&P)
surgery consent
blood transfusion consent or refusal
admission service agreement
nursing preoperative checklist
MAR
diagnostic test results

8. a. name of surgery for surgery consent
b. enemas
c. shaves, scrubs, or showers
d. name of anesthesiologist or anesthesiology group
e. miscellaneous orders
f. diet
g. preoperative medications
9. a. diet
b. intake and output
c. intravenous fluids
d. vital signs
e. catheters, tubes, and drains
f. activity
g. positioning
h. observation of the operative site
i. medications
10. (See Procedure 19–3, page 391)
11. documents that intend to indicate a patient's wishes in the event that the patient becomes incapacitated.
12. Any eight of the following:
copy insurance cards.
verify insurance (may be done in advance when admission is scheduled).
ask patient or patient guardian to sign appropriate insurance forms.
interview patient or family to obtain personal information.
prepare admission forms (condition of admission agreement and facesheet) and obtain signatures.
ask patient if he or she has advanced directives or would they like to create one. (Required in most States).
prepare patient's identification bracelet.
enter information into computer for patient identification labels
secure patient valuables if necessary. (may be done on nursing unit by admitting nurse)
supply and explain required information including a copy of the Patient's Bill of Rights
include any test results, prewritten orders or consents that have been previously sent to the admitting department in the packet that accompanies the patient to the nursing unit
13. A *living will* is a declaration made by the patient to family, medical staff, and all concerned with the patient's care stating what is to be done in the event of a terminal illness; it directs the withholding or withdrawing of life-sustaining procedures. A *power of attorney* for health care is when the patient appoints a person (called a proxy or agent) to make health care decisions should the patient be unable to do so.
14. An advanced directive becomes effective when the patient becomes incapacitated.

CHAPTER 20

Exercise 1

1. AMA
2. ECF

Exercise 2

1. against medical advice
2. extended care facility

Review Questions

1. (See Procedure 20–1, pages 396–397)
2. Ask the patient to be seated until his or her nurse is advised.

3. (See Procedure 20–1, Task #14, page 397)
4. (See Procedure 20–2, page 401)
5. (See Procedure 20–3, page 401)
6. a. an illness ending in death
   b. a death
   c. after death
   d. care and services of a nonmedical nature that consist of feeding, bathing, watching and protecting the patient
   e. an examination of the body after death
   f. donating one's organs and/or tissues after death
   g. a signed consent authorizing a specific funeral home to remove a deceased patient's body from a health care facility
   h. a death that occurs due to sudden , violent or unexplained circumstances
   i. a medical facility caring for patients requiring some expert care or custodial care
   j. a meeting that will include the physician or physicians caring for the patient, the primary nurses, the case manager or social worker and other care givers involved with the patient's care
   k. centralized, coordinated, multidisciplinary process that ensures that the patient has a plan for continuing care after leaving the hospital.
7. (See Procedure 20–4, page 407)
8. (See Procedure 20–6, page 410)
9. (See Procedure 20–5, page 410)
10. (See Procedure 20–7, page 411)

CHAPTER 21

Review Questions

1. The vital signs should be recorded as soon as they are all written on the TPR sheet so that they are available to the doctor when he or she makes hospital rounds.
2. The doctor may use vital signs data to prescribe treatment for the patient.
3. Write "mistaken entry" on the incorrect connecting line, then graph the correct value.
4. Recopy the entire record showing the correct data – draw a diagonal line through the old record in ink and write "mistaken entry" on the line. Write recopied in ink with your name, status and the date on both the old record and the recopied record.
5. The original would be placed behind the recopied record under the graphic divider in the chart; it remains a permanent part of the patient's chart.
6. a. 37.0°
   b. 38.5°
   c. 37.6°
   d. 35.9°
7. a. 100.8°
   b. 103.1°
   c. 97.5°
   d. 100.0°
8. a. to have the records available for the attending physician and other health care personnel
   b. to assist the health records department in assembling all patient records for storage
9. a. file at the same time each day.
   b. separate the records according to the patient's name so that you need obtain and open the chart binder only once.
   c. always check the patient's name on the chart back with the name on the record before filing it.
   d. place the record behind the correct chart divider.
   e. initial all records you file.

10. a. purchasing department: nonnursing items, such as pens and pencils
    b. central service department: items used for nursing procedures, such a catheterization tray
    c. pharmacy: all medications
    d. dietary department: food items, such as milk and crackers
    e. laundry department
11. a. the difference between the radial pulse and the apical heartbeat
    b. a scale used to measure temperature in which the freezing point of water is 0° and the boiling point is 100°
    c. the body wastes from the digestive tract that are discharged from the body through the anus
    d. a scale used to measure temperature in which 32° is the freezing point of water and 212° is the boiling point
12. a. bowel movement
    b. temperature, pulse, respiration
    c. Celsius
    d. Fahrenheit
    e. postpartum
    f. postoperative day

CHAPTER 22

Review Questions

1. a. acquired immunodeficiency syndrome
   b. AIDS related complex
   c. Centers for Disease Control and Prevention
   d. hepatitis B virus
   e. human immunodeficiency virus
   f. Occupational Safety and Health Administration
   g. personal protective equipment
   h. tuberculosis
   i. *Rescue* individuals in danger; *Alarm:* sound the alarm; *Confine* the fire by closing all doors and windows; *Extinguish* the fire with the nearest suitable fire extinguisher
2. a. accidents
   b. thefts from persons on hospital property
   c. errors of omission of patient treatment or errors of administration of patient treatment
   d. exposure to blood and body fluids such as caused by a needle-stick
3. The health unit coordinator may be expected to assist with the evacuation of patients who are endangered by the fire. If the fire is not on the unit, the health unit coordinator may help the nursing personnel to close the doors to the patient rooms.
4. a. avoid the use of extension cords
   b. do not overload electrical circuits
   c. inspect cords and plugs for breaks and fraying
   d. unplug equipment when servicing
   e. unplug equipment that has liquid spilled in it
   f. unplug and do not use equipment that is malfunctioning
5. a. *Streptococcus*
   b. *Staphylococcus*
   c. *Pseudomonas*
6. a. division of the U.S. Public Health Service that investigates and controls diseases that have epidemic potential
   b. a precautionary measure taken to prevent a patient with low resistance to disease from becoming infected
   c. when the patient ceases to breathe or when respirations are so depressed that the blood cannot receive sufficient oxygen and therefore the body cells die (may also be referred to as *code arrest*)
   d. another term for isolation
   e. disease-carrying organisms too small to be seen with the naked eye

f. an emergency that is life-threatening

g. the placement of a patient apart from other patients insofar as movement and social contact are concerned, for the purpose of preventing the spread of infection

h. an episode that does not normally occur within the regular hospital routine

i. a disease that may be transmitted from one person to another

j. a basic hazard communication tool wich gives details on chemical dangers and safety procedures.

k. the patient's heart contractions are absent or insufficient to produce a pulse or blood pressure (may also be referred to as *code arrest*)

l. a planned procedure that is carried out by hospital personnel when a large number of persons have been injured

m. infections that are acquired from within the health care facility

n. the creation of a barrier between the health care worker and the patient's blood and body fluids (may also be called universe precautions).

o. a department in the hospital that addresses the prevention and containment of liability regarding patient care incidents.

p. required use of mask and ventilated room, in conjunction with standard precautions.

7. a. notify the hospital telephone operator to announce the code

b. direct the code arrest team to the patient's room

c. remove the patient information sheet from the patients chart and take or send the chart to the patient's room.

d. notify all physicians connected with the patients case when requested to do so by nurse or doctor

e. notify the patient's family of the situation if requested to do so

f. label any laboratory specimens with the patient's ID label, enter the test ordered in the computer and send the specimen to the laboratory stat.

g. call the appropriate departments for treatments and supplies as needed

h. alert the admissions department and the ICU for possibility of transfer to ICU.

i. for a successful code, follow the procedure for a transfer to another unit; for an unsuccessful code procedure, follow the procedure for postmortem care.

8. The health unit coordinator should wear gloves and wash hands after handling specimens (even when bagged).

9. For statistical purposes, records must be kept of infectious diseases; infection control is essential to provide a safe environment for both patients and health care workers.

10. a. infectious agent or pathogen (bacteria)

b. a reservoir or source for pathogen to live and grow (human body, contaminated water or food, animals, insects, etc)

c. means of escape (blood, urine, feces, wound drainage, etc)

d. route of transmission (direct contact, airborne)

e. entry way (mouth, nostrils, and breaks in the skin)

f. susceptible host (individual who does not have adequate resistance to the invading pathogen).

11. a. air

b. personal contact

c. body excretions

12. a. organ transplant recipients

b. burn victims

c. patients receiving chemotherapy

13. a. gloves

b. gowns

c. goggles

d. masks

14. an infection in which the infecting organisms take advantage of the patient's weakened immune system

15. a. pneumocystis carinii pneumonia (PCP)

b. Kaposi's sarcoma (KS)

16. a. Mail is checked and the patient's room and bed numbers are written on each envelope. If patient has been discharged, write, "discharged" in pencil on the envelope and send back to mail room. Deliver when able or designate to a hospital volunteer.

b. Sign the receipt slip for flowers only if the patient is still in the hospital and can receive flowers. Send back or give flowers to family if the patient has been discharged or cannot receive them. Pediatric patients cannot receive rubber balloons and they would need to be sent back or given to family members.

CHAPTER 23

UNIT 1

Exercise 1

1. WR   CV   S
   cyt / o / logy

2. WR   S
   gastr / ectomy

3. P   WR   S
   sub / hepat / ic

4. WR   CV   WR   CV   S
   electr / o / cardi / o / gram

5. WR   CV   S
   cardi / o / logy

6. P   WR   S
   trans / hepat / ic

Exercise 2

1. cardiology
2. cytology
3. gastrectomy
4. gastroenteritis
5. gastric
6. intragastric
7. nephrectomy

Review Questions

1. a. languages past and present: Greek (e.g., *nephrology*), Latin (e.g., *maternal*), and modern languages, such as *lavage* from the French.

b. eponyms – generally named after discoverer, e.g. *Pap smear*

c. acronyms – words formed from first letter of a descriptive phrase, e.g., *laser*

2. a. word root: the basic part of a word (*Example:* gastr/ic)

b. prefix: the part of the word placed *before* the word root to alter its meaning (*Example:* intra/gastric)

c. suffix: the part of the word added at the *end* of the word to alter its meaning (*Example:* gastr/ic)

d. combining vowel: usually an *o* used between word roots or between a word root and a suffix (*Example:* gastr/o/enteritis)

3. a. A combining vowel is *not used* when connecting a prefix and word root.

b. When connecting *two word roots*, the combining vowel is usually *used* even if the second root begins with a vowel.

c. When connecting a *word root* to a *suffix*, a combining vowel is usually *not used* if the suffix begins with a *vowel*.

4. a. dividing medical terms into word parts and identifying each word part

b. when given a definition of a medical condition, using word parts to build corresponding medical terms.

Unit 2
Review Questions

1. a. the basic unit of all living things
   b. a group of similar cells that work together to perform particular functions
   c. made up of two or more tissue types to perform one or more common functions
   d. a group of organs working together in a common purpose to perform complex body functions
2. a. epithelial
   b. connective
   c. muscle
   d. nerve
3. a. cranial—brain
   b. thoracic—heart
   c. abdominal—stomach
   d. pelvic—bladder
   e. spinal—spinal cord
   (*Note:* Other organs may be correct answers.)
4. 1. e   6. b   11. l
   2. d   7. g   12. j
   3. h   8. f   13. n
   4. c   9. k   14. m
   5. a   10. i
5. a. protects the underlying tissues
   b. assists in regulating body temperature
   c. passes messages of pain, cold, and touch to the brain
   d. synthesis of Vitamin K
6. epidermis / dermis / subcutaneous (or hypodermis)
7. melanin / albinism
8. oil (sebaceous)
9. sweat glands (sudoriferous)
10. cell membrane—keeps the cell intact and is selectively porous; cytoplasm—main body of the cells and cell activities take place here; nucleus—control center and plays an important role in reproduction
11. 1. b   4. f   7. h
    2. a or h   5. d   8. g
    3. e   6. c

Exercise 1

1. internal organs   7. disease   12. cancer
2. skin   8. cancer   13. skin
3. cell   9. connective tissue, flesh   14. cancer
4. tissue   15. nail
5. skin   10. epithelium
6. hair   11. fat

Exercise 2

1. pertaining to
2. study of
3. one who specializes in the diagnosis and treatment of (specialist, physician)
4. resembling
5. inflammation
6. tumor
7. producing, originating, causing
8. through, across, beyond
9. pertaining to
10. under or below

Exercise 3

1. WR   cyt/o
2. WR   derm/o, dermat/o, cutane/o
3. S   -logist
4. S   -oid
5. WR   viscer/o
6. WR   hist/o
7. S   -al
8. S   -logy
9. P   trans-
10. WR   carcin/o, cancer/o. onc/o
11. P   sub-

Exercise 4

1. WR CV S
   cyt / o / logy   study of cells
2. WR S
   trich / oid   resembling hair
3. WR CV S
   path / o / logy   study of (body changes caused by) disease
4. WR CV S
   path / o / genic   producing disease
5. WR S
   dem / al   pertaining to skin
6. WR S
   cyt / oid   resembling a cell
7. WR S
   viscer / al   pertaining to internal organs
8. WR CV S
   hist / o / logy   study of tissue
9. WR CV S
   dermat / o / logist   one who specializes in the diagnosis and treatment of skin (diseases)
10. WR S
    dermat / itis   inflammation of the skin
11. WR CV S
    carcin / o / genic   producing cancer
12. WR S
    epitheli / al   pertaining to epithelium
13. WR S
    carcin / oma   cancerous tumor
14. WR S
    epitheli / oma   tumor composed of epithelial (cells)
15. WR S
    sarc / oma   tumor composed of connective tissue
16. WR S
    lip / oma   tumor (containing) fat
17. WR CV S
    path / o / logist   one who specializes in the diagnosis and treatment of disease
18. WR S
    dermat / oid   resembling skin
19. WR CV S
    dermat / o / logy   study of skin (branch of medicine that deals with skin diseases)
20. P WR S
    trans / derm / al   pertaining to (entering) through the skin

21. WR CV S
   onc / o / logy   study of cancer
22. P   WR   S
   sub / ungu / al   pertaining to under the nail
23. P   WR   S
   sub / cutane / ous   pertaining to under the skin

Exercise 5

1. cytoid
2. trichoid
3. a. dermoid
   b. dermatoid
4. pathologist
5. dermatologist
6. a. dermal
   b. cutaneous
7. visceral
8. histology
9. pathology
10. dermatology
11. pathogenic
12. cytology
13. dermatitis
14. lipoma
15. epithelioma
16. epithelial
17. carcinogenic
18. sarcoma
19. carcinoma
20. a. transdermal
    b. transcuta-
       neous
21. oncology
22. subungual
23. subcutaneous

Exercise 6

Spelling exercise

UNIT 3

Review Questions

1. a. protects the internal organs
   b. provides the framework for the body
   c. acts with muscles to produce movement
   d. produces blood cells
   e. stores calcium and phosphorus
2. periosteum
3. cranium (8 bones).
   a. frontal, 1
   b. parietal, 2
   c. temporal, 2
   d. ethmoid, 1
   e. sphenoid, 1
   f. occipital, 1

   face (14 bones):
   a. maxilla, 2
   b. mandible, 1
   c. nasal, 2
   d. lacrimal, 2
   e. zygomatic, 2
   f. vomer, 1
   g. inferior nasal concha (2)
   h. palatine (2)

4. hyoid (1 bone)
5. a. malleus(2)
   b. incus (2)
   c. stapes (2)
6. a. cervical (7)
   b. thoracic (12)
   c. lumbar (5)
   d. sacrum (1)
   e. coccyx (1)
7. a. scapula
   b. clavicle
   c. humerus
   d. radius
   e. ulna
   f. carpals
   g. metacarpals
   h. phalanges
8. a. ilium
   b. ischium
   c. pubis
9. a. femur
   b. patella
   c. tibia
   d. fibula
   e. tarsal
   f. metatarsal
   g. phalanges
10. a. skeletal muscles / biceps (voluntary)
    b. cardiac / heart (involuntary)
    c. smooth / stomach (involuntary)

11. a. a place on the skeleton where two or more bones meet
    b. attaches muscles to bones
    c. tough band of tissues that connect bone to bone at a joint
12. a. osteoarthritis
    b. rheumatoid arthritis
13. a. laminectomy
    b. diskectomy
14. a. broken bone, no open wound
    b. broken bone, open wound
    c. bone has been twisted apart
    d. bone is splintered or crushed
    e. bone is partially bent and partially broken
    f. occurs when the vertebra collapse by trauma or pathology
15. total (name of joint) arthroplasty
16. osteoclasts / osteoblasts
17. a. headaches
    b. ringing in the ears
    c. hearing loss
    d. dizziness
18. osteoporosis
19. Any of the following:
    calcium supplements and Vitamin D
    weight bearing exercise
    hormonal replacement therapy (if appropriate)
    correct posture
    drugs to slow down the dissolving process of the osteoclasts

Exercise 1

Note: Not all of the combining forms will be labeled on the diagram.

3. clavic/o
4. clavicul/o
5. cost/o
6. crani/o
7. femor/o
8. humer/o
12. patell/o
13. phalang/o
14. scapul/o
15. stern/o
16. vertebr/o

Exercise 2

1. joint
2. bone
3. rib
4. skull
5. femur
6. muscle
7. humerus
8. patella
9. sternum
10. clavicle
11. scapula
12. phalange
13. vertebra(e)
14. clavicle
15. electrical activity, electricity
16. lamina
17. cartilage
18. meniscus

Exercise 3

1. phalang/o
2. arthr/o
3. oste/o
4. femor/o
5. patell/o
6. scapul/o
7. vertebr/o
8. a. clavic/o
   b. clavicul/o
9. crani/o
10. stern/o
11. humer/o
12. cost/o
13. my/o
14. lamin/o
15. chondr/o
16. menisc/o

Exercise 4

1. -plasty
2. -algia
3. a. -ar
   b. -ic
   c. -al
   d. -ous
4. -tomy
5. -ectomy
6. -graph
7. -graphy
8. -gram
9. -trophy
10. -osis
11. -scope
12. -scopy
13. -centesis

Exercise 5

1. pain
2. instrument to record
3. record, x-ray image
4. process of recording, x-ray imaging
5. surgical incision or to cut into
6. development, nourishment
7. pertaining to
8. surgical repair
9. surgical removal
10. pertaining to
11. abnormal condition
12. visual examination
13. instrument used for visual examination
14. surgical puncture to aspirate fluid

Exercise 6

1. intra-
2. dys-
3. sub-
4. a. a-
   b. an-
5. inter-
6. supra-

Exercise 7

1. within
2. above
3. below
4. difficult, painful, labored, abnormal
5. without
6. between

Exercise 8

1. WR   CV   WR   CV   S
    electr / o / my / o / gram   record of electrical activity of muscle

2. WR   S
    my / oma   a tumor (formed of) muscle (tissue)

3. WR   CV   WR   S
    stern / o / clavicul / ar   pertaining to the sternum and clavicle

4. WR   S
    crani / al   pertaining to the cranium

5. WR   CV   WR   S
    vertebr / o / cost / al   pertaining to the vertebrae and ribs

6. WR   S
    arthr / itis   inflammation of a joint

7. P   WR   S
    inter / vertebr / al   pertaining to between the vertebrae

8. WR   S
    humer / al   pertaining to the humerus

9. P   S/WR
    dys / trophy   abnormal development

10. P   WR   S
    sub / scapul / ar   pertaining to below the scapula

11. WR   S
    arthr / osis   abnormal condition of a joint

12. WR   CV   WR   CV   S
    electr / o / my / o / graphy   process of recording the electrical activity of muscle

13. WR   CV   S
    arthr / o / gram   x-ray image of a joint

14. WR   CV   WR   CV   S
    electr / o / my / o / graph   instrument to record the electrical activity of muscle

15. WR   CV   WR   S
    stern / o / cost / al   pertaining to the sternum and ribs

16. WR   S
    arthr / algia   pain in a joint

17. P   WR   S
    sub / cost / al   pertaining to below a rib (or ribs)

18. WR   S
    femor / al   pertaining to the femur

19. WR   CV   S
    clavic / o / tomy   surgical incision into the clavicle

20. WR   CV   S
    arthr / o / tomy   surgical incision of a joint

21. P   WR   S
    intra / crani / al   pertaining to within the cranium

22. P   WR
    a / trophy   without development (or decrease in size of a normally developed organ)

23. WR   CV   S
    arthr / o / plasty   surgical repair of a joint

24. WR   S
    oste / oma   tumor (composed of) bone

25. WR   S
    cost / ectomy   excision of a rib

26. WR   CV   S
    crani / o / plasty   surgical repair of the cranium

27. WR   S
    patell / ectomy   excision of the patella

28. WR   S
    vertebr / ectomy   excision of a vertebra

29. WR   CV   S
    crani / o / tomy   surgical incision into the cranium

30. P   WR   S
    supra / scapul / ar   pertaining to above the scapula

31. WR   S
    stern / oid   resembling the sternum

32. WR   CV   S
    chondr / o / genic   producing cartilage

33. WR   CV   S
    arthr / o / scopy   visual examination of the inside of a joint

34. WR   S
    chondr / itis   inflammation of the cartilage

35. WR   CV   S
    arthr / o / scope   instrument used to visualize a joint

36. WR   S
    chondr / ectomy   excision of cartilage

37. WR   S
    lamin / ectomy   excision of the lamina

38. WR   S
    stern / al   pertaining to the sternum

39. WR   S
    menisc / ectomy   excision of the meniscus

40. WR CV S
    arthr / o / centesis   surgical puncture to aspirate fluid from a joint

41. WR S
    menisc / itis   inflammation of the meniscus

Exercise 9

1. cranial
2. sternoid
3. subscapular
4. femoral
5. arthrotomy
6. chondrectomy
7. arthralgia
8. arthritis
9. arthrosis
10. humeral
11. atrophy
12. vertebrocostal
13. craniotomy
14. costectomy
15. subcostal
16. arthrogram
17. vertebrectomy
18. electromyogram
19. clavicotomy
20. electromyography
21. dystrophy
22. myoma
23. electromyograph
24. sternoclavicular
25. intervertebral
26. intracranial
27. sternocostal
28. patellectomy
29. cranioplasty
30. osteoma
31. clavicotomy
32. chondrogenic
33. arthroscopy
34. arthroscope
35. chondritis
36. chondrectomy
37. laminectomy
38. sternal
39. arthrocentesis
40. meniscectomy
41. meniscitis

Exercise 10

1. branch of medicine dealing with the diagnosis and treatment of diseases, fractures, or abnormalities of the musculoskeletal system
2. doctor specializing in orthopedics
3. progressive, crippling disease of the muscles
4. insertion of a hollow needle into the sternum to obtain bone marrow sample for laboratory study

Exercise 11

Spelling exercise

Exercise 12

1. orthopedics / orthopedist
2. sternal puncture
3. electromyography
4. a. lower inner leg bone
   b. upper arm bone
   c. neck bone
   d. pelvic bone
   e. collar bone
   f. arm bone, thumb side
5. a. costectomy
   b. (correct)
   c. laminectomy
   d. clavicotomy
   e. (correct)
   f. patellectomy
   g. osteoarthrotomy
   h. (correct)
6. arthrogram / arthrocentesis

UNIT 4
Review Questions

1. a. nerves: transmit impulses from one part of the body to another
   b. brain: the main center for coordinating body activity
   c. spinal cord: the pathway for conducting sensory impulses to the brain and motor impulses down from the brain
2. neuron / sensory / motor
3. a. cerebrum: contains sensory, motor, sight, and hearing centers; memory, judgment, and emotional reactions also take place in the cerebrum
   b. cerebellum: assists in coordination of voluntary muscles and maintains balance
   c. brain stem: contains the control centers for blood pressure, respiration, and heartbeat
4. Extends from the brain stem passing through the spinal cavity to between the first and second lumbar vertebrae. It is the pathway for conducting sensory and motor impulses to and from the brain.
5. dura mater / arachnoid / pia mater
6. 1. a
   2. f
   3. d
   4. c
   5. b
7. a. preictal
   b. interictal
   c. postictal

Exercise 1

Note: Not all of the combining forms will be labeled on the diagram.

1. cerebell/o
2. cerebr/o
3. encephal/o
4. mening/o
5. myel/o
6. neur/o

Exercise 2

1. cerebrum
2. brain
3. nerve
4. gray matter
5. meninges
6. spine
7. spinal cord or bone marrow
8. cerebellum
9. air
10. speech
11. mind

Exercise 3

1. neur/o
2. cerebr/o
3. mening/o
4. myel/o
5. cerebell/o
6. encephal/o
7. spin/o
8. pneum/o
9. poli/o
10. phas/o
11. psych/o

Exercise 4

1. -oma
2. -plasty
3. -ar, -al, -ic, -ous
4. -rrhaphy
5. -rrhea
6. -itis
7. -logist
8. -gram
9. -logy
10. -rrhagia
11. -cele
12. -ectomy
13. -tomy
14. -algia

Exercise 5

1. record, x-ray image
2. inflammation
3. the study of
4. discharge
5. rapid discharge
6. to suture
7. herniation, protrusion
8. pertaining to
9. surgical removal
10. surgical repair
11. surgical incision
12. pain
13. abnormal condition

Exercise 6

1. WR CV S
    neur / o / logy   study of nerve (branch of medicine that deals with the nervous system)

2. WR CV WR S
    cerebr / o / spin / al   pertaining to the brain and spine

3. WR   S
    neur / algia   pain in a nerve

4. WR CV WR   S
    poli / o / myel / itis   inflammation of the gray matter and the spinal cord

5. WR CV   S
    neur / o / plasty   surgical repair of a nerve

6. WR   S
    encephal / itis   inflammation of the brain

7. WR   S
    mening / itis   inflammation of the meninges

8. WR CV WR CV S
    pneum / o / encephal / o / gram   x-ray image of the (ventricles in the) brain using air

9. WR CV   S
    neur / o / rrhaphy   suture of a nerve

10. WR CV   S
    neur / o / logist   one who specializes in the diagnosis and treatment of nerves

11. WR CV   S
    encephal / o / cele   herniation of brain tissue through (a gap in) the skull

12. WR CV WR CV S
    electr / o / encephal / o / gram   recording of electrical activity of the brain

13. WR CV WR CV S
    mening / o / myel / o / cele   protrusion of the spinal cord and meninges through the vertebral column

14. WR   S
    cerebell / itis   inflammation of the cerebellum

15. WR   S
    cerebr / osis   abnormal condition of the brain

16. WR   S
    neur / oma   tumor of nerve (cells)

17. WR CV   S
    myel / o / rrhagia   hemorrhage into the spinal cord

18. WR CV   S
    myel / o / gram   x-ray image of the spinal cord using dye

19. WR   S
    neur / itis   inflammation of a nerve

Exercise 7

1. a disease characterized by hardening patches along the brain and spine
2. convulsive disorder of the nervous system marked by recurrent or chronic seizures
3. partial paralysis and lack of muscle coordination from a defect, injury, or disease of the brain present at birth or shortly after.
4. impaired blood supply to parts of the brain

5. a process of recording brain structures by use of sound recorded on a graph
6. paralysis of the right or left side of the body
7. paralysis of the legs and/or lower part of the body
8. paralysis that affects all four limbs
9. removal of cerebrospinal fluid for diagnostic purposes
10. accumulation of blood in the subdural space
11. radiologic imaging that produces images of "slices" of the body
12. a noninvasive nuclear procedure for imaging tissues
13. loss of expression or understanding of speech or writing

Exercise 8

1. neuritis
2. encephalitis
3. meningitis
4. neuroplasty
5. neurologist
6. neurorrhaphy
7. neuroma
8. neuralgia
9. cerebrospinal
10. meningomyelocele
11. cerebellitis
12. encephalocele
13. pneumoencephalogram
14. myelorrhagia
15. electroencephalogram
16. myelogram

Exercise 9

Spelling exercise

Exercise 10

Spelling exercise

Exercise 11

1. neurology / neurologist
2. cerebrovascular / accident / CVA / hemiplegia
3. meningitis / spinal puncture / (lumbar puncture) / spinal puncture (lumbar puncture)
4. a. electroencephalogram
   b. myelogram
   c. pneumoencephalogram
   d. echoencephalogram

UNIT 5
Review Questions

1. a. skull bones
   b. eyelashes
   c. eyelids
   d. lacrimal apparatus
   e. conjunctiva
2. Sound enters the pinna, travels through the auditory canal, and strikes the tympanic membrane, which sends the ossicles into motion. The stapes vibrate the oval window, the waves continue to travel via the fluid in the cochlea to the auditory nerve and on to the brain.
3. 1. f   4. i   7. k
   2. h   5. b   8. a
   3. j   6. d
4. a. conjunctiva
   b. cornea
   c. aqueous humor
   d. pupil
   e. lens
   f. vitreous humor

5. a. cones; adaptation to bright light and color vision
   b. rods; adaptation to dim light
6. a. pinna and auditory canal
   b. tympanic membrane, eustachian tube, malleus, incus, stapes
   c. oval window, cochlea, semicircular canals
7. cloudiness of the lens of the eye
8. abnormal increase of intraocular pressure
9. a. chronic infections
   b. head injuries
   c. prolonged exposure to environmental noise
   d. hypertension
   e. cardiovascular disease
   f. ototoxic drugs
10. a. masking the noise by using music
    b. biofeedback
11. separation of the retina from the choroid
12. a. photocoagulation
    b. crysosurgery
    c. scleral buckling

Exercise 1

1. 1. blephar/o
   2. conjunctiv/o
   3. irid/o
   4. kerat/o
   5. ophthalm/o
   6. retin/o
   7. scler/o
2. 1. miring/o
   2. ot/o
   3. staped/o

Exercise 2

1. retina	5. conjunctiva	8. eyelid
2. cornea	6. ear	9. iris
3. sclera	7. tympanic	10. stapes
4. eye	membrane	

Exercise 3

1. ophthalm/o	5. myring/o	9. kerat/o
2. blephar/o	6. scler/o	10. staped/o
3. retin/o	7. conjunctiv/o	
4. ot/o	8. irid/o	

Exercise 4

1. WR   CV   S
    ophthalm / o / scope   instrument used for visual examination of the eye

2. WR   CV   S
    ophthalm / o / logist   one who specializes in the diagnosis and treatment of the eye

3. WR   S
    ophthalm / ectomy   excision of the eye

4. WR CV   S
    ot / o / rrhea   discharge from the ear

5. WR CV   S
    ot / o / scope   instrument used for visual examination the ear

6. WR CV WR CV   S
    irid / o / scler / o / tomy   incision into the iris and sclera

7. WR   S
    irid / ectomy   excision of (part of) the iris

8. WR   CV   S
    blephar / o / plasty   surgical repair of the eyelid

9. WR   CV   S
    blephar / o / rrhaphy   suture of an eyelid

10. WR   CV   WR   S
    kerat / o / conjunctiv / itis   inflammation of the cornea and conjunctiva

11. WR   CV   S
    kerat / o / cele   herniation of (a layer of the) cornea

12.   WR   S
    conjunctiv / itis   inflammation of the conjunctiva

13. WR   CV   S
    myring / o / tomy   incision of the tympanic membrane

14. WR   CV   S
    myring / o / plasty   surgical repair of the tympanic membrane

15. WR   CV   S
    kerat / o / tomy   incision into the cornea

Exercise 5

1. otitis media	10. ophthalmectomy
2. ophthalmoscope	11. sclerotomy
3. blepharorrhaphy	12. blepharoplasty
4. otorrhea	13. myringotomy
5. iridosclerotomy	14. myringoplasty
6. scleroplasty	15. keratoconjunctivitis
7. iridectomy	16. conjunctivitis
8. keratocele	17. keratotomy
9. otoscope	

Exercise 6

1. cloudiness of the lens of the eye
2. removal of the clouded lens of the eye
3. separation of the retina from the choroid
4. surgical removal of the eyeball
5. weakness of the eye muscle (crossed eyes)
6. eye disease caused by increased pressure from within the eye
7. a professional person trained to examine the eyes and prescribe glasses.
8. transplantation of a donor cornea into the eye of a recipient

Exercise 7

Spelling exercise

Exercise 8

1. ophthalmoscope / otoscope
2. otitis media / myringotomy
3. cataract / cataract extraction
4. enucleation / ophthalmectomy
5. strabismus

Unit 6
Review Questions

1 and 2. See page 505 for labeled diagram.
3. a. artery: carries blood away from heart
   b. arterioles: connect arteries to capillaries
   c. capillaries: exchange of substances between the blood and the body cells
   d. venules: connect capillaries to veins
   e. veins: carry blood back to the heart
4. plasma:
   a. transports nutrients and waste material
   b. transports hormones
   c. assists in blood clotting
5. a. erythrocytes: carry oxygen and carbon dioxide
   b. leukocytes: fight against pathogenic microorganisms
   c. platelets: aid in blood clotting
6. a. O
   b. A
   c. B
   d. AB
7. a. destroys old red blood cells, bacteria, and germs
   b. stores blood for an emergency
8. 1. g   4. a   7. e
   2. b   5. d   8. i
   3. c   6. h

Exercise 1

	Type	Meaning
1.	P	below normal
2.	P	without
3.	WR	blood
4.	WR	spleen
5.	WR	cell
6.	S/WR	narrowing
7.	P	inside
8.	WR	white
9.	WR	red
10.	WR	blood vessel
11.	WR	heart
12.	WR	artery
13.	P	surrounding (outer)
14.	P	between
15.	P	within
16.	S/WR	hardening
17.	S/WR	condition of the blood
18.	S	enlargement
19.	WR	vein
20.	WR	aorta
21.	WR	clot
22.	P	above normal
23.	P	fast, rapid
24.	P	slow

Exercise 2

	Type	Word Elements
1.	WR	aort/o
2.	S	-megaly
3.	S/WR	-sclerosis
4.	P	inter-
5.	WR	arteri/o
6.	WR	angi/o

7.	WR	leuk/o
8.	S/WR	-stenosis
9.	WR	splen/o
10.	P	a-, an-
11.	S	-pexy
12.	P	endo-
13.	WR	hem/o
14.	WR	cyt/o
15.	P	hypo-
16.	WR	erythr/o
17.	WR	cardi/o
18.	P	peri-
19.	S/WR	-emia
20.	WR	phleb/o
21.	WR	thromb/o
22.	P	tachy
23.	P	brady

Exercise 3

1. WR   S
   aort / ic   pertaining to the aorta
2. WR   CV   S
   splen / o / megaly   enlargement of the spleen
3. WR   CV   S
   hem / o / rrhage   rapid flow of blood (from a blood vessel)
4. WR   S
   thromb / osis   abnormal condition (formation) of a blood clot
5. WR   CV   WR
   leuk / o / cyte   white blood cell
6. WR   CV   WR
   erythr / o / cyte   red blood cell
7. WR   CV   S
   cardi / o / logist   one who specializes in the diagnosis and treatment of the heart
8. WR   CV   S
   cardi / o / megaly   enlargement of the heart
9. WR   CV   S
   phleb / o / tomy   incision into the vein (to withdraw blood)
10. WR   CV   S
   angi / o / rrhaphy   suturing of a blood vessel
11. WR   S
   splen / ectomy   excision of the spleen
12. WR   CV   S
   splen / o / pexy   surgical fixation of the spleen
13. P   WR   S
   endo / card / itis   inflammation of the inner (lining) of the heart
14. WR   CV   S
   arteri / o / sclerosis   hardening of the arteries
15. WR   CV   S
   arteri / o / stenosis   constriction (narrowing) of the arteries
16. WR   CV   WR   S
   thromb / o / phleb / itis   inflammation of a vein due to a clot

17. WR   S
hemat / oma   tumor-like mass formed from
                               blood in the tissues

18. WR   CV   S
hemat / o / logy   study of blood

19. WR   S
leuk / emia   blood condition of white (dis-
                               ease characterized by rapid, ab-
                               normal production of white
                               blood cells)

20. P   S(WR)
an / emia   blood condition of without
                               (deficiency of erythrocytes)

21. WR   CV WR   CV   S
electr / o / cardi / o / gram record of electrical activity of
                               the heart

22. WR   CV WR   CV   S
electr / o / cardi / o / graph machine used to record electri-
                               cal activity of the heart

23. WR   CV WR   CV   S
electr / o / cardi / o / graphy process of recording electrical
                               activity of the heart

24. WR   CV   S
angi / o / gram   x-ray image of blood vessels

25. WR   CV   S
arteri / o / gram   x-ray image of an artery

26. WR   CV   S
aort / o / gram   x-ray image of the aorta

27. P   WR   S
peri / card / itis   inflammation of the outer
                               (sac) of the heart

28. P   WR   S
tachy / card / ia   condition of rapid heart (rate)

29. P   WR   S
brady / card / ia   condition of slow heart (rate)

30. WR   CV   S
angi / o / plasty   surgical repair of a blood
                               vessel

Exercise 4

1. aortogram
2. arteriogram
3. angiogram
4. electrocardiogram
5. endocarditis
6. arteriosclerosis
7. thrombophlebitis
8. hematology
9. cardiology
10. cardiologist
11. cardiomegaly
12. phlebotomy
13. splenectomy
14. splenopexy
15. hemorrhage
16. leukocyte
17. erythrocyte
18. pericarditis

Exercise 5

1. laboratory test that measures the volume percentage of red blood cells in whole blood
2. laboratory procedure that measures the oxygen-carrying pigment of the red blood cells
3. sudden stopping of the heartbeat
4. pertaining to the heart and blood vessels
5. excision of hemorrhoids
6. heart attack (damage of the heart muscle from insufficient blood supply to the area)

7. enlarged veins in the rectal area
8. within a vein
9. diagnostic procedure to visualize the heart and to determine the presence of heart disease or heart defects
10. dilation of a weak area of the arterial wall
11. floating mass that blocks a blood vessel
12. high blood pressure
13. low blood pressure
14. inability of the heart to pump enough blood to the body parts
15. blood vessels that supply blood to the heart
16. abnormal accumulation of fluid in the intercellular spaces of the body
17. variation from a normal rhythm
18. condition of rapid heart rate

Exercise 6

Spelling exercise

Exercise 7

1. hematology / hematocrit / hemoglobin
2. a. myocardial infarction
   b. coronary occlusion
   c. coronary thrombosis
3. splenectomy, hemorrhoidectomy
4. cardiovascular
5. cardiologist
6. cardiac arrest / cardiac arrest (or "code")
7. electrocardiography / electrocardiograph
8. angiogram
9. cardiac catheterization
10 a. WBC
   b. RBC
   c. platelets
11. plasma

UNIT 7
Review Questions

1. a. taking nutrients into the digestive tract through the mouth
   b. the chemical and mechanical breakdown of food for use by the body cells
   c. transfer of digested food from the small intestine to the bloodstream
   d. the removal of solid waste from the body
2. ingestion, digestion, absorption, and elimination
3. mouth; pharynx; esophagus (upper and lower esophageal sphincter); stomach (pyloric sphincter); small intestine—duodenum, jejunum, ileum (ileocecal sphincter between small and large intestine); large intestine—cecum, colon (ascending colon, transverse colon, descending colon, sigmoid colon); rectum (anal sphincter)
4.

Name of Digestive Enzyme	Organ of Secretion	Organ of Function
a. hydrochloric acid	gastric glands	stomach
b. saliva	salivary glands	mouth
c. bile	liver	small intestine (duodenum)
d. pancreatic enzymes	pancreas	small intestine (duodenum)
e. intestinal enzymes	small intestine	small intestine

5. a. salivary glands
   b. teeth
   c. tongue
   d. liver
   e. gallbladder
   f. pancreas
   6. pyloric sphincter
7. a. mastication of food, mixing with salivary juices to start digestion
   b. container for food, and chemically and mechanically aids in the digestive process
   c. digestion is completed
   d. absorption of water and elimination of solid waste from the body
   e. stores bile from the liver and secretes it to the duodenum
8. 1. e
   2. a
   3. b
   4. f
   5. d

Exercise 1

Note: Not all of the combining forms will be labeled in the diagram.
2. appendic/o
4. chol/o or chol/e
5. col/o
6. duoden/o
8. esophag/o
9. gastr/o
10. gloss/o or lingu/o
11. hepat/o
13. ile/o
15. pancreat/o
18. stomat/o

Exercise 2

1. mouth
2. tongue
3. stomach
4. rectum
5. pancreas
6. intestine
7. liver
8. lip
9. esophagus
10. condition of / S
11. bile, gall
12. bladder
13. duodenum
14. colon
15. ileum
16. abdomen
17. appendix
18. abdomen
19. stone or calculus
20. creation of an artificial opening into / S
21. hernia
22. sigmoid

Exercise 3

1. -tomy—incision into a body part; *laparotomy:* incision into the abdomen
2. ectomy—surgical removal (of a body part) *appendectomy:* surgical removal of the appendix
3. stomy—creation of an artificial opening into; *colostomy:* creation of an artificial opening into the colon

Exercise 4

1. WR CV S
   gloss / o / plegia   paralysis of the tongue
2. WR S
   append / ectomy   surgical removal of the appendix
3. R CV WR S
   chol / e / cyst / ectomy   surgical removal of the gallbladder
4. WR CV S
   gastr / o / stomy   creation of an artificial opening into the stomach (for feeding purposes)
5. WR CV S
   hepat / o / megaly   enlargement of the liver
6. WR CV S
   ile / o / stomy   creation of an artificial opening into the ileum

7. WR CV S
   pylor / o / plasty   surgical repair of the pyloric sphincter
8. WR CV S
   proct / o / rrhea   excessive discharge from the rectum
9. WR CV WR S
   chol / e / cyst / itis   inflammation of the gallbladder
10. WR S
    gastr / itis   inflammation of the stomach
11. P WR S
    sub / lingu / al   pertaining to under the tongue
12. WR S
    ile / itis   inflammation of the ileum
13. WR CV WR CV S
    chol / e / cyst / o / gram x-ray image of the gallbladder
14. WR CV S
    sigmoid / o / scopy   visual examination of the sigmoid colon
15. WR S
    gastr / ectomy   surgical removal of the stomach
16. WR CV S
    gastr / o / scopy   visual examination of the stomach
17. WR CV S
    gastr / o / scope   instrument used for visual examination of the stomach
18. WR S
    col / itis   inflammation of the colon
19. WR S
    hepat / itis   inflammation of the liver
20. WR CV S
    col / o / stomy   creation of an artificial opening into the colon
21. WR CV S
    herni / o / rrhaphy   surgical repair of a hernia (by suturing of the containing structure)
22. WR CV S
    colon / o / scope   instrument used for visual examination of the colon
23. WR CV S
    colon / o / scopy   visual examination of the colon
24. WR CV WR CV
    esophag / o / gastr / o /-
    WR CV S
    duoden / o / scopy   visual examination of the esophagus, stomach, and duodenum

Exercise 5

1. stomatitis
2. cholecystitis
3. cholelithiasis
4. cholecysto<u>gram / D</u>
5. cholecyst<u>ectomy / S</u>
6. pancreatitis
7. proctoscope
8. procto<u>scopy</u> / D
9. abdomino<u>centesis</u> / D
10. colo<u>stomy</u> / S
11. ileo<u>stomy</u> / S
12. esophago<u>scopy</u> / D
13. gastroscope
14. esophagoenterostomy / S

15. gastritis
16. glosso<u>rrhaphy</u> / S
17. cheilo<u>plasty</u> / S
18. col<u>ectomy</u> / S
19. glossoplegia
20. stomatogastric
21. sublingual
22. proctorrhea
23. hepatomegaly
24. hepatoma
25. pancreatic
26. appendicitis
27. append<u>ectomy</u> / S
28. colono<u>scopy</u> / D
29. colonoscope
30. esophagogastroduodeno<u>scopy</u> / D

Exercise 6

1. condition of painful intestines accompanied by diarrhea
2. x-ray image of the esophagus and the stomach
3. x-ray image of the colon
4. x-ray image of the gallbladder
5. yellowness of the skin and eyes
6. inflammation of the colon with the formation of ulcers
7. ulcer in the stomach
8. chronic inflammatory disease that can affect any part of the bowel

Exercise 7

Spelling exercise

Exercise 8

1. b. ileostomy: <u>Ile</u> is the word root for the small intestine; -stomy is the suffix that means artificial opening.
2. cholelithiasis / cholecystogram / cholecystectomy
3. subligual
4. a. esophagoscopy, esophagoscope
   b. gastroscopy, gastroscope
   c. proctoscopy, proctoscope
5. upper gastrointestinal (UGI) / barium enema (BE)
   a. gastrectomy
   b. pyloroplasty
   c. vagotomy
6. a. laparotomy
   b. (correct)
   c. herniorrhaphy
   d. colectomy
   e. gastrostomy

UNIT 8
Review Questions

1. oxygen / carbon dioxide
2. oxygen / carbon dioxide
3. a. nose
   b. pharynx
   c. larynx
   d. trachea
   e. bronchus
   f. bronchioles
   g. alveoli

4. pharynx / epiglottis
5. a. warmed and moistened
   b. pathogenic microorganisms removed
   c. foreign particles removed
   6. larynx
7. Cone-shaped organs located in the thoracic cavity. The right is larger and divided into three lobes, whereas the left has only two lobes. The bronchus, after entering the lung, continues to subdivide into smaller tubes called bronchioles. At the end of each is a cluster of air sacs or alveoli. The pleura is a double sac that surrounds each lung.
8. a. hemothorax
   b. pneumothorax
   c. atelectasis
   d. pulmonary embolism
9. chronic obstructive pulmonary disease
10. a. cigarette smoking
    b. environmental pollution
    c. occupational hazards
    d. chronic infections

Exercise 1

1. bronch/o
2. laryng/o
3. pharyng/o
4. pleur/o
6. pneum/o
7. pneumon/o
8. pulmon/o
9. rhin/o
12. trache/o

Exercise 2

1. pneum/o, pneumon/o, pulmon/o
2. pharyng/o
3. laryng/o
4. trache/o
5. tonsill/o
6. bronch/o
7. pleur/o
8. rhin/o
9. pnea/o
10. thorac/o

Exercise 3

1. P   WR
   dys / pnea — difficulty breathing
2. WR   CV   S
   pharyng / o / cele — abnormal protrusion in the pharynx
3. P   S
   a / pnea — without breathing (temporary stopping of breathing)
4. WR   CV   WR   S
   bronch / o / trache / al — pertaining to the bronchi and trachea
5. WR   CV   WR   S
   trache / o / esophag / eal — pertaining to the trachea and esophagus
6. P   WR   S
   endo / trache / al — pertaining to within the trachea
7. WR   CV   S
   pharyng / o / plegia — paralysis of the pharynx
8. WR   CV   WR   S
   rhin / o / pharyng / itis — inflammation of the nose and throat
9. WR   CV   S
   rhin / o / rrhagia — rapid flow of blood from the nose (nosebleed)
10. WR   CV   S
    bronch / o / scope — instrument used for visual examination of the bronchi
11. WR   CV   S
    bronch / o / scopy — visual examination of the bronchi

Exercise 4

1. bronchitis
2. laryngitis
3. tracheostomy
4. pneumonectomy or pneumectomy
5. lobectomy
6. pleuropexy
7. rhinoplasty
8. thoracotomy
9. thoracentesis or thoracocentesis
10. tonsillitis
11. adenoiditis

Exercise 5

1. pneumothorax
2. emphysema
3. pneumonia
4. pleuropexy
5. pharyngitis

Exercise 6

1. chronic obstructive pulmonary disease
2. upper respiratory infection
3. pulmonary embolism

Exercise 7

1. tissue in the nasopharynx
2. excision of a lobe of the lung
3. disease of the alveoli of the lung
4. (infection or) inflammation of a lung
5. (infection or) inflammation of the pharynx, larynx, or bronchi
6. without breathing (temporary stopping of breathing)
7. difficulty breathing
8. abnormal protrusion in the pharynx
9. excision of the larynx
10. air in pleural cavity (that causes lung to collapse)
11. rapid flow of blood from the nose (nosebleed)
12. x-ray image of the lung and bronchi
13. instrument used for visual examination of the larynx
14. a chronic disease characterized by attacks of dyspnea, wheezing, and coughing
15. a chronic obstruction of the airway
16. a chronic infectious disease that commonly affects the lungs

Exercise 8

Spelling exercise

Exercise 9

1. thoracocentesis
2. laryngoscope / endotracheal
3. tracheostomy / tracheostomy / tracheostomy
4. bronchoscopy / bronchoscope
5. pneumothorax / dyspnea / thoracotomy / thoracotomy
6. tonsillectomy, adenoidectomy

Unit 9
Review Questions

1. urethra
2. to monitor and regulate extracellular fluids and to remove some of the waste material from the blood and to excrete it from the body
3. nephron, to remove waste materials and water from the blood. The process of filtration begins at the entrance of the nephron in the glomeruli.
4. Two ureters drain the urine to the bladder, and then it passes from the bladder through the urethra to the outside.
5. water / waste material
6. antidiuretic hormone / anterior pituitary gland
7. a. produce sperm
   b. produce testostcrone
8. The sperm passes from the seminiferous tubules to the epididymis through the vas deferens, and then through the urethra to the outside of the body. The seminal vesicles and prostate gland add solution to the sperm along the passageway.
9. 1. c
   2. e
   3. b
   4. g

Exercise 1

1. a. 1. cyst/o
      2. nephr/o or ren/o
      3. pyel/o
      4. nephr/o or ren/o
      6. ureter/o
      7. urethr/o
   b. 6. ureter/o
      7. urethr/o
      9. orchi/o or orchid/o
      10. orchi/o or orchid/o
      11. prostat/o
      12. vas/o

Exercise 2

1. ur/o, urin/o	5. cyst/o	8. urethr/o
2. pyel/o	6. orchi/o, orchid/o	9. urin/o
3. ren/o, nephr/o	7. vas/o	10. prostat/o
4. ureter/o		

Exercise 3

1. WR S ur / emia	urine in the blood
2. WR CV S ur / o / logist	doctor specializing in the diagnosis and treatment of diseases of the urinary tract and of the male reproductive organs
3. WR CV WR CV S nephr / o / lith / o / tomy	incision into the kidney to remove a stone
4. WR S prostat / ectomy	surgical removal of the prostate gland
5. WR S nephr / itis	inflammation of the kidney

6. WR   CV   S
  ur / o / logy   study of urine (branch of medi-
                         cine dealing with the urinary sys-
                         tem and the male reproductive
                         system)

7. WR   S
  orchi / ectomy   excision of a testis

8. WR   CV   WR   S
  nephr / o / lith / iasis   condition of kidney stone

9. WR   CV   S
  cyst / o / cele   herniation of the urinary bladder

10. WR   CV   S
  cysts / o / scopy   visual examination of the bladder

11. WR   S
  nephr / ectomy   excision of a kidney

12. WR   CV   S
  nephr / o / pexy   surgical fixation of a kidney

13. WR   CV   WR   S
  pyel / o / nephr / itis   inflammation of the kidney and
                         renal pelvis

14. WR   S
  ureter / algia   pain in the ureter

15. WR   S
  urethr / al   pertaining to the urethra

16. WR   CV   WR   CV   S
  ureter / o / lith / o / tomy   incision into the ureter to re-
                         move a stone

17. WR   S
  cyst / itis   inflammation of the bladder

18. WR   CV   S
  urethr / o / plasty   surgical repairof the urethra

19. WR   CV   S
  urethr / o / rrhaphy   suture of a urethral tear

Exercise 4

1. cystoscope   10. ureteralgia
2. nephritis   11. cystocele
3. nephrectomy   12. cystogram
4. urologist   13. pyelonephritis
5. hematuria   14. nephrolithotomy
6. uremia   15. urethroplasty
7. urethrorrhaphy   16. nephropexy
8. vasectomy   17. urology
9. prostatectomy   18. orchiectomy or orchidectomy

Exercise 5

1. a laboratory test to analyze urine to assist in the diagnosis of disease
2. kidney stone
3. swelling of the scrotum caused by the collection of fluid
4. removal of the prostate gland through the urethra
5. surgical removal of the foreskin of the penis
6. pertaining to the urine
7. passage of urine from the body

Exercise 6

1. intravenous pyelogram
2. kidneys, ureters, and bladder
3. blood urea nitrogen

4. transurethral resection
5. benign prostatic hyperplasia
6. urinalysis

Exercise 7

Spelling exercise

Exercise 8

1. urinary catheterization / urinalysis
2. cystitis
3. KUB / blood urea nitrogen / BUN
4. urologist
5. cystoscopy / he may be anesthetized

UNIT 10
Review Questions

1. estrogen / progesterone / estrogen
2. fallopian tubes
3. cervix
4. to produce the female reproductive cell, to provide hormones, to provide for conception, and to provide for pregnancy
5. a. The uterus contains and nourishes the fetus. It also plays a role in
      menstruation and labor.
   b. The ovaries produce the female reproductive cell, called the
      ovum. They produce the hormones estrogen and progesterone.
   c. The fallopian tubes are a passageway for the ovum from the
      ovaries to the uterus. Fertilization takes place in the tubes.
   d. The vagina connects the uterus to the outside of the body. It re-
      ceives the penis during intercourse and is part of the birth canal
      through which the baby passes from the uterus to the outside of
      the body.
6. follicle-stimulating hormone
7. pelvic inflammatory disease
8. ectopic pregnancy
9. endometriosis

Exercise 1

1. cervic/o   8. metr/o   12. uter/o
2. colp/o   9. oophor/o   13. vagin/o
4. hyster/o   11. salping/o

Exercise 2

1. men/o   5. salping/o   8. cervic/o
2. gynec/o   6. oophor/o   9. mast/o or
3. colp/o or vagin/o   7. hyster/o, metr/o, or   mamm/o
4. perine/o   uter/o

Exercise 3

1. WR   CV   S
  gynec / o / logy   study of women (branch
                         of medicine dealing
                         with female reproductive
                         organs)

2. WR CV   S
  colp / o / rrhaphy   suture of the vagina

3.   WR   S
    oophor / ectomy   surgical removal of an ovary

4.   WR   S
    oophor / itis   inflammation of an ovary

5.   WR   CV   WR   S
    salping / o / oophor / ectomy   excision of a fallopian tube and an ovary

6.   WR   CV   S
    salping / o / pexy   surgical fixation of a fallopian tube

7.   WR   S
    hyster / ectomy   surgical removal of the uterus

8.   P   WR   CV   S
    dys / men / o / rrhea   painful menstrual discharge

9.   WR   CV   S
    colp / o / scope   instrument used for visual examination of the vagina (and cervix)

10.   WR   CV   S
    mamm / o / plasty   surgical repair of the breast(s)

11.   P   WR   CV   S
    a / men / o / rrhea   without menstrual discharge

12.   WR   CV   S
    mamm / o / gram   x-ray image of the breast

13.   WR   CV   WR   CV   S
    hyster / o / salping / o / gram   x-ray image of the uterus and fallopian tubes

14.   WR   CV   S
    colp / o / scopy   visual examination of the vagina and cervix

Exercise 4

1. oophorectomy
2. gynecology
3. salpingopexy
4. oophoritis
5. colposcope
6. metrorrhea
7. cervicectomy
8. hysterosalpingo-oophorectomy
9. salpingocele
10. ureterovaginal
11. cervicitis
12. hysterectomy
13. colporrhaphy
14. perineoplasty
15. vaginal
16. mastectomy
17. salpingo-oophorectomy
18. dysmenorrhea
19. hysterosalpingogram
20. amenorrhea
21. mammogram
22. mammoplasty
23. colposcopy

Exercise 5

1. physician specializing in the diagnosis and treatment of women
2. pertaining to the uterus
3. instrument used for expanding the vagina to allow for visual examination of the vagina and cervix
4. excessive uterine bleeding during and between periods.
5. surgical procedure to scrape the uterus and the inner walls
6. female reproductive cell

Exercise 6

a. dilation and curettage
b. hysterosalpingo-oophorectomy
c. perineoplasty
d. colporrhaphy
e. salpingopexy

Exercise 7

Spelling exercise

Exercise 8

1. f
2. a
3. b
4. c
5. g
6. h
7. d
8. e

Exercise 9

1. a doctor who practices obstetrics
2. source of nourishment for the unborn child
3. fluid that surrounds the fetus
4. incision into the uterus through the abdominal wall to deliver the fetus

Exercise 10

1. gynecology / obstetrics
2. vaginal speculum / cervical Pap smear

Unit 11
Review Questions

1. iodine
2. a. 2, 3, 4, 6, 10
  b. 7
  c. 11
  d. 5, 12
  e. 1
  f. 9
  g. 8
3. The hormones it produces stimulate the functions of the other endocrine glands. The hypothalamus directly regulates the secretory activity of the pituitary gland.
4. communication, integration, and control
5. islets of Langerhans / pancreas
6. necessary for the metabolism of carbohydrates in the body
7. a. polyuria
  b. polydipsia
  c. glycosuria
  d. hyperglycemia
  e. polyphagia
8. hyperthyroidism

Exercise 1

1. aden/o
2. thyr/o, thyroid/o
3. adren/o, adrenal/o
4. parathyroid/o

Exercise 2

1. adenitis
2. thyroidectomy
3. parathyroidectomy
4. adenoid
5. adenoma
6. adenosis
7. adrenalitis

Exercise 3

1. islets of Langerhans (pancreas)
2. thyroid gland
3. adrenal gland
4. thyroid gland
5. adrenal gland
6. pituitary gland

Exercise 4

1. diabetes insipidus
2. Addison's disease
3. Cushing's disease
4. hypothyroidism
5. secretions

Exercise 5

Spelling exercise

Exercise 6

1. diabetes mellitus / islets of Langerhans / Ua / FBS / GTT / HbA_{1c} / blood glucose monitoring
2. a. pituitary
   b. adrenal cortex
   c. islets of Langerhans
   d. adrenal medulla
   e. ovary
   f. testes
   g. thyroid gland
3. a. protein-bound iodine
   b. T_3, T_4, T_7 uptake
   c. thyroid scan

Index

Page numbers followed by *f* indicate figures; those followed by *t* indicate tables; those followed by *b* indicate boxes.